T0251397

# PREVENTION OF RESPIRATORY DISEASES

# LUNG BIOLOGY IN HEALTH AND DISEASE

*Executive Editor*

**Claude Lenfant**
*Director, National Heart, Lung and Blood Institute*
*National Institutes of Health*
*Bethesda, Maryland*

The opinions expressed in these volumes do not necessarily represent the views of the National Institutes of Health.

# PREVENTION OF RESPIRATORY DISEASES

*Edited by*

## Albert Hirsch

*Service de Pneumologie
Hôpital Saint-Louis
Paris, France*

## Marcel Goldberg

*Institut National de la
Santé et de la
Recherche Médicale (INSERM)
Paris, France*

## Jean-Pierre Martin

*Institut National de la
Santé et de la
Recherche Médicale (INSERM)
Rouen, France*

## Roland Masse

*Commissariat a l'Energie Atomique
Fontenay-aux-Roses, France*

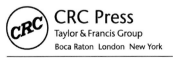

CRC Press
Taylor & Francis Group
Boca Raton London New York

CRC Press is an imprint of the
Taylor & Francis Group, an **informa** business

CRC Press
Taylor & Francis Group
6000 Broken Sound Parkway NW, Suite 300
Boca Raton, FL 33487-2742

© 1993 by Taylor & Francis Group, LLC
CRC Press is an imprint of Taylor & Francis Group, an Informa business

No claim to original U.S. Government works

**Visit the Taylor & Francis Web site at**
**http://www.taylorandfrancis.com**

**and the CRC Press Web site at**
**http://www.crcpress.com**

# INTRODUCTION

*An ounce of prevention is worth a pound of cure.*

It is hard to know when this old English proverb was first recorded, but an expert librarian assured me that it was before the eighteenth century.

There is some sort of mystique about the word "prevention." Perhaps it is because of the ancientness of the concept it expresses. Indeed, we know that the Yellow Emperor (2697–2597 B.C.) in his *Classic of Internal Medicine* already advocated prevention:

> Hence the sages did not treat those who were already ill; they instructed those who were not yet ill. . . . To administer medicines to diseases which are already developed is comparable to the behavior of those persons who begin to dig a well after they have become thirsty, and of those who begin to cast weapons after they have already engaged in battle.

It is of great interest that today's textbooks of internal medicine hardly speak of prevention. Instead, they teach us to "administer medicines to diseases which are already developed."

The reality is that good medicine should cover the entire spectrum, that is, from prevention to cure! As H. Sigerist said, "The barriers between preventive and curative medicine must be broken down" (1959).

Of course, prevention is more than a word. It is a science, and, like all sciences, it has greatly benefited from the vast discoveries in biology and medicine that have characterized the last decades. For years, the greatest minds of medicine have known that to prevent a disease one must understand its course and its mechanism. The best examples are to be found in the realm of infectious diseases.

But what about respiratory diseases? There is no doubt that since the end of World War II we have seen extraordinary discoveries about their cause and their mechanisms. As Dr. S. S. Fitch, of Philadelphia, said, "At one moment, (they) obtrude upon our notice in a gentle light; at another, they burst forth with the most brilliant meteoric glare, dazzling us with their splendor and awaking profound and wondrous anticipations of the future" (1853).

Thus, it comes as no surprise that the Lung Biology in Health and Disease series should include a volume on prevention of respiratory diseases. Ever since the publication of the first Surgeon General's Report on Smoking and Health, in 1964, we have known that one of the most powerful ways to alleviate, if not suppress, the enormous human and economical toll of respiratory disease would be to ban smoking. But we have also learned how difficult it is to reach this goal. However, investigations have uncovered other ways to prevent many lung diseases. This volume, edited by Drs. Hirsch, Goldberg, Martin, and Masse, offers the readers a panoply of approaches that cover a great number of respiratory diseases. Truly, it brings the reader to the forefront of current knowledge and provides opportunities to reduce the severe public health problems that these diseases constitute.

In his foreword, Sir Richard Doll says "Respiratory disease, perhaps more than any other type of disease, is able to be prevented more easily than cured." It is our hope that this volume will help to give prevention the visibility and weight it deserves. The editors and authors deserve much gratitude for making such a valuable contribution.

Claude Lenfant, M.D.
Bethesda, Maryland

# FOREWORD

Cast out one devil and seven others may enter. If those of us who are concerned with preventive medicine did not know it before, we know it now that reduced mortality rates have led to such an expansion in the population of the world that it threatens future well-being with damage to the natural environment and destruction of the world's resources. We see it, too, on a smaller scale in the subject of this book, for the pattern of respiratory disease has changed greatly in the last hundred years, not just because of the conquest of silicosis, lobar pneumonia, and respiratory tuberculosis (the erstwhile captain of the kings of death), but also because of the emergence of new epidemics as a result of increased cigarette consumption, the widespread use of asbestos, and the substitution of air-conditioning for natural ventilation of buildings.

Not all the diseases that have become more prominent have necessarily done so because of a real increase in incidence. The new devils have not completely replaced the old, and the greater prominence of some diseases may have arisen simply because their incidence has persisted unchanged while the total incidence of respiratory disease has been reduced, and others may have become more prominent because the improvement in public health has lowered the threshold for the recognition of disease and made us aware of levels of disease that would formerly have been accepted as within the range of normal variation. The greater prominence of some diseases is not always clear, and the establishment of the trends in incidence of diseases such as asthma is an urgent problem for research if their causes are to be fully identified and controlled.

That a monograph in the series on lung biology in health and disease be dedicated to prevention was obligatory, because respiratory disease, perhaps more than any other type of disease, can be prevented more easily than cured. Emphysema and all the respiratory cancers (nasal, laryngeal, bronchial, alveolar, and pleural) could all be rare if only society applied the knowledge that it already has to prevent them. They cannot be eliminated completely, as some infectious diseases can be, because some cases of emphysema are due to genetic defects so serious that, no matter how ideal the environment, degeneration occurs early in life, while some cancers in all organs are due to natural radioactivity that cannot be avoided.

Disease in some instances cannot be avoided until further research has clarified the environmental and behavioral causes. In others, it may not be possible to avoid the external factors, and the possibility of prevention depends on a better understanding of the mechanisms by which the disease is produced. For some diseases, particularly for those produced by occupational hazards and the public use of asbestos, prevention has been or can be achieved simply by government regulation and the voluntary action of industrial companies. There is, however, no similar simple method for the prevention of the vast number of tobacco-related diseases (respiratory and other) that are now estimated to be responsible for nearly 20 percent of all deaths in developed countries, and, probably, for more in the future, as the use of tobacco spreads among women. General education, professional advice, and government action all have a part to play, but there is much still to be learned about the pharmacological dependence that makes cessation of smoking so difficult for some people, and the social factors that make its adoption by the young so attractive.

**Sir Richard Doll**
Imperial Cancer Research Fund Cancer Studies Unit
Radcliffe Infirmary
Oxford, England

# PREFACE

Health is determined by many factors: intrinsic factors of genetic heritage and aging, extrinsic factors present in the communal environment, such as physical pollutants in water and air and microbiologic agents, social and work environment factors, and finally, access to health care and social support delivery systems. Prevention can be defined as actions converging on changeable factors to promote health for individuals and for the community. The purpose of preventive medicine is to reduce the risk of contracting a disease, or to identify an early manifestation of disease, if early treatment can reduce the risk of subsequent disability or death (1). The latter purpose can merge into that of curative medicine. For example, the management of a cigarette smoker who presents symptoms of chronic bronchitis would include advice to stop smoking in order to decrease or delay the risk of chronic obstructive pulmonary disease (COPD). Different levels of prevention are currently categorized as: primary prevention—to detect and change factors so as to avoid disease; secondary prevention—to detect and cure disease at a stage prior to the occurrence of any symptoms; and tertiary prevention—to minimize the consequences for a patient who already has the disease. (Tertiary prevention applies particularly to the elderly, for whom prevention of disability and handicap depends largely on recognition and treatment of symptoms already present.)

The role of pneumology in preventive medicine is historically linked to the control of tuberculosis infection, which was one of the most fatal pandemics of the industrialized countries, and which remains one of the major causes of morbidity and mortality in the developing world. That a large part of the decline of the death rate from tuberculosis in England and Wales occurred before the introduction of streptomycin in 1947 underlines the role of intrinsic and social determinants in the trend of this epidemic. On the assumption that without streptomycin the decline in mortality would have continued at about the same rate after as prior to 1946, it has been estimated that treatment by streptomycin reduced the number of deaths in the period since it was introduced (1948–1971) by 51 percent, but if one examines the total period since cause of death was first recorded (1848–1971), the reduction was 3.2 percent (2). Drug therapy of tuberculosis is, nevertheless, the best example of therapeutic efficacy demonstrated by randomized controlled trial (3).

In the second half of the twentieth century, with the decrease in infectious diseases, chronic disease and cancers are responsible for most premature deaths in the industrialized world. Lung cancer, COPD, and asthma play a large part in total morbidity and mortality. This volume illustrates the role of most of the known extrinsic and potentially preventable determinants in respiratory diseases.

Part One, edited by Marcel Goldberg, discusses the relationship between respiratory diseases and occupation, an association made since the earliest times. One of the earliest occupations, mining, was known to be hazardous not only because of accidents but also because of respiratory diseases. While many of the classic occupational diseases have now been virtually eliminated, the introduction of new technology and changing patterns of employment have led to new problems such as occupational asthma and occupational respiratory cancers. To further the prevention of occupational respiratory diseases, there is a need for more information from improved occupational mortality data, and from a more comprehensive system of reporting of industrial diseases by employers and medical practitioners. Better evaluation of possible control measures should be established, and urgent measures need to be taken to improve the awareness and knowledge of the medical profession.

Part Two, edited by Roland Masse, devoted to environmental sources of respiratory disease, discusses the evidence of individual sensitivity or susceptibility to the effects of air pollutants. Such sensibility may be limited to specific pollutants or classes of pollutants. The U.S. Clean Air Act specially recognizes that some individuals in the population are sensitive to air pollutants and need to be protected by air quality standards (4). It is usually difficult to determine the cause of sensitivity, although various biological mechanisms have been studied. Asthmatics are excellent examples of individuals who are susceptible to the effects of many environmental agents. The conditions defining populations at risk and the methodology to study the respiratory risks have to be clearly assessed.

Part Three edited by Jean-Pierre Martin, reviews the difficult problem of biological markers of risk. The markers for cancers can be separated into markers of exposure to a specific substance and markers of early lesions which usually are not specific for a particular substance and do not indicate the dose of exposure (5). In epidemiological research on cancer etiology, biological markers can be used in cases with either early lesions or invasive cancers. These two approaches should be considered in the framework of two basic problems: What is the advantage of measuring exposure at the individual level? and What is the advantage of a biological marker as compared to traditional epidemiological methods?

The last part is devoted to the relationship between tobacco and respiratory diseases. From the first official report in 1962 by the Royal College of Physicians in the U.K. (5), up to the 25-year progress report of the U.S. Surgeon General (6), a mass of data concerning the health consequences of tobacco smoking and their mechanisms—as well as the social, behavioral, and pharmacological factors involved in starting or stopping tobacco use—have been obtained. In order to promote respiratory health, a number of general recommendations can be made, followed by specific suggestions concerning the role of health professionals, and particularly pneumologists. These recommendations are: 1) all forms of promotion of tobacco should be prohibited, 2) price rises of tobacco products should exceed the rate of inflation to discourage increasing sales, 3) restrictions on smoking in public places and workplaces should be extended, 4) public education about the importance of tobacco as a major risk to health should be maintained and enhanced, both for the general population and as part of the school curriculum, public educatiuon could be funded by a special levy on tobacco products, 5) all health care professionals should offer smoking cessation advice in any consultation with smokers, 6) more support services should be available to help those involved in smoking cessation work, 7) research on more effective ways to stop smoking should be conducted, and 8) nonsmoking should be established as the norm on all healthcare premises.

The editors would like to thank Karen Slama, Ph.D., for her assistance in coordinating the editing of this book.

**Albert Hirsch**

### References

1. Preventive medicine. A report of a working party of the Royal College of Physicians. Royal College of Physicians of London, 1991.
2. McKeown T. The role of medicine. Dream, mirage, or nemesis? Nuffield Provincial Hospital Trust 1976.
3. Cochrane AL. Effectiveness and efficiency. Random reflections on health services. Nuffield Provincial Hospital Trust 1972.

4. Lebowitz MD. Population at risk: addressing health effects due to complex mixtures with a focus on respiratory effects. Environmental Health Perspectives, 1991; 95:35–38.

5. Riboli E, Saracci R. Markers of exposure and of early lesions in cancer epidemiology. Revue d'Epidemiologie et de Santé Publique, 1985; 33:304–311.

6. Royal College of Physicians. Smoking and health. London: Pitman Medical, 1962.

7. U.S. Department of Health and Human Services. Reducing the health consequences of smoking: 25 years of progress. A Report of the Surgeon-General. USDHHS, PHS, CDC Office on Smoking and Health, DHHS Publication No. (CDC) 89–8411, 1989.

# CONTRIBUTORS

**Isabella Annesi, D.Sc.**   Epidemiological Research Unit, INSERM U169, Villejuif, France

**Margaret R. Becklake, M.D., F.R.C.P.(London)**   Professor and Career Investigator, Medical Research Council of Canada and Department of Epidemiology and Biostatistics and Department of Medicine, McGill University, Montreal, Quebec, Canada

**Simone Benhamou, Ph.D.**   INSERM U351 and Institut Gustave Roussy, Villejuif, France

**Franco Berrino**   Istituto Nazionale Tumori, Milan, Italy

**Joseph G. Bieth, Ph.D.**   Research Director, Laboratory of Enzymology, INSERM U237, Illkirch, France

**Kjell Bjartveit, M.D.**   Chairman, National Council on Tobacco and Health, National Health Screening Service, Oslo, Norway

**Paolo Boffetta, M.D., M.P.H.**    Unit of Analytical Epidemiology, International Agency for Research on Cancer, Lyon, France

**Catherine Bonaiti-Pellié, M.D., Ph.D.**    Directeur de Recherches, Unité de Recherche d'Epidémiologie Génetique, INSERM U155, Paris, France

**Denis A. Charpin, M.D., M.P.H.**    Professor of Chest Diseases and Allergy, Department of Chest Diseases, Marseille School of Medicine, Marseille, France

**Caroline Cohen, Ph.D.**    Pharmacologist, Groupe Pharmacology SNC, Synthelabo Recherche, L.E.R.S., Bagneux, France

**J. Cosme**    Biopathologie et Toxicologie Pulmonaire, INSERM U139, Créteil, France

**Robert E. Dales, M.D., M.Sc.**    Associate Professor, Department of Medicine and Department of Epidemiology and Community Medicine, University of Ottawa, Ottawa, Ontario, Canada

**James H. Day, M.D., F.R.C.P.(C), F.A.C.P.**    Professor and Head, Division of Allergy and Immunology, Department of Medicine, Queen's University, Kingston, Ontario, Canada

**Marie-Hélène Dizier, Ph.D.**    Genetic Markers in Complex Diseases, Unité de Recherches de Epidémiologie Génetique, INSERM U155, Paris, France

**Donald A. Enarson, M.D.**    Professor, Pulmonary Division, Department of Medicine, University of Alberta, Alberta, Canada

**Josué Feingold, M.D.**    Genetic Markers in Complex Diseases, Unité de Recherches d'Epidémiologie Génetique, INSERM U155, Paris, France

**Marcel Goldberg, M.D., Ph.D.**    Professor, INSERM U88, Paris, France

**Paquerette Goldberg, Ph.D.**    INSERM U88, Paris, France

**John P. Hanrahan, M.D., M.P.H.**    Assistant Professor in Medicine, Channing Laboratory, Brigham and Women's Hospital and Harvard Medical School, Boston, Massachusetts

**D. J. Hartmann, Ph.D.**    Centre de Radioanalyse and CNRS URA 1459, Institut Pasteur de Lyon, Lyon, France

**Dick Heederik, Ph.D.** Epidemiology and Public Health, University of Wageningen, Wageningen, The Netherlands

**Denis Hémon** Directeur de Recherche, Department of Environmental Epidemiology, INSERM U170, Villejuif, France

**Jack E. Henningfield, Ph.D.** Chief, Clinical Pharmacology Branch, Addiction Research Center, National Institute on Drug Abuse, Baltimore, Maryland

**Catherine Hill, M.B., Ch.B., M.S.** INSERM U351 and Institut Gustave Roussy, Villejuif, France

**Gerry B. Hill, M.B., Ch.B., M.Sc.** Medical Consultant, Bureau of Chronic Disease Epidemiology, Laboratory Centre for Disease Control, Ottawa, Ontario, Canada

**Albert Hirsch, M.D.** Professor of Pneumology and Head, Service de Pneumologie, Hôpital Saint-Louis, Paris, France

**Dietrich Hoffmann, Ph.D.** Associate Director, Environmental Carcinogenesis, American Health Foundation, Valhalla, New York

**Ilse Hoffmann, B.S.** Research Coordinator, American Health Foundation, Valhalla, New York

**M. P. Jacob, Ph.D.** Chargée de Recherches (CR 1) CNRS, Laboratoire de Biochimie du Tissu Conjonctif, CNRS (UA CNRS 1460), Créteil, France

**Serge Karsenty, Ph.D.** Sociologist, Unité Mixte CNRS-INSERM "Recherches en Economie de la Santé," Centre National de la Recherche Scientifique, Paris, France

**Francine Kauffmann, M.D.** Research Director, Epidemiological Research Unit, INSERM U169, Villejuif, France

**Serge Koscielny, Ph.D.** Statistician, Department of Biostatistics and Epidemiology, Institut Gustave Roussy, Villejuif, France

**C. Lafuma, Ph.D.** Chargée de Recherches CNRS (CR 1), Laboratoire de Biochimie du Tissu Conjonctif, CNRS (UA CNRS 1460), Créteil, France

**P. A. Laurent, M.D., Ph.D.** Biopathologie et Toxicologie Pulmonaire, INSERM U139, Créteil, France

**Michael D. Lebowitz, Ph.D.** Professor of Medicine and Associate Director, Respiratory Sciences Center, University of Arizona College of Medicine, Tucson, Arizona

**Annette Leclerc, Ph.D.** Researcher, INSERM U88, Paris, France

**Danièle Luce, Ph.D.** Researcher, INSERM U88 Paris, France

**Jean-Luc Malo, M.D.** Chest Physician, Chest Department, Faculty of Medicine, Sacre-Coeur Hospital, and University of Montreal, Montreal, Quebec, Canada

**Jean-Pierre Martin, M.D.** Scientist, Pneumology, INSERM U295, Rouen, France

**Roland Masse, Ph.D.** Director of the Department of Experimental Pathology and Toxicology, Commissariat à l'Energie Atomique, Fontenay-aux-Roses, France

**J. C. McDonald, M.D., F.R.C.P.** Professor Emeritus, Epidemiology Research Unit, National Heart and Lung Institute, London Chest Hospital, London, England

**Claude Molina, M.D.** Professor of Pneumology, President, French Lung Association, and University of Clermont-Ferrand, Paris, France

**J. M. Mur, M.D.** Head, Epidemiology Department, Institut National de Recherche et de Sécurité, Vandoeuvre, France

**J. C. Pairon, M.D.** Biopathologie Pulmonaire et Renale, INSERM U139, Créteil, France

**Taeke M. Pal, M.D.** Department of Social Medicine and Epidemiology, State University, Groningen, The Netherlands

**Linda L. Pederson, Ph.D.** Department of Epidemiology and Biostatistics and Department of Medicine, University of Western Ontario, London, Ontario, Canada

**Wallace B. Pickworth, Ph.D.** Pharmacologist, Clinical Pharmacology Branch, Addiction Research Center, National Institute on Drug Abuse, Baltimore, Maryland

**Martin Raw, Ph.D.** Honorary Research Fellow, Department of Public Health, Kings College School of Medicine and Dentistry, London, England

**Jonathan M. Samet, M.D., M.S.** Chief, Pulmonary and Critical Care Division, and Professor, Department of Medicine, University of New Mexico School of Medicine, Albuquerque, New Mexico

**Rodolfo Saracci, M.D.** Chief, Unit of Analytical Epidemiology, International Agency for Research on Cancer, Lyon, France

**Richard Sesboüé, M.D.** Scientist, INSERM U295, Rouen, France

**Karen Slama, Ph.D.** Behavioral Scientist, Service de Pneumologie, Hôpital Saint-Louis, Paris, France

**John D. Spengler, M.S., Ph.D.** Professor of Environmental Health and Director for the Exposure Assessment and Engineering Program, Department of Environmental Health, Harvard University School of Public Health, Boston, Massachusetts

**Walter O. Spitzer, M.D., F.R.C.P.** Strathcona Professor and Chairman, Department of Epidemiology and Biostatistics, McGill University, Montreal, Quebec, Canada

**Isabelle Stücker** Chargé de Recherches, Department of Environmental Epidemiology, INSERM U170, Villejuif, France

**Margot Tirmarche, M.Sc.** Epidemiologist, Departement de Protection de la Santé de l'Homme et de Dosimetrie/SEGR, Institut de Protection et de Sûreté Nucleaire, Fontenay-aux-Roses, France

**Daniel Vervloet, M.D.** Professor of Pneumology and Head, Allergy Division, Department of Chest Diseases, Marseille School of Medicine, Marseille, France

**Scott T. Weiss, M.D., M.S.** Associate Professor in Medicine, Channing Laboratory, Brigham and Women's Hospital and Harvard Medical School, Boston, Massachusetts

# CONTENTS

# Part One

## OCCUPATIONAL DISEASES

MARCEL GOLDBERG

In this part, which is devoted to respiratory occupational diseases, we deal only indirectly with prevention. This is a deliberate choice based on the fact that most preventive measures that can be used at the workplace are very familiar: The toxic effects of airborne pollutants result from their being inhaled, and most preventive measures consist of reducing the quantity of pollutants inhaled, or even eliminating them altogether by individual or collective methods of protection not specifically related to the nature of the pollutants or to the disease prevented. However, this is not always the only approach to prevention, particularly in the presence of individual susceptibility, which could favor development of the disease, since in such a situation it is possible to organize an individually made-to-measure system of primary or secondary prevention, as we shall see in Chapter 6.

We focus on the epidemiology of respiratory occupational diseases. This is because it is an epidemiological study of respiratory occupational diseases which will enable us to identify the causes of diseases and organize prevention on a scientific basis. Epidemiological investigation of the occupational risks of respiratory disease has a long history, and much of the established knowledge we have today has been obtained in this way. Occupational factors weigh heavily in respiratory disease and a large number of toxic agents have been identified and measured in the workplace. However, much remains to be done in identifying other toxic agents, about which we have little or no knowledge, in determining their exact nature and their effects and in analyzing their interactions and relationships with the individual characteristics of workers exposed. Epidemiological research is currently very active in all these areas, and in this part we provide an overview of the main aspects of what is known about the primary respiratory diseases, with an emphasis on the main problems now facing us and the principal avenues of future research.

The section about occupational diseases includes a general presentation of the main trends of current epidemiological research into respiratory diseases, in terms of the main types of risk factors and including a general discussion of the general problem of taking tobacco into account in an epidemiological analysis of respiratory diseases (Chapter 1), followed by a detailed review of established data and the perspectives for epidemiological research about the occupational factors involved in the main diseases and various organs of the respiratory system; the main respiratory cancers are first investigated: pulmonary (Chapter 2), pleural (Chapter 3), upper respiratory tract (Chapter 4), and sinonasal cancer (Chapter 5). There are also two chapters on chronic nonneoplastic diseases: occupational asthma (Chapter 6) and chronic nonspecific lung disease (Chapter 7). The section ends with two chapters dealing with the main methodological problems which will determine to a great extent future research into occupational diseases: analysis of interactions between environmental factors and genetic susceptibility (Chapter 8) and measurement of occupational exposure (Chapter 9).

# 1

## Epidemiology of Occupational Respiratory Hazards: Recent Advances

**J. M. MUR**

Institut National de Recherche et de Sécurité
Vandoeuvre, France

## I. Introduction

A bibliographical review of epidemiological studies published over the last 5 years has led us to individualize the themes that have been the subject of the most numerous publications. These research themes are not new, which shows a certain continuity in epidemiological research on respiratory risks of occupational origin.

Few studies are devoted to the identification of unrecognized respiratory risks; nevertheless, the methodology used and the indicators of effects studied contribute to a better knowledge of the respiratory effects of known occupational exposure factors. Among these effects, the most frequent publications concern exposure to asbestos fibers, silica, isocyanates, and organic dusts. The role of smoking is taken into consideration increasingly in these studies. The themes retained and the publications cited here are not exhaustive, and this bibliographical review does not pretend to represent a complete appraisal of recent developments of the epidemiological respiratory risks of occupational origin.

## II.  Exposure to Asbestos

### A.  Pleural Plaques and Pulmonary Function

Among the diverse nonmalignant radiological abnormalities associated with asbestos exposure, the most frequent are pleural plaques. These develop slowly and, in general, only appear at least 20 years after the onset of exposure. Afterward, their prevalence increases 3% after 20 to 30 years, 14% after 30 to 39 years, and 57% after 40 years, according to Marcus et al. [1]; and from 5.4% before 10 years to 21.2% after 40 years, according to Selikoff et al. [2]. The prevalence of these pleural abnormalities increases with the duration of exposure to asbestos as well; in a survey of 534 boilermakers, Demers et al. [3] observed less than 2% among the workers who had been exposed less than 20 years, and about 20% among those who had a higher exposure duration.

Several studies have been carried out to determine whether these pleural plaques are only a radiological mark of prior exposure to asbestos or whether they are associated with pulmonary function alterations, which could announce the progression of asbestosis. Marcus et al. [1] compared 925 car mechanics who had been exposed to asbestos (in brake repair, notably) with 109 unexposed subjects (office workers from car repair firms). Forty-one mechanics (i.e., 4.4%) had pleural plaques, but none of the comparisons did. The authors did not observe any significant difference in the spirometric tests (FVC, FEV1) between the two subject groups.

In a longitudinal study carried out over almost 10 years, Jones et al. [4] analyzed the progress of radiographic and functional pulmonary abnormalities in 167 workers from two asbestos cement factories (exposure to crocidolite and chrysotile). Through the logistic regression technique they observed a larger decrease in total lung capacity (TLC) and residual volume (RV) in workers whose radiographic pleural abnormalities had worsened than in those whose abnormalities had not progressed. However, the authors question the biological significance of this observation, as it is not associated with a decrease in forced vital capacity (FVC). Velonakis et al. [5] analyzed by multiple regression the relationships between radiological and functional pulmonary abnormalities in a survey of 141 merchant marine seamen. They observed negative associations (nonsignificant) between the existence of pleural abnormalities and vital capacity (FVC) and expiratory flows (FEF 25% and FEF 50%).

In a survey of 202 shipyard workers, Jävholm and Sanden [6] observed a decrease in vital capacity among 87 workers with pleural plaques in comparison with the other workers; this effect was even more important with an extended exposure to asbestos. In 79 shipyard workers with diaphragmatic pleural plaques, Kilburn and Warshaw [7] observed a decrease in expiratory flows (FEV1, FEV1/FVC, FEF 75–85%) and greater total lung capacity (TGV) and residual volume (RV/TGV) than in reference values.

Some of these studies seem therefore to suggest that the existence of pleural plaques, even when limited (e.g., to the diaphragm), is accompanied by functional pulmonary changes of a restrictive or obstructive type. However, the results of these studies are not sufficiently corroborative to conclude that the existence of pleural plaques announces a progression toward asbestosis. Other studies, which include gaseous transfer tests as well, are necessary to research the early signs of pulmonary fibrosis.

### B.  Asbestos and Lung Cancer: Dose–Response Relationships

Many studies have brought to the fore a dose–response relationship between the cumulative exposure over time to asbestos and the relative risk of lung cancer. As Amandus and Wheeler [8] and Neuberger and Kundi [9] present it, the slopes of these relationships are variable according to the studies; this variability may be due to differences in effect according to the nature of the fibers and to methodological differences (cohort effect, confounding factors, definition of exposures, pathology, etc.). Thus in a cohort of 2816 subjects exposed to chrysotile in the asbestos cement industry, Neuberger and Kundi [10] did not observe any increase in the risk of lung cancer for concentrations lower than 25 fibers/mL-year as well as for those higher concentrations after adjustment for smoking.

Despite these differences, it is likely that the risk of lung cancer is connected to a cumulative exposure to asbestos fibers. However, is there a dose below which the risk does not increase? Browne [11] analyzed the results of several epidemiological studies and deduced from them that the threshold of an increase in the risk of lung cancer would be placed between 25 and 100 f/cm$^3$-years. Later studies seem to confirm the existence of a threshold.

In a cohort study of 6391 workers in two asbestos cement factories, Hughes et al. [12] put forward a significant excess in respiratory cancers only among the workers in one of the two factories, the one where crocidolite was used, for a cumulative exposure above 25 mppcf-y and after an exposure delay above or equal to 20 years [relative risk (RR) = 2.00]. However, they also observed in the two factories a significantly higher number of respiratory cancers among workers who had a short exposure time [from 3 to 6 months; standardized mortality rate (SMR) = 1.40].

Amandus and Wheeler [8] and Neuberger and Kundi [9] observed a significant increase in the risk of lung cancer in a cohort of 575 subjects exposed to tremolite–actinolite whose cumulative exposure was above or equal to 400 f/cm$^3$- year and a latency period above or equal to 20 years (SMR = 5.76). In a cohort of 6506 workers from a crocidolite milling firm, Armstrong et al. [13] observed that the level of respiratory cancers grew significantly 15 to 20 years after a cumulative exposure above 100 f/cm$^3$- years. However, the notion of an exposure threshold seems weakened by a study by Seidman et al. [14] on a cohort of 820 workers in an amosite asbestos factory having been exposed to strong concentrations of asbestos within a relatively short period. They observed that mortality from lung cancer is connected to exposure duration (and cumulated dose) and that the latency period of overmortality from lung cancer is all the shorter when the exposure dose is high.

The relationship of dose × latency period in the risk of lung cancer could explain why the exposure threshold put forth in several epidemiological studies is no more than an artifact, connected to short follow-up periods. Let us make the hypothesis that overmortality through lung cancer is connected to the exposure dose of asbestos and to the latency period, as represented in Figure 1. The overmortality through lung cancer for a follow-up period below $t$ only appears for an exposure dose above or equal to $d$, which appears as a threshold value.

This hypothesis seems confirmed in a study by Enterline et al. [15] on a cohort of 1074 workers in an asbestos production factory having retired between 1941 and 1967. A first analysis of mortality between 1941 and 1961 revealed a significant increase of the risk of lung cancer for an exposure above or equal to 250 mppcf-y (SMR = 2.92); a second analysis of the same cohort over a longer period (1941–1980) revealed, in fact, that the increase of incidence was significant for an exposure below 125 mppcf-y (SMR = 2.58). This study illustrates the importance of follow-up length in the estimation of a threshold effect. To determine if there really is a critical exposure threshold, it is therefore necessary to follow over a long period (at least 40 years) subjects having had a weak exposure.

### C. Relationships Between Lung Cancer and Asbestosis

It is well established that asbestos exposure provokes pulmonary fibrosis, called *asbestosis*, and increases the incidence of bronchial cancer. However, we do not for the moment know whether these two affections provoked by asbestos are independent, or whether, on the contrary, bronchial cancers due to asbestos are simply developed (or encouraged) by asbestosis. Epidemiological studies to test this hypothesis are difficult and few in number, as they have to rely on histopathological data for authenticate both pulmonary fibrosis and bronchial cancers.

In a cohort of 17,800 insulation workers, Kipen et al. [16] identified 450 cases of lung cancer, of which 219 had had a pulmonary radiography allowing a diagnosis of pulmonary fibrosis; among these 219 cases, histopathological examinations could be conducted on noncancerous lung tissue in 138 cases. In every case there were histopathological signs of diffuse interstitial fibrosis, although radiological abnormalities (small irregular opacities $\geq 1/0$) were visible in only 82% of these cases. Wagner et al. [17] conducted a histopathological

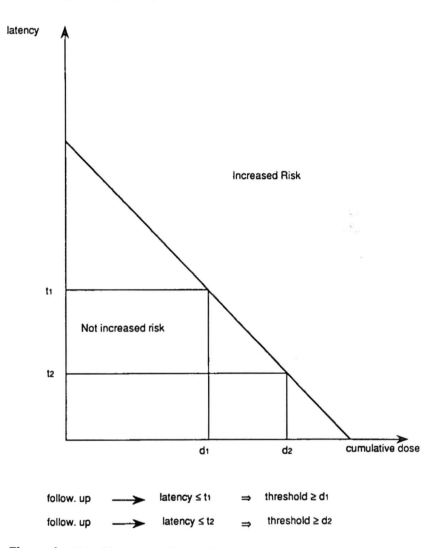

**Figure 1**   Risk of lung cancer due to asbestos exposure.

study of 36 deaths due to asbestos exposure. Among the deaths were 14 cases of lung cancer associated with moderate or severe asbestosis. The 19 cases of pleural mesothelioma were associated with minimal or mild asbestosis.

Sluis-Cremer and Bezuidenhout [18,19] carried out a study on a group of 427 deceased asbestos miners (crocidolite and asbestos), on whom histopathological examinations had been done. There were 35 cases of lung cancer which they compared, using the logistic regression technique, with 364 subjects who were free of lung cancer. Among the various independent factors introduced into the model (smoking, age, asbestos exposure, asbestosis), asbestosis appeared to be the most important explanatory factor of lung cancer; according to the model used, the relative risk of bronchial cancer was 4.45 for mild asbestosis and 10.40 for moderate or large asbestosis. The role of asbestosis persisted when in a complementary step-by-step logistic regression analysis, the signs of asbestos exposure were taken into account beforehand. The standardized proportional mortality rate (SPMR) for bronchial cancer was 417 in mild asbestosis cases and 563 in moderate or severe asbestosis.

Although certainly too few in number, these epidemiological studies on the relationships between asbestosis and lung cancer seem to suggest that the incidence of lung cancer is increased in cases of asbestosis.

### D.  Risk of Larynx Cancer Connected to Asbestos

The risk of larynx cancer connected to asbestos exposure has been brought up in several epidemiological studies reviewed by Edelman [20]. Only two of 13 cohort studies and two case-control studies suggested such a risk; however, consumption of alcohol and tobacco was not taken into account in these studies. According to Edelman [20], the larynx cancer–asbestos exposure relationship has not been established. Several studies were carried out later. These were cohort studies which, for the most part, did not bring to the fore an increased risk of larynx cancer either: Hughes et al. [12] (SMR = 0.56; 0 = 3), Armstrong et al. [13] (0.68 ≤ SMR ≤ 1.09; 0 = 2), Seidman et al. [14] (SMR = 1.92; 0 = 7: VADS cancers), Enterline et al. [15] (SMR = 1.14; 0 = 2), Finkelstein [21] (SMR = 0; 0 = 0). However, these studies have poor statistical power as a result of the small numbers of larynx cancer cases observed.

The study conducted by Raffn et al. [22] on a cohort of 7996 workers in the asbestos cement industry is more powerful. For the 8.44 expected cases of larynx cancer in the total cohort, 14 were observed; the SMR = 1.66 was at the limit of signification [95% confidence interval (CI): 0.91 to 2.78]. The risk of larynx cancer appeared significantly increased in the subcohort of workers employed before 1940 (SMR = 5.50; 0 = 5). However, the authors did not give any indication on the consumption of alcohol and tobacco in this cohort.

In the same way, for a cohort of 1058 chrysotile miners, Piolatto et al.

[23] observed eight cases of laryngeal cancer for an expected 33 (SMR = 2.7; $p < 0.05$). The SMR was higher, but not significant, in the subcohort of longer exposure (SMR = 4.6; 0 = 5). Although the SMR in this study were equally high for affections associated with alcohol consumption (cancer of the oral cavity and pharynx: SMR = 2.3; cirrhosis of the liver: SMR = 2.9), the possible role of asbestos exposure could not be discounted in the increased risk for larynx cancer.

These two studies do not clearly bring to the fore a risk of larynx cancer connected with asbestos, but they incite us the think that this risk cannot be excluded. However, research on this effect requires more powerful studies, especially taking into consideration more closely such confounding factors as the consumption of alcohol and tobacco.

### E. Mesotheliomas

Mesotheliomas (pleural, peritoneal, pericardial) are rare cancers connected with asbestos exposure. The latency period after the onset of exposure is at least 20 years. The frequency of these cancers seems connected with the duration or amount of asbestos exposure. In a case-control study (eight cases) included in a cohort study, Hughes et al. [12] observed odds ratios that grew with exposure duration: 1.6 from 1 to 15 years, 9.0 from 15 to 25 years, and 12.0 beyond 25 years of exposure.

In the same way, Armstrong et al. [13], in a cohort of 6505 crocidolite miners, observed, after a latency period of 20 years, an incidence rate increase of mesotheliomas in relationship with cumulative exposure to asbestos. However, mesothelioma cases can appear with low exposure durations. In the cohort study by Raffn et al. [22], two cases in 10 were exposed for less than 5 years (SMR = 3.77; CI = 0.42 - 13.62). In a study by Hughes et al. [12], three cases in 10 were exposed less than 1 year. In a study by Enterline et al. [15], three cases in eight had a cumulative exposure under 100 mppcf-y.

Moreover, prior asbestos exposure is not always identified and, in certain cases, may be ruled out. In 124 pleural mesothelioma cases, Van Gelder et al. [24] were not able to show prior asbestos exposure in 29 cases. Mowé and Gylseth [25] identified, through the Norwegian cancer registry, 117 male and 29 female cases of mesothelioma (pleural and peritoneal). For 18% of the men and 83% of the women, prior asbestos exposure was most improbable. In 36 cases of histologically confirmed pleural and peritoneal mesothelioma, Hirsch et al. [26] were able to eliminate prior asbestos to exposure in 10 cases (27.8%). In 68 cases of pleural mesothelioma in western Glasgow, Hulks et al. [27] did not show prior asbestos exposure in 14 cases (20.6%).

In a study conducted in Switzerland by Minder and Vader [28], of 203 cases of pleural mesothelioma that occurred to men aged from 30 to 74, 12 concerned furniture workers; according to the authors, it was unlikely that these workers had any prior asbestos exposure. Thus if there is no doubt that asbestos exposure is responsible for a large number of mesotheliomas, the role of other factors (e.g., ionizing radiations) can be suspected. The mesothelioma registries, as they exist in several countries (Great Britain, Sweden, Norway, France, etc.), will make it possible to carry out case-control epidemiological studies in the research of these factors.

## III.  Artificial Mineral Fibers

Because of the risks associated with asbestos use, other fibrous materials (man-made mineral fibers) have been developed for some time. A review of epidemiological studies to evaluate possible risks connected with these fibers was carried out by Saracci [29]. According to the author, prior studies do not permit removal of the hypothesis of an excess risk of lung cancer connected with exposure to these fibers. Of eight analyzed mortality studies, four did not present evidence of such a risk, and the results of the four others were compatible with the hypothesis of such a risk.

This explains why a vast multicentric European study was carried out by Simonato et al. [30] on a cohort of 21,967 workers in 13 factories producing man-made mineral fibers. Analyzing 189 deaths (151.2 expected) in this cohort, mortality by lung cancer seemed associated with time since first exposure but not duration. There was an excess of mortality through lung cancer among workers exposed to rock wool and slag wool at the beginning of production of these fibers before the introduction of health measures. On the other hand, there was no such risk for glass-wool production workers.

Other man-made mineral fibers are presently being developed (ceramic fibers). Although no epidemiological study has yet been published on the risks connected with exposure to these fibers, experimental data (still unpublished) may create the fear of a risk of bronchial cancer and mesothelioma. In agreement with the profession, epidemiological studies will be undertaken to evaluate the reality of this risk.

## IV.  Silica Exposure and Lung Cancer

The hypothesis of an association between silica exposure and the risk of lung cancer was advanced more than 50 years ago. Since then numerous epidemiological studies have been conducted to test this hypothesis, but their results disagree. In fact, two hypotheses on the pulmonary carcinogenic role of silica can be formulated.

## A.  First Hypothesis

Is silica exposure, alone or associated with other substances (e.g., aromatic polycyclic hydrocarbons), a risk factor of lung cancer?

### Cohort Studies

Cohort studies have been conducted in diverse sectors of activity (mines, quarries, foundries, etc.). Silica exposure is not always defined with precision, and other risk factors (occupational or nonoccupational) are rarely taken into consideration. Their results are conflicting. Fletcher [31] studied the mortality of a cohort of 11,048 foundry workers in Great Britain. He observed an overmortality from lung cancer (SMR = 1.49), which was greater among workers directly exposed to silica (SMR = 1.71); this risk was associated with length of employment but increased with the date of first exposure, whereas at the same time exposure to silica decreased. The author deduced from this that the excess of lung cancers could not be directly attributable to silica exposure. In the same article Fletcher reports the results of an analysis of the causes of death of 1540 foundry workers. The standardized proportional mortality ratios (SPMRs) for lung cancer were high for skilled (SPMR = 125) and unskilled (SPMR = 154) molders; however, in this last group, there appeared an inverse relationship with length of employment.

Steenland and Beaumont [32] also carried out a proportional mortality study on a cohort of granite cutters, of which 1905 were dead. They observed only a slight, nonsignificant excess of mortality from lung cancer [proportional mortality ratio (PMR) = 1.09], but they indicated that the risk of lung cancer could be high among silicotic subjects. Thomas and Stewart [33] studied the mortality of 2055 pottery workers exposed to silica and talc. There was an excess of mortality from lung cancer (64 observed, 37 expected), more particularly among those workers exposed to the highest concentrations of silica and nonfibrous talc. The overmortality from lung cancer increased with exposure length to nonfibrous talc.

Neuberger et al. [34] studied the mortality of a cohort of 1630 workers exposed to nonfibrous dusts of an ill-defined nature, but very likely containing, for some, crystalline silica in diverse industrial sectors. They observed, in this cohort, a lung cancer mortality 45 times higher than in the comparison cohort of the same size, made up of workers unexposed to dusts.

Costello and Graham [35] followed a cohort of 5414 granite workers, of which 1932 died between 1950 and 1982. They did not observe an overmortality through lung cancer. Archer et al. [36] compared rates of silicosis and lung cancer among five mining groups selected on the basis of degrees of their exposure to silica and radon. When silica exposure levels were high (without exposure to radon), silicosis rates were high but lung cancer rates were not increased; lung cancer rates increased only in the case of radon exposure.

Brown et al. [37] conducted a retrospective mortality study on a cohort of 3328 gold mine workers. They observed a slight overmortality from lung cancer only among workers employed before 1930, when the levels of exposure to dusts were higher. However, they could not provide evidence of a relationship between cumulative exposure to dusts and the risk of lung cancer.

### Case-Control Studies

A large case-control study was carried out by Siemiatycki et al. [38] to research the relationships between 20 types of cancer and exposure to inorganic dusts. The job histories of the cases and controls were obtained by interview and analyzed by experts to evaluate exposures. After adjustment for potential confounders, a significant association between lung cancer and exposure to silica [odds ratios (OR) = 1.4], to excavation dust (OR = 1.9), to cement dust (OR = 2.5), and abrasives dust (OR = 1.4) appeared.

Another case-control study, more particularly centered on the relationships between lung cancer and exposure to coal mine dusts, was conducted by Ames et al. [39]: A one-to-one matched case analysis (to evaluate the risk of coal mine dusts and smoking) and a 2:1 matched case analysis (to evaluate the risk of coal mine dusts independent of smoking) were employed on 317 cases of lung cancer. No evidence of a coal mine dust exposure/lung cancer risk was found, nor was there evidence of an interactive effect with smoking.

Meijers et al. [40] conducted a study on 381 Danish coal miners with lung cancer matched with controls (smoking, unknown, was not taken into consideration in the matching). The length of work underground was not significantly different between cases and controls.

### Other Studies

A geographic epidemiological study was carried out by Frazier and Sundin [41] in the United States, comparing maps of potential silica exposure and maps of mortality. There was some coincidence in the geographical distribution of mortality through silicosis and lung cancer in coal mining areas.

### B. Second Hypothesis

Does silicosis increase the risk of lung cancer? Numerous cohort and case-control studies have been carried out over the last few years to test this hypothesis. These studies generally take the possible effects of smoking into consideration more closely than do precedent studies. On the whole their results seem more concordant.

### Cohort Studies

We are dealing with cohort subjects having a recognized pneumoconiosis. Of seven studies analyzed, six seem to indicate an increased lung cancer risk for silicotic subjects. Only the study by Meijers et al. [42] of 334 Danish miners with pneumoconiosis does not present evidence of overmortality through lung cancer (SMR = 1.31).

Schuler and Ruttner [43] observed a relative lung cancer risk of 2.2 in a cohort of 2399 silicotic subjects; this overmortality did not seem to be attributed only to smoking, which was not taken into consideration in this study. In the same way, Finkelstein et al. [44], Westerholm et al. [45], and Kurppa et al. [46] observed an overmortality through lung cancer among silicotic subjects whose smoking habits were not known.

In the following two cohort studies, smoking was taken into consideration. Tze Pin et al. [47] studied a cohort of 1419 silicotic men not having been exposed to asbestos or aromatic polycyclic hydrocarbons. The risk of lung cancer was high among underground (SMR = 3.41) and surface (SMR = 1.87) miners and increased with the severity of silicosis. Zambon et al. [48] observed a doubling of mortality from lung cancer in a cohort of 1234 silicotics. The risk of lung cancer increased with time since the onset of silica exposure, in particular after 20 years.

### Case-Control Studies

Of three recent case-control studies, most of which took smoking into consideration, two seemed to indicate a relationship between silicosis and lung cancer. Hessel and Sluis-Cremer [49] compared 127 South African gold miners with lung cancer with other cancer-free miners, matched for age and smoking. They did not observe an association between exposure to silica or silicosis and lung cancer.

Forastière et al. [50] carried out a case (72 lung cancers)-control (319 subjects matched on age and smoking) study in a region of Italy where there is a large ceramic industry. In this study 45.8% of the cases and 32.6% of the controls were ceramic workers (absolute risk:1.8). 21% of the cases and 7.8% of the controls had silicosis (absolute risk: 3.4). The relative risk of lung cancer was 3.9 for the silicotic ceramic workers and 1.4 for the nonsilicotic. In an analogous study of 309 lung cancer cases and 309 controls, Mastrangelo et al. [51], observed that silica exposure increased the risk of lung cancer only when in the presence of pulmonary silicosis. This risk tended to increase with the length of silica exposure and heavy smoking.

### Other Studies

Two studies dealt with the analysis of dead silicotic subjects. Forastière et al. [52] analyzed the causes of death of 595 silicotics. The proportion of deaths from lung cancer was increased in comparison with that of the regional population (OR = 4.1). However, this overmortality did not seem to be associated with the intensity of silicosis. The prevalence of smoking was not different between the dead lung cancer subjects and those who died from silicosis.

James [53] analyzed the autopsy results of 1827 coal miners and 1531 controls who were not miners. There were 5.1% of lung cancers among the miners that had simple pneumoconiosis and 1.4% among those that had massive fibrosis. Moreover, the incidence of lung cancer was weaker among the miners than among those that were not miners. Recent epidemiological studies do not provide corroborating results on the pulmonary carcinogenic role of silica exposure. On the other hand, several studies present evidence of a heightened risk of lung cancer among silicotic subjects. The hypothesis of a silicosis–lung cancer association appears more and more likely.

## V.  Respiratory Pathology of Farmers

Exposure to organic dusts and microorganisms in agricultural areas is responsible for frequent and diverse pathological respiratory impairments, which have been the object of numerous epidemiological studies over the last few years. The diseases observed can be divided into three categories: toxic syndrome due to organic dusts; allergic diseases, among which are asthma and extrinsic allergic alveolitis ("farmer's lung); and chronic obstructive bronchopneumopathies.

### A.  Toxic Syndrome Due to Organic Dusts

Toxic syndrome due to organic dusts appears a few hours after exposure to organic dusts (grain, hay, straw, etc.) and is revealed by a transitory syndrome that can last several days, accompanied by fever, myalgies, thoracic oppression, cough, and headache. Because of the transitory character of these syndromes, their incidence rate is difficult to evaluate. In a study of 2866 Finnish farmers, Husman et al. [54] identified 13.6% of organic dust toxic syndromes. They noticed that these appearances happened more frequently among cattle farmers (14%) than among pig farmers (8.5%). The organic dust toxic syndrome seemed to be a factor predisposing the development of chronic bronchitis. These syndromes are generally attributed to endotoxin inhalation; however, Rask-Andersen et al. [55] did not observe a significant difference in the endotoxin concentrations between 27 farms where such syndromes appeared and 18 comparison farms.

Several studies have been carried out to research the possible inplication of immunological mechanisms. Pratt et al. [56] did not present evidence of precipitant antibodies against the usual antigens of farmer's lung, nor even of specific precipitant antibodies of agricultural produces handled by 29 subjects unloading silos. Rask-Andersen [57] identified 80 cases of organic dust toxic syndrome among 390 Swedish farmers. He did not observe a significant difference in the frequency of positive prick tests, in the total concentration of IgE, and in the existence of precipitant antibodies between the subjects presenting this syndrome and those who were free of it.

Malmberg and Rask-Andersen [58] compared 470 Swedish farmers with 20 cattle breeders. Of the farmers, 128 presented at least one febrile symptom, diagnosed as organic dust toxic syndrome; 29% of these subjects had precipitant antibodies, although the proportion was 53% among farmers with extrinsic allergic alveolitis (farmer's lung) and 11% among the cattle breeders. On the other hand, Warren et al. [59] presented evidence of a relationship between respiratory symptomatology, the frequency of positive prick tests, the increase in total IgE concentration, and the level of exposure to grain dusts in a study of 424 men working regularly on a farm, 237 men working occasionally on a farm, and 266 men not working on a farm.

Malmberg et al. [60] carried out an epidemiological study of 289 Swedish farmers; among them, 2% had asthma, 4% had experienced bronchial obstructive symptoms associated with the inhalation of organic dusts, 4% had intrathoracic wheezing, and 6% had febrile responses to the handling of moldy hay (organic dust toxic syndrome?). The spirometry and the level of IgE among the latter was normal; however, the presence of precipitant antibodies was higher (7%) than among those who had not had a febrile response (4%). It would seem that febrile responses occur when the atmospheric concentration of microorganisms is above $10^9$ microorganisms/m$^3$. In another study, Malmberg et al. [61] identified 6.1% of febrile responses among 2174 Swedish farmers. The subjects having these symptoms had precipitant antibodies and an immunoglobin IgG increase more frequently than subjects never having had these symptoms.

### B. Farmer's Lung

According to Rylander [62], this affection is due to an acute and chronic inflammation of the distale bronchia and alveoli. The illness starts suddenly with respiratory symptoms (cough, thoracic oppression) associated with general signs: shivers, fever, headache, nausea, arthralgia, and myalgia. The illness generally appears following repeated exposure, most notably to moldy hay. The length of the illness is variable (a few days to a few weeks) and stops when exposure ceases. However, the illness can progress toward pulmonary fibrosis. At the acute stage, a chest x-ray may reveal small nodular parenchyma infiltrations resembling pneumonia or miliara.

According to Terho et al. [63], the annual incidence rate of farmer's lung disease is 44 per 100,000 of the Finnish agricultural population. In another study of 9483 Finnish farmers, Terho et al. [64] observed a prevalence of 1.7% and an annual incidence level of 540 per 100,000 of farmer's lung disease among cattle breeders. Among 381 Irish farmers, Stanford [65] identified 4.9% of certain cases and 10.4% of probable ones. Tao et al. [66] counted 11.4% among 1054 subjects handling hay. According to Terho et al. [67], this infection is more frequent among cattle breeders. In several studies there was evidence of antibodies with variable frequency. The proportion of positive serologic tests to antigens of thermoactinomyces vulgaris was high in a survey of farmers' studies by Tao et al. [66].

Belin and Malmberg [68] researched the presence of antibodies among farmers. Of 250 serums from Icelandic farmers, 150 of whom presented symptoms of farmer's lung illness, they observed a significant correlation between the symptoms and the existence of precipitant antibodies to *Micropolyspora faeni*. In another group of Swedish farmers, they noticed higher levels (through the DIG-ELISA method) of IgG antibody (*Rhizopus* and *Aspergillus fumigatus*) and IgA antibodies (*M. faeni*) among farmers presenting symptoms of farmer's lung disease than among those who were free of it.

Brouwer et al. [69] researched the presence of IgE and IgG4 antibodies against pig fodder and biological pig extract (urine, hair) antigens in a group of 57 pig farmers. None of the subjects had IgE antibodies against pig extracts; but IgG antibodies against pig fodder was frequent, particularly in a subgroup of farmers that fattened pigs in enclosed spaces. In a survey of 339 poultry farmers, Müller et al. [70] counted 5% having farmer's lung disease, and 22% of all the subjects had precipitant antibodies (against biological hen extract). The presence of antibodies was connected to exposure length. Intracutaneous testing with hen serum provoked an Arthus reaction in 28.6% and a delayed reaction in 26.2% of the subjects having antibodies; no reaction was observed in those who had no antibodies.

In the study by Malmberg and Rask-Andersen [58] cited earlier, 35 of 470 farmers had a farmer's lung disease; 53% of these subjects had precipitant antibodies. On the other hand, in the study by Marx et al. [71], the presence of antibodies specific to agents of farmer's lung disease was associated with the existence of asthma and chronic bronchitis, but not to extrinsic allergic alveolitis.

### C.  Chronic Obstructive Bronchopneumopathies

Several studies show chronic bronchitis and/or alteration in lung function among farmers. In the study by Terho et al. [64] cited earlier, the prevalence of chronic bronchitis was 8% in the entire set of 9483 studied farmers and 7.6% among cattle breeders; the annual incidence rate was 2047 and 2017 per 100,000, respectively. The prevalence and incidence of chronic bronchitis was twice as high in smokers than in nonsmokers and twice as high in atopic subjects than in nonatopic ones. De Haller [72] observed a higher prevalence of chronic bronchitis in dairy farmers (43%) than in a control group (5%). This difference was greater in nonsmokers (31% vs. 2%). Among 824 agricultural workers, Milosevic [73] observed a variable prevalence of chronic bronchitis based on type of activity: it was higher in cattle breeders (39.3%).

Hurst et al. [74] compared 1939 farmers to 556 controls. Respiratory symptomatology (cough, expectoration, shortness of breath) and functional lung abnormalities (reduction of FVC, $FEV_1$, and MMFR) were more frequent in farmers than in controls. Among 1175 farmers, Iversen et al. [75] observed asthma appearances (5.5% in dairy farmers and 10.9% in pig farmers), shortness of breath, thoracic wheezing, and cough (7.4% in dairy farmers and 28.3% in pig farmers). Iversen et al. [76] individualized three groups of farmers. Those who had asthma (47) had a reduced $FEV_1$ (forced expired volume in 1 s value), and bronchial hyperreactivity, not, however, associated with length of employment. Among those who presented thoracic wheezing symptoms, shortness of breath, and cough (63), the reduction in $FEV_1$ was associated with histamine concentration and the length of employment in pig farming. Among the asymptomatic subjects (34), the $FEV_1$ value and bronchial reactivity were not connected to any of these factors.

In another study, Iversen et al. [77] observed that among 103 pig farmers with normal lung function, 37% had bronchial hyperreactivity to histamine, connected to the existence of lung symptoms. Rylander et al. [78] compared bronchial reactivity to metacholine in 36 pig farmers, 23 dairy farmers, and 16 controls. They observed that bronchial reactivity was higher in farmers than in the controls and that it was connected to job length. Dosman et al. [79] observed a reduction of vital capacity (FVC), of $FEV_1$, and of midexpiratory flow rate in 1824 farmers compared to 556 controls.

In the study by Dalphin et al. [80] the prevalence of chronic bronchitis was 12% among cattle breeders and 6% among a same-sized control group. All the spirometric signs were lower in the farmers when compared with the controls. In the same way, Musk et al. [81] observed a reduction in $FEV_1$, and a nonspecific cutaneous (prick test) and bronchial reactivity among the women most exposed to flour dust in a commercial bakery. Respiratory effects (reduction of FVC, $FEV_1$, respiratory symptomatology) were observed as well in pig farmers by Haglind and Rylander [82], Wilhelmsson et al. [83], and Donham et al. [84]. Studies have also been conducted on the functional pulmonary effects of short-term exposure to grain dusts.

Revsbech and Andersen [85] observed, in 132 grain-handling subjects, a relationship between the daily variations in peak expiratory flow rate (PEFR) and the exposure level. James et al. [86] studied the ventilation function of 41 grain-handling subjects and 10 controls for 4 weeks. They observed a reduction in $FEV_1$ greater in exposed subjects than in the controls at the end of the first week, followed by a return to normal. On the other hand, Manfreda et al. [87]

did not observe, in a group of 1892 people (of which 968 women) living in a rural community, a relationship between exposure to grain dusts and respiratory symptomatology or function.

Heederik et al. [88] studied the progress, over a week, of respiratory function of 33 pig farmers. There was no evidence of a significant relationship between the functional pulmonary signs of these subjects and the grain or endotoxin concentrations to which they were exposed. Donham et al. [84] compared the respiratory symptomatology and function of 57 pig farmers and 55 matched controls. Among the farmers the prevalence of chronic cough was greater (68% vs. 24%) and the expiratory flow rates (FEF$_{50}$ and FEF$_{75}$) weaker than in the controls. There was a significant correlation between the reduction of expiratory flow rates (FEF$_{50}$ and FEF$_{75}$) of the farmers throughout the workday and atmospheric concentrations of endotoxins and bacteria. In another study, Donham et al. [89] observed that the reduction of FEV$_1$ and FEF$_{25-75}$ throughout the workday was significantly larger among 257 poultry farmers compared to 150 controls. These many epidemiological studies testify to the large prevalence and diversity of respiratory effects in rural communities.

## VI.  Respiratory Pathology Connected to Exposure to Cotton Dusts

### A.  Byssinosis

This disease was described by Schilling in 1955 as a thoracic oppression coming on Monday morning. According to Rylander [90], this symptomatology may be attributable to gram-negative bacteria endotoxins contaminating cotton. Several recent epidemiological studies have been conducted to evaluate the frequency of this illness in association with the exposure level to cotton dusts. In a study of 4656 workers employed in spinning and weaving man-made fiber and cotton, Cinkotai et al. [91,92] observed that the prevalence of byssinosis (3.9% in total) was related to cotton dust concentration, exposure length, and cotton quality.

Ong et al. [93] observed a global byssinosis prevalence of 2.3%, associated with cotton dust concentrations in 2317 cotton workers. In the study conducted by Takam and Nemery [94] in a textile industry in Cameroun, byssinosis prevalence was 18% in 125 subjects exposed to mean dust concentration of 6.4 mg/m$^3$. In 1375 cotton industry workers in Jakarta, Baratawidjaja [95] observed a byssinosis prevalence of 30% in spinners and 19.25% in weavers. The dust concentrations were high and associated with byssinosis prevalence. However, the latter did not appear connected to exposure length.

Certain authors have tried to objectivize the symptomatic manifestations of byssinosis using functional pulmonary tests at both the beginning and end of work shifts. Dehong et al. [96] evaluated byssinosis prevalence in two cotton industries. In one of them, where cotton dust concentration levels were high (57 to 159 mg/m$^3$), byssinosis prevalence was 22.2%. In the other factory, where dust concentrations were lower (6.8 mg/m$^3$), byssinosis prevalence was 1.2%. These authors observed a significant relationship between byssinosis prevalence and cotton dust exposure length. Measurements of FEV$_1$ were carried out at the beginning and end of Monday work shifts. Only subjects with byssinosis had a significant reduction of FEV$_1$, a mean of 177 mL. In the study conducted by Mu-Zhen [97] on 289 cotton workers, byssinosis prevalence was 4.2% and connected to cotton dust concentrations (mean atmospheric respirable dust concentrations of 0.2 to 3.5 mg/m3). Reduction of at least 5% of FEV$_1$ between the beginning and end of work shifts, as well as the prevalence of reduced FEV$_1$ values (<80% of reference values), was highest among subjects with at least 15 years of exposure (42.3% and 73.8%, respectively).

In their study of 2317 cotton industry workers in Hong Kong, Ong et al. [93] observed that reduction of at least 10% of FEV$_1$, between the beginning and end of work shifts, was more frequent among carders (13%) than among weavers (7%). Rastogi [98] also observed a larger decrease of FEV$_1$ between the beginning and end of work shifts in workers with byssinosis (294.1 ± 28.2 mL) than in those free from it (66.3 ± 8.3 mL). Awad Elkarim and Onsa [99] carried out a study on 186 spinners in two Sudanese textile factories. Byssinosis prevalence was 37% in one factory where coarse cotton was processed and 1% in the other where fine cotton was processed. Mean respirable dust concentrations in the two factories were 0.43 and 0.23 mg/m$^3$, respectively. The proportion of subjects in whom FEV$_1$ reduced by more than 0.2 mL between the beginning and end of work shifts was higher in the first factory (48%) than in the second (11%).

Christiani et al. [100,101] compared symptomatology and pulmonary function of 448 workers from two cotton mills with 439 silk mill workers in China. Byssinosis prevalence was 8% in workers exposed to cotton but did not appear connected to work duration or exposure level. The reduction of FEV$_1$ over the work shift was greater in cotton workers when exposure duration was longer and was larger in byssinotic subjects than in cotton workers without byssinosis. Bazas et al. [102] compared 41 cotton workers (bale opening and carders) to 39 controls. Among subjects exposed to cotton (mean atmospheric respirable dust concentration of about 0.2 mg/m$^3$), byssinosis prevalence was 5%. A reduction of FEV$_1$ > 0.2l over the work shift was observed in 39% of workers exposed to cotton and 25% of controls. Massin et al. [103] carried out a study on 774 French cotton industry workers and 464 controls. Byssinosis prevalence was 6.2% in subjects exposed to cotton and was connected to exposure duration. A reduction of 10% in peak expiratory flow (PEF) over the work shift was observed in 8.1% of exposed subjects and 2.1% of controls; however, the manifestations of bronchial reactivity appeared but were only weakly connected to the existence of byssinosis.

### B. Pulmonary Function Changes and Chronic Obstructive Bronchopneumopathies

Rastogi et al. [104] observed that the prevalence of obstructive syndromes was 15.7% in 133 byssinotic subjects, 6.8% in cotton-exposed subjects without symptomatology, and 2.3% in controls. Among byssinotics, the prevalence of obstructive syndromes was connected to the degree of byssinosis: 9.6% for grade I and 31.5% for grade II. Moreover, the prevalence of obstructive syndromes for cotton-exposed subjects (with or without byssinosis) was connected to exposure duration. Similarly, Lu et al. [105] observed a prevalence of chronic bronchitis of 14.4% in 861 cotton-exposed subjects and 5.1% in 822 controls. The $FEV_1$ value decreased by 32.1% and 16.5%, respectively, for subjects from these two groups.

In a study conducted by Takam and Nemery [94], cotton-exposed subjects had a PEF value significantly below that of controls. In the exposed subjects, the prevalence of chronic bronchitis was 52% in byssotics and 6% in subjects without byssinosis. According to Awad Elkarim and Onsa [99], the prevalence of chronic bronchitis was 29% in coarse cotton–exposed workers and 2% in those exposed to fine cotton. According to Christiani et al. [100,101], the relative risk of chronic bronchitis connected to employment in cotton industries was 3.3.

Chronic bronchitis and obstructive syndromes seem to persist after exposure stops. Thus Elwood et al. [106] noticed a reduction of 2 to 8% of FVC and $FEV_1$, and a heightened prevalence of chronic bronchitis in 472 retired subjects exposed to cotton compared with 418 controls. The reduction of functional pulmonary signs was in relation to the level of prior cotton exposure. In their study, Lu et al. [105] individualized among retired subjects (from 1 to 10 years), 173 having been exposed to cotton and 373 controls. The pulmonary function of subjects having been exposed to cotton was less good (with the exception of vital capacity) than that of retired controls, among smokers.

## VII.  Respiratory Effects Connected to Isocyanate Exposure

Exposure to isocyanates is more and more frequent as a result of the growing use of these substances in the composition of paints, varnishes, polyurethane foam, and so on, Asthmatic pathology connected to toluylene–diisocyanate (TDI) and methylene–diisocyanate (MDI) exposure has been known for more than 50 years and led to the substitution of isocyanates with a higher molecular weight and of prepolymers supposed less toxic. Epidemiological studies are continued, on the one hand, to evaluate respiratory risks connected to these isocyanates and, on the other hand, to improve knowledge of the sensitization mechanisms to these substances.

### A. Acute Respiratory Effects to Isocyanates Exposure

Studies have been conducted to evaluate pulmonary function changes of workers exposed to isocyanates throughout the day or the week of work. Alexandersson et al. [107] studied functional pulmonary changes (spirometry, nitrogen washout) between the start and end of the work week in 41 automobile industry painters exposed to HDI-BT, to a mean concentration of 115 $\mu$g/m$^3$ (Swedish TWA = 90 $\mu$g/m$^3$) and in 70 controls (mechanics) matched on sex, age, size, and smoking habits. Base values (Monday morning) of closing volume (CV/VC) were higher in painters than in controls, but the progression over the week of spirometric signs and nitrogen washout evaluation was not significantly different between the painters and controls.

Holness et al. [108] carried out a similar study on 95 workers exposed to TDI (mean exposure = 1.2 ± 1.4 ppb) and 35 controls. Spirometric indices values were not significantly different on Monday morning between subjects and controls. Reduction in spirometric indices over the work week was greater in the exposed workers than in the controls: 44% of exposed workers and 22% of controls had a reduction of at least 5% in spirometric indices values between the beginning and end of the work shift. However, the authors were not able to present evidence of a relationship between TDI exposure level and spirometric indices changes.

### B. Research on Bronchial Reactivity

Hjortsberg et al. [109] carried out a test of bronchial reactivity to methacholine on 20 subjects exposed to isocyanates without respiratory syndromes, five subjects with occupational isocyanate asthma, and 10 controls. They observed a larger small airways reactivity among exposed subjects and asthmatics than among controls. Bronchial reactivity intensity was not significantly different between the symptomless exposed subjects and asthmatics. Among 51 aeroplane industry spray painters exposed to diverse isocyanates (TDI, HDI, MDI, IDPI, PPI), Seguin et al. [110] identified 10 subjects with respiratory symptoms (nocturnal cough, intrathoracic wheezing, shortness of breath, etc.). They submitted these subjects to nonspecific (histamine) and specific (PPI and MDI) challenge tests. All the symptomatic subjects presented a positive reaction to histamine, and six of them had a positive reaction to the isocyanate specific provocation test.

A similar study was carried out by Paggiaro et al. [111] on 20 painters with TDI occupational asthma. A TDI specific challenge test allowed the subjects to be split up into three groups in accordance with the concentration level of TDI triggering off a bronchial reaction: nine subjects reacted to a mild TDI concentration (0.02 ppm), seven to a moderate concentration, and four to a higher concentration (0.25 ppm). However, no relationship appeared between the threshold of bronchial reactivity and spirometric indices changes at the time of exposure to the mildest concentration, between TDI concentration and bronchial reactivity intensity (for subjects reacting to at least two different TDI concentrations), or between TDI bronchial reactivity and nonspecific bronchial reactivity to methacholine.

## C.  Immunological Studies

Keskinen et al. [112] measured out concentrations in total and specific immunoglobulins (IgE) to TDI (RAST) in 35 subjects with occupational asthma due to isocyanates (TDI, MDI, HDI), confirmed by a specific challenge test. The authors also carried out cutaneous challenge tests (prick test) to common allergens; at least one of these tests was positive for 11 of the 35 subjects: seven of them had an immediate reaction to the bronchial specific challenge test and four had a late reaction. Less than 50% of the immediate reactions to the bronchial challenge test were associated with an IgE mediation. None of the late reaction subjects to the bronchial provocation test had specific antiisocyanates IgE. Total IgE concentration was higher in subjects having specific antibodies (185 KV/I). The authors concluded that specific antibody research using the RAST method is useful in confirming occupational asthma due to isocyanates but cannot replace bronchial specific provocation tests because of false negatives.

Grammer et al. [113] measured out IgE and IgG specific antiisocyanate antibodies using the ELISA method in 150 subjects exposed to HDI and THDI. Specific IgG antibodies were identified in 7 to 18% subjects and specific IgE in 6 to 9% (following the workplace). The proportion of subjects with specific antibodies seemed higher in the most exposed subjects (IgG: 15%; IgE: 6 to 9%) than in the least exposed subjects (IgG: 7%). However, there was no relationship between specific antibodies concentrations and exposure duration to isocyanates, or in the existence of respiratory symptoms.

Game [114] researched IgE specific antibodies (*p*-tolylisocyanate/human serum albumin: PTI-MSA) in 70 TDI exposed subjects and 20 nonexposed blood donors. Three subjects with asthma or chronic bronchial obstruction connected to isocyanates and one exposed subject, but without symptomatology, had abnormally high antibody values. However, the authors indicated that this technique does not identify the antigenic determinant.

## D.  Long-Term Pulmonary Effect of Exposure to Isocyanates

Banks et al. [115] followed six subjects with asthma due to TDI. The respiratory symptoms of these subjects did not improve and nonspecific bronchial reactivity persisted 5 years after exposure to isocyanates had ceased. Other studies seem to indicate that prolonged exposure to isocyanates may lead to chronic obstructive bronchopneumopathy. Among 180 subjects exposed to HDI, Saia et al. [116] found 19% with chronic bronchitis. About 50% of these workers had a reduction of vital capacity and $FEV_1$; these functional changes were connected to exposure length to isocyanates.

For 6 years Tornling et al. [117] studied the pulmonary function of 36 automobile industry painters exposed to HDI and HDI-BT, and 115 controls. Reduction in FVC, $FEV_1$, and closing volume (CV) was significantly larger in smoking painters than in smoking controls (no significant difference for nonsmokers). It would seem that this progression was connected to the frequency of high peak exposures to HDI-BT and not the mean concentration of isocyanates. These studies confirm the risk of bronchial sensitization to isocyanates. However, as a result of exposures being frequently joined to different isocyanates, it remains difficult to evaluate their specific effects. Nonspecific (methacholine) and specific bronchial challenge tests seem the most reliable method in proving the occupational origin of isocyanate asthmas. Immunological determinations are delicate and their interpretation difficult. Long-term effects (chronic obstructive bronchopneumopathies) are likely. Some of the recent epidemiological studies on the effects of exposure to isocyanates are contested methodologically because of the small size of the study groups and the absence of comparison controls.

## VIII. Tobacco, Occupational Exposure, and Respiratory Diseases

Smoking is an important and frequent risk factor in some respiratory diseases (chronic bronchitis, lung cancer). As a result of this effect, the interpretation of epidemiological studies on the risks of occupational respiratory diseases is disturbed. The problems posed by smoking in epidemiological enquiries have two natures.

### A. Smoking as a Bias Factor in Epidemiological Studies on Occupational Risks

Smoking can be a bias in epidemiological surveys on occupational respiratory risks. Smoking is connected to certain ethnic, social, and occupational characteristics, and this fact may constitute a confounding factor with regard to the studied occupational exposure factors. Brackbill et al. [118], Siematycki et al. [119], and Sterling and Weinham [120] have shown that smoking habits differ according to race, occupational status (working or unemployed), and occupation. However, the importance of this bias risk must not be overestimated. Thus, in their study, Siematycki et al. [119] did not present evidence of the relationship between smoking habits and exposure to 10 industrial pollutants. Furthermore, Blair et al. [121] observed very good correlation coefficients between crude and smoking-adjusted SMR values for different affections connected to smoking: lung cancer ($r = 0.88$), bladder cancer ($r = 0.98$), and intestinal cancer ($r = 0.97$).

However, it is preferable, when possible, to take smoking habits into consideration in epidemiological surveys. In certain cases the information can be had directly from the subjects medical or administrative files. As Marsh et al. [122] indicated, this information is more difficult to obtain in retrospective cohort surveys. In cases like these, Axelson and Steenland [123] proposed the use of indirect methods such as mortality analysis of other illnesses connected to smoking, use of an internal reference cohort, use of an adjustment factor corresponding to hypothesized differences in smoking between the exposed and nonexposed groups, or dose–response analysis of the occupational data studied.

## B.  Interactions Between Smoking and Occupational Respiratory Hazards

### Methodological Aspects

It may be that smoking modifies the relationship between exposure to an occupational factor and its effect on health. This action, often called *interaction,* has an ambiguous meaning in the publications of epidemiological studies. According to Thomas and Whittemore [124], the definition of interaction between two factors is in fact linked to the statistical model used to explain the joint effects of these two factors. The most frequently used models are the additive and the multiplicative. The agreement of observations with the multiplicative model is frequently wrongly called interaction or synergistic. In fact, according to these authors, interaction can be defined as a discrepancy between the data observed and the chosen statistical model. For example, there is interaction when the relative risk (in the case of a multiplicative model) or the risk difference (in the case of an additive model) linked to one of the factors depends on exposure to the other factor.

### Examples

#### Asbestos and Tobacco

Saracci [125] applied three models (additive, multiplicative, synergistic) to data from several epidemiological studies on the risks of cancer connected with asbestos. He observed that the multiplicative model was the most suitable. In a cohort study of 12,051 asbestos-exposed workers, Selikoff and Hammond [126] observed a multiplicative effect of exposure to asbestos (RR = 5) and smoking (RR = 10) in a lung cancer risk. Dave et al. [127] also observed a multiplicative effect in a case (62 lung cancers)-control (198 subjects) study; however, the relative risks of these two factors were different from the preceding study: asbestos (RR = 2), smoking (RR = 8).

On the other hand, in a study by Kjuus et al. [128], the relative risk values of lung cancer observed were intermediary between values calculated according to an additive model and a multiplicative model. Furthermore, in their study, Berry et al. [129] observed a higher SMR value by lung cancer linked to asbestos exposure in nonsmokers than in smokers, contrary to most of the other studies. Lilis et al. [130] studied radiological pulmonary abnormalities in a cohort of 1117 asbestos-exposed workers. They noticed a greater prevalence of small parenchymal opacities among smokers than among nonsmokers; this difference decreased when duration since onset of exposure increased and had no significance after 40 years. They observed no significant relationship between the development of pleural abnormalities (pleural fibrosis, pleural plaques) and smoking.

### Silicosis and Tobacco

In a case-control study Mastrangelo et al. [51] observed an increase in lung cancer risk connected to silicosis and smoking; these two seemed to act according to an additive model. Sadler and Roy [131] studied mortality, all causes together, in a cohort of 1193 coal miners with pneumoconiosis. The degree of pneumoconiosis and smoking intensity seemed to interfere according to an additive model on mortality. In the same way, Hnizdo [132] studied mortality through chronic bronchopneumopathy in a cohort of 2209 South African gold miners. The additive model used to explain smoking effect and exposure to dusts required an interaction term, which led the author to estimate that exposure joined to these two factors probably had a multiplicative effect.

Marini et al. [133] studied the effects of exposure to coal dusts and smoking on the symptomatology and respiratory function of 3380 coal miners. The effects of exposure on the $FEV_1$ value expressed in ratio prevalence terms were identical for smokers and nonsmokers (multiplicative effect?); on the other hand, the prevalance ratios for chronic bronchitis were higher among nonsmokers than among smokers (interaction relative to the multiplicative model?).

The large number of epidemiological studies on occupational risks that take smoking into consideration is not surprising because of the major effects of this nonoccupational factor on respiratory pathology. It is to be hoped that this factor will be included even more in later studies so as to better present evidence of occupationally derived respiratory risk factors, of which a certain number probably have lesser effects than those of smoking.

## IX.  Conclusions: Epidemiology and Prevention of Occupational Respiratory Risks

The recent epidemiological studies on occupational respiratory risks appear directed more toward the prevention of known risks than toward the identification of unknown risks. This evolution manifests itself through the following characteristics:

1.  *STUDY of dose × effect relationships.* These studies analyze the relationships between the exposure level to occupational factors and the risk intensity of the exposed subjects (e.g., asbestos and lung cancer); they bring objective elements in the definition of exposure limit values.

2.  *RESEARCH of early indicators of effects.* These studies bring to the fore biological and/or functional infrapathological deviations which can be used for the biomonitoring of exposed subjects so that they may be removed from the risk before the installation of an occupational pathology.

3.  *EXPLORATION of the physiopathology of occupational respiratory diseases.* These studies focus on the mechanisms of occupational respiratory diseases (e.g., relationships between pneumoconiosis and lung cancer, immunological aspects of the respiratory pathology of farmers or of subjects exposed to isocyanates). Knowledge of these mechanisms can contribute to a better prevention of occupation risks.

4.  *RESEARCH of the predictive value of certain abnormalties and the study of their progress over time.* For example: pleural plaques linked to asbestos exposure: Do they announce a progression towards abestosis? The functional respiratory abnormalities observed in farmers and in subjects exposed to isocyanates: Do they develop into chronic obstructive bronchopneumopathies? These data allow us to individualize subjects at risk and put a deliberate medical supervision in place.

5.  *TAKING INTO account of nonoccupational factors in the determining of occupation illnesses* (e.g., smoking). These studies allow us to evaluate the importance of the occupational component in multifactorial diseases (bronchopulmonary cancer, chronic obstructive bronchopneumopathies) and to determine possible interactions between these factors. Besides the reduction of exposure to occupational factors, these studies can lead to suggesting measures of hygiene so as to preserve the health of exposed subjects.

Although epidemiology seems to be developing more toward occupational risks prevention than toward their identification, there are still few epidemiological studies of prevention in the strict sense of the word, allowing us to evaluate the efficiency of prevention measures able to be put to work. Despite the difficulties of carrying out such studies, their development would be a very useful additional contribution of epidemiology to the prevention of occupational risks, notably respiratory.

## References

1. Marcus K, Jarvholm BG, Larsson S. Asbestos-associated lung effects in car mechanics. Scand J Work Environ Health, 1987;13:252–54.
2. Selikoff IJ, Lilis R, Levin G. Asbestotic radiological abnormalities among United States Merchant Marine Seamen. Br J Ind Med 1990;47:292–97.
3. Demers RY, Neale AV, Robins T, et al. Asbestos-related pulmonary disease in boilermakers. Am J Ind Med 1990;17:327–39.
4. Jones RN, Diem JE, Hughes JM, Hammad YY, Glindmeyer HW, Weill H. Progression of asbestos effects: a prospective longitudinal study of chest radiographs and lung function. Br J Ind Med 1989;46:97–105.
5. Velonakis EG, Tsorva A, Tzonou A, Trichopoulos D. Asbestos-related chest x-ray changes among Greek merchant marine seamen. Am J Ind Med 1989;15:511–16.
6. Järvholm B, Sanden A. Pleural plaques, respiratory function. Am J Ind Med 1986;10:419–26.
7. Kilburn KH, Warshaw RH. Abnormal pulmonary function associated with diaphragmatic pleural plaques due to exposure to asbestos. Br J Ind Med 1990;47:611,614.
8. Amandus HE, Wheeler R, Jankovic J, Tucker J. The morbidity and mortality of vermiculite miners and millers exposed to tremolite-actinolite. I. Exposure estimates. Am J Ind Med 1987;11:1–14.
9. Amandus HE, Wheeler R. The morbidity and mortality of vermiculite miners and millers exposed to tremolite-actinolite. II. Mortality. Am J Ind Med 1987;11:15–26.
10. Neuberger M, Kundi M. Individual asbestos exposure: smoking and mortality—a cohort study in the asbestos cement industry. Br J Ind Med 1990;47;615–20.
11. Browne K. A threshold for asbestos related lung cancer. Br J Ind Med 1986;43:556–58.
12. Hughes JM, Weill H, Hammad YY. Mortality of workers employed in two asbestos cement manufacturing plants. Br J Ind Med 1987;44:161–74.
13. Armstrong BK, de Klerk NH, Musk AW, Hobbs MST. Mortality in miners and millers of crocidolite in Western Australia. Br J Ind Med 1988;45:5–13.
14. Seidman H, Selikoff IJ, Gelb SK. Mortality experience of amosite asbestos factory workers: dose–response relationships 5 to 40 years after onset of short-term work exposure. Am J Ind Med 1986;10:479–514.
15. Enterline PE, Hartley J, Henderson V. Asbestos and cancer: a cohort followed up to death. Br J Ind Med 1987;44:396–401.
16. Kipen HM, Lilis R, Suzuki Y, Valciukas JA, Selikoff IJ. Pulmonary

fibrosis in asbestos insulation workers with lung cancer: a radiological and histopathological evaluation. Br J Ind Med 1987;44:96–100.

17. Wagner JC, Newhouse ML, Corrin B, Rossiter GE, Griffiths DM. Correlation between lung fibre content and disease in East London asbestos factory workers. In: Bignon J, Peto J, Saracci R, eds. Non-occupational exposure to mineral fibres. IARC Scientific Publication 90. Lyon, France: IARC, 1989:444–48.

18. Sluis-Cremer GK, Bezuidenhout BN. Relation between asbestosis and bronchial cancer in amphibole asbestos miners. Br J Ind Med 1989;46:537–40.

19. Sluis-Cremer GK, Bezuidenhout BN. Relation between asbestosis and bronchial cancer in amphibole asbestos miners (reply). Br J Ind Med 1990;47;215–16.

20. Edelman DA. Laryngeal cancer and occupational exposure to asbestos. Int Arch Occup Environ Health 1989;61:223–27.

21. Finkelstein MM. Analysis of mortality patterns and workers' compensation awards among asbestos insulatin workers in Ontario. Am J Ind Med 1989;16:523–28.

22. Raffn E, Lynge E, Juel K, Korsgaard B. Incidence of cancer and moratlity among employees in the asbestos cement industry in Denmark. Br J Ind Med 1989;46:90–96.

23. Piolatto G, Negri E, la Vecchia C, Pira E, Decarli A, Peto J. An update of cancer mortality among chrysotile asbestos miners in Balangero, Northern Italy. Br J Ind Med 1990; 47;810–14.

24. Van Gelder T, Hoogsteden HC, Versnel MA, van Hezik J, Vandenbroucke JP, Planteydt HT. Malignant pleural mesothelioma in the southwestern part of the Netherlands. Eur Respir J 1989;2:981–84.

25. Mowé G, Gylseth B. Occupational exposure and regional variation of malignant mesothelioma in Norway, 1970–79. Am J Ind Med 1986;9:323–32.

26. Hirsch A, Brochard P, de Cremoux J, et al. Features of asbestos-exposed and unexposed mesothelioma. Am J Ind Med 1982;3:413–22.

27. Hulks G, Thomas J ST J, Waclawski E. Malignant pleural mesothelioma in western Glasgow 1980–86. Thorax 1989;44:496–500.

28. Minder CE, Vader JP. Malignant pleural mesothelioma among Swiss furniture workers. A new high-risk group. Scand J Work Environ Health 1988;14:252–56.

29. Saracci R. Ten years of epidemiologic investigations on man-made mineral fibers and health. Scand J Work Environ Health 1986;12:5–11.

30. Simonato L, Fletcher AC, Cherrie J, et al. The man-made fiber European historical cohort study. Extension of the follow-up. Scand J Work Environ Health 1986;12;34–47.

31. Fletcher AC. The mortality of foundry workers in the United Kingdom. In: Goldsmith DF, Winn DM, Shy CM, eds. Silica, silicosis, and cancer: controversy in occupational medicine. Cancer Research Monographs, Vol. 2. New York: Praeger, 1986:385–401.

32. Steenland K, Beaumont J. A proportionate moratlity study of granite cutters. Am J Ind Med 1986;9:189–201.

33. Thomas TL, Stewart PA. Mortality from lung cancer and respiratory disease among pottery workers exposed to silica and talc. Am J Epidemiol 1987;125:35–43.

34. Neuberger M, Kundi M, Westphal G, Grundorfer W. The Viennese dusty worker study. In: Goldsmith DF, Winn DM, Shy SM, eds. Silica, silicosis, and cancer: controversy in occupational medicine. Cancer Research Monographs. Vol. 2. New York: Praeger, 1986:415–22.

35. Costello J, Graham WGB. Vermont granite workers' mortality study. In: Goldsmith DF, Winn DM, Shy CM, eds. Silica, silicosis, and cancer: controversy in occupational medicine. Cancer Research Monographs. Vol. 2. New York: Praeger, 1986:437–40.

36. Archer VE, Roscoe JR, Brown D. Is silica or radon daughters the important factor in the excess lung cancer among underground miners? In:Goldsmith DF, Winn DM, Shy CM, eds. Silica, silicosis, and cancer: controversy in occupational medicine. Cancer Research Monographs. Vol. 2. New York: Praeger, 1986:375–84.

37. Brown DP, Kaplan SD, Zumwalde RD, Kaplowitz M, Archer VE. Retrospective cohort mortality study of underground gold mine workers. In: Goldsmith DF, Winn DM, Shy CM, eds. Silica, silsicosis, and cancer: controversy in occupational medicine. Cancer Research Monographs. Vol. 2. New York: Praeger, 1986:335–50.

38. Siemiatycki J, Dewar R, Lakhani R, et al. Cancer risks associated with 10 inorganic dusts: results from a case-control study in Montreal. Am J Ind Med 1989;16:547–67.

39. Ames RG, Amandus H, Attfield M, Green FY, Vallyathan V. Does coal mine dust present a risk for lung cancer? A case-control study of U.S. coal miners. Arch Environ Health 1983;38:331–33.

40. Meijers JMM, Swaen GMH, Slangen JJM, van Vliet C. Lung cancer among Dutch coal miners: a case-control study. Am J Ind Med 1988;14:597–604.

41. Frazier TM, Sundin DS. Industrial demographics and population at risk for silica exposures. In: Goldsmith DF, Winn DM, Shy CM, eds. Silica, silicosis, and cancer: controversy in occupational medicine Cancer Research Monographs. Vol. 2. New York: Praeger, 1986:3–9.

42. Meijers JMM, Swaen GMH, Slangen JJM, van Vliet K, Sturmans F. Long-term mortality in miners with coal workers' pneumoconiosis in the Netherlands: a pilot study. Am J Ind Med 1991;19:43–50.

43. Schuler G, Ruttner JR. Silicosis and lung cancer in Switzerland. In: Goldsmith DF, Winn DM, Shy DM, eds. Silica silicosis, and cancer: controversy in occupational medicine. Cancer Research Monographs. Vol. 2. New York: Praeger, 1986:357–66.

44. Finkelstein MM, Muller J, Kusiak R, Suranyi G. Follow-up of miners and silicotics in Ontario. In: Goldsmith DF, Winn DM, Shy CM, eds. Silica, silicosis, and cancer: controversy in occupational medicine. Cancer Research Monographs. Vol. 2. New York: Praeger, 1986:321–25.

45. Westerholm P, Ahlmark A, Maasing R, Segelberg I. Silicosis and lung cancer—a cohort study. In: Goldsmith DF, Winn DM, Shy CM, eds. Silica, silicosis, and cancer: controversy in occupational medicine. Cancer Research Monographs. Vol. 2. New York: Praeger, 1986:327–33.

46. Kurppa D, Gudbergsson H, Hannunkari I, et al. Lung cancer among silicotics in Finland. In: Goldsmith DF, Winn DM, Shy CM, eds. Silica, silicosis, and cancer: controversy in occupational medicine. Cancer Research Monographs. Vol. 2. New York: Praeger, 1986:311–19.

47. Tze Pin Ng, Shiu Lun Chan, Lee J. Mortality of a cohort of men in a silicosis register: further evidence of an association with lung cancer. Am J Ind Med 1990;17;163–71.

48. Zambon P, Simonato L, Mastrangelo G, et al. Mortality of workers compensated for silicosis during the period 1959–1963 in the Veneto region of Italy. Scand J Work Environ Health 1987;13:118–23.

49. Hessel PA, Sluis-Cremer GK. Case-control study of lung cancer and silicosis. In: Goldsmith DF, Winn DM, Shy CM, eds. Silica, silicosis, and cancer: controversy in occupational medicine. Cancer Research Monographs. Vol. 2. New-York: Praeger, 1986:351–55.

50. Forastière F, Lagorio S, Michelozzi P, et al. Silica, silicosis and lung cancer among ceramic workers: a case-referent study. Am J Ind Med 1986;10:363–70.

51. Mastrangelo G, Zambon R, Simonato L, Rizzi P. A case-referent study investigating the relationship between exposure to silica dust and lung cancer. Int Arch Occup Environ Health 1988;60:299–302.

52. Forastière F, Lagorio S, Michelozzi P, Perucci CA, Axelson O. Mortality pattern of silicotic subjects in the Latium region, Italy. Br J Ind Med 1989;46:877–80.

53. James WRL. Primary lung cancer in South Wales coal-workers with pneumoconiosis. Br J Ind Med 1955;12:87–91.

54. Husman K, Terho EO, Notkola V, Nuutinen J. Organic dust toxic syndrome among English farmers. Am J Ind Med 1990; 17:79–80.

55. Rask-Andersen A, Malmberg P, Lundholm M. Endotoxin levels in farming: absence of symptoms despite high exposure levels. Br J Ind Med 1989;46:412–16.

56. Pratt DS, Stallones L, Darrow D, May JJ. Acute respiratory illness associated with silo unloading. Am J Ind Med 1986;10:328.
57. Rask-Andersen A. Organic dust toxic syndrome among farmers. Br J Ind Med 1989;46:233–38.
58. Malmberg P, Rask-Andersen A. Natural and adaptive immune reactions to inhaled microorganisms in the lungs of farmers. Scand J Work Environ Health, 1988; 14(Suppl 1):68–71.
59. Warren CPW, Holford-Strevens V, Manfreda J. Respiratory disorders among Canadian farmers. Eur J Respir Dis 1987;71(Suppl 154):10–14.
60. Malmberg P, Palmgren U, Rask-Andersen A. Relationship between symptoms and exposure to mold dust in Swedish farmers. Am J Ind Med 1986;10:316–17.
61. Malmberg P, Rask-Andersen A, Palmgren U, Hoglund S, Kolmodin-Hedman B. Respiratory problems among Swedish farmers. Correlation between symptoms and environment. Eur J Respir Dis 1987;71(Suppl 154):22–27.
62. Rylander R. Lung diseases caused by organic dust in the farm environment. Am J Ind Med 1986;10:221–27.
63. Terho EO, Heinonen OP, Lammi S. Incidence of clinically confirmed farmer's lung disease in Finland. Am J Ind Med 1986;10:330.
64. Terho EO. Husman K, Vohlonen I. Prevalence and incidence of chronic bronchitis and farmer's lung with respect to age, sex, atopy, and smoking. Eur J Respir Dis 1987;71:19–28.
65. Stanford CF, Hall G, Chivers A, Martin B, Nicholls DP, Evand J. Farmer's lung in Northern Ireland. Br J Ind Med 1990;47:314–16.
66. Tao BG, Chen GX, Wu AL, et al. An epidemiological study on farmer's lung among hay grinders in Dafeng County. Occup Health Bull 1985;1:51–58.
67. Terho EO, Vohlonen I, Husman K. Prevalence and incidence of chronic bronchitis and farmer's lung with respect to socioeconomic factors. Int Arch Occup Environ Health 1987;71:29–36.
68. Belin L, Malmberg P. Antibodies to microbial antigens in various farmer populations. Am J Ind Med 1986;10:277–80.
69. Brouwer R, Heederik D, van Swieten P. IgG4 antibodies against pig-derived antigens. Am J Ind Med 1990;17:96–98.
70. Müller S, Bergmann K-Ch, Kramer H, Wuthe H. Sensitization, clinical symptoms, and lung function disturbances among poultry farm workers in the German Democratic Republic. Am J Ind Med 1986;10:281–82.
71. Marx JJ, Guernsey J, Emanuel DA, et al. Cohort studies of immunologic lung disease among Wisconsin's dairy farmers. Am J Ind Med 1990;18:263–68.
72. de Haller R. Respiratory symptoms, preventive aspects in farmers chronically exposed to moldy hay. Am J Ind Med 1986;10:288.

73.  Milosevic M. The prevalence of chronic bronchitis in agricultural workers of Slavonia. Am J Ind Med 1986;10:319–22.

74.· Hurst TS, Dosman JA, Graham BL, et al. Respiratory symptoms and pulmonary function in Saskatchewan Farmers. Am J Ind Med 1990, 17, 59.

75.  Iversen M, Dahl R, Korsgaard J, Jensen EJ, Hallas T. Cross-sectional study of respiratory symptoms in 1,175 Danish farmers. Am J Ind Med 1990;17:60–61.

76.  Iversen M, Dahl R, Korsgaard J, Jensen EJ, Hallas T. Study of bronchial hyperreactivity and loss of lung function in farmers. Am J Ind Med 1990;17:62–63.

77.  Iversen M, Pedersen B, Dahl R. Relationship between respiratory symptoms and bronchial hyperreactivity in pig farmers. J Occup Med 1990;17:64–65.

78.  Rylander R, Essle N, Donham KJ. Bronchial hyperreactivity among pig and dairy farmers. Am J Ind Med 1990;17:66–69.

79.  Dosman JA, Graham BL, Hall D, van Loon P, Bhasin P, Froh F. Respiratory symptoms and pulmonary function in farmers. Am J Ind Med 1987;29:38–43.

80.  Dalphin JC, Bildstein F, Pernet D, Dubiez A, Depierre A. Prevalence of chronic bronchitis and respiratory function in a group of dairy farmers in the French Doubs Province. Chest 1989;95:1244–47.

81.  Musk AW, Venables KM, Crook B, et al. Respiratory symptoms, lung function, and sensitisation to flour in a British bakery. Br J Ind Med 1989;46:636–42.

82.  Haglind P, Rylander R. Occupational exposure and lung function measurements among workers in swine confinement buildings. J Occup Med 1990;1987;29:904–7.

83.  Wilhelmsson J, Bryngelsson IL, Ohlson CG. Respiratory symptoms among Swedish swine producers. Am J Ind Med 1989;15:311–18.

84.  Donham KJ, Haglind P, Peterson Y, Rylander R. Environmental and health studies in swine confinement buildings. Am J Ind Med 1986;10:289–93.

85.  Revsbech P, Andersen G. Diurnal variation in peak expiratory flow rate among grain elevator workers. Br J Ind Med 1989;46:566–69.

86.  James AL, Zimmerman MJ, Ryan G, Musk AW. Exposure to grain dust and changes in lung function. Br J Ind Med 1990;47:466–72.

87.  Manfreda J, Cheang M, Warren CPW. Chronic respiratory disorders related to farming and exposure to grain dust in a rural adult community. Am J Ind Med 1989;15:7–19.

88.  Heederik D, van Zwieten R, Brouwer R. Across-shift lung function changes among pig farmers. Am J Ind Med 1990;17:57–58.

89. Donham KJ, Leistikow B, Merchant J, Leonard S. Assessment of U.S. poultry workers respiratory risks. Am J Ind Med 1990;17:73–74.
90. Rylander R. The role of endotoxin for reactions after exposure to cotton dust. Am J Ind Med 1987;12:687–97.
91. Cinkotai EF, Rigby A, Pickering CAC, Seaborn D, Faragher E, Recent trends in the prevalence of byssinotic symptoms in the Lancashire textile industry. Br J Ind Med 1988;45:782–89.
92. Cinkotai FF, Seaborn D, Pickering CAC, Faragher E. Airborne dust in the personal breathing zone and the prevalence of byssinotic symptoms in the Lancashire textile industry. Ann Occup Hyg 1988;32:103–13.
93. Ong SG, Lam TH, Wong CM, et al. Byssinosis and other respiratory problems in the cotton industry of Hong Kong. Am J Ind Med 1987;12:773–77.
94. Takam J, Nemery B. Byssinosis in a textile factory in Cameroon: a preliminary study. Br J Ind Med 1988;45:803–9.
95. Baratawidjaja KG. Byssinosis study in Jakarta, Indonesia. Am J Ind Med 1987;12:784.
96. Dehong L, Shixuan L, Maobo D, Cuijuan Z. Preliminary approach to the diagnosis of byssinosis. Am J Ind Med 1987;12:731–35.
97. Mu-Zhen L. The health investigation of cotton textile workers in Beijing. Am J Ind Med 1987;12:759–64.
98. Rastogi SK. Pulmonary function evaluation in Indian textile workers. Am J Ind Med 1987;12:782.
99. Awad Elkarim MA, Onsa SH. Prevalence of byssinosis and respiratory symptoms among spinners in Sudanese cotton mills. Am J Ind Med 1987;12:281–89.
100. Christiani DC, Eisen EA, Wegman DH, et al. Respiratory disease in cotton textile workers in the People's Republic of China. I. Respiratory symptoms. Scand J Work Environ Health 1986;12:40–45.
101. Christiani DC, Eisen EA, Wegman DH, et al. Respiratory disease in cotton textile workers in the People's Republic of China. II. Pulmonary function results. Scand J Work Environ Health 1986;12:46–50.
102. Bazas T, Harrington JM, Bazas B. An investigation on the prevalence of byssinosis in three Greek spinning mills. Med Lav 1984;75:478–85.
103. Massin N, Moulin JJ, Wild P, Meyer-Bisch C, Mur JM. A study of the prevalence of acute respiratory disorders among workers in the textile industry. Int Arch Occup Environ Health 1991;62:555–60.
104. Rastogi SK, Gupta BN, Mathur N, Husain T. A study of the prevalence of ventilatory obstruction in textile workers exposed to cotton dust. Environ Res 1989;50:56–67.
105. Lu PL, Christiani DC, Ye T-T, et al. The study of byssinosis in China: a comprehensive report. Am J Ind Med 1987;12:743–53.

106. Elwood PC, Sweetnam PM, Bevan C, Saunders MJ. Respiratory disability in ex-cotton workers. Br J Ind Med 1986;43:580–86.
107. Alexandersson R, Plato N, Kolmodin-Hedman B, Hedenstierna G. Exposure, lung function, and symptoms in car painters exposed to hexamethylendiisocyanate and biuret modified hexamethylendiisocyanate. Int Arch Environ Health 1987;42:367–73.
108. Holness DL, Broder I, Corey PN, et al. Respiratory variables and exposure–effect relationships in isocyanate-exposed workers. J Occup Med 1984;26:449–55.
109. Hjortsberg U, rbæk P, Arborelius M. Small airway hyperreactivity among lifelong non-atopic non-smokers exposed to isocyanates. Br J Ind Med 1987;44:824–28.
110. Seguin P, Allard A, Cartier A, Malo JL. Prevalence of occupational asthma in spray painters exposed to several types of isocyanates, including polymethylene polyphenylisocyanate. J Occup Med 1987;29:340–44.
111. Paggiaro PL, Lastrucci L, Pardi F, Rossi O, Bacci E, Talini D. Specific bronchial reactivity to toluene diisocyanate: dose–response relationship. Respiration 1986;50:167–73.
112. Keskinen H, Tupasela O, Tiikkainen U, Nordman H. Experiences of specific IgE in asthma due to diisocyanates. Clin Allergy 1988;18:597–604.
113. Grammer LC, Eggum P, Silverstein M, Shaughnessy MA, Liotta JL, Patterson R. Prospective immunologic and clinical study of a population exposed to hexamethylene diisocyanate. J Allergy Clin Immunol 1988;82:627–33.
114. Game CJA. Australian TDI workers sera assayed for IgE against a *p*-tolyl-isocyanate-human serum albumin conjugate. Am Ind Hyg Assoc J 1982;43:759–63.
115. Banks DE, Rando RJ, Barkman HW. Persistence of toluene diisocyanate-induced asthma despite negligible workplace exposures. Chest 1990;97:121–25.
116. Saia B, Fabbri L, Mapp C, Marcer G, Mastrangelo G. Epidemiology of chronic non-specific lung disease in a population exposed to isocyanate. I. Analysis of symptoms. II. Analysis of respiratory impairment. Med Lav 1976;67:278–284, 305–314.
117. Tornling G, Alexandersson R, Hedenstierna G, Plato N. Decreased lung function and exposure to diisocyanates (HDI and HDI-BHT) in car repair painters: observations on re-examination 6 years after initial study. Am J Ind Med 1990;17:299–310.
118. Brackbill R, Frazier T, Shilling S. Smoking characteristics of U.S. workers, 1978–1980. Am J Ind Med 1988;13:5–41.
119. Siemiatycki J, Wacholder S, Dewar R, et al. Smoking and degree of

occupational exposure: are internal analyses in cohort studies likely to be confounded by smoking status? Am J Ind Med 1988;13:59–69.

120. Sterling TD, Weinkam JJ. Comparison of smoking-related risk factors among black and white males. Am J Ind Med 1989;15:319–33.
121. Blair A, Hoar SK, Walrath J. Comparison of crude and smoking-adjusted standardized mortality ratios. J Occup Med 1985;27:881–84.
122. Marsh GM, Sachs DPL, Callahan C, Leviton LC, Ricci E, Henderson V. Direct methods of obtaining information on cigarette smoking in occupational studies. Am J Ind med 1988;13:71–103.
123. Axelson O, Steenland K. Indirect methods of assessing the effects of tobacco use in occupational studies. Am J Ind Med 1988;13:105–118.
124. Thomas DC, Whittemore AS. Methods for testing interactions, with applications to occupational exposures, smoking, and lung cancer. Am J Ind Med 1988;13:131–47.
125. Saracci R. Asbestos and lung cancer: an analysis of the epidemiolgical evidence on the asbestos–smoking interaction. In: Lemen R, Dement JM, eds. Dusts and disease. Proceedings of the Conference on Occupational Exposures to Fibrous and Particulate Dust and Their Extension into the Environment. Park Forest South, IL: Pathofox Publishers, 1979:157–69.
126. Selikoff IJ, Hammond EC. Asbestos and smoking JAMA 1979;242:458–59.
127. Dave SK. Edling C, Jacobsson P, Axelson O. Occupation, smoking, and lung cancer. Br J Ind Med 1988;45:790–92.
128. Kjuus H, Skjæerven R, Langard S, Lien JT, Aamodt T. A cast-referent study of lung cancer, occupational exposures and smoking. Scand J Work Environ Health 1986;12:193–202.
129. Berry G, Newhouse ML, Antonis P. Combined effect of asbestos and smoking on mortality from lung cancer and mesothelioma in factory workers. Br J Ind Med 1985;42:12–18.
130. Lilis R, Selikoff IJ, Lerman Y, Seidman H, Gelb SK. Asbestosis: interstitial pulmonary fibrosis and pleural fibrosis in a cohort of asbestos insulation workers: influence of cigarette smoking. Am J Ind Med 1986;10:459–70.
131. Sadler RL, Roy TJ. Smoking and mortality from coalworkers' pneumoconiosis. Br J Ind Med 1990, 47, 141–142.
132. Hnizdo E. Combined effect of silica dust and tobacco smoking on mortality from chronic obstructive lung disease in gold miners. Br J Ind Med 1990;47:656–64.
133. Marini WM, Gurr D, Jacobsen M. Clinically important respiratory effects of dust exposure, smoking in British coal miners. Am Rev Respir Dis 1988;137:106–12.

# 2

# Occupational Factors of Lung Cancer

**PAOLO BOFFETTA and RODOLFO SARACCI**

International Agency for Research on Cancer
Lyon, France

## I.  Introduction

Lung cancer was considered to be a rare disease as late as at the beginning of the twentieth century. Today, it is the commonest cancer worldwide. In 1980 it was estimated that 660,500 cases occurred in the world, accounting for 10.4% of all new cancers, and this number is increasing at a rate of about 0.5% per year [1].

Squamous cell carcinoma is the most frequent histological type of lung cancer in males, whereas adenocarcinoma is the most frequent type in females. Although smoking is associated with all types of lung cancer cells, squamous cell carcinoma is seen mainly among smokers, and adenocarcinoma among nonsmokers. An increase observed in various regions of the United States in adenocarcinomas in both males and females has been attributed to a combination of factors (including occupational exposures) other than cigarette smoking [2]. However, available information is seldom sufficient to conclude that specific occupational exposures are associated with the occurrence of cancer of a specific cell type.

Although it is true that the majority of lung cancer is related etiologically to cigarette smoking, there are a number of factors that in occupationally or otherwise exposed persons can be an important determinant of the cancers in the respiratory tract [3]. In this chapter we review known and suspected occupational causes of lung cancer. Risk factors that occur primarily in the general environment (e.g., air pollution), as well as tobacco smoking (e.g., exposure to passive smoking in the workplace), are not discussed in detail; however, aspects such as interaction between tobacco smoking and occupational exposures are addressed briefly.

## II.  Occupational Risk Factors of Lung Cancer

Although tobacco smoking is the major determinant of lung cancer, other respiratory exposures can induce tumors on their own or enhance the carcinogenic effect of tobacco smoke. Most notable among these are certain chemical and physical agents that are found in the workplace and often, at lower levels, in the general environment. In fact, the lung is one of the preferred target organs for those agents and complex exposures that have been established as being carcinogenic to humans [4,5]. Apart from tobacco smoke, a causal association with lung cancer has been demonstrated according to the International Agency for Research on Cancer (IARC) for 11 agents or mixtures and seven exposure circumstances (see Table 1) [6]. Furthermore, there are 11 agents, mixtures, or exposure circumstances which according to IARC are probably carcinogenic to the human lung (Table 2) [6]. All but azathioprine, an immunosuppressant drug, are primarily occupational exposures. These factors are reviewed briefly below; for each of them, the current IARC evaluation [6] is reported.

### A.  Arsenic and Arsenic Compounds (IARC Group 1)

Inorganic arsenic was suspected of being carcinogenic to the skin and possibly to other tissues of smelter workers in Cornwall in the United Kingdom as early as 1820, but definitive evidence linking exposure to arsenic compounds with lung cancer accrued only by the late 1960s and 1970s. Workers employed in hot metallurgical processes, particularly nonferrous smelters, are the major occupationally exposed groups that have been demonstrated to be at increased risk of lung cancer [7]. Other occupational groups demonstrating an increased risk of lung cancer following exposure to arsenic compounds include fur handlers, manufacturers of sheep-dip compounds, and vineyard workers [7,8].

### B.  Chromium[VI] Compounds (IARC Group 1)

The first clear indication that chromium compounds could induce lung tumors in humans came in the 1940s from studies of workers in chromate-producing

**Table 1** Established Human Lung Carcinogens According to IARC

| | |
|---|---|
| Individual agents | Asbestos |
| | Arsenic and arsenic compounds |
| | Bis(chloromethyl) ether |
| | Chloromethyl methyl ether (technical grade) |
| | Chromium[VI] compounds |
| | Mustard gas |
| | Nickel compounds |
| | Talc containing asbestiform fibers |
| Complex mixtures | Coal tars |
| | Coal-tar pitches |
| | Soots |
| | Tobacco smoke |
| Exposure circumstances | Aluminum production |
| | Coal gasification |
| | Coke production |
| | Iron and steel founding |
| | Painters (occupational exposure as) |
| | Radon and its decay products |
| | Underground hematite mining (with exposure to radon) |

*Source:* Ref. 6.

**Table 2** Probable Human Lung Carcinogens According to IARC

| | |
|---|---|
| Individual agents | Acrylonitrile |
| | Azathioprine |
| | Beryllium and beryllium compounds |
| | Cadmium and cadmium compounds |
| | Silica (crystalline) |
| Complex mixtures | Diesel engine exhaust |
| | Mineral oils (untreated and mildly treated) |
| | Welding fumes |
| Exposure circumstances | Boot and shoe manufacture and repair |
| | Rubber industry |
| | Spraying and application of insecticides (occupational exposures in) |

*Source:* Ref. 6.

plants [9]. Since that time a large number of epidemiological studies have been carried out on the association between chromates and the occurrence of lung cancer [10]. The consistency of findings and the magnitude of the excesses demonstrated the carcinogenic potential of chromium[VI] compounds.

### C.  Nickel Compounds (IARC Group 1)

Nickel refinery workers from many countries have shown substantial increased risks of lung cancer [11,12]. Other occupational groups exposed to nickel among which an increased risk of lung cancer has been detected include sulfide nickel ore miners and high-nickel-alloy manufacture [11].

### D.  Beryllium (IARC Group 2A)

Workers exposed to beryllium are probably at elevated risk of lung cancer [7,13,14]. The most informative data are those derived from the U.S. Beryllium Case Registry, in which cases of beryllium-related lung diseases were collected from different industries. A recent report from this population confirmed the excess of lung cancer [15].

### E.  Cadmium (IARC Group 2A)

An increase in lung cancer occurrence have been found in some cohorts of cadmium smelter and nickel–cadmium battery workers [7,16]. Concurrent exposure to arsenic among smelters and to nickel among battery workers, as well as inconsistencies in the results of these studies, do not yet allow a final conclusion on the carcinogencity of cadmium to humans [17].

### F.  Asbestos (IARC Group 1)

Asbestos is an important occupational lung carcinogen. Strong evidence that inhalation of asbestos fibers could increase the risk of lung cancer was reported in 1955 when a ten-fold excess of lung cancer among asbestos workers was found [18]. Lung cancer and mesothelioma are the major asbestos-related neoplasms, but cancers from other sites, such as gastrointestinal tract, larynx, and kidney, have been reported in asbestos workers. All different forms of asbestos have been causally related to lung cancer and mesothelioma. In addition, talc containing asbestiform fibers has been shown to be carcinogenic to human lung in talc miners and millers and pottery workers [7,19].

   A distinctive characteristic of asbestos-induced lung cancer is its synergistic relationship with cigarette smoking (see Section IV). Because the bulk of excess lung cancer results from the synergism between smoking and asbestos, breaking either causal pathway may result in a reduction in risk for asbestos workers.

### G. Crystalline Silica (IARC Group 2A)

A number of studies among miners, quarry workers, foundry workers, ceramic workers, granite workers, and stonecutters have shown that people diagnosed as having silicosis after exposure to dust containing crystalline silica have an increased risk of lung cancer [7,20]. Coal miners, on the other hand, do not appear to be at higher risk of lung cancer [21]. In all the industries studied, with the exception of the granite and stone industry, exposure to silica occurs with concomitant exposure to other lung carcinogens, such as polynuclear aromatic hydrocarbons.

### H. Polynuclear Aromatic Hydrocarbons (IARC Group 2A)

Polynuclear aromatic hydrocarbons (PAHs) are formed mainly as a result of pyrolytic processes, especially the incomplete combustion of organic materials, as well as from natural processes, such as carbonization. There are several hundred PAHs, the best known of which is benzo[a]pyrene. In addition, a number of heterocyclic aromatic compounds (e.g., carbazole, acridine), as well as PAHs with a $NO_2$ group (nitroarenes), can be generated by incomplete combustion [22].

Suspicions during the first half of the century of increased risks of lung cancer among workers exposed to PAHs in coal carbonization processes (gas retort houses, coke ovens, gas generators) were confirmed in the 1950s and 1960s (see Section II.I) [7]. The most prominent finding was an increased death rate from lung cancer among workers at coke plants, especially among those working topside of the coke ovens. Increased lung cancer risk has also been observed among workers exposed to mixtures of PAHs, many of which are carcinogenic to animals (Table 3). The most important mixtures are reviewed briefly in (Sections II.I, II.J, II.K).

### I. Soots, Coal Tars, Coal-Tar Pitch (IARC Group 1)

Soots are by-products of the incomplete combustion or pyrolysis of carbon-containing materials: their composition and properties are therefore highly variable. Coal tars are by-products of coal carbonization, and coal-tar pitch is a residue produced during the distillation of coal tars: their composition varies depending on the temperature of carbonization or distillation as well as on the composition of coal, but in general PAHs represent the major group of constituents [24,25].

Cohort studies of mortality among chimney sweeps in various European countries have shown an increased risk of lung cancer, which has been attributed

**Table 3**   Polynuclear Aromatic Hydrocarbons That Are Established to Be
Carcinogenic in Experimental Animals According to IARC

Polynuclear aromatic hydrocarbons [22]
   Benz[*a*]anthracene
   Benzo[*a*]pyrene
   Dibenz[*a,h*]anthracene
   Benzo[*b*]fluoranthene
   Benzo[*j*]fluoranthene
   Benzo[*k*]fluoranthene
   Dibenzo[*a,e*]pyrene
   Dibenzo[*a,h*]pyrene
   Dibenzo[*a,i*]pyrene
   Dibenzo[*a,l*]pyrene
   Indeno[1,2,3-*cd*]pyrene

Polynuclear nitroaromatic hydrocarbons [23]
   1,6-Dinitropyrene
   1,8-Dinitropyrene
   6-Nitrochrysene
   2-Nitrofluorene
   1-Nitropyrene
   4-Nitropyrene

to soot exposure [7,25]. Several epidemiological studies have shown excesses
of lung cancer among workers exposed to pitch fumes in aluminum production
[26], calcium carbide production [27], roofing [24], and millwrighting and
welding in a stamping plant [28]. In these industries, exposure to tar, particularly
coal tar, does also occur [7,24]. Another industry in which an excess of lung
cancer is due to exposure to coal-tar fumes is coal gasification and coke
production [29,30].

### J.   Diesel Engine Exhaust (IARC Group 2A)

A possible carcinogenic risk of engine exhaust is related to inhalation of
particulate, which is composed mainly of elemental carbon, adsorbed organic
material, including PAHs and nitroarenes, and traces of metallic compounds.
Diesel engine exhaust shares similar physical and chemical characteristics with
gasoline engine exhaust as well as airborne materials from many other combustion
sources. This makes it difficult to quantify the individual's exposure in both the
environment and the workplace. An increased risk of lung cancer was found in
some but not all studies that tried to analyze diesel engine exhaust exposure

separately from other combustion products. The occupational groups studied include railroad workers, dockers, bus garage workers, bus company employees, and professional lorry drivers [31].

### K.   Other Mixtures of Polynuclear Aromatic Hydrocarbons

Carbon blacks, gasoline engine exhaust, mineral oils, shale oils, and bitumens have been studied as for carcinogenicity in humans. Shale oils and untreated and mildly treated mineral oils are carcinogenic to humans (IARC group 1), whereas gasoline engine exhaust is possibly carcinogenic (IARC group 2B) and highly refined mineral oils, bitumens, and carbon blacks are not classifiable as to their carcinogenicity to humans (IARC group 3) [7,31]. Although these mixtures do contain PAHs, a carcinogenic effect on the human lung has not been demonstrated for any of them, and the evidence of carcinogenicity for untreated and mildly treated mineral oils and for shale oils is based on increased risk of cancers from sites other than lung (mainly, skin and scrotum) among exposed workers. However, some suggestions of increased risk of lung cancer are derived from studies of printing pressmen exposed to mineral oils [32], workers in the asphalt industry exposed to bitumens [33], and carbon black workers [34]. The concomitant exposure to agents with high concentration of PAHs, such as coal tars, makes difficult the interpretation of these studies. No indication of an increased risk of lung cancer can be derived from the few studies that have tried to analyze specificity occupational exposure to gasoline engine exhaust. However, there is some evidence of an increased risk of lung cancer among drivers and other workers exposed to exhaust from engines that were not defined but were likely to include gasoline as well as diesel engines [31].

### L.   Mustard Gas (IARC Group 1)

Bis($\beta$-chloroethyl)sulfide, known as mustard gas, was widely used during World War I, and studies of soldiers exposed to mustard gas as well as of workers employed in its manufacture have revealed subsequent development of lung cancer [7,35]. Some antineoplastic drugs used clinically are derivatives of mustard gas.

### M.   Bis(chloromethyl) Ether and Chloromethyl Methyl Ether (Technical Grade) (IARC Group 1)

Numerous epidemiological studies from around the world have demonstrated that workers exposed to chloromethyl methyl ether and/or bis(chloromethyl) ether have an increased risk of lung cancer, primarily of the small-cell type [7,36].

### N.  Acrylonitrile (IARC Group 2A)

Workers exposed to acrylonitrile have been found to be at higher risk of lung cancer in some but not all studies conducted among workers in textile fiber manufacture, acrylonitrile polymerization, and the rubber industry [7,37].

### O.  Radon and Its Decay Products (IARC Group 1)

Lung cancer has been common among miners in certain areas of central Europe, accounting for as many as 30 to 50% of all deaths in the early twentieth century. The cancers have also occurred in excess among uranium miners in various countries as well as among underground hematite miners and metal miners [38,39]. A common factor among each of these occupational groups is exposure to ionizing radiation from $\alpha$-rays emitted by inhaled radon particles. The concentration of radon in indoor air in most buildings is likely to be much higher than outdoor concentrations. The main sources of radiation indoors are the ground of the construction site and the building materials used.

### P.  Ionizing Radiation (Not Evaluated by IARC)

Although humans have evolved in an environment of ionizing radiation contributed by cosmic rays, radon, and radioactive nuclides, it was not until man-made sources were developed that the effects of ionizing radiation started to become known. The doses and dose rates of environmental (other than occupational) radiation are low, and the detection of effects at such low doses is very difficult. Occupationally exposed people are those employed in nuclear power, medical radiology, industrial radiology, and a number of other activities that are mainly associated with research.

The main source of data on radiation and cancer is follow-up studies of atomic bomb survivors [40,41]. The risk of lung cancer is elevated among atomic bomb survivors as well as among people who have received radiation therapy [42]. No convincing evidence, however, is currently available on the existence of an elevated lung cancer risk among workers exposed to low-level ionizing radiation, such as those occurring in the nuclear industry [43,44].

### Q.  Occupational Exposure as a Painter (IARC Group 1)

Elevated risk of lung cancer among painters was found in three large cohort studies and in eight small cohort and census-based studies, as well as 11 case-control studies from various countries [45]. Five of these studies took smoking into account and showed an increase of 30% or more in lung cancer risk. On the other hand, little evidence of an increase in lung cancer risk was found among workers involved in the manufacture of paint (IARC Group 3) [45].

### R. Other Exposures and Occupations

A number of other chemicals, mixtures, occupations, and industries that have been evaluated by IARC to be carcinogenic to humans (IARC Group 1) do not have lung cancer as the primary target organ. Nonetheless, the possibility of an increased risk of lung cancer has been raised for some of these chemicals, such as vinyl chloride [7,46], and industries, such as boot and shoe manufacture and repair [7,47], the rubber industry [7,48], and furniture making and cabinetmaking [7,49], but the evidence is not consistent.

Furthermore, several agents, which have the lung as one of the main targets, have been considered to be possible human carcinogens (IARC Group 2B), on the basis of carcinogenic activity in experimental animals and/or limited epidemiological evidence. They include chemicals such as lead [7], cobalt [50], and man-made vitreous fibers (rock wool, slag wool, and glass wool) [51], as well as complex mixtures such as bitumes [7] and welding fumes [52].

## III. Proportion of Lung Cancers Attributable to Occupational Exposures

The estimation of the proportion of lung cancer attributable to occupational exposures has been based on the relative risks of various occupations, adjusted for smoking, in case-control studies. Simonato and co-workers [53] reviewed a number of epidemiological studies and found estimates of population attributable risk ranging from 1 to 40% (Table 4). The variability depended on the geographical location of the study (i.e., the proportion of people occupationally exposed to carcinogens) and the method used to define occupational exposure. Therefore, it does not seem advisable to provide a single figure of the proportion of lung cancers attributable to occupational exposures.

## IV. Interaction Between Smoking and Occupational Risk Factors

Interaction between two risk factors occurs when the relative risk among subjects exposed to two factors is different from the sum (additive model) or the product (multiplicative model) of relative risks of subjects exposed to each of the two factors separately [66]. In practice, however, the terms *additive interaction* and *multiplicative interaction* are used when the relative risk among subjects exposed to both factors is close to the value derived according to the additive or multiplicative model, respectively [67]. Epidemiological studies have seldom been detailed enough to enable a thoughtful analysis of possible interactions: even in these cases, data did not usually permit to discriminate between the additive and multiplicative models [67]. Among the occupational risks factors of lung cancer that have been studied for interaction are smoking, asbestos, ionizing radiations, nickel, and arsenic.

**Table 4** Proportion of Lung Cancer Attributable to Occupational Exposures from Selected Epidemiologic Studies

| Study reference, location | Proportion of lung cancers attributable to occupational exposures | | |
| | Based on job exposure matrix[a] | Exposure to known lung carcinogens[b] | Exposure to known and suspected lung carcinogens[b] |
| --- | --- | --- | --- |
| Blot et al., 1978 [54], U.S. | — | 8.8 | 8.8 |
| Blot et al., 1980 [55], U.S. | — | 16.0 | 16.0 |
| Blot et al., 1982 [56], U.S. | — | 15.4 | 15.4 |
| Blot et al., 1983 [57], U.S. | — | 11.3 | 12.5 |
| Pastorino et al., 1984 [58], Italy | 21.0–33.0 | — | — |
| Pannett et al., 1985 [59], U.K. | 0.6–15.3 | — | — |
| Vena et al., 1985 [60], U.S. | 3.9–6.3 | — | — |
| Damber and Larsson, 1985 [61], Sweden | — | 40.0 | 40.0 |
| Buiatti et al., 1985 [62], Italy | — | 0 | 1.3 |
| Kvale et al., 1986 [63], Norway | 14.3—27.0 | — | — |
| Kjuus et al., 1986 [64], Norway | 22.2—35.1 | — | — |

*Source:* Derived from ref. 53.
[a]The lower estimate refers to exposure to known or probable carcinogens, the upper estimate refers to exposure to possible carcinogens as well.
[b]Based on the list provided by Simonato and Saracci [65].

Most of the studies on asbestos-exposed workers, which included data on smoking, suggested a multiplicative interaction between the two factors in the causation of lung cancer. However, no uniform pattern was seen among the studies: the differences may be due to the effect of various types of asbestos fibers, to the fact that both asbestos and smoking may act at different stages of the carcinogenic process, to the variability in exposure circumstances (e.g., miners vs. millers), and to the definition of exposed categories (e.g., combination of ex-smokers and never-smokers) [67].

The interaction between smoking and ionizing radiations has been studied in two situations: underground mining involving exposure to inhaled radon emission and atomic bomb explosions involving exposure to gamma and neutron radiations. The studies on the interaction between tobacco smoking and radon exposure indicate a multiplicative interaction in U.S. uranium miners and interactions close to the additive model in Swedish nonuranium miners. The average radon doses and dose rates were lower in the Swedish studies that in the U.S. studies, and there might have been qualitative differences between the two mining situations (e.g., dustiness) [67]. An analysis of a large cohort of atomic bomb survivors was not able to discriminate between an additive and a multiplicative model of interaction between smoking and estimated radiation exposure on lung cancer [68].

Less information is available on the interaction between smoking and exposure to nickel or arsenic. The interaction appears to be additive for nickel, between additive and multiplicative for arsenic [67].

## V. Carcinogenic Effects of Lung Carcinogens on Other Organs

A number of lung carcinogens have been related to increased risk of cancer in other organs [4]. Table 5 provides a list of established and suspected associations: among the sites more frequently involved are skin, bladder, other organs in the respiratory tract, and organs in the gastrointestinal tract. The ultimate mechanisms of action of human carcinogens are not known [69], and it is not clear whether mechanisms of carcinogenicity in different organs involve steps, such as metabolic activation, formation of DNA adducts, and oncogene activation, which may be different from organ to organ. This might be the case for nonrespiratory organs, such as urinary bladder, whereas the carcinogenic process in tissues anatomically close to lung, such as pleural mesothelium and larynx epithelium, may be similar to that occurring in the lung. In particular, biopersistence of carcinogenic fibres, such as man-made mineral fibers, in the lung, and migration to pleura is a field of active research in current years [70].

**Table 5**  Known or Suspected Lung Carcinogens That Are Established or Suspected Carcinogens in Other Organs

| Carcinogen | Other target organs |
| --- | --- |
| Arsenic | Liver (angiosarcoma), skin |
| Asbestos | Gastrointestinal tract, peritoneum, larynx, pleura |
| Cadmium | Prostate |
| Mustard gas | Nose and nasal sinuses |
| Nickel | Nose and nasal sinuses, larynx |
| Soots, tars, mineral oils | Gastrointestinal tract, larynx, skin, bladder |
| Vinyl chloride | Gastrointestinal tract, liver (angiosarcoma), brain, lymphohematopoietic system |
| Rubber manufacture | Stomach, skin, bladder, leukemia |

*Source:* Derived from ref. 4.

## VI.   Current Methodological Issues in the Study of Occupational Risk Factors for Lung Cancer

Many known occupational lung carcinogens have been identified between 1950 and 1979. During the last decade, most of the epidemiological work has been done on clarification of the role of agents suspected to be carcinogenic, for which a final conclusion can hardly be drawn at present. Several reasons explain the easiness in the "early" identification of occupational lung carcinogens.

First, many of the carcinogens detected in the past are fairly potent; that is, they cause substantial augmentation of the risk of lung cancer among exposed workers, even when these workers were exposed to other potent lung carcinogens, such as tobacco smoke. Furthermore, it has been possible to identify occupational populations with definite exposure to the agent of interest and relatively low concomitant exposure to other carcinogens (e.g., nickel refinery workers [12]). Finally, the carcinogens that were identified occurred only to a limited extent outside the occupational environment; that is, the "general" population, which was used as a comparison in many occupational studies, was practically free of the exposure of interest.

During the last decade, however, it became clear that such relatively easy research conditions no longer existed, and that most of the suspected lung carcinogens, such as those listed in Table 2, present more complex methodological problems to investigators. A first problem is represented by the low levels of exposure to suspected lung carcinogens. One example is exposure to man-made vitreous fibers in the production industry. Current airborne fiber exposure levels in the European rock wool and glass wool production industry are generally below 0.1 fiber/mL, and in the continuous filament production industry are one order of magnitude lower [71]. It is known that past exposure was generally higher, a fact that justifies the conduction of retrospective cohort studies, but the actual levels are not known. A simulation exercise suggested levels as high as 5 fibers/mL [72], whereas a mathematical model provided estimates rarely exceeding 1 fiber/mL [73]. Exposure to low levels of carcinogens will result in small elevation of lung cancer risk.

A second problem is the concomitant exposure to other carcinogens, which occurs in many occupational settings entailing exposure to a suspected carcinogen. An increased risk of lung cancer has been found in several epidemiological studies on cadmium-exposed workers in the smelting and nickel–cadmium battery industries [16]. In these industries, there is the possibility of exposure to arsenic and nickel, respectively, which makes the interpretation of results difficult [16,17]. This problem may be overcome by improving the refinement of methods for exposure assessment, through extensive review of available industrial hygiene data, mathematical modeling of past exposure, and use of biological markers of exposure [74]. In many situations, however, it is nearly impossible to disentangle the various exposures even if the data for each individual exposure may be good.

Furthermore, the study of suspected occupational lung carcinogens, which also occur in the general environment, creates special methodological problems. An example is the investigation of the health effects of exposure to diesel engine exhaust: in industrial urban populations, virtually everybody is exposed to it or to similar agents, such as gasoline engine exhaust and products of other combustion processes. It is therefore very difficult to identify a truly unexposed population, which may serve as an appropriate referent group. The most convincing studies in this area have been conducted within an industrial population (railroad workers) by identifying groups of workers with high and low exposure to diesel exhaust [75,76].

## VII. Use of Biological Markers in Occupational Lung Cancer Research

During the last decade, molecular epidemiology, an area of research that applies biochemical markers to epidemiological studies, has been proposed to overcome some of the methodological problems presented above [77]. Some of the markers might be useful to better define the exposure of interest: methods have been developed to measure the covalent binding products of carcinogens with DNA and proteins. The background for these methods is that binding of a chemical to DNA is thought to be an early event in the cascade of biochemical changes eventually leading to the neoplasm [78,79]. In target tissues of experimental animals, the levels of adducts correlate with tumor response [80,81], but only sparse data are available for target tissues, such as lung, in humans. Generally, DNA adducts in nontarget tissues, such as lymphocytes, or protein (usually, hemoglobin or albumin) adducts are used as a surrogate measure of DNA binding [82].

An interesting example of application of DNA adducts among workers exposed to lung carcinogens is a series of studies conducted among foundry workers in Finland and coke workers in Poland [83–86]. The studies from Finland showed that adducts in white blood cell DNA correlate with estimated exposure to PAHs, in terms of both individual exposure and job. In the study from Poland, higher levels of aromatic DNA adducts in white blood cells were found among battery coke workers than among nonbattery workers, again reflecting a gradient in estimated PAH exposure and lung cancer risk.

A second field of application of biological markers are early effects of carcinogens. Cytogenetic endpoints, chromosomal aberrations, sister chromatid exchanges, and micronuclei have been used extensively in occupational monitoring [87]. Recently, at least two new methods of investigating early events in carcinogenesis, which are relevant to occupational carcinogens, have been developed. Point mutations in the human hypoxanthine guanine phosphorobosyltransferase (HPRT) genes have been associated with exposure to ionizing radiation [88] and increased levels of *ras* and *fes* oncoproteins have been detected in plasma of foundry workers exposed to PAHs [89].

A third field of application of biological markers is lung cancer susceptibility. The interindividual variability of enzymes implicated in the metabolism of lung carcinogens, such as aryl hydrocarbon hydroxylase (AHH), epoxide hydrolase, and glutathione transferase, has been shown to be as high as 50- to 500-fold [90]. Lung cancer risk has been reported to be increased among extensive debrisoquine metabolizers [91] and in people with high induction levels of AHH [92]. Both enzymes are part of the cytochrome P450 complex. In the only study that took occupational exposures to carcinogens into account, an apparent synergism in lung cancer risk between the ability to metabolize extensively debrisoquine and occupational exposure to asbestos and PAHs was noted [91]. However, phenotypic characterization of polymorphism suffer from many limitations, and recently DNA-based assays have been developed for the genotyping of debrisoquine [93] and AHH [94] polymorphism.

The new techniques may become very valuable in improving the specificity and sensitivity of exposure assessment, in allowing the investigation of intermediate steps in the carcinogenic process, and in helping to prevent occupationally induced lung cancer. However, at present they still suffer from several limitations. Only a few studies have been conducted to ensure standardization of methods among different laboratories and across similar methods. One example is an interlaboratory comparison for two techniques of measuring DNA adducts, the postlabeling technique and immunoassay, in which good correlations have been found [83]. The cost of these analyses is usually high, which hampers their application to full-scale epidemiological studies. Furthermore, the relevance of some markers is questionable (e.g., use of surrogate tissues), and current knowledge is lacking on important steps of the carcinogenic process, such as DNA repair activities.

## VIII.  Occupational Lung Cancer in Developing Countries

Little information is available on occupational lung cancer in developing countries. Among the industries for which more data are available are asbestos mining, asbestos goods manufacturing, and mining. Two cohort studies of asbestos miners and asbestos product manufacturing workers have been conducted in China [95]. A six- to ninefold excess risk of lung was found in these populations. The association between asbestos exposure and pleural mesothelioma was first reported in South Africa [96]. Reports of mesothelioma cases from other developing countries, such as Mexico, Singapore, and Zimbabwe, are suggestive of extensive exposure to asbestos fibers [97–99]. The sparse industrial hygienic data suggest exposure levels higher than those currently present in developed countries [100–104]. However, it is unclear whether the plants that have been surveyed form a representative or "clean" sample.

Increased risk of lung cancer was found among South African gold miners [105,106], which was related to silica exposure. Underground tin miners from Yunnan, a Chinese region, are at very high risk of lung cancer [107,108]. The risk was attributed to exposure to radon [109] and arsenic [110]. Similarly, tin miners from Guangxi, another Chinese region, were found at higher risk of lung cancer [111]. An increase in lung cancer was also found among Chinese hematite miners [112]. Increased risk of lung cancer were found in two cohorts of silicotic patients from Hong Kong [113] and Singapore [114].

Workers in metal smelting and refining were found at higher risk of lung cancer in a population-based study from Shenyang, China [115], as were members of a iron molder union from South Africa [116]. A series of studies have been conducted among Chinese workers employed in PAH-related industries: coke manufacturing, coal gasification, shale refining, and synthetic oil manufacture [95]. In all these industries, an increased risk of lung cancer was detected. Other studies from China indicate increased risk among benzene-exposed workers [117], arsenic smelters [95], chromate manufacture workers [95], chloromethyl methyl ether exposed workers [95], rubber workers exposed to curing agents or talc powder [118], fur workers [119], and detergent and cosmetic manufacture [120]. A suggestion of increased risk of lung cancer among tobacco farmers comes from a study from Zimbabwe [121].

Taxi drivers from Singapore were not at higher risk of lung cancer [122], nor were diagnostic x-ray workers from China [123], fishermen from Singapore [124], textile workers from China [120], or vinyl chloride–exposed workers from China [95]. Two studies based on routinely collected records were conducted in Hong Kong [125] and Singapore [126]. The study from Hong Kong found increased risks of lung cancer among fishermen and construction workers, whereas the study in Singapore found increased risks among construction workers and transport equipment operators.

In conclusion, little information is available on occupational lung cancer in developing countries, with a few exceptions, such as selected industries in China, Singapore, and Hong Kong, as well as asbestos industries from Zimbabwe and South Africa. The available evidence, however, strongly points toward the presence of a large number of occupationally related lung cancer cases in developing countries. Special efforts should be devoted to improve the amount of information available and to implement preventive measures.

## IX. Prevention of Occupational Lung Cancer

Prevention of occupational lung cancer has occurred where protection of a work force potentially exposed to known lung carcinogens has been implemented sufficiently to ensure that appreciable increased risk has never occurred. Thus data on workers of the nuclear industry have not so far suggested any increased risk of cancer of the respiratory tract [43,44].

Another instance of successful prevention is where an occupation has disappeared or been abolished. Such examples include mustard gas manufacture, which caused a large excess of cancer of the respiratory tract among workers employed during World War II in Japan and England [127,128]. This production ceased in these countries after the end of the war. Other examples include the great reduction in size of uranium miners in Ontario [129] and the cessation of gas manufacture by coal carbonization in developed countries [130].

The most common prevention of occupational lung cancer, however, is connected with decreased exposure levels in the workplace. This phenomenon will lead to a lower risk of cancer among workers employed recently than in workers employed longer ago. Respiratory cancer standardized mortality ratios in a U.S. cohort of workers exposed to chloromethyl ethers was 5.3 for those employed in jobs considered exposed during 1960–1964, and 4.1, 3.8, and 1.8 for each subsequent quinquennium, respectively [131]. Following the implementation of preventive measures, similar results were found among other chloromethyl methyl ether workers [132], as well as in iron ore miners [133] and workers exposed to arsenic [134–137], nickel [12,138,139], chromium [140–143], and asbestos [144–146].

On the other hand, the decreasing exposure levels might have different effects on workers who had been exposed to higher levels, depending on the mechanism of action of the carcinogen. According to the multistage model of carcinogenesis [147], if an agent is acting early in the carcinogenic process, reduction or cessation of exposure over time will not substantially affect the risk of subsequent development of cancer [148]. If, on the other hand, the agent is acting on a late step or is a complete carcinogen, a reduction in exposure will lead to a decrease in cancer risk [148]. There are too few data at present to identify the mechanisms of action of occupational lung carcinogens and to predict the effect of reduction or cessation of exposure on the risk of lung cancer among workers exposed to high levels in the past. It is obvious that current scientific uncertainties should not refrain from implementing all measures aimed to reduce exposure wherever a carcinogen is identified in the workplace.

### References

1. Parkin DM, Läärä E, Muir CS. Estimates of the worldwide frequency of sixteen major cancers in 1980. Int J Cancer 1988;41:184–97.
2. Dodds L, Davis S, Polissar L. A population-based study of lung cancer incidence trends by histologic type, 1974–81. J Natl Cancer Inst 1986;76:21–9.

3. Doll R, Peto R. The causes of cancer: quantitative estimates of avoidable risks of cancer in the United States today. Oxford: Oxford University Press, 1981.

4. Merletti F, Heseltine E, Saracci R, Simonato L, Vainio H, Wilbourn J. Target organs for carcinogenicity of chemicals and industrial exposures in humans: a review of results in the IARC monographs on the evaluation of the carcinogenic risk of chemicals to humans. Cancer Res 1984;44:2244–50.

5. Tomatis L, Aitio A, Wilbourn J, Shuker L. Human carcinogens so far identified. Jpn J Cancer Res 1989;80:795–807.

6. IARC monographs on the evaluation of the carcinogenic risks to humans. Vols. 1–53. Lyon, France: IARC, 1972–1991.

7. IARC monographs on the evaluation of the carcinogenic risks to humans. Overall evaluations of carcinogenicity. An updating of IARC monographs, Vols 1–42. (Suppl. 7). Lyon, France: IARC, 1987.

8. Frank AL. Occupational cancers of the respiratory system. Semin Occup Med 1987;2:257–66.

9. Machle W, Gregorius F. Cancer of respiratory system in the United States chromate-producing industry. Public Health Rep 1948;63:114–27.

10. Chromium and chromium compounds, IARC monographs on the evaluation of the carcinogenic risks to humans. Vol. 49. Chromium, nickel and welding. Lyon, France: IARC, 1990:49–256.

11. Nickel and nickel compounds. IARC monographs on the evaluation of the carcinogenic risks to humans. Vol. 49. Chromium, nickel and welding. Lyon, France: IARC, 1990:257–445.

12. Report of the international committee of nickel carcinogenesis in man. Scand J Work Environ Health 1990;16:1–82.

13. Beryllium and beryllium compounds. IARC monographs on the evaluation of the carcinogenic risk of chemicals to humans. Vol. 23. Some metals and metallic compounds. Lyon, France: IARC, 1980:143–204.

14. Saracci R. Beryllium and lung cancer: adding another piece to the puzzle of epidemiologic evidence. J Natl Cancer Inst 1991;83:1362–63.

15. Steenland K, Ward E. Lung cancer incidence among patients with beryllium disease: a cohort mortality study. J Natl Cancer Inst 1991;83:1380–85.

16. Boffetta P. Methodological aspects of the epidemiological association between cadmium and cancer in humans. In: Nordberg G, Alessio L, Herber RFM, eds. Cadmium in the human environment: toxicity and carcinogenicity. IARC Scientific Publication 118. Lyon, France: IARC, 1993 (in press).

17. Doll R. Cadmium in the human environment. Concluding remarks. In: Nordberg G, Alessio L, Herber RFM, eds. Cadmium in the human environment: toxicity and carcinogenicity. IARC Scientific Publication 118. Lyon, France: IARC, 1993 (in press).

18. Doll R. Mortality from lung cancer among asbestos workers. Br J Ind Med 1955;12:81–86.
19. Talc not containing asbestiform fibres and talc containing asbestiform fibres. IARC monographs on the evaluation of the carcinogenic risks to humans. Vol. 42. Silica and some silicates. Lyon, France: IARC, 1987:185–224.
20. Silica. IARC monographs on the evaluation of the carcinogenic risks to humans. Vol. 42. Silica and some silicates. Lyon, France: IARC, 1987:39–143.
21. Boffetta P, Cardis E, Vainio H, et al. Cancer risks related to electricity production. Eur J Cancer 1991;27:1504–19.
22. IARC monographs on the evaluation of the carcinogenic risk of chemicals to humans. Vol. 32. Polynuclear aromatic compounds. Part 1: Chemical, environmental and experimental data. Lyon, France: IARC, 1984.
23. IARC monographs on the evaluation of the carcinogenic risks to humans. Vol. 46. Diesel and gasoline engine exhausts and some nitroarenes. Lyon, France: IARC, 1989.
24. Coal-tars and derived products. IARC monographs on the evaluation of the carcinogenic risk of chemicals to humans. Vol. 35. Polynuclear aromatic compounds. Part 4: Bitumens, coal-tars and derived products, shale-oils and soots. Lyon, France: IARC, 1985:83–159.
25. Soots. IARC monographs on the evaluation of the carcinogenic risk of chemicals to humans. Vol. 35. Polynuclear aromatic compounds. Part 4: Bitumens, coal-tars and derived products, shale-oils and soots. Lyon, France: IARC, 219–46.
26. Aluminum production. IARC monographs on the evaluation of the carcinogenic risk of chemicals to humans. Vol. 34. Polynuclear aromatic compounds. Part 3: Industrial exposures in aluminum production, coal gasification, coke production, and iron and steel founding. Lyon, France: IARC, 1984:37–64.
27. Kjuus H, Andersen A, Langard S. Incidence of cancer among workers producing calcium carbide. Br J Ind Med 1986;43:237–42.
28. Silverstein M, Maizlish N, Park R, Mirer F. Mortality among workers exposed to coal tar pitch volatiles and welding emissions: an exercise in epidemiologic triage. Am J Public Health 1985;75:1283–87.
29. Coal gasification. IARC monographs on the evaluation of the carcinogenic risk of chemicals to humans. Vol. 34. Polynuclear aromatic compounds. Part 3: Industrial exposures in aluminum production, coal gasification, coke production, and iron and steel founding. Lyon, France: IARC, 1984;65–99.
30. Coke production. IARC monographs on the evaluation of the carcinogenic risk of chemicals to humans. Vol. 34. Polynuclear aromatic compounds.

Part 3: Industrial exposures in aluminum production, coal gasification, coke production, and iron and steel founding. Lyon, France: IARC, 1984;101–31.

31. Diesel and gasoline engine exhausts. IARC monographs on the evaluation of the carcinogenic risks to humans. Vol. 46. Diesel and gasoline engine exhausts and some nitroarenes. Lyon, France: IARC, 1989:41–185.

32. Mineral oils. IARC monographs on the evaluation of the carcinogenic risk of chemicals to humans. Vol. 33. Polynuclear aromatic compounds. Part 2: Carbon blacks, mineral oils and some nitroarenes. Lyon, France: IARC, 1984:87–168.

33. Bitumens. IARC monographs on the evaluation of the carinogenic risk of chemicals to humans. Vol. 35. Polynuclear aromatic compounds. Part 4: Bitumens, coal-tars and derived products, shale-oils and soots. Lyon, France: IARC, 1985:39–81.

34. Carbon blacks. IARC monographs on the evaluation of the carcinogenic risk of chemicals to humans. Vol. 33. Polynuclear aromatic compounds. Part 2: Carbon blacks, mineral oils and some nitroarenes. Lyon, France: IARC, 1984:35–85.

35. Case RAM, Lea AJ. Mustard gas poisoning, chronic bronchitis and lung cancer. An investigation into the possibility that poisoning by mustard gas in the 1914–18 war might be a factor in the production of neoplasia. Br J Prev Soc Med 1955;9:62–72.

36. Bis(chloromethyl)-ehter and chloromethyl methyl ether (technical-grade). IARC monographs on the evaluation of the carcinogenic risk of chemicals to man. Vol. 4. Some aromatic amines, hydrazine and related substances, *N*-nitroso compounds and miscellaneous alkylating agents. Lyon, France: IARC, 1974:231–38, 239–45.

37. Acrylonitrile. IARC monographs on the evaluation of the carcinogenic risk of chemicals to humans. Vol. 19. Some monomers, plastics and synthetic elastomers, and acolein. Lyon, France: IARC, 1979:73–113.

38. Radon. IARC monographs on the evaluation of the carcinogenic risks to humans. Vol. 43. Man-made mineral fibres and radon. Lyon, France: IARC, 1988:173–259.

39. BEIR IV, Committee on the Biological Effects of Ionizing Radiation. Health risks of radon and other internally deposited alpha-emitters. Washington, DC: National Academy of Sciences, 1988.

40. Preston DL, Kato H, Kopecky KJ, Fujita S. Life span study report 10. Part 1: Cancer mortality among A-bomb survivors in Hiroshima and Nagasaki, 1950–82. Technical Report RERF TR 1986:1–86.

41. Shimizu Y, Kato H, Schull WJ, Preston DL, Fujita S, Pierce DA. Life span study report 11. Part 1. Comparison of risk coefficients for site-spe-

cific cancer mortality based on the DS86 and T65DR shielded kerma and organ doses. Technical Report RERF TR 1987:12–87.

42. Smith PG, Doll R. Mortality among patients with ankylosing sponchylitis after a single treatment course with x-rays. Br J Med 1982;284:449–60.

43. Beral V, Fraser P, Booth M, Carpenter L. Epidemiological studies of workers in the nuclear industry. In: Russell Jones R, Southwood R, eds. Radiation and health: the biological effects of low-level exposure to ionizing radiation. Chichester, West Sussex, England, Wiley, 1987:97–106.

44. BEIR V, Committee on the Biological Effects of Ionizing Radiation. Health effects of exposure to low levels of ionizing radiation. Washington, DC: National Academy of Sciences, 1990.

45. Occupational exposures in paint manufacture and painting. IARC monographs on the evaluation of the carcinogenic risks to humans. Vol. 47. Some organic solvents, resin monomers and related compounds pigments and occupational exposures in paint manufacture and painting. Lyon, France: IARC, 1989:327–442.

46. Vinyl chloride. IARC monographs on the evaluation of the carcinogenic risk of chemicals to humans. Vol. 19. Some monomers, plastics and synthetic elastomers, and acrolein. Lyon, France: IARC, 1979:377–438.

47. Boot and shoe manufacture and repair. IARC monographs on the evaluation of the carcinogenic risk of chemicals to humans. Vol. 25. Wood, leather and some associated industries. Lyon, France: IARC, 1981:249–77.

48. IARC monographs on the evaluation of the carcinogenic risk of chemicals to humans. Vol. 28. The rubber industry. Lyon, France: IARC, 1982.

49. Furniture and cabinet-making. IARC monographs on the evaluation of the carcinogenic risk of chemicals to humans. Vol. 25. Wood, leather and some associated industries. Lyon, France: IARC, 1981:99–138.

50. Cobalt and cobalt compounds. IARC monographs on the evaluation of carcinogenic risks to humans. Vol. 52. Chlorinated drinking-water; chlorination by-products; some other halogenated compounds; cobalt and cobalt compounds. Lyon, France: IARC, 1991;363–472.

51. Man-made mineral fibres. IARC monographs on the evaluation of the carcinogenic risks to humans. Vol. 43. Man-made mineral fibres and radon. Lyon, France: IARC, 1988:39–171.

52. Welding. IARC monographs on the evaluation of the carcinogenic risks to humans. Vol. 49. Chromium, nickel and welding. Lyon, France: IARC, 1990:447–525.

53. Simonato L, Vineis P, Fletcher AC. Estimates of the proportion of lung cancer attributable to occupational exposure. Carcinogenesis 1988;9:1159–65.

54. Blot WJ, Harrington JM, Toledo A, Hoover R, Heath CW, Fraumeni JF. Lung cancer after employment in shipyards during World War II. N Engl J Med 1978;21:620–24.
55. Blot WJ, Morris LE, Stroube R, Tagnon I, Fraumeni JF. Lung and laryngeal cancers in relation to shipyard employment in coastal Virginia. J Natl Cancer Inst 1980;65:571–75.
56. Blot WJ, Davies JE, Brown LM, et al. Occupation and the high risk of lung cancer in northeast Florida. Cancer 1982;50:364–71.
57. Blot WJ, Brown LM, Pottern LM, Stone BJ, Fraumeni JF. Lung cancer among long-term steel workers. Am J Epidemiol 1983;117:706–16.
58. Pastorino U, Berrino F, Gervasio A, Pesenti V, Riboli E, Crosignani P. Proportion of lung cancers due to occupational exposure. Int J Cancer 1984;33:231–37.
59. Pannett B, Coggon D, Acheson ED. A job-exposure matrix for use in population based studies in England and Wales. Br J Ind Med 1985;42:777–83.
60. Vena JE, Byers TE, Cookfair D, Swanson M. Occupation and lung cancer risk. An analysis by histologic subtypes. Cancer 1985;56:910–17.
61. Damber L, Larsson LG. Underground mining, smoking, and lung cancer: a case-control study in the iron ore municipalities in northern Sweden. J Natl Cancer Inst 1985;74:1207–13.
62. Buiatti E, Kriebel D, Geddes M, Santucci M, Pucci N. A case-control study of lung cancer in Florence, Italy. I. Occupational risk factors. J Epidemiol Community Health 1985;39:244–50.
63. Kvale G, Bjelke E, Heuch I. Occupational exposure and lung cancer risk. Int J Cancer 1986;37:185–93.
64. Kjuus H, Skjaerven R, Langard S, Lien JT, Aamodt T. A case-referent study of lung cancer, occupational exposures and smoking. I. Comparison of title-based and exposure-based occupational information. Scand J Work Environ Health 1986;12:193–202.
65. Simonato L, Saracci R. Cancer, occupational. In: Parmeggiani L, ed. Encyclopedia of occupational health and safety. 3rd revision. Geneva: ILO, 1983:369–75.
66. Rothman KJ. Synergism and antagonism in cause–effect relationships. Am J Epidemiol 1974;99:385–88.
67. Saracci R. The interactions of tobacco smoking and other agents in cancer etiology. Epidemiol Rev 1987;9:175–93.
68. Prentice RL, Yoshimoto Y, Mason MW. Relationship of cigarette smoking and radiation exposure to cancer mortality in Hiroshima and Nagasaki. J Natl Cancer Inst 1983;70:611–22.
69. Vainio H, Magee PN, McGregor D, McMichael AJ, eds. Mechanisms of

carcinogenesis in risk identification. IARC Scientific Publication 116. Lyon, France: IARC, 1992.

70. Scholze H. Durability investigations on siliceous man-made mineral fibres. A critical review. Glastech Ber 1988;61:161–71.

71. Cherrie J, Dodgson J. Past exposures to airborne fibers and other potential risk factors in the European man-made mineral fiber production industry. Scand J Work Environ Health 1986;12(suppl.):26–33.

72. Cherrie J, Krantz S, Schneider T, Öhberg I, Kamstrup O, Linander W. An experimental simulation of an early rock wool/slag wool production process. Ann Occup Hyg 1987;31:583–93.

73. Krantz S, Cherrie JW, Schneider T, Öhberg I, Kamstrup O. Modelling of past exposure to MMMF in the European rock/slag wool industry. Arb Halsa 1991;1:1–42.

74. Stewart PA, Herrick RF. Issues in performing retrospective exposure assessment. Appl Occup Environ Hyg 1991;6:421–27.

75. Garshick E, Schenker MB, Muñoz A, et al. A case-control study of lung cancer and diesel exhaust exposure in railroad workers. Am Rev Respir Dis 1987;135:1242–48.

76. Garshick E, Schenker MB, Muñoz A, et al. A retrospective cohort study of lung cancer and diesel exhaust exposure in railroad workers. Am Rev Respir Dis 1988;137:820–25.

77. Perera FP. Molecular cancer epidemiology: a new tool in cancer prevention. J Natl Cancer Inst 1982;78:887–98.

78. Miller JA, Miller EC. Ultimate chemical carcinogens as reactive mutagenic electrophiles. In: Hiatt HH, Watson JD, Winsten JA, eds. Origins of human cancer. Cold Spring Harbor, NY: Cold Spring Harbor Laboratory, 1977:605–27.

79. Weinstein IB. The origins of human cancer: molecular mechanisms of carcinogenesis and their implications for cancer prevention and treatment. Cancer Res 1988;48:4135–43.

80. Beland FA, Fullerton NF, Kinouchi T, Poirier MC. DNA adducts formation during continuous feeding of 2-acetylaminogluorene at multiple concentrations. In: Bartsch H, Hemminki K, O'Neill IK, eds. Methods of detecting DNA damaging agents in humans: applications in cancer epidemiology and prevention. IARC Scientific Publication 89. Lyon, France: IARC, 1988:175–80.

81. Wogan GN. Detection of DNA damage in studies on cancer etiology and prevention. In: Bartsch H, Hemminki K, O'Neill IK, eds. Methods for detecting DNA damaging agents in humans: applications in cancer epidemiology and prevention. IARC Scientific Publication 89. Lyon, France: IARC, 1988:32–51.

82. Perera FP, Santella RM, Breuner D, Young TL, Weinstein IB. Application

of biological markers to the study of lung cancer causation and prevention. In: Bartsch H, Hemminki K, O'Neill IK, eds. Methods for detecting DNA damaging agents in humans: applications in cancer epidemiology and prevention. IARC Scientific Publication 89. Lyon, France: IARC, 1988:451–59.

83. Hamminki K, Perera FP, Phillips DH, Randerath K, Reddy MV, Santella RM. Aromatic DNA adducts in white blood cells of foundry workers. In: Bartsch H, Hemminki K, O'Neill IK, eds. Methods for detecting DNA damaging agents in humans: applications in cancer epidemiology and prevention. IARC Scientific Publication 89. Lyon, France IARC, 1988:190–95.

84. Perera FP, Hemminki K, Young TL, Brenner D, Kelly G, Santella RM. Detection of polycyclic aromatic hydrocarbon–DNA adducts in white blood cells of foundry workers. Cancer Res 1988;48:2288–91.

85. Phillips DH, Hemminki K, Alhonen A, Hewer A, Grover PL. Monitoring occupational exposure to carcinogens: detection by $^{32}$P-postlabeling or aromatic DNA adducts in white blood cells from iron foundry workers. Mutat Res 1988;204:531–41.

86. Hemminki K, Grzybowska E, Chorazy M, et al. DNA adducts in humans environmentally exposed to aromatic compounds in an industrialized area of Poland. Carcinogenesis 1990;7:1229–31.

87. Sorsa M. Monitoring of sister chromatid exchanges and micronuclei as biological endpoints. In: Berlin A, Draper M, Hemminki K, Vainio H, eds. Monitoring human exposure to carcinogenic and mutagenic agents. IARC Scientific Publication 59. Lyon, France: IARC, 1984:339–49.

88. Messing K, Bradley WEC. In vivo mutant frequency rises among breast cancer patients after exposure to high doses of gamma radiation. Mutat Res 1985;152:107–12.

89. Brandt-Rauf P, Smith S, Perera F, et al. Serum oncogene proteins in foundry workers. J Soc Occup Med 1990;40:11–14.

90. Vähäkangas K, Pelkonen O. Host variations in carcinogen metabolism and DNA repair. In: Lynch HT, Hirayama R, eds. Genetic epidemiology of cancer. Boca Raton, FL: CRC Press, 1989:6–40.

91. Caporaso N, Hayes RB, Dosemeci M, et al. Lung cancer risk, occupational exposure, and the debrisoquine metabolic phenotype. Cancer Res 1989;49:3675–79.

92. Bartsch H, Hietanen E, Petruzelli S, et al. Possible prognostic value of pulmonary AH-locus-linked enzymes in patients with tobacco-related lung cancer. Int J Cancer 1990;46:185–88.

93. Gough AC, Miles JS, Spurr NK, et al. Identification of the primary gene defect at the cytochrome P450 CYP2D locus. Nature 1990;347:773–76.

94. Spurr NK, Wolf CR. Genetic analysis of the cytochrome P450 system. In: Waterman MR, Johnson EF, eds. Methods in enzymology. New York: Academic Press 1992.
95. Wu W. Occupational cancer epidemiology in the People's Republic of China. J Occup Med 1988;30:968–74.
96. Wagner JC, Sleggs CA, Marchand P. Diffuse pleural mesothelioma and asbestos exposure in the North Western Cape Province. Br J Ind Med 1960;17:260–71.
97. Ho SF, Lee HP, Phoon WH. Malignant mesothelioma in Singapore. Br J Ind Med 1987;44:788–89.
98. Mendez Vargas MM, Maldonado Torres L, Stanislawski EC, Mendoza Ugalde HC. Mesotelioma maligno en un trabajador del asbesto. Rev Med Inst Mex Seguro Soc 1982;20:249–57.
99. Cullen MR, Baloyi RS. Chrysotile asbestos and health in Zimbabwe. I. Analysis of miners and millers compensated for asbestos-related diseases since independence (1980). Am J Ind Med 1991;19:161–69.
100. Mohamed IY. Asbestos-cement pneumoconiosis: first surgically confirmed case in Kuwait. Am J Ind Med 1990;17:241–45.
101. Berman DM. Asbestos and health in the Third World: the case of Brazil. Int J Health Serv 1986;16:253–62.
102. Huang JQ. A study on the dose–response relationship between asbestos exposure level and asbestosis among workers in a Chinese chrysotile product factory. Biomed Environ Sciences 1990;3:90–98.
103. Oleru UG. Polmonary function of control and industrially exposed Nigerians in asbestos, textile, and toluene diisocyanate-foam factories. Environ Res 1980;23:137–48.
104. Cullen MR, Baloyi RS. Prevalence of pneumonoconiosis among coal and heavy metal miners in Zimbabwe. Am J Ind Med 1990;17:677–82.
105. Wyndham CH, Bezuidenhout BN, Greenacre MJ, Sluis-Cremer GK. Mortality of middle aged white South African gold miners. Br J Ind Med 1986;43:677–84.
106. Hnizdo E, Sluis-Cremer GK. Silica exposure, silicosis, and lung cancer: a mortality study of South African gold miners. Br J Ind Med 1991;48:53–60.
107. Sun SQ. Etiology of lung cancer at the Gejiu tin mine, China. Int Symp Princess Takamatsu Cancer Res Fund 1987;18:103–15.
108. Xuan XZ, Schatzkin A, Mao BL, et al. Feasibility of conducting a lung cancer chemoprevention trial among tin miners in Yunnan, P.R. China. Cancer Causes Control 1991;2:175–82.
109. Qiao YL, Taylor PR, Yao SX, et al. Relation of radon exposure and tobacco use to lung cancer among tin miners in Yunnan Province, China. Am J Ind Med 1989;16:511–21.
110. Taylor PR, Qiao YL, Schatzkin A, et al. Relation of arsenic exposure to

lung cancer among tin miners in Yunnan Province, China. Br J Ind Med 1989;46:881–86.

111. Wu KG, Fu H, Mo CZ, Yu LZ. Smelting, underground mining, smoking, and lung cancer: a case-control study in a tin mine area. Biomed Environ Sci 1989;2:98–105.

112. Chen SY, Hayes RB, Liang SR, Li QG, Stewart PA, Blair A. Mortality experience of haematite mine workers in China. Br J Int Med 1990;47:175–81.

113. Ng TP, Chan SL, Lee J. Mortality of a cohort of men in a silicosis register: further evidence of an association with lung cancer. Am J Ind Med 1990;17:163–71.

114. Chia SE, Chia KS, Phoon WH, Lee HP. Silicosis and lung cancer among Chinese granite workers. Scand J Work Environ Health 1991;17:170–74.

115. Xu ZY, Blot WJ, Xiao HP, et al. Smoking, air pollution, and the high rates of lung cancer in Shenyang, China. J Natl Cancer Inst 1989;81:1800–1806.

116. Sitas F, Douglas AJ, Webster EC. Respiratory disease mortality patterns among South African iron moulders. Br J Ind Med 1989;46:310–15.

117. Yin SN, Li GL, Tain FD, et al. A retrospective cohort study of leukemia and other cancers in benzene workers. Environ Health Perspect 1989;82:207–13.

118. Zhang ZF, Yu SZ, Li WX, Choi BC. Smoking, occupational exposure to rubber, and lung cancer. Br J Ind Med 1989;46:12–15.

119. Wang HL. Cancer among fur workers. Chung Hua Yu Fang I Hsueh Tsa Chih 1987;21:129–32.

120. Levin LI, Zheng W, Blot WH, Gao YT, Frameni JF. Occupation and lung cancer in Shanghai: a case-control study. Br J Ind Med 1988;45:450–58.

121. Kusemamariwo T, Neill P. Carcinoma of the bronchus in tobacco farm workers. An unrecognized high risk group. Trop Geogr Med 1990;42:261–64.

122. Koh D, Guanco-Chua S, Ong CN. A study of the mortality patterns of taxi drivers in Singapore. Ann Acad Med Singapore 1988;17:579–82.

123. Wang JX, Inskip PD, Boice JD, Li BX, Zhang JY, Fraumeni JF. Cancer incidence among medical diagnostic x-ray workers in China, 1950 to 1985. Int J Cancer 1990;45:889–95.

124. Jeyaratnam J, Lee J, Lee HP, Phoon WO. Stomach cancer incidence in a cohort of fishermen in Singapore. Scand J Work Environ Health 1987;13:524–26.

125. Ng TP. Occupational mortality in Hong Kong, 1979–1983. Int J Epidemiol 1988;17:105–10.

126. Lee HP. Cancer incidence in Singapore by occupational groups. Ann Acad Med Singapore 1984;13:366–70.

127. Wada S, Miyanishi M, Nishimoto Y, Kambe S, Miller RW. Mustard gas as a cause of respiratory neoplasia in man. Lancet 1968;1:1161–63.
128. Easton DF, Peto J, Doll R. Cancers of the respiratory tract in mustard gas workers. Br J Ind Med 1988;45:652–59.
129. Chovil A. The epidemiology of primary lung cancer in uranium miners in Ontario. J Occup Med 1981;23:417–21.
130. Doll R, Vessey MP, Beasley RWR, et al. Mortality of gas workers. Final report of a prospective study. Br J Ind Med 1972;29:394–406.
131. Maher KV, DeFonso LR. Respiratory cancer among chloromethyl ether workers. J Natl Cancer Inst 1987;78:839–43.
132. McCallum RI, Woolley V, Petrie A. Lung cancer associated with chloromethyl methyl ether manufacture: an investigation at two factories in the United Kingdom. Br J Ind Med 1983;40:384–89.
133. Kinlen LJ, Willows AN. Decline in the lung cancer hazard: a prospective study of the mortality of iron ore miners in Cumbria. Br J Ind Med 1988;45:219–24.
134. Sandström AIM, Wall SGI, Taube A. Cancer incidence and mortality among Swedish smelter workers. Br J Ind Med 1989;46:82–89.
135. Lee-Feldstein A. Arsenic and respiratory cancer in humans: follow-up of copper smelter employees in Montana. J Natl Cancer Inst 1983;70:601–9.
136. Mabuchi K, Lilienfield AM, Snell LM. Lung cancer among pesticide workers exposed to inorganic arsenicals. Arch Environ Health 1979;34:312–20.
137. Tokudome S, Kuratsune M. A cohort study on mortality from cancer and other causes among workers at a metal refinery. Int J Cancer 1976;17:310–17.
138. Magnus K, Andersen A, Høgetveit AC. Cancer of respiratory organs among workers at a nickel refinery in Norway. Second report. Int J Cancer 1982;30;681–85.
139. Chovil A, Sutherland RB, Halliday M. Respiratory cancer in a cohort of nickel sinter plant workers. Br J Ind Med 1981;38:327–33.
140. Enterline PE. Respiratory cancer among chromate workers. J Occup Med 1974;16:523–26.
141. Davies JM. Lung cancer mortality among workers making lead chromate and zinc chromate pigments at three English factories. Br J Ind Med 1984;41:158–69.
142. Alderson MR, Rattan NS, Bidstrup L. Health of workmen in the chromate-producing industry in Britain. Br J Ind Med 1981;38:117–24.
143. Hayes RB, Lilienfield AM, Snell LM. Mortality in chromium chemical production workers: a prospective study. Int J Epidemiol 1979;8:365–74.
144. Acheson ED, Gardner MF, Winter PD, Bennett C. Cancer in a factory using amosite asbestos. Int J Epidemiol 1984;13:3–10.

145. Newhouse ML, Berry G, Skidmore JW. A mortality study of workers manufacturing friction materials with chrysotile asbestos. Ann Occup Hyg 1982;26:899–909.
146. Blot WJ, Fraumeni JF. Time-related factors in cancer epidemiology. J Chron Dis 1987;40:1S–8S.
147. Day NE, Brown CC. Multistage models and the primary prevention of cancer. J Natl Cancer Inst 1980;64:977–89.
148. Kaldor JM, Day NE. Interpretation of epidemiological studies in the context of the multistage model of carcinogenesis. In: Barrett JC, ed. Mechanisms of environmental carcinogenesis. Vol. II. Multisteps models of carcinogenesis. Boca Raton, FL: CRC Press, 1990:21–57.

# 3

# Epidemiology of Pleural Cancer

**J. C. McDONALD**

National Heart and Lung Institute
London Chest Hospital
London, England

## I. Introduction

Malignant mesothelial tumors, mainly affecting the pleura, and less often the peritoneum, pericardium, and tunica vaginalis testis, have been the subject of intensive etiological research over the past 30 years. This flood of activity was initiated by the reported evidence of the causal association with asbestos exposure, before which the disease was considered little more than a puzzling pathological curiosity. Much concerning the epidemiology of the disease is now fairly clear, but there remain important questions unanswered. The former is dealt with quite briefly and the latter discussed more fully to help identify priority areas for the research still needed.

## II. What Is Now Clear

### A. Incidence

Malignant mesothelioma was once a rare tumor and remains so in women; however, in industrialized countries, the incidence in men has been rising at 5 to 10% per year since the 1950s, and perhaps earlier [1]. Difficulties in diagnosis and uneven levels of ascertainment reduce the reliability of the available data on incidence, due largely to the low and decreasing frequency of autopsy, without which there is always doubt about the site of the primary tumor. The most extensive information on long-term trends is provided by the SEER program in the United States [2], by pathologists in Canada [3], and by mortality statistics in the United Kingdom [4] and Scandinavia [5].

It has long been evident that there are large differences in the geographical distribution of the disease both within and between countries. Wagner et al. [6] in 1960 were the first to focus attention on the remarkable occurrence of cases in the crocidolite mining area of the North West Cape Province of South Africa. In 1979, Baris et al. [7] reported an extremely high frequency in a localized area of central Turkey, where a particular type of fibrous zeolite was a common geological feature. The concentration of cases in major naval dockyard cities of Western Europe and North America has long been documented [8]. Other studies have demonstrated a high incidence of the disease in South Africa and Western Australia, probably attributable to the crocidolite mining industries in these countries. Less dramatic but conceivably as important is evidence from the United States that the incidence is relatively high in the Rocky Mountain states of Wyoming, Colorado, and some predominantly rural counties of New York [9].

## B. Etiology

From the outset it has been evident that the occurrence of mesothelioma in workers exposed to asbestos was probably related strongly to the type of fiber with which they had worked. Wherever the exposure has been predominantly crocidolite, the proportion of persons affected has been high. This has been documented in both South African and Australian crocidolite miners and millers, in British and Canadian gas mask filter assembly, and in American cigarette filter manufacture [10]. It has also been evident in two asbestos textile plants where some crocidolite was used [11,12] in contrast to one where it was not [13]. It can explain the high rates of the disease in naval dockyard areas, where crocidolite was common in naval insulation materials. It is reflected in the aggregation of cases in the vicinity of large crocidolite-using plants in east London [14] and Hamburg [15]. It is supported by lung burden analyses where crocidolite fibers are found in much greater concentrations in cases than controls [16–18].

The status of chrysotile is much more confusing for two primary reasons, discussed further in Section III. The first is that chrysotile, although accounting for over 90% of all asbestos fiber produced, has seldom been used without admixture of crocidolite or amosite. Moreover, even as mined and subsequently sold commercially, it usually contains a small amount (perhaps 1 to 2%) of another amphibole fiber, tremolite. Second, chrysotile is less able to penetrate and much less durable than most amphibole fibers in lung tissue. Body burden analyses at autopsy are thus more difficult to interpret for chrysotile than for durable fibers.

Although there can be no reasonable doubt that amosite asbestos is an important cause of mesothelioma, the epidemiological data present some anomalies. In particular, there is still little evidence that the mining and milling of this fiber in South Africa, the only place where it has been produced, is associated with many cases of the disease. On the other hand, workers were badly affected in a large insulation products plant in New Jersey that used only amosite [19]. For many years it was maintained that the high incidence of mesothelioma in North American insulation workers was due to the chrysotile content of insulation materials rather than to a high, or higher, content of amosite. This hypothesis is less easy to sustain in the light of experience in the New Jersey plant and the result of controlled lung burden studies in North America [17,18], which have shown an amosite excess of order similar to that for crocidolite.

The two remaining amphibole fiber types—anthophyllite and tremolite—have always been of minor commercial value and have received correspondingly little epidemiological investigation. Anthophyllite, mined and milled only in Finland but now no longer, has produced few if any cases of mesothelioma [20]. Fibrous tremolite is widespread in the earth's crust but mined commercially on only a limited scale. With the exception of small cohorts of mine workers in Montana engaged in the exploitation of a vermiculite deposit, heavily contaminated with amphibole fiber in the tremolite series, there is no direct evidence that such exposure has caused mesothelioma [21]. However, the fact that tremolite fibers are commonly found in close association with many minerals of commercial importance, including chrysotile, talc, zeolites, and fibrous clays, has made this issue a pressing one.

The possibility that mesothelioma might occur in workers exposed to man-made mineral fibers (MMMFs) was investigated in three large cohorts totaling 41,185 workers employed in their manufacture in Europe and North America. Only four deaths were ascribed to the disease in a total of 7862 deaths from all causes, one in a man also exposed to amosite [22]. Exposure levels in MMMF manufacture are extremely low, however. Apart from fibrous erionite there is little or no evidence that other natural or man-made mineral fibers have caused the disease.

### C. Occupational Risks

Surveys of mesothelioma in specific occupations, whether prospective or retrospective in type, provide measurements of risk in these occupations within defined circumstances. These studies are highly selective, not comprehensive, and do not easily allow comparison between occupations. Few surveys have attempted to assess the relative contribution of various jobs on a large or national scale. One such was based on all fatal cases ascertained through pathologists in Canada, 1960–1972, and in the United States, 1972 [23]. Matched controls were selected from the same pathology department and detailed employment histories obtained by interview with the next of kin. An occupational analysis of 10 or more years before death was made for 344 male cases and their controls. This showed that by far the greatest relative risk (46.0) was for insulation work, following in descending order by asbestos production and manufacture (6.1), heating trades (4.4), shipyard work (2.8), and construction work (2.6). Mining and asbestos cement work made little contribution to the first category and demolition very little to the last. Occupations for which no increased risk was detected included, notably, garage work, building maintenance, carpentry, and transport, together with several other named jobs for which the numbers were smaller.

### D. Latency and Tumor Location

Malignant mesothelial tumors, whatever their location, appear equally associated with asbestos exposure, with time since first exposure and in rapidity of fatal outcome. Little can be said about tumors of the pericardium and tunica vaginalis, but substantial and largely unexplained differences do exist in the epidemiology of pleural and peritoneal tumors. It has been suggested that only pleural tumors are associated with chrysotile exposure, but a peritoneal case was diagnosed in Quebec chrysotile production workers, and remarkably few have been found among Australian crocidolite miners. Whereas in the 1960s peritoneal tumors comprised up to 30% of the total, in recent years it has not been more than about 10%. It is not that peritoneal tumors are now less frequent but rather that the steady increase has been in pleural tumors. It is suggested that the explanation may lie in the intensity of exposure but on little objective evidence.

Time between first (relevant) exposure and death from mesothelioma has been recorded in several studies. This latency period or, more correctly, lapse time varies with species and is not understood. In humans the median interval lies between 30 and 40 years with only 5 to 10% under 20 years and very few, if any, under 14 years [10].

### III. What Remains Unclear

### A. Background Incidence

The question of whether and to what extent malignant mesothelioma occurred before the industrial exploitation of asbestos is of much scientific interest. Without this knowledge it is possible to assess the absolute risk of the disease under specified conditions of exposure, but not the attributable risk. This is not a serious matter when dealing with potent causes of the disease such as crocidolite, but it is of concern in studies of weaker or more questionable agents, such as chrysotile or man-made mineral fibers. Although not conclusive, evidence recently reviewed all suggests that there is and has been a background incidence of the disease, very low in childhood but rising with age, and perhaps more common in males than females [24]. The cause of these cases is quite unknown but a number of reasons for believing that they exist follow.

### Historical Reports

The production of asbestos for industrial use began at the end of the nineteenth century and remained at a low level until World War I. It is unlikely that exposure resulting from this activity could have produced any detectable increase in mesothelioma until about 1950, which is indeed when asbestos-related case reports began to appear, culminating in the paper by Wagner et al. in 1960 [6]. However, a search through earlier publications reveals that many cases and quite large case series, all based on autopsy study, were reported in the journals from about 1870 on. As stated in 1943 by Saccone and Coblenz [25], "as knowledge of the existence of the tumour spread, it came to be reported with increasing frequency." These authors also refer to an often-quoted but elusive paper published in 1767, attributed to Lieutaud, describing two pleural tumors in a study of 3000 autopsies. The historical evidence is confused by the large number of diagnostic labels used in the past to describe these tumors, due mainly to controversy over which cell line or tissue was the site of origin. The name *pleuroma* was suggested, but mesothelioma prevailed. There seems little doubt from clinical and pathological descriptions that these tumors would today be classified by pathologists as malignant pleural mesotheliomas. It would thus appear that during the long period under review, about one such case was found on average per 1000 autopsies in Europe and North America, with a male to female ratio of up to 1.8 and a steady increase in frequency with age. Unfortunately, no reliable estimate of disease incidence can be derived from these data.

### Cases in Childhood

Even in the Turkish villages where there was exposure to fibrous erionite from birth, cases of mesothelioma were not seen in childhood. The rarity of cases with onset less than 20 years from first exposure to asbestos at work or in the household of asbestos workers also implies that cases under the age of 20 years are most unlikely to have resulted from such exposure, and even less likely if the exposure was of very low intensity, as in the general environment. Nevertheless, there is little doubt that mesothelioma in children does occur. A series of 80 cases in children up to 19 years of age (mean 9.7 years) was systematically collected and analyzed, 38 from the United States and 42 from 15 other countries [26]. The ratio of males to females was 1.4, and in only two cases (aged 3 and 17 years) was there a history of possible exposure to asbestos. Tissue samples from 22 cases were reviewed by a panel of pathologists that accepted 10 and classified three as possible. Again, it is difficult to move from a case series of this kind to estimates of incidence; however, data from these and other sources were in approximate agreement with an annual rate in North America of about one case per 10 million population under 20 years of age [24].

### Mortality Trends

Backward extrapolation from the sharply deviating trends for male and female mortality, seen in North America and Europe, suggest that in the 1950s, or perhaps rather earlier, the background incidence in both sexes may have been about 1 per million population [3]. This is corroborated by two other analyses. Age-adjusted rates for nine regions of the United States included in the SEER surveillance program (1979–1984) indicate that male to female ratios fall in a similar manner in relation to incidence [24]. In a survey of cases recorded in the Los Angeles County cancer registry for 1974–1978, an equal number of cases in both sexes were without history of asbestos exposure. The incidence rate for these cases was also about 1 per million [27].

### Fibrous Zeolites

The zeolite family of aluminosilicate minerals is widespread in nature and some may occur in fibrous habit. In the mountain states of the western United States and some 40 other countries there are many known deposits of erionite or other zeolites, but at present it appears that none are mined commercially [28]. In the Cappadocia region of central Turkey where fibrous erionite (a zeolite variety) is a prominent feature of the landscape, its presence is associated in certain small villages with a disastrous level of malignant mesothelioma. Inhalation studies with fibrous erionite in experimental animals have resulted in extremely high rates of pleural tumor. The question of whether this group of fibrous minerals can account for any general background incidence in humans is an important one on which to date there is little evidence. In our own survey of mesothelioma cases and controls in North America in 1972 [23], 17 cases and 12 controls lived for 20 to 40 years before death near a zeolite deposit in the United States. After allowance for asbestos exposure, the relative risk was 1.60 (95% confidence interval, 0.58 to 4.93). Reference was made earlier to the relatively high incidence recorded in two Rocky Mountain states [9].

### Lung Burden Analyses

Studies of asbestos and other mineral fibers in lung tissue at autopsy on mesothelioma cases and controls provide highly specific evidence, but their sensitivity is handicapped mainly by the small numbers of subjects and also by limits of detection. However, these studies have shown that in a few cases no asbestos fibers of any kind are seen and, in a larger number, no long fibers (>8μm) [24].

### B. The Tremolite Question

In a recently published review and synthesis of current knowledge relating to asbestos in buildings by the Health Effects Institute, Wagner made the following dissenting statement: "I do not accept that pure chrysotile will cause mesotheliomas." He went on to say: "I agree with the workers on lung tissue burden who have demonstrated that certain tremolite asbestos fibres of the right length and diameter, because of their durability, are the cause of mesotheliomas in the majority of cases in Quebec" [29]. This in essence is the tremolite question, sometimes considered as academic because chrysotile and tremolite cannot be separated but of considerable scientific importance, nevertheless, and perhaps in the longer term, practically.

The extensive program of epidemiological research in the Quebec chrysotile mining industry begun in 1965 was conducted largely because it was believed that exposure was to a single asbestos fiber type. While investigating the uneven distribution of pleural changes among workers in the various mines and mills, Gibbs [30] was probably the first to suggest that minerals other than chrysotile might account for them. However, he did not specify tremolite fibers, and at that time the fact that these might be present in or near the ore body was not generally appreciated. It was only when Pooley [31] examined by electron microscopy lung tissue taken at autopsy from a small number of former miners that chrysotile and tremolite fibres were seen in surprisingly similar concentrations. More systematic examination soon raised the question of the extent to which the fibrogenic and carcinogenic consequences of exposure were attributable to tremolite, chrysotile, or both [32]. In the last decade several investigations have thrown further light on the question but failed so far to answer it. Virtually all the evidence comes from lung burden studies which effectively use the human lung as a sampling device. The present level of contamination of chrysotile by tremolite is still not known, let alone in the past or in other mining areas. Formidable problems face the investigator who wishes to use lung burden analyses for epidemiological research [33].

Four points require consideration:

1. Fibers present in lung tissue at death do not necessarily reflect the past, qualitatively or quantitatively. Amphibole fibers are not only retained

more readily than chrysotile but for much longer. Thus only studies well controlled for time-related variables can be interpreted.

2.  Studies depend on the availability of tissue obtained postmortem or by surgery, both of which are liable to many types of selection bias. This problem is compounded by the need for similar tissue from comparable referents.

3.  Inhaled and retained fibers are not evenly distributed throughout the lung. Samples of any kind are difficult to get, and this source of variation (error) can seldom be taken into account.

4.  The significance of fibers in lung tissue at death will depend on the nature of the probable cancer-producing mechanism. If the fibers act as the primary carcinogen, retention may be of critical importance. If they act as a transport medium for chemical carcinogens (e.g., polycyclic hydrocarbons from tobacco smoke) or by activating some latent virus already present, long-term retention may have little relevance.

The fact that some but not necessarily all chrysotile is accompanied by trace amounts of tremolite fiber and that the latter, either because it is more durable or penetrates the lower respiratory tract more readily, is disproportionately concentrated in lung may have little epidemiological significance unless there is independent evidence of its greater pathogenicity. Animal experiments have failed to demonstrate any important difference between tremolite and chrysotile, and probably cannot having regard for the short life-span of small mammals and the time required for significant removal of the more soluble type of fiber. Direct epidemiological evidence in humans is also scanty, mainly because there are so few opportunities for pure tremolite exposure. It was suggested some years ago that tremolite might be responsible for lung cancer and mesothelioma in New York State talc miners [34,35], but this has always been disputed. The only clear evidence comes from cohort studies of the Montana vermiculite miners mentioned earlier [21]. Even here, the number of employees was small and there is no certainty that the amphibole fibers to which they were exposed, although classified geologically as in the tremolite series, were idential to those found in association with Quebec chrysotile. There seems little doubt, however, that among 165 deaths observed in this cohort of 406 vermiculite workers, four were probably due to mesothelioma.

In the very much larger cohort of male Quebec miners, only 10 cases of mesothelioma were identified in 3291 deaths before 1976 in a cohort of some 10,000 men. A further follow-up is in progress, and although the proportional mortality from this disease will certainly be higher, some 70% of the cohort members have died, leaving survivors now aged 70 to 100 years. Although there is some reason to believe that the proportion of tremolite in asbestos as produced in the Thetford Mines region of Quebec is higher than in the Asbestos region, the cases of mesothelioma have been distributed fairly equally. However, the question is seriously complicated by the fact that the mining company in Asbestos also operated a manufacturing plant in which substantial amounts of crocidolite were used in the production of asbestos cement pipe and for military gas mask filters [36]. Lung burden studies based on deaths in the general population in and near Asbestos showed that crocidolite was quite widespread [37].

Despite problems in the interpretation of mineral fibers in tissue at autopsy, we believe it unreasonable to discount the results of well-controlled studies. Such investigations have consistently failed to show any important difference in chrysotile fiber concentration between mesothelioma cases and controls. On the other hand, chrysotile concentrations at autopsy correlate reasonably well with lifetime exposure estimates in both mine workers and in textile plant workers [38]. The substantially higher concentrations of amphibole fibers, including tremolite, in cases than in controls is equally consistent. It is hard to escape the conclusion that amphibole fibers are the major cause of mesothelioma and that a proportion of the few cases in chrysotile workers could be well explained by tremolite [18].

### C. Exposure-Response

Because occupational asbestos exposure has seldom been to a single pure fiber type and is in any case most difficult to quantify, precise information on risk in relation to duration and intensity is lacking. However, certain rather general points are clear enough. Unlike asbestos-related lung cancer, for example, mesothelioma commonly occurs in the absence of pulmonary fibrosis, especially where exposure has been mainly to amphibole fiber and not chrysotile. Unlike lung cancer, there is no evidence that cigarette smoking is a cofactor of any importance [10].

Reflections of intensity and duration are evident in two other types of data. Even in situations of high risk, for example in gas mask assembly and amosite insulation product manufacture, there is a deficiency of cases with exposure of less than about 6 months [39]. A descending gradient in exposure intensity is probable in (1) household members of an asbestos worker, (2) persons who live in the immediate vicinity of an asbestos mine or factory, (3) residents in large industrial cities, and (4) rural residents. Studies of mesothelioma have demonstrated risk in the first two categories, but only where the exposure entailed crocidolite, and no evidence of excess in the latter two categories [10].

An element of quantification is obtainable from the dozen or so cohort studies where individual estimates of exposure were made in terms of intensity and duration. More might have been made of these data had the investigators felt less intimidated by problems of fiber type and conversion from dust particle to fiber concentrations. An early attempt by Newhouse and Berry, later updated [40], used only subjective estimates of intensity, from low through moderate to high, and simple division of employment into less than or more than 2 years. They showed, nevertheless, that risk of mesothelioma was systematically related to these crude variables. In the Quebec chrysotile mining cohort, among seven cases at Thetford Mines, uncomplicated by the possible contribution of crocidolite at Asbestos, risk was also related to accumulated exposure [39]. The case with the lowest exposure was in a man who had experienced an estimated exposure of 59 fiber-years. If the mesothelioma risk was dominated by a tremolite content of about 1.5%, this might suggest evidence of risk, from the amphibole component, at around 1 fiber-year.

In textile workers with chrysotile obtained primarily from Thetford Mines, one mesothelioma was recorded among 570 deaths [13]. The exposure for this worker lay between about 200 and 400 fiber-years, roughly equivalent to about 4 fiber-years in terms of tremolite, if the tremolite content were similar to that in the mines. However, lung burden analyses suggest that the tremolite content of the chrysotile to which mine workers were exposed was about 2.5 times greater than for the textile workers [38]. Correcting for this factor, the relevant exposure in this case might have been about 2 fiber-years. In the Montana vermiculite cohort, the case of mesothelioma with least exposure was in a man employed for 1.9 years at an average of 7.8 fibers/mL (14.8 fiber-years). While less than the gross figures for chrysotile miners and textile workers, the latter exposure is higher than might be expected if tremolite fibers were entirely responsible for mesothelioma in these two groups. This type of speculation indicates how difficult it will be to answer the underlying question without better information on exposure–response relationships, in particular for tremolite.

The problems associated with chrysotile in lung burden analyses apply less obviously to amphibole fibers. If it be assumed that what is found in the lung at death reflects the accumulated exposure in life, well-controlled studies probably give a more accurate and type-specific estimate of risk than anything based solely on environmental measurements. Ways may eventually be found whereby fiber concentrations in lung, together with data on duration, might be used to estimate the average intensity to which a person had been exposed, but this has not yet been attempted. The main achievement of such research to date has been to strengthen the evidence that risk of mesothelioma is systematically related to amphibole fiber concentration in lung tissue. This was clearly shown for crocidolite by the Nottingham cohort of military gas mask assembly workers [41] and Australian miners and millers [42]. It was also seen in surveys of mesothelioma cases from Canada, the United States, and the United Kingdom [17,41]. The last three studies, though large, were not sufficiently so to differentiate reliably between the risks attributable to crocidolite, amosite, and tremolite, nor to give any indication as to the occupational or other environmental source of the fibers. Two of the lung burden studies, however, indicated that discrimination between cases and controls rested on fibers more than 8 μm in length, with little or no contribution from shorter fibers [18,42].

There are pressing political and administrative needs for a rational yardstick to guide decision making, particularly in situations with very low levels of exposure. Several attempts have been made to meet this requirement by providing risk estimates based on statistical modeling. Public health decisions can seldom await scientific certainty, so these efforts are obviously justified. As the subject is too large and technical for discussion here, the reader is referred to the recent report of the Health Effects Institute [29] for a well-balanced account of this approach. The reliability of statistical risk assessment procedures depends wholly on the epidemiological data available, the assumptions that must be made, and the biological concepts on which they are based. The conclusions reached are thus essentially hypothetical and require periodic review in the light of developing knowledge.

## IV. Direction for Future Research

The three main areas where there is need for better understanding are quite closely linked. Clarification of the role of fibrous tremolite and other naturally occurring mineral fibers will throw light on the question of background incidence and also help assess the risk of mesothelioma from chrysotile exposure. Without this knowledge it is difficult to obtain any precise concept of quantitative relationships between exposure to any of the commercial types of asbestos and risk of mesothelioma. In addition, there is a need for adequate surveillance of risk resulting from exposure to the rapidly developing range of man-made fibers; this requirement would also be largely met by the same research.

Well-designed epidemiological studies, which must include lung fiber analyses, are now required. No air sampling device can conceivably equal the sensitivity, specificity, and direct biological relevance of the human lung. The difficulties of interpretation, outlined in Section III, deserve study in their own right so that proper allowance can be made for confounding effects in design or analysis. These problems are not insuperable given the appropriate research.

Two main types of study are needed, the first based on cohorts of asbestos workers where there is reliable information on individual estimates of past occupational exposure and the second based on the ascertainment of mesothelioma deaths in defined populations. Both approaches are heavily dependent on access to lung tissue at autopsy; control for the selective forces that operate will therefore require much thought. More extensive studies, with lung tissue analyses in cases of accidental death, where autopsies are often mandatory, could help assess bias associated with selection for autopsy in deaths from natural causes.

The primary purpose of cohort-based research is to calibrate environmental estimates of exposure more exactly in terms of intensity and fiber type. This may best be achieved by focusing both microscopic and statistical analyses on lung tissue samples that reflect documented exposure in specific work locations. Given a sufficient amount of such data, it should be possible to estimate more accurately both exposure and mesothelioma risk, even in the absence of direct observation on the cases themselves.

Systematic research on mesothelioma cases in the general population has considerable scope and potential. Ideally, such studies should include panel review of autopsy material, detailed occupational and residential histories, and comparable investigation of appropriate controls. However, these features may cause difficulty over cost and confidentiality; only the controls are essential. The main purpose of this approach is the search for causes of mesothelioma unrelated to occupational asbestos exposure; economy may therefore be achieved by excluding cases probably explained in that way. Choice of controls is not easy; while it is desirable that they should be selected from the same autopsy series, this may lead to undesirably close geographical matching. As the distribution of occupations, geological factors, and many social characteristics are all related to locality, case-control differences may be lost as a result. This problem might be overcome by selecting two controls for each case, one from the same department of pathology and one from a department of similar standing from elsewhere.

### References

1.  McDonald JC. Health implications of environmental exposure to asbestos. Environ Health Perspect 1985;62:319–28.
2.  Connelly RR, Spirtas R, Myers MH, Percy CL, Fraumeni JF. Demographic patterns for mesothelioma in the United States. J Natl Cancer Inst 1987;78:1053–59.
3.  McDonald JC, Sébastien P, McDonald AD, Case BW. Epidemiological observations on mesothelioma and their implications for non-occupational exposure. In: Davis N, ed. Mineral fibres in non-occupational environment. Vol. 90. Lyon, France: IARC, 1989:420–427.
4.  Jones RD, Smith DM, Thomas PG. Mesothelioma in Great Britain in 1968–1983. Scand J Work Environ Health 1988;14:145–52.
5.  Anderson M, Olsen JH. Trend and distribution of mesothelioma in Denmark. Br J Cancer 1985;51:699–705.
6.  Wagner JC, Sleggs CA, Marchand P. Diffuse pleural mesothelioma and asbestos exposure in the North Western Cape Province. Br J Ind Med 1960;17:260–71.
7.  Baris YI, Artvinli M, Sahin AA. Environmental mesothelioma in Turkey. Ann NY Acad Sci 1979;330:423–32.

8. McDonald JC, McDonald AD. Epidemiology of mesothelioma from estimated incidence. Prev Med 1977;6:426–46.
9. Enterline PE, Henderson VL. Geographic patterns for pleural mesothelioma deaths in the United States, 1968–81. J Natl Cancer Inst 1987;79:31–37.
10. McDonald JC, McDonald AD. Epidemiology of mesothelioma. In: Liddell DK, Miller K, eds. Mineral fibers and health. Boca Raton, FL: CRC Press, 1991:143–64.
11. McDonald AD, Fry JS, Woolley AJ, McDonald JC. Dust exposure and mortality in an American factory using chrysotile, amosite and crocidolite in mainly textile manufacture. Br J Ind Med 1983;40:368–74.
12. Peto J, Doll R, Hermon C, Binns W, Clayton R, Goffe T. Relationship of mortality to measures of environmental asbestos pollution in an asbestos textile factory. Ann Occup Hyg 1985;29:305–55.
13. McDonald AD, Fry JS, Woolley AJ, McDonald JC. Dust exposure and mortality in an American chrysotile textile plant. Br J Ind Med 1983;40:361–67.
14. Newhouse ML, Thompson H. Mesothelioma of pleura and peritoneum following exposure to asbestos in the London area. Br J Ind Med 1965;22:261–69.
15. Bohlig H, Dabbert AF, Dalquen P, Hain E, Hinz I. Epidemiology of malignant mesothelioma in Hamburg. Preliminary report. Environ Res 1970;3:365–72.
16. Jones JSP, Roberts GH, Pooley FD, Clark NJ, Smith PG, Owen WG, Wagner JC, Berry G, Pollock DJ. The pathology and mineral content of lungs in cases of mesothelioma in the United Kingdom in 1976. In: Wagner JC, ed. Biological effects of mineral fibers 2. IARC Scientific Publication 30. Lyon, France: IARC, 1980:187–99.
17. McDonald AD, McDonald JC, Pooley FD. Mineral fibre content of lung in mesothelial tumours in North America. Ann Occup Hyg 1982;26:417–22.
18. McDonald JC, Armstrong B, Doell D, McCaughey WTE, McDonald AD, Sébastien P. Mesothelioma and asbestos fiber type: evidence from lung tissue analysis. Cancer 1989;63:1544–47.
19. Seidman H, Selikoff IJ, Hammond EC. Short-term asbestos work exposure and long-term observation. Ann NY Acad Sci 1979;330:61–89.
20. Meurman LO, Kiviluoto R, Hakama M. Mortality and morbidity among the working population of anthophyllite asbestos miners in Finland. Br J Ind Med 1974;31:105–12.
21. McDonald JC, McDonald AD, Armstrong B, Sébastien P. Cohort study of mortality of vermiculite miners exposed to tremolite. Br J Ind Med 1986;43:436–44.
22. McDonald JC, Case BW, Enterline PE, Henderson V, McDonald AD,

Plourde M, Sébastien P. Lung dust analysis in the assessment of past exposure of man-made mineral fibre workers. Ann Occup Hyg 1990;34:427–41.

23. McDonald AD, McDonald JC. Malignant mesothelioma in North America. Cancer 1980;46:1650–56.

24. McDonald JC, McDonald AD. Mesothelioma: is there a background? In: Proceedings of the International Conference, Mesothelial Cell and Mesothelioma Past, Present and Future, Paris, 1991. Eur Respir Rev (in press).

25. Saccone A, Coblenz A. Endothelioma of the pleura. Am J Clin Pathol 1943;13:188–207.

26. Fraire AE, Cooper S, Greenberg SD, Buffler P, Langston C. Mesothelioma in childhood. Cancer 1988;62:838–47.

27. Peto J, Henderson BE, Pike MC. Trends in mesothelioma incidence and the forecast epidemic due to asbestos exposure during World War II. In: Peto R, Schneiderman M, eds. Quantification of occupational cancer. Banbury Report 9. Cold Spring Harbor Laboratory 1981:51–72.

28. Baris YI. Asbestos and erionite related chest diseases. Ankara, Turkey: Semih Ofset Matbaacilik, 1987:113–17.

29. Asbestos in public and commercial buildings: a literature review and synthesis of current knowledge. Cambridge MA: Health Effects Institute, 1991.

30. Gibbs GW. Etiology of pleural calcification: a study of chrysotile asbestos miners and millers. Arch Environ Health 1979;34:76–83.

31. Pooley FD. An examination of the fibrous mineral content of asbestos lung tissue from the Canadian chrysotile mining industry. Environ Res 1976;12:281–98.

32. Churg A. Analysis of lung asbestos content. Br J Ind Med 1991;48:649–52.

33. McDonald JC. Tremolite, other amphiboles and mesothelioma. Am J Ind Med 1988;14:247–49.

34. Kleinfeld M, Messite J, Zaki MH. Mortality experiences among talc workers: a follow-up study. J Occup Med 1974;16:345–49.

35. Brown DP, Dement JM, Wagoner JK. Mortality patterns among miners and millers occupationally exposed to asbestiform talc. In: Lemon R, Dement JM, eds. Dust and diseases. Park Crescent, IL: Pathotox, 1979:317–24.

36. McDonald AD, McDonald JC. Mesothelioma after crocidolite exposure during gas mask manufacture. Environ Res 1978;17:340–46.

37. Case BW, Sébastien P. Biological estimation of environmental and occupational exposure to asbestos. Ann Occup Hyg (Suppl 1) 1988;32:181–86.

38. Sébastien P, McDonald JC, McDonald AD, Case R, Harley R. Respiratory

cancer in chrysotile textile and mining industries: exposure inferences from lung analysis. Br J Ind Med 1989;46:180–87.

39. Liddell D. Epidemiological observations on mesothelioma and their implications for nonoccupational exposure to asbestos. In: Spengler JD, Ozkaynak H, McCarthy JF, Lee H, eds. Proceedings of Symposium on Health Effects of Exposure to Asbestos in Buildings, December 14–16, 1988. Cambridge, MA: Harvard University Energy and Environmental Policy Centre, 1989.

40. Newhouse ML, Berry G, Wagner JC. Mortality of factory workers in East London 1933–1980. Br J Ind Med 1985;42:4–11.

41. Jones JSP, Pooley FD, Sawle GW, Smith PG, Berry G, Wignall BK, Aggarwal A. The consequences of exposure to asbestos dust in a wartime gas-mask factory. In: Wagner JC, ed. Biological effects of mineral fibers 2. IARC Scientific Publication 30. Lyon, France: IARC, 1980:637–53.

42. Rogers AJ, Leigh J, Berry G, Ferguson DA, Mulder HB, Ackad M. Relationship between lung asbestos fiber type and concentration and relative risk of mesothelioma. Cancer 1991;67:1912–20.

# 4

# Occupational Factors of Upper Respiratory Tract Cancers

**FRANCO BERRINO**

Istituto Nazionale Tumori
Milan, Italy

## I. Introduction

The relationship between occupational exposure and the occurrence of oral, pharyngeal, and laryngeal cancer has been addressed with a variety of methodologies: hospital- and population-based case-control studies, historical perspective (retrospective cohort) studies based on the follow-up of exposed workers or on the record linkage between census occupational data and cancer registry files, proportional mortality studies, and case reports.

With the exception of southern European countries and a few developing countries, the incidence of upper aerodigestive tract cancer is relatively low with respect to lung cancer and cancer of the lower digestive organs. Table 1 shows the highest incidence rates observed in the United States, the United Kingdom, Scandinavia, and Latin-speaking European countries for tongue, oral cavity, oropharynx, nasopharynx, hypopharynx, and larynx cancer, as reported in *Cancer Incidence in Five Continents*, Volume 5 (1978–1982), by Cancer Registries [1]. Lung cancer rates are shown for comparison. The relatively low incidence of cancer for specific upper respiratory and digestive sites explains why most studies have been carried out on small groups, usually less than 100 or 200 cases. Low power is actually one of the major limits of the available

**Table 1** Age-Standardized Incidence of Upper Digestive and Respiratory Tract Cancers[a]

| Site:<br>ICD-IX: | Tongue<br>141 | Mouth<br>143–5 | Oroph.<br>146 | Nasoph.<br>147 | Hypoph.<br>148 | Larynx<br>161 | Lung<br>162 |
|---|---|---|---|---|---|---|---|
| U.S. white | 3.4 | 4.7 | 2.5 | 1.3 | 1.8 | 10.0 | 84.5 |
| U.S. black | 4.9 | 10.1 | 5.6 | 1.6 | 5.2 | 12.6 | 110.0 |
| Scandinavia | 1.3 | 1.6 | 1.1 | 1.2 | 0.7 | 5.3 | 74.2 |
| U.K. | 1.4 | 2.1 | 1.1 | 0.6 | 0.8 | 5.1 | 100.4 |
| Latin Europe | 7.9 | 13.5 | 13.9 | 1.3 | 16.5 | 17.2 | 80.5 |

*Source:* Ref. 1.
[a]Maximum world standardized rates per 100,000 men per year observed in five Western populations.

studies. In southern European countries, however, the incidence is relatively high, and larger studies are feasible.

The anatomy of the upper respiratory and digestive tract is complex for the nonspecialist. Actually, the exact definition of the borders between contiguous organs is also rather subjective among specialists, and the oncological classifications for this region are not consistent [2]. The border between the pharynx and larynx, in particular, sometimes called the epilarynx, is frequently misclassified. According to the International Classification of Disease, for instance, the anterior surface and free border of the epiglottis, as well as the "carrefour" between the epiglottic border, the ariepiglottic, and the pharyngoepiglottic fold, belong to the oropharynx (ICD 146), and the border of the ariepiglottic fold to the hypopharynx (ICD 148), but tumors originating in these sites are frequently referred to as larynx cancer (ICD 161). The term *extrinsic larynx* is still used, which sometimes refers to supraglottic lesions (ICD 161), sometimes to lesions overlapping the larynx and pharynx (which should be coded at ICD 149), and sometimes to obvious pharyngeal lesions.

Misclassification of cancer sites may be quite substantial; in northern Italy, for instance, where these tumors are very frequent, the Lombardy Cancer Registry has shown that up to one-third of deaths coded to ICD 161 were not due to laryngeal cancers but to cancers of other sites. Table 2 shows the distribution of the presumably correct cancer sites in 410 patients whose death certificates reported larynx cancer as the underlying cause of death.

Moreover, due to the small number of cases, most epidemiological studies group oral and pharyngeal cancer together, sometimes even without giving details of the specific sites that are included, even though there are reasons to think that the etiology of cancer for different anatomical subsites of this region may be substantially different. There is evidence, for example, that alcoholic beverages affect the hypopharynx and epilarynx more than the endolarynx [2].

As a whole, however, the etiology of cancer at these sites, at least in Occidental countries, is widely explained by exposure to tobacco and alcohol

**Table 2** Lombardy Cancer Registry[a]

| ICD-IX | Primary site | n | Percent |
|--------|--------------|-----|---------|
| 161 | Larynx | 279 | 68.0 |
| 148 | Hypopharynx | 59 | 14.4 |
| 146 | Oropharynx | 27 | 6.6 |
| 141 | Tongue | 8 | 2.0 |
| 162 | Lung | 8 | 2.0 |
| 150 | Oesophagus | 7 | 1.7 |
| 144 | Floor of mouth | 4 | 1.0 |
| 149 | Pharynx NOS | 4 | 1.0 |
| 145 | Oral cavity | 2 | 0.5 |
| 193 | Thyroid | 1 | 0.2 |
| 143 | Gum | 1 | 0.2 |
| 195.0 | Head and neck, NOS | 9 | 2.2 |
| | Total not larynx | 131 | 32.0 |

[a]Distribution by primary site of 410 deaths for whom death certificate underlying cause was larynx cancer.

[2]. The relative risks (RRs) of heavy drinkers and smokers is on the order of 5 and 10, respectively, and the effect of combined exposure on the RR is multiplicative [3]. Other dietary factors, such as foods rich in β-carotene, α-tocopherol, or ascorbic acid, may help in preventing these diseases [4]. Tobacco and diet may be determined by social and cultural factors, which in turn may be associated with occupational exposures. The occupational studies in which they are not taken into account are therefore difficult to interpret. One must consider, however, that with a few exceptions, such as bartenders, tobacco manufacturers, or occupations where smoking is forbidden, the association of jobs with tobacco and alcohol consumption has usually proven to be minor.

Whatever the design of the study, discovering and quantifying occupational hazards require assessment of occupational exposures among study subjects, including exposure that occurred many years before the onset of cancer. With the exception of prospective cohort studies, carrying out measurements is impossible, and workplaces usually do not retain hygiene records long enough to cover the relevant period. Most studies have therefore relied solely on proxy measures such as job title, industry, and duration of employment, thus resulting in substantial underestimation of risk. As has recently been pointed out [5]: "These crude types of assessments may be useful in surveillance systems or in hypothesis generating studies. They should rarely be used, however, in hypothesis testing."

Most case-control studies have collected lifetime occupational histories (or the occupational history after a given date) with details on industry, department, and job title, which have been variously grouped in the analysis. In addition, some investigators have used checklists covering a number of specific occupational exposures [6,7], while others have classified job titles and industries for potential exposure to specific substances [8,9]. The latter procedure, performed by industrial hygienists, is usually more rewarding than use of a checklist, as workers may be unaware of the nature of many chemicals to which they have been exposed. Burch et al. [8] and Morris Brown et al. [9], for instance, found a relationship between larynx cancer and asbestos that Ahrens et al. [6] and Zagraniski et al. [7] were not able to find using checklists. Job exposure matrices (JEMs) are being used, too, in which a panel of occupational hygienists and physicians blindly establish a judgment regarding exposure to a list of occupational titles or codes [10]. A JEM may be less costly than the approach of evaluating each job history by a specially trained team of chemists and hygienists, but their statistical power is lower [11].

A number of studies have used clever proxies to classify exposure. Ahrens et al. [6], for instance, classified as exposed to asbestos those occupations with the highest rate of compensated disease due to asbestos in Germany (rate of asbestosis, mesothelioma, and lung cancer associated with asbestosis more than 20 times above the average). With such a categorization the tobacco- and alcohol-adjusted odds ratio (OR) for asbestos was 5.7 [95% confidence limit (CL) 1.1, 28.7], while the OR based on the checklist was 1.1 (95% CL 0.5, 2.4). In a review of the relationship of asbestos and larynx cancer observed in cohort studies [12], the presence of a significant exposure has been judged on the basis of the existence of an excess of lung cancer, which is to be expected in the presence of a significant exposure to asbestos.

The two basic approaches to the analysis of case-control studies, however, remain the job-title and the JEM methodology. Two large studies on larynx cancer are summarized briefly here to illustrate these methodologies; then the occupational associations that have been published are described and discussed.

## II. IARC International Case-Control Study

In the early 1980s a large population-based incidence case-control study was carried out in six areas of southern Europe where larynx and hypopharynx cancer incidence was known to be especially high [2,13]. The major aim of the study was to clarify the role of tobacco smoking and intake of alcohol beverages, and their interaction. Information on alcoholic beverages was collected within the framework of a thorough documentation of the normal diet, the effect of which has also been analyzed. A total of 1010 incident cases were accurately described and classified according to the site of origin of the tumor (glottic, supraglottic, epilarynx, hypopharynx) and compared with 2176 controls drawn from the general population from which the cases arose. The occupational history was recorded starting from 1945. For each job lasting at least 6 months, information was collected on job title, activity of the plant, type of production, and specific tasks of the interviewee. Job titles and economic activities were coded according to the International Standard Classification of Occupations of the International Labour Office (ILO) [14], revised edition 1968, and to the four-digit International Standard Industrial Classification (ISIC) [15] of all economic activities of the United Nations. Ten percent of the questionnaires were double checked for coding accuracy. A job exposure matrix for 13 agents that are or may be related to respiratory cancer (asbestos, polycyclic aromatic hydrocarbons (PAH), chromium and compounds, nickel and compounds, arsenic and compounds, manmade mineral fibers, wood dust, leather dust, isopropyl alcohol, diethylsulfate, naphthalene, sulfuric acid, and formaldehyde) and three nonspecific exposures (dust, gas or fumes, and solvents) was applied to this data base [10]. Each ILO–ISIC combination was assessed with regard to probability and intensity of exposure to the 16 agents in three different periods, 1945–1955, 1956–1965, and 1966 onward, by a panel of industrial hygienists and occupational epidemiologists. The exposures were grouped into the following categories: (1) job-related exposure not higher than that of the general population; (2) possible cumulative exposure (job-related) slightly higher than that of the general population; (3) possible job-related exposure to levels definitely higher than that of the general population, but available information not sufficient to discriminate between exposed and unexposed; (4) job-related exposure to the specific agent; and (5) job-related exposure to the specific agent with known instances of particularly high exposure. Category 3 was further divided into three subgroups: (a) less than one-third, (b) between one-third and two-thirds, and (c) greater than two-thirds of the workers in the ILO–ISIC combinations likely to be exposed. Preliminary results are shown in Table 3, where glottic and supraglottic cancers are grouped as endolarynx, while epilarynx is included in hypopharynx. The analysis is confined to 315 cases and 819 controls aged less than 55 years at interview for which occupational history was complete. The data suggest that inhaled formaldehyde or solvents may affect the upper respiratory tract more than the digestive tract. Dusty exposures, with or without asbestos, and fumes or mists, which may contain PAH, seem to have a greater effect on the pharyngeal side of the channel. Older subjects, whose occupational history was truncated in 1945, did not show any significent association except with wood dust (data not shown).

## III. Danish Cancer Registry Linkage Study

To identify high- and low-risk groups for laryngeal cancer in Denmark, all persons aged 30 to 74 in the 1970 census were followed up over 10 years [16]. Census data, which included several sociodemographic characteristics concerning residence, dwelling, education, and occupation, were linked with the Central

**Table 3**  Associations Between Selected Occupational Exposures and Endolarynx and Hypopharynx Cancer in IARC Collaborative Case-Control Study[a]

|                        | *Endolarynx*   | *Hypopharynx*  |
|------------------------|----------------|----------------|
| Asbestos               | 1.7 (1.1–2.5)  | 2.1 (1.2–3.8)  |
| Chromium compounds     | 1.4 (0.9–2.0)  | 1.4 (0.8–2.5)  |
| Formaldehyde           | 1.7 (1.1–2.5)  | 1.4 (0.8–2.4)  |
| PAH[b]                 | 1.2 (0.7–1.9)  | 2.2 (0.9–5.2)  |
| Dust (except asbestos) | 1.5 (0.9–2.4)  | 1.9 (0.9–3.9)  |
| Gas, fumes, and vapors | 1.3 (0.8–2.0)  | 2.5 (1.1–5.6)  |
| Solvents               | 1.9 (1.3–2.8)  | 1.5 (0.9–2.5)  |

[a]Relative risks (and 95% confidence intervals) adjusted for tobacco, alcohol, social class, and dietary vitamins, for exposed (any category) versus unexposed subjects.
[b]Polycyclic aromatic hydrocarbons.

Population Register to identify persons who died or emigrated and with the Danish Cancer Registry, where over 1000 incident cases were identified that could be analyzed.

The study showed that demographic factors and broad occupational groups were strongly related to the occurrence of larynx cancer. For example, the risk for skilled workers living in Copenhagen was estimated to be five times higher than the risk for self-employed agricultural workers. This kind of study typically lacks information on the individual consumption of tobacco and alcohol, the major potential confounders. Information on the regional and sociodemographic distribution of these two factors, however, was available from other surveys. The data were sufficient to conclude that the major occupational variation in the risk of larynx cancer could not be fully explained by variations in tobacco and alcohol consumption.

To pinpoint specific high-risk occupations, the study was also analyzed for 492 occupational groups defined by the census codes for occupation and industry. Fifty-eight groups for which the observed number of cases exceeded the expected number plus one were tabulated. A number of groups, such as workers in restaurants and breweries, who may be exposed to high alcohol consumption, and workers in shipyards and the building industry, who may be exposed to asbestos, were expected to be at high risk because of exposure to known risk factors. Others, however (e.g., butchers), were not, and can be considered genuinely data generated. For other occupational groups also at high risk, such as various categories of drivers, metal workers (including smiths, mechanics, fitters, and repair shop owners), seamen, chemical workers, and to a lesser extent, perhaps, bakers, stone, clay, or glass workers, various porters, and with only four cases each, self-employed cleaners, firemen, draftsmen, and newspaper typographers, some reasonable explanations can be offered a posteriori but were not explicitly hypothesized.

Observational studies such as the Danish record linkage study serve to generate hypotheses about etiology. The authors therefore did not perform any statistical tests on the aforementioned specific occupational groups. The value of this kind of generating hypothesis study has just been revealed by analysis of the IARC multicentric case-control study. After careful control for alcohol, tobacco, and social class, it has been confirmed, for instance, that butchers, clay workers, and blacksmiths have a significantly high risk [13].

## IV. Occupational Associations

### Asbestos

Asbestos exposure has fairly consistently been found associated with larynx cancer. As reviewed by Smith et al. [12], in prospective studies a clear excess of larynx cancer was almost invariably present whenever the level of exposure was sufficiently high to increase the risk of lung cancer. Case-control studies are usually positive, too, with the exception of a few studies with a poor categorization of exposure. A very high relative risk (RR) value observed in the first published case-control study [crude RR = 14.5; 95% confidence interval (CI) 5 to 39) [17] was not confirmed in subsequent studies, most of which provided RR estimates of between 1.5 and 2 [12]. Several studies that did not explicitly classify the subjects in terms of asbestos exposure have provided evidence of high risk in asbestos-related occupations, such as boilermakers [9], plumbers and pipefitters [8,9], asbestos cement production workers [18], in port services, marine transportation, and the shipyard industry [6,9,13,19,20], railroad workers [13,21], and in a number of occupations where asbestos exposure may be only minimal, such as welders [22] and other metal workers [6,8,20,21,23], masons and other construction workers [13,20,21,23–25], automobile mechanics [21], and drivers [9,18,21,24,26].

Nevertheless, the relationship between asbestos and larynx cancer remains a highly controversial issue. According to Liddell [27], "the evidence on the link between exposure to asbestos and laryngeal cancer definitely fails to satisfy the criteria for causation set by Bradford Hill." According to Edelman [28], "neither case control nor cohort studies have established an increased risk of laryngeal cancer for asbestos workers." According to Chan and Gee [29], "the available epidemiological evidence does not support a causal association." The main reasons for these contrary views are the following: (1) most studies do not reach statistical significance (as one would expect from small studies with major sources of misclassification of both the exposure and the outcome), (2) observed RR values are mutually inconsistent (as one would expect from studies with different definitions and different levels of exposure), and (3) tobacco and alcohol have not always been taken into account (but in several cases have, and whenever they have, the association persisted [8,9,18, and the IARC study]. Better studies would certainly be welcomed, but one cannot reject a repeatedly observed association on the basis of low power and low-quality negative studies.

One should be prepared to acknowledge that the observed relationship between asbestos exposure and larynx cancer is one of the soundest results that can be achieved when occupational epidemiology is based on retrospective assessment of exposure. Those who are not prepared to do so need go no further in reading this chapter, as no sounder risk factor is going to be considered.

As for pharynx cancer, in the IARC study the relationship of asbestos with hypopharynx was higher than that with larynx (Table 3). On the contrary, no relationship with asbestos was elicited in a study on oral or oropharyngeal cancer carried out in northern Italy and analyzed with the same JEM as that developed for the international IARC study (RR = 1.1) [30]. There was, however, a significant relationship with work in the construction industry (RR = 2.5; 95% CI 1.3 to 4.5), mainly plumbers, pipefitters, and electrical workers. The study did not provide separate analyses of oral and oropharyngeal cancer because of the small numbers (74 and 12 cases, respectively). A high risk of oro- or hypo-pharyngeal cancer for a number of jobs in the construction industry has also been reported, after proper adjustment for tobacco and alcohol, by Vaughan [31], especially for carpenters and painters, and by Haguenoer et al. [20], especially for jobs involving heavy dust exposure, such as masonry, tile laying, and plastering. In conclusion, it seems that working in the construction industry entails a high risk of pharyngeal cancer, but it is not clear whether it depends on specific jobs of on the general environment. A high risk for carpenters in the construction industry and for motor vehicle operators has also been reported for nasopharynx cancer [31].

### Beryllium; Bis(chloromethyl)Ether

Suspected because of their role in lung cancer, a nonsignificant positive association with larynx cancer has been found in a small hospital-based case-control study in which exposure was sought with the aid of a checklist of substances [7].

### Chromium Compounds

Recognized as causing lung cancer, the role of chromium compounds in larynx cancerogenesis has been under investigation in three population based case-control studies which failed to provide convincing evidence [9,18,52]. Exposure was defined by grouping occupations possibly exposed; in the Morris Brown et al. study [9] a significant association was present only when potential exposures to both chromium and paint were considered, but paint may indicate exposure to other substances, too, such as solvents and asbestos. Merletti et al. [30] did not find any relationship with cancer of the oral cavity or oropharynx.

### Diethylsulfate

*See Sulfuric Acid.*

### Dust

Occupations involving dust (of whatever type) have been found associated with larynx cancer in several case-control studies [7,18,52]. Dust is unlikely to be carcinogenic per se; it might just be an indicator of an unclean environment (i.e., of a higher exposure to any other carcinogenic substance that may be present in the workplace), but it might also enhance the effect of other substances. No relationship has been found with oral or oropharyngeal cancer [30].

### Formaldehyde

The carcinogenicity of formaldehyde for the upper respiratory tract is well established in rodents but is conflicting for humans. Blair et al. [32] have reported the mortality experience of 26,561 workers (600,000 person-years) of the 10 largest U.S. plants producing or using formaldehyde. Six deaths from nasopharyngeal cancer among exposed workers were observed versus two expected based on population death rates. A nonsignificant excess for larynx (12 observed vs. 8 expected) and oropharynx (5 observed vs. 2.6 expected), but not for hypopharynx cancer (1 observed vs. 1.7 expected) was also observed. Exposure levels were estimated for each job title using work environment monitoring data for recent years and discussing previous plant operations with experienced personnel. None of the upper respiratory tract cancers, however, showed any clear relationship with intensity or cumulative exposure.

In a population-based study where formaldehyde exposure was assessed by application of a JEM, Vaughan et al. [33] did not find any significant association with nasopharyngeal cancer (27 cases), nor with oropharyngeal or hypopharyngeal cancer (205 cases); however, slightly elevated RR values were associated with the highest exposure score categories and a significant association was present between residential exposure and nasopharyngeal carcinoma [34]. In the IARC study the association was statistically significant for the endolarynx but not for the epilarynx-hypopharynx (Table 3). A JEM-based positive relationship (RR = 1.8 for probable or definitive exposure, not statistically significant) was also found by Merletti et al. [30] for oral or oropharyngeal cancer. Excess mortality from larynx cancer has been reported for barbers and hairdressers

[13,35,36]; this finding created the suspicion that hair dyes could be carcinogenic, but hairdressers are also exposed to formaldehyde.

### Gasoline and Diesel Fuel

Borderline significant associations with larynx cancer have been reported by Ahrens et al. [6] and Morris Brown et al. [9]. In most studies drivers have been found to be high risk (see "Asbestos").

### Hair Dyes

*See Formaldehyde.*

### Isopropylic Alcohol Manufacture

*See Sulfuric Acid.*

### Man-made Mineral Fibers

The follow-up on 22,000 workers, producing rock, slag, or glass wool in 13 European factories [37] showed a 64% increase in the incidence of buccal cavity and pharynx cancer (ICD 140 to 149): 28 observed vs. 17.0 expected [standardized mortality rate (SMR) = 164; CI 109 to 238], but not of larynx cancer. However, the excess was not consistent across factories. A significant association with hypopharynx cancer, greater than for endolarynx, is also present in the IARC international case-control study. One should remember, however, that in code-based JEM the distinction between asbestos and man-made mineral fibers may be very difficult because the latter has progressively been substituted for asbestos in many occupations; in this case a specific checklist might be more specific.

### Mineral Oil

A positive nonsignificant association of mineral oil with larynx cancer was reported by Ahrens et al. [6] and Wynder et al. [24] (oil and grease), but no association was found by Morris Brown et al. [9] (oil and grease) and Zagraniski et al. [7] (cutting oils). In an incident series reported from northern Italy [38], lathe operators, who are exposed to cutting oils, were more frequent victims of larynx cancer than in the general census data.

### Mustard Gas

A definite increased risk for mustard gas producers was reported by Wada et al. [39] and Manning et al. [40].

### Nickel

Five cases of larynx cancer (vs. 1.3 expected), together with a clear excess of nasal and lung cancer, were observed in a Norwegian factory where Canadian nickel ore was roasted, smelted, and refined [41]. However, no association with larynx cancer was observed in a population-based case-control study carried out in Ontario, where there are large nickel mining and processing industries (tobacco-adjusted RR = 1.0, based on 23 exposed cases) [8]. Grouping potential exposures to nickel compounds (alloys, battery, plastic production), a Danish population-based case-control study elicited a tobacco-adjusted RR value of 1.7 (95% CI 1.2 to 2.5) [22], but no relationship was found in the JEM-based IARC study or in a checklist-based analysis of a hospital case-control study carried out in Connecticut (7). No association was detected with oral or oropharyngeal cancer [30].

### Polycyclic Aromatic Hydrocarbons

Many jobs in the metal and transportation industries, in heating facilities, and in maintenance work, which have repeatedly been found associated with upper digestive and respiratory tract cancer (see "Asbestos"), may involve exposure to polycyclic aromatic hydrocarbons (PAHs). Most workers exposed to asbestos are actually exposed to PAHs, too. The IARC JEM attempted to group all potential sources of PAH exposure to study these cancer sites (Table 3). A significant excess risk following at least 10 years of probable or certain PAH exposure was observed for hypopharyngeal cancer only. When a 20-year induction period was taken into account, the RR value was 3.3 (95% CI 1.2 to 8.7). No effect was discovered when the same matrix was applied to oral cancer [30].

### Solvents

In the IARC study the JEM analysis showed a significant relationship with endolarynx cancer but not with hypopharynx cancer (Table 3). A nonsignificant excess of 1.3 (95% CI 0.7 to 2.5), based on self-reported exposure, has been reported by Ahrens et al. [6] for larynx cancer; no excess was found by Merletti et al. [30], based on JEM, for buccal or oropharyngeal cancer. Solvent exposure might actually be the reason why a number of studies have reported elevated risks for painters [9,23] and metal workers (see "Asbestos").

### Sulfuric Acid

Weil et al. [42] reported an excess of nasal and vocal cord cancers among workers who used the strong sulfuric acid process in isopropyl alcohol production. Strong sulfuric acid was also implicated in a study of ethanol production workers [43].

As recently reviewed by Soskolne et al. [44], diethylsulfate was then suspected as the carcinogen in the strong acid process, but subsequently, an excess of upper respiratory cancers was reported among workers exposed to a variety of processes using sulfuric acid in a petroleum and chemical plant [45], metal pickling [46,47], and in washing soap production [48]. It was then suggested that sulfuric acid itself could be responsible, but one may easily hypothesize that the inhalation of any acidic pollutant would increase the risk. The association seems too strong to be explained by life-style cofounders: Soskolne et al. [45] actually controlled for tobacco and alcohol with a case-control design nested within the cohort without detecting any significant confounding effect on the estimated RR value, which ranged from over 4 when all upper respiratory cancers were considered, to 13 (95% CI 2 to 86) when the analysis was confined to the larynx.

The relationship with sulfuric acid seems difficult to capture in case-control studies, possibly because of the poor validity of retrospective categorization of exposure [9,18,52]; however, a significant association has been reported by Cookfair et al. [49]. Sulfuric acid is one of the most widely used chemicals, and its use might explain why several studies have observed an excess of larynx cancer in the chemical [16,36] and leather industries [50], sulfuric acid being common in both.

### Wood Dust

Wynder et al. [24], reported a significant association of larynx cancer with wood dust among nonsmokers or long-term exsmokers (4 of 18 cases (22%), compared with 1.2% among hospital controls) but not among smokers. After adjusting for tobacco and alcohol use, Olsen and Sabroe [18] and Bonassi et al. [19] found nonsignificant RR values, of 1.4 and 1.5, repectively; the latter authors, however, warned that most of the woodworkers also had exposure to glues, lacquers, varnishes, and dyes, which showed a RR value of 1.4. A higher than expected risk has also been reported (inconsistently) for the lumber industry [21,51] and for woodworkers [7]. The IARC study showed a higher risk for both laryngeal and hypopharyngeal cancer only among subjects older than 55 years at diagnosis.

### Other Factors

A number of occupational groups that have been found repeatedly to be at high risk of upper digestive or respiratory tract cancer are not easily classified in the specific exposure categories above. Drivers and other road transportation workers, vehicle mechanics, other mechanics, welders, precision metal workers, machine tool operators, other machinists, and painters, for instance, may be exposed to a number of the specific substances above, mostly in low doses, such as asbestos, polycyclic aromatic hydrocarbons, and other toxic substances in fuel vapors and exhaust, or metal dust, solvents, cutting oils, and formaldehyde, but one cannot exclude that other relevant factors may be part of the cause.

Textile workers have repeatedly been found associated with both larynx and pharynx cancer. Actually, since the associaton was first reported in the 1930s (Kennaway, 1936, quoted in [52]) for textile spinners, a complex pattern of positive and negative studies has been reported, reviewed in ref. 52, the analysis of which is beyond the scope of the present work. Textile workers may be exposed to formaldehyde, solvents, dyes, oil mists, acid mists and, obviously, to textile dust. A small minority may also be exposed to asbestos, but the information available does not make it possible to disentangle which, if any, of these substances may be responsible for the effects observed. A more in-depth analysis of specific tasks for cases and controls should be carried out than that which has been possible to date.

### References

1. Muir C, Waterhouse J, Mack T, Powell J, Whelan S. Cancer incidence in five continents. Vol. 5. IARC Scientific Publication 88. Lyon, France: IARC, 1987.

2. Tuyns AJ, Estève J, Raymond L, Berrino F, Benhamou E, Blanchet F, Boffetta P, Crosignani P, Del Moral A, Lehmann W, Merletti F, Pequignot G, Riboli E, Sancho Garnier H, Terracini B, Zubiri A, Zubiri L. Cancer of the larynx/hypopharynx, tobacco and alcohol: IARC international case-control study in Turin and Varese (Italy), Zaragoza and Navarra (Spain), Geneva (Switzerland) and Calvados (France). Int J Cancer 1988;41:483–91.

3. Estève J, Tuyns AJ. Models for combined action of tobacco and alcohol on risk of cancer. In: Feo F, Pani P, Columbano A, eds. Chemical carcinogenesis. New York: Plenum Press, 1988: 649–55.

4. Estève J, Pequignot G, Riboli E, Merletti F, Crosignani P, Ascunce N, Zubiri L, Raymond L, Repetto F, Tuyns AJ. Cancer of the larynx/hypopharynx and diet: an IARC international case-control study in South Western Europe. 1992 (submitted for publication).

5. Stewart PA, Herrick RF, Blair A, Checkoway H, Droz P, Fine L, Fischer L, Harris R, Kauppinen T, Saracci R. Highlights of the 1990 Leesburg, Virginia, international workshop on retrospective exposure assessment for occupational epidemiology studies. Scand J Work Environ Health 1991;17:281–85.

6. Ahrens W, Jockel KH, Patzak W, Elsner G. Alcohol, smoking and occupational factors in cancer of the larynx: a case-control study. Am J Ind Med 1991;20:477–93.

7.  Zagraniski RT, Kelsey JL, Walter SD. Occupational risk factors for laryngeal carcinoma: Connecticut, 1975–1980. Am J Epidemiol 1986;124:67–76.

8.  Burch JD, Howe GR, Miller AB, Semenciw R. Tobacco, asbestos, and nickel in the etiology of cancer of the larynx: a case-control study. J Natl Cancer Inst 1981;67:1219–24.

9.  Morris Brown LM, Mason TJ, Pickle LW, Stewart PA, Buffler PA, Burau K, Ziegler RG, Fraumeni JF. Occupational risk factors for laryngeal cancer on the Texas Gulf Coast. Caner Res 1988;48:1960–64.

10. Ferrario F, Continenza D, Pisani P, Magnani C, Merletti F, Berrino F. Description of a job-exposure matrix for sixteen agents which are or may be related to respiratory cancer. In: Hogstedt C, Reuterwall C, eds. Progress in occupational epidemiology. Amsterdam: Excerpta Medica, 1988:379–82.

11. Dewar R, Siemiatycki J, Gerin M. Loss of statistical power associated with the use of a job-exposure matrix in occupational case-control studies. Appl Occup Environ Hyg 1991;6:508–15.

12. Smith AH, Handley MA, Wood R. Epidemiological evidence indicates asbestos causes laryngeal cancer. J Occup Med 1990;32:499–507.

13. Berrino F, Boffetta P, Estève J, Merletti F, Pisani P, Raymond L, Tuyns A. Larynx cancer and occupation: preliminary results from the IARC multicentric case control study. 9th International Symposium on Epidemiology in Occupational Health. Cincinnati, OH: NIOSH, 1992.

14. Classification internationale type des professions, ed. rev. Geneva: International Labour Office. 1968.

15. Index de la classification internationale type par industrie, de toutes les branches d'activité économique. New York: United Nations, 1975.

16. Guenel P, Engholm G, Lynge E. Laryngeal cancer in Denmark: a nationwide longitudinal study based on register linkage data. Br J Ind Med 1990;47:473–79.

17. Stell PM, McGill T. Asbestos and laryngeal carcinoma. Lancet 1973;2:416–17.

18. Olsen J, Sabroe S. Occupational causes of laryngeal cancer. J Epidemiol Community Health 1984;38:117–21.

19. Bonassi S, Ceppi M, Puntoni R, Valeria F, Vercelli M, Belli S, Biocca M, Comba P, Ticchiarelli L, Mariotti F, Taddeo D, Zuccherelli D, Casalini A, Perini C, Nelli L, Sansoni G, Pupp N, Farina M, Luciani A. Mortality studies of dockyard workers (longshoremen) in Italy. Am J Ind Med 1985;7:219–27.

20. Haguenoer JM, Cordier S, Morel C, Lefebvre JL, Hemon D. Occupational risk factors for upper respiratory tract and upper digestive tract cancers. Br J Ind Med 1990;47:380–83.

21. Flanders WD, Rothman KJ. Occupational risk for laryngeal cancer. Am J Public Health 1982;72:369–72.
22. Olsen J, Sabroe S, Lajer M. Welding and cancer of the larynx: a case-control study. Eur J Clin Oncol 1984;20:639–43.
23. Coggon D, Pannett B, Osmond C, Acheson ED. A survey of cancer and occupation in young and middle aged men. I. Cancers of the respiratory tract. Br J Cancer 1986;43:332–38.
24. Wynder EL, Covey LS, Mabuchi K, Mushinski M. Environmental factors in cancer of the larynx. A second look. Cancer 1976;38:1591–1601.
25. Williams RR, Stegens NL, Goldsmith JR. Associations of cancer site and type with occupation and industry from the Third National Cancer Survey interview. J Natl Cancer Inst 1977;59:1147–85.
26. Flanders WD, Cann CI, Rothman KJ, Fried MP. Original contributions work-related risk factors for laryngeal cancer. Am J Epidemiol 1984;119:23–32.
27. Liddell FDK. Laryngeal cancer and asbestos (editorial). Br J Ind Med 1990;47:289–91.
28. Edelman DA. Laryngeal cancer and occupational exposure to asbestos. Int Arch Environ Health 1989;61:223–27.
29. Chan CK, Gee BL. Asbestos exposure and laryngeal cancer: an analysis of the epidemiologic evidence. J Occup Med 1988;30:23–27.
30. Merletti F, Boffetta P, Ferro G, Pisani P, Terracini B. Occupation and cancer of the oral cavity or oropharynx in Turin, Italy. Scan J Work Environ Health 1991;17:248–54.
31. Vaughan TL. Occupation and squamous cell cancers of the pharynx and sinonasal cavity. Am J Ind Med 1989;16:493–510.
32. Blair A, Stewart P, O'Berg M, Gaffey W, Walrath J, Ward J, Bales R, Kaplan S, Cubit D. Mortality among industrial workers exposed to formaldehyde. J Natl Cancer Inst 1986;76:1071–84.
33. Vaughan TL, Strader C, Davis S, Dling JR. Formaldehyde and cancers of the pharynx, sinus and nasal cavity. I. occupational exposures. Int J Cancer 1986;38:677–83.
34. Vaughan TL, Strader C, Davis S, Daling JR. Formaldehyde and cancer of the pharynx, sinus and nasal cavity. II. Residential exposures. Int J Cancer 1986;38:685–88.
35. Alderson M. Cancer mortality in male hairdressers. J Epidemiol Community Health, 1980;34:182–85.
36. Viadana E, Bross I, Houten L. Cancer experience of men exposed to inhalation of chemicals or to combustion products. J Occup Med 1976;18:787–92.
37. Simonato L, Fletcher AC, Cherrie J, Andersen A, Bertazzi PA, Charnay N, Claude J, Dodgson J, Esteve J, Frentzel-Beyme R, Gardner MJ, Jensen

OM, Olsen JH, Saracci R, Teppo L, Winkelmann R, Westlerholm P, Winter PD, Zocchetti C. The man-made mineral fiber European historical cohort study. Scand J Work Environ Health 1986;12(Suppl 1):34–47.

38. Assi A, Turolla E, Berrino F. Epidemiologia del carcinoma laringeo nell'Alto Milanese. Epidemiol Prev. 1977;2:43–50.

39. Wada S, Mujanishi M, Nashimoto Y, et al. Mustard gas as a cause of respiratory neoplasia in man. Lancet 1968;1:1161–63.

40. Manning KP, Skegg DCG, Stell PM, Doll R. Cancer of the larynx and other occupational hazards of mustard gas workers. Clin Otolaryngol 1981;6:165–67.

41. Pedersen E, Hogetveit AC, Andersen A. Cancer of the respiratory organs among workers at a nickel refinery in Norway. Int J Cancer 1973;12:32–41.

42. Weil CS, Smith HF, Nale TW. Quest for a suspected industrial carcinogen. Arch Ind Hyg 1952;5:535–47.

43. Lynch J, Hanis NM, Bird MG, Murray KJ, Walsh JP. An association of upper respiratory cancer with exposure to dietyl sulfate. J Occup Med 1979;21:333–41.

44. Soskolne CL, Pagano G, Cipollaro M, Beaumont J, Giordano GG. Epidemiologic and toxicologic evidence for chronic health effects and the underlying biologic mechanisms involved in sub-lethal exposures to acidic pollutants. Arch Environ Health 1989;44:180–91.

45. Soskolne CL, Zeighami EA, Hanis MN, Kupper LL, Herrmann N, Amsel J, Mausner JS, Stellman JM. Laryngeal cancer and occupational exposure to sulfuric acid. Am J Epidemiol 1984;120:358–69.

46. Ahlborg G, Hogstedt C, Sundell L, Aman G. Laryngeal cancer and pickling house vapors. Scand J Work Environ Health 1981;7:239–40.

47. Steenland K, Schnorr T, Beaumont J, Halperin W, Bloom T. Incidence of laryngeal cancer and exposure to acid mists. Br J Ind Med 1988;45:766–76.

48. Forastiere F, Valesini S, Salimei E, Magliola ME, Perucci CA. Respiratory cancer among soap production workers. Scand J Work Environ Health 1987;13:258–60.

49. Cookfair DL, Wende KE, Michalek AM, Vena JE. A case-control study of laryngeal cancer among workers exposed to sulfuric acid (abstract). Am J Epidemiol 1985;122:521.

50. Decouflé P. Cancer risks associated with employment in the leather and leather products industry. Arch Environ Health 1979;34:33–37.

51. Elwood JM, Pearson JCG, Skippen DH. Alcohol, smoking, social and occupational factors in the etiology of cancer of the oral cavity, pharynx and larynx. Int J Cancer 1984;34:603–12.

52. Exposures in the textile manufacturing industry. IARC monographs on the evaluation of the carcinogenic risk of chemicals to humans. Vol. 48. Lyon, France: IARC, 1990.

# 5

# Occupational Factors of Sinonasal Cancers

**ANNETTE LECLERC and DANIÈLE LUCE**

INSERM U88
Paris, France

## I. Sinonasal Cancers: General Aspects

This chapter deals with cancers of the nasal cavity and paranasal sinuses, also called sinonasal cancers (SNCs). The corresponding codes in the ninth revision of the International Classification of Diseases are 160.0, nasal cavity; 160.2, maxillary sinus; 160.3, ethmoidal sinus; 160.4 to 160.9, other and unspecified. Nasopharyngeal cancers (ICD-9 147) are not studied in this chapter. Skin cancers of the external nose are also excluded.

Sinonasal cancers are rare diseases. The annual incidence rate adjusted for age and sex ranges from 0.3 to 1 case per 100,000 subjects in most countries [1,2]. The male/female ratio is about 2:1. Incidence is higher in several East Asian countries than in North America or Europe. This rare cancer has often been associated with occupational exposure. Roush [3] suggested that the percentage of SNC attributable to occupational agents might approach 50% in some regions. The relationship between sinonasal cancer and occupational risk factors varies according to histological type. The most frequent type is squamous cell carcinoma. Adenocarcinomas are the second largest group in many studies, at least among men. Other histologic types are less frequent. It is worth noting that insofar as reliable data on histological types are available, the percentages of cases with adenocarcinomas and squamous cell carcinomas differ according to country. These differences may be related to differences in occupational risk factors. No major risk factor of nonoccupational origin is widely recognized, although tobacco consumption has been found to be related to SNC in several studies [4–7].

Due to the rarity of the disease, most epidemiologic results are provided by case-control studies. The number of cases in a cohort study is generally too small to be informative, except in cohorts of woodworkers, who present a high risk of SNC. The tables in this chapter show data for the main occupational exposures (woodwork, leather and textile dust, formaldehyde). Data presented include the country of the study, the period of diagnosis of the cases, and values of relative risks (RRs). For simplicity, we used the term *relative risk* whether the measurement of association was the odds ratio (for case-control study), the standardized incidence ratio (SIR) or standardized proportional incidence ratio (SPIR), or a proportional mortality ratio. Significantly elevated RR values are indicated with an asterisk. The term *no association* is used in the table when the authors concluded that there was no excess, or when the relative risk was not significant and less than 2.

## II.  Woodwork

### A.  Epidemiologic Results

The clinical observation that nasal cancer was particularly frequent among woodworkers was recorded as early as 1923 [8]. The first epidemiologic approach was from Acheson, based on observations from Macbeth in the region of High Wycombe in the United Kingdom, where chair making had been the main industry for many years [9,10]. Around 1970, similar observations on the association between nasal sinus tumors and the furniture industry were made in Belgium and the Netherlands [11]. This association was not observed during the same period in Canada [12]. Several other studies have been published on the relationship between nasal cancer (especially adenocarcinoma) and occupational exposure in the furniture industry [11]. Other wood exposures were less well documented, at least until 1980 [13].

A summary of selected results from epidemiologic studies published after 1980 is presented in Tables 1 and 2. The studies are classified according to the exposure variable. Most often, the analysis was made using the job title, or branch of activity. Details regarding the type of wood (hardwood, softwood) were sometimes given, especially in more recent papers. In some studies results were given separately for adenocarcinomas and squamous cell carcinomas, which is useful since some occupational factors are specific to one histologic type.

As can be seen in Table 1, all the studies on the association with the furniture industry and cabinetmaking show that the association is specific to adenocarcinomas. The intensity of the relationship varies according to country. Very high values of relative risk were observed in case-control studies in European countries: 140 in the Netherlands [14], 90 in Italy [15], and 35 in France [16]. Record linkage studies in the United Kingdom, Denmark, and Sweden provide figures for SIR or SPIR comparable to the relative risk, but based on less precise data concerning the occupation and histologic type [17–19]. In a cohort study of 8141 furniture workers in Sweden, the risk of adenocarcinoma was multiplied by 44 among those workers (compared to the general population). No excess was observed for squamous cell carcinoma [20].

The figures observed in North America contrast with these high values. Brinton found a relative risk of 5.7 for adenocarcinoma in North Carolina [5]. This relatively low value was observed in a region that accounts for approximately one-third of the total U.S. population engaged in furniture manufacturing. Other studies from Canada and the United States show similar results [21–24].

The situation in East Asia is particular in that the association between the furniture industry and nasal cancer has not always been observed [7,25,26]. Ng (Hong Kong) and Takasaka (Japan) found no association with the furniture industry. It is worth noting that in these studies the percentages of adenocarcinomas was very low (less than 7%). Fukuda (Japan) found a relatively low but significant relative risk (2.9) for woodworkers (not only furniture workers) in a study limited to squamous cell cancer of the maxillary sinus.

The situation of carpenters and joiners is less clear than that of cabinetmakers. This occupational group was not considered at risk in the United Kingdom [17]. On the other hand, in the Netherlands and France their situation was similar to that of cabinetmakers, although the risk of adenocarcinoma was lower [14,16]. This could not be explained by the fact that some of them had also worked as cabinetmakers. Woodworking machine operators also presented an elevated risk in the United Kingdom [17], United States [27], and France [16]. The association was not limited to one histologic type. Elwood showed a significant excess of sinonasal cancer of all histologic types for wood exposure in general, in a Canadian region where jobs involving wood are found mainly in the forestry industry and in sawmills [6]. Another Canadian study indicated an excess of mortality from sinonasal cancer among loggers but not among other woodworkers [22]. Similar results were observed in the United States [23]. No excess risk was observed for sawmill workers in Sweden [19] or for loggers in France [16].

Part of the differences between countries could be due to the type of wood. Hardwood (e.g., beech, oak) is used more often in Europe, especially in the southern countries. For that reason some studies focused on the type of wood (Table 2). Specific associations between hardwood (or "hardwood and mixed

**Table 1** Sinonasal Cancer and Wood Dust Exposure According to Job Titles

| Exposure | Country | Author | Ref. | Type of study | Period | Results | | |
|---|---|---|---|---|---|---|---|---|
| | | | | | | Sinonasal cancer in general | Adenocarcinoma | Squamous cell carcinomas |
| Furniture industry, cabinetmaker | Netherlands | Hayes | [14] | Case-control: 91 male cases, 195 controls | 1978–81 | RR = 12.5[a] | RR = 140[a] | No association |
| | Italy | Battista | [15] | Case-control: 36 male cases, 164 controls | 1963–81 | RR = 4.7[a] | RR = 90[a] | b |
| | France | Luce | [16] | Case-control: 207 cases, 409 controls | 1986–88 | b | Males: RR = 35[a] | No association |
| | U.K. | Acheson | [17] | National record linkage (incidence); 1602 cases; analysis by occupation limited to men (925) | 1963–67 | RR = 6.2[a] (chair maker) RR = 9.7[a] (cabinetmaker) | c | No association |
| | Denmark | Olsen | [18] | Record linkage (incidence): 382 cases | 1970–84 | Males: RR = 3.6[a,d] | b | b |
| | Sweden | Malker | [19] | National record linkage (incidence):770 cases | 1961–79 | Males: RR = 4.1[a] | Males: RR = 17[a] | No association |
| | Sweden | Gerhardsson | [20] | Cohort study (incidence): 8141 furniture workers | 1960–79 | RR = 7.1[a] | RR = 44[a] | No association |
| | U.S. | Viren | [23] | Mortality case-control study: 322 male cases, 664 controls | 1962–77 | No association(e) | b | b |
| | U.S. | Brinton | [5] | Case-control: 160 cases, 290 controls | 1970–80 | No association | Males: RR = 5.7[a] | No association |
| | Hong Kong | Ng | [25] | Case-control: 225 cases, controls: 224 nasopharyngeal cancer, 226 other malignancies | 1974–81 | No association | b | b |
| | Japan | Takasaka | [26] | Case-control: 107 male cases, 413 controls | 1971–82 | No association | b | b |

| Occupation | Country | Author [ref] | Study | Years | Result 1 | Result 2 | Result 3 |
|---|---|---|---|---|---|---|---|
| Carpenters, joiners | U.K. | Acheson [17] | National record linkage: 925 male cases | 1963–67 | No association | c | No association |
| | Netherlands | Hayes [14] | Case-control: 91 male cases, 195 controls | 1978–81 | RR = 2.1 | RR = 16.3[a] | No association |
| | France | Luce [16] | Case-control: 207 cases, 409 controls | 1986–88 | b | Males: RR = 25[a] | No association |
| Woodworking machine operators | U.K. | Acheson [17] | National record linkage: 925 male cases | 1963–67 | RR = 2.9[a] | No association | No association |
| | U.S. | Vaughan [27] | Case-control: 27 cases, 552 controls | 1979–83 | b | b | RR = 7.5[a] |
| | France | Luce [16] | Case-control: 207 cases, 409 controls | 1986–88 | b | Males: RR = 7.4[a] | No association |
| Sawmill industry | Sweden | Malker [19] | National record linkage (incidence): 770 cases | 1961–79 | No association | No association | RR = 2.9 |
| Loggers | France | Luce [16] | Case-control: 207 cases, 409 controls | 1986–88 | b | No association | b |
| | Canada | Gallagher [22] | Proportionate mortality study: 5457 loggers | 1950–78 | RR = 3.6[a,d] | b | b |
| | U.S. | Viren [23] | Mortality case-control study: 322 male cases, 664 controls | 1962–77 | RR = 3[a,e] | b | b |
| Loggers, carpenters | Canada | Elwood [6] | Case-control: 121 male cases, 120 controls | 1939–77 | RR = 2.5[a] | Increased risk | Increased risk |
| Wood related occupation, other than furniture making, joinery, and carpentry | Netherlands | Hayes [14] | Case-control: 91 male cases, 195 controls | 1978–81 | No association | No association | No association |

a RR significantly higher than 1.
b Information not available.
c Significant excess in male woodworkers.
d Based on proportional ratios.
e Based on occupation on the death certificate.

**Table 2**  Sinonasal Cancer and Wood Dust Exposure According to Kind of Wood

| | | | | | | Results | | |
| | | | | | | Sinonasal cancer in general | Adenocarcinoma | Squamous cell carcinomas |
| Exposure | Country | Author | Ref. | Type of study | Period | | | |
|---|---|---|---|---|---|---|---|---|
| Hardwood + softwood | Denmark, Finland, Sweden | Hernberg | [28] | Case-control: 167 cases, 167 controls | 1977–80 | RR = 12.0[a] | Significant association | Positive association, nonsignificant |
| Hardwood dust | Denmark, Finland, Sweden | Hernberg | [28] | Case-control: 167 cases, 167 controls | 1977–80 | RR = 2 | Positive association nonsignificant | No association |
| | France | Martinez-Cortés | [29] | Case-control: 207 cases, 409 controls | 1986–88 | [b] | RR = 168[a] | No association |
| Softwood dust | Denmark, Finland, Sweden | Hernberg | [28] | Case-control: 167 cases, 167 controls | 1977–80 | RR = 3.3[a] | No association | RR = 2.5 |
| | France | Martinez-Cortés | [29] | Case-control: 207 cases, 409 controls | 1986–88 | [b] | [b] | Elevated risk only for beginning of exposure before 1946 |
| Predominantly softwood dust | Canada | Elwood | [6] | Case-control: 121 male cases | 1939–77 | RR = 2.5[a] | Association for both histologic types | Association for both histologic types |
| | U.S. | Vaughan | [30] | Case-control: 27 squamous cell cases, 552 controls | 1979–83 | [b] | [b] | RR = 3.1[a]: restricted to exposure 15 or more years before diagnosis |

[a]RR significantly higher than 1.
[b]Information not available.

wood") and adenocarcinoma have been observed in Scandinavian countries [28] and France [29]. Exposure to softwood might increase the risk of squamous cell carcinoma, with a long interval between first exposure and the occurrence of cancer [27–32]. Elwood is the only author who noticed an excess of adenocarcinoma among workers exposed mainly to softwood. However, in his study there was no individual assessment of exposure. Moreover, possibility of misclassification of histologic type is probably greater with retrospective information on histologic type, as in this study (with some cases diagnosed as early as 1939).

### B. Factors Related to the Occurrence of Sinonasal Cancer in Woodworkers; Causal Explanations

The excess of sinonasal cancer was observed predominantly among furniture-makers. The association with woodworking in the furniture industry appears to be specific to adenocarcinoma. However, recent studies indicated that woodworkers outside the furniture industry presented a slight excess of sinonasal cancer and that wood exposure (hard and soft wood) also increased the risk of squamous cell carcinoma.

The mean latency period for adenocarcinomas (time between first exposure to wood dust and diagnosis) is about 40 years [13]. It is similar for squamous cell carcinomas. It is widely accepted that the causal agent in wood exposure is wood itself. The main argument in favor of this hypothesis is that the risk has remained high over time, even in countries in which various additional exposures have existed in different periods especially in the furniture industry (glues, varnishes, lacquers, and paints) [13,33].

Differences according to the job performed or the type of wood (hard or soft) might be related to the size of wood particles. Small particles produced in cabinetmaking and from hardwood might more harmful [34]. Some differences between countries might be due to differences in systems for removing wood dust from the workplace. In small shops and factories in Europe, the level of exposure is probably higher than in large factories, which are predominant in the United States [21].

The mechanisms by which wood may cause sinonasal cancer are not clear. However, prolonged inhalation of wood dust by furniture workers has been shown to impair mucociliary clearance and lead to squamous metaplasia [3,33,35]. Small particles of wood dust reach nasal sinuses. They contain various biologically active substances, one or several of which could be carcinogenic. Such substances include flavonols, other phenolic compounds, and many terpenoids, some of which probably exert a protective function on timber by acting as natural insecticides and fungicides [33]. In addition to constituents of wood dust, other substances are produced, due to the high temperatures of some machine operations, such as sanding. Hardell suggested that chlorophenol exposure, frequent among woodworkers, could increase the risk due to wood dust alone [36].

## III.  Leather Work

Table 3 gives results from different studies on leather exposure (leather dust or surrogate for leather dust exposure, such as footwear industry, or shoemakers). An excess of nasal cancer among leather workers has been observed in the United Kingdom [17,37], Denmark [18], and Italy [38–40]. The most striking results were from Merler, with a clear dose–effect relationship between the level of exposure to leather dust and the relative risk of adenocarcinoma. The excess was observed mainly for adenocarcinomas, although Merler also indicated an elevated risk for squamous cell carcinomas. The latency period for adenocarcinoma to develop was comparable to that observed for woodworkers [38].

Other studies in the Netherlands [14], the United States [5], Japan [26], and France [16] did not confirm these results. This does not necessarily imply that there is no risk. Because leather exposure is rare in many regions, only small numbers of exposed cases and controls are observed. This limits the statistical power of the studies. Another explanation could be that the risk may decrease over time in some occupational environments, since the number of studies showing an excess risk was relatively high before 1981 [11]. This appears to be consistent with comments from both Merler and Cecchi, who stressed that cases were heavily exposed to leather dust in poor working conditions.

As in the wood industry, no definite carcinogenic agent has been identified in the leather industry, although solvents, dyes, chromate salts, and tannic acid used in leather tanning have been suspected by various authors. These hypotheses are supported by the observation of an excess of SNC among workers exposed to chromates in the manufacture of chromates and to chromate products in other industrial branches [5]. However, leather dust itself might be the causal agent. In one of the Italian studies, the author stressed that the major occupational risk did not concern the tannery but rather, boot and shoes factories and the use of leather milling machines [40]. Pippard also concluded that the increased risk of nasal cancer was largely confined to workers employed in the finishing department [37].

## IV.  Textile Work

Positive associations between textile work and nasal cancer have been found in the United States [41], United Kingdom [17], Sweden [19], Italy [42], France [16], and Hong Kong [24] (Table 4). In some studies the excess was limited to women, which might be due to a higher frequency of exposure among women.

**Table 3** Sinonasal Cancer and Leather Work

| Exposure | Country | Author | Ref. | Type of study | Period | Results | | |
|---|---|---|---|---|---|---|---|---|
| | | | | | | Sinonasal cancer in general | Adenocarcinoma | Squamous cell carcinomas |
| Leather dust | Italy | Merler | [39] | Case-control: 21 cases, 39 controls | 1968–82 | RR = 15.7[a] | Clear dose-effect relation: RR = 41[a] | b |
| Exposure to leather | U.S. | Brinton | [5] | Case-control: 160 cases, 290 controls | 1970–80 | No association | b | b |
| Leather industry | Netherlands | Hayes | [14] | Case-control: 91 male cases, 195 controls | 1978–81 | No association | No association | No association |
| | Sweden | Malker | [19] | National record linkage (incidence): 770 cases | 1961–79 | No association | No association | No association |
| | Italy | Loi | [40] | Case-control: 38 male cases, 186 controls | 1972–83 | RR = 8.1[a] | Significant excess | No association |
| Shoe and leather workers | France | Luce | [16] | Case-control: 207 cases, 409 controls | 1986–88 | b | No association | RR = 2.12 |
| Leather workers | U.K. | Acheson | [17] | National record linkage (incidence): 925 male cases | 1963–67 | RR = 4.36[a] | RR = 3.2[a] | No association |
| | Japan | Takasaka | [26] | Case-control: 107 male cases, 413 controls | 1971–82 | No association | b | b |
| Manufacture of leather products including footwear | Denmark | Olsen | [18] | Record linkage (incidence): 382 cases | 1970–84 | Males: RR = 12.3[a,c] | b | b |
| Shoemaker | Italy | Cecchi | [38] | Case-control: 11 cases of adenocarcinoma, 22 controls | 1963–77 | b | Significant excess | b |
| Boot and shoe makers | U.K. | Pippard | [37] | Cohort study (mortality): 5017 men | 1939–82 | RR = 5.3[a] | b | b |

[a]RR significantly higher than 1.
[b]Information not available.
[c]Based on proportional ratios.

**Table 4** Sinonasal Cancer and Textile Work

| Exposure | Country | Author | Ref. | Type of study | Period | Results | | |
|---|---|---|---|---|---|---|---|---|
| | | | | | | Sinonasal cancer in general | Adenocarcinoma | Squamous cell carcinomas |
| Textile or clothing industry | U.S. | Brinton | [41] | Case-control: 160 cases, 290 controls | 1970–80 | RR = 0.8 (males), RR = 2.1[a] (females) | RR = 2.5 (males), RR = 2.5 (females) | RR = 0.7 (males), RR = 2.2 (females)[b] |
| | Italy | Bimbi | [42] | Case-control: 53 cases, 217 controls | 1982–85 | RR = 2.9[a] | No exposed adenocarcinomas | |
| Textile and clothing workers | U.K. | Acheson | [17] | National record linkage (incidence): 1602 cases | 1963–67 | RR = 2.1[a] for male clothing workers; no excess among male textile workers | Excess among females for textile (RR = 2.2) and clothing workers (RR = 2.5), no association among males | No association |
| | France | Luce | [16] | Case-control: 207 cases, 409 controls | 1986–88 | [b] | RR = 4 (females), no association (males) | RR = 9.5[a] (females), no association (males) |
| Textile workers | Sweden | Malker | [19] | National record linkage (incidence): 770 cases | 1961–79 | RR = 2.4[a] (males) | RR = 2.3 (males) | RR = 1.4 (males), RR = 3 (females)[b] |
| | Hong Kong | Ng | [25] | Case-control: 225 cases | 1974–81 | RR = 3.5[a] (males), RR = 2.1[a] (females) | [b] | |

[a]RR significantly higher than 1.
[b]Information not available.

Cases were seen among tailors and dressmakers (self-employed and employees) and workers in the textile industry. The small number of cases and controls did not permit a detailed analysis. In a study from Tola (Finland), leisure-time knitting and sewing was significantly more common among the female cases, with a relative risk of 4.9 [43].

Excess risk was not limited to one histologic type. Some authors noticed a higher risk among persons employed for more than 15 years [25] and among those with heavy dust exposure [41]. Brinton noticed in several studies, including her own, that a large proportion of cases were exposed to cotton. The findings of a study performed in an Italian region where the wool industry is predominant indicated that there was no relationship with SNC [44]. Concerning the causal agents, Ng suggested that exposures specific to secondary processes that produce treated textile fibers from raw fibers could possibly increase the risk due to heavy exposure to textile dust [25]. It has been suggested that exposure to formaldehyde in the textile industry might increase the risk of nasal cancer. However, in her study Brinton noticed that few individuals reported such exposure. Instead, the excess risk seemed more closely related to occupations with significant exposure to dust [5].

## V. Formaldehyde

Formaldehyde is a widely used chemical, well known for acute toxic effects. During the past years, some controversy has arisen over a possible carcinogenic effect, subsequent to studies in which rats and mice exposed to formaldehyde developed squamous cell carcinomas of the nasal passages [45–47]. The first epidemiologic studies were cohort studies focused on professional groups with a high level of exposure, such as embalmers and anatomists. Other cohort studies have been performed in industrial environments, and focused mainly on chemical workers. A review of these studies was presented by Blair et al. [48]. The observed and expected number were summed up to create combined relative risk estimates. The value of the combined relative risk for industrial workers was 1.1 for nasal cavity. Only one death from nasal cancer occurred among the professionals, the number of expected deaths being less than 1.

Due to the rarity of sinonasal cancer (the number of observed cases does not exceed 2 in any study), cohort studies are not suitable for detecting an excess. More recent studies (Table 5) have been case-control studies, using approaches of varying sophistication for assessing occupational exposure to formaldehyde among cases and controls. The exposure assessment was generally done by an expert, since formaldehyde exposure is not specific to a limited list of occupations. The expert relied only on job titles or on a detailed questionnaire on job history.

**Table 5**  Sinonasal Cancer and Formaldehyde Study Results

| Country | Author | Refs. | Type of study | Period | Nasal cancer in general | Adenocarcinoma | Squamous cell carcinomas |
|---|---|---|---|---|---|---|---|
| U.S. | Roush | [50] | Case-control: 198 cases, 605 controls | 1935–75 | No association | b | b |
|  | Vaughan | [49] | Case-control: 53 cases, 552 controls | 1979–83 | No association | b | b |
| Denmark | Olsen | [51,52] | Case-control: 525 cases 2465 controls | 1970–82 | RR = 1.6: adjusted on wood exposure (men only) | RR and 95% confidence limits adjusted on wood exposure (men only) 2.2 (0.7;7.2) | 2.3 (0.9;5.8) |
| Netherlands[c] | Hayes | [53] | Case-control: 91 male cases, 195 controls | 1978–81 | No exposure to wood dust, or low level of exposure RR = 2.5[a] (expert A), RR = 1.6 (expert B) Moderate or high level of exposure to wood dust RR = 1.9 (expert A), could not be studied (expert B) | Could not be studied   No association | RR = 3[a] (expert A), RR = 1.9[a] (expert B) Could not be studied |
| France | Luce | [54] | Case-control: 207 cases 409 controls | 1986–88 | b | among males exposed to medium or high levels of wood dust, significantly elevated RR for highest exposure categories of formaldehyde | no association |

[a] RR significantly higher than 1.
[b] Information not available.
[c] Two independent assessment of exposure (experts A and B).

The results from four case-control studies were published in 1986 and 1987. Vaughan et al. [49] and Roush et al. [50] found no excess of nasal cancer. In a Danish study, Olsen et al. showed an elevated but not significant excess among males for both adenocarcinomas and squamous cell carcinoma [51,52]. The analysis took into account wood exposure, often associated with formaldehyde exposure. The increased risk of 2.3 for squamous cell carcinoma was based on 13 cases exposed to formaldehyde, of which only four were unexposed to wood dust. Only one case of adenocarcinoma was exposed to formaldehyde and unexposed to wood.

Hayes et al. [53] found a significant association for squamous cell carcinoma among the subgroup of cases and controls with low levels of wood dust exposure. No such relationship was found for the adenocarcinomas, which could only be examined in the moderate-to-high wood dust exposure group. Luce et al. did not confirm these results for squamous cell carcinoma. For adenocarcinoma it was not possible to study the relationship with formaldehyde independently from wood exposure (only one case exposed to formaldehyde and unexposed to wood). However, among those exposed to medium or high levels of wood dust, significantly elevated RR were found for highest exposure categories of formaldehyde.

## VI.  Other Occupational Exposures

### A.  Nickel and Chromium

Nickel refining has been strongly correlated with sinonasal cancer mainly in the United Kingdom [55], Norway, and Canada [56,57]. Tumors were most often squamous carcinomas. In the United Kingdom the excess risk occurred in workers first employed before 1930. The main studies on nickel refining and sinonasal cancer were discussed by Doll et al. [58]. According to this review, the risk of SNC decreased with a more recent date of first employment, most certainly due to a drastic decrease in exposure levels. It was not clear whether a specific nickel compound was the carcinogenic agent, and the opinion of Doll et al. was that it might be nickel itself, whether present in the working environment in sulfide, oxide, metallic, or soluble compounds.

Animal experiments have shown that various nickel compounds may produce sarcomas at the site of injection [3]. However, manufacturing with nickel has not been shown to carry an excess risk, as indicated by Roush et al. [59] and Grandjean et al. [60]. Hernberg studied nickel and chromium exposure arising from occupations such as welding, in which exposures are often mixed (nickel + chromium) [28]. He found a significant excess for the category "welding, flame cutting, and soldering" and for chromium. Exposure to nickel showed an excess that nearly reached statistical significance at the 5% level. Other authors did not confirm these results. However, Grandjean concludes that exposure levels for all nickel and inorganic nickel compounds should be kept as low as reasonably achievable [60]. An excess of sinonasal cancer was found in a cohort of chromate production workers (4 observed deaths, 0.26 expected) [61].

### B.  Basic Metal Industry

A Danish national study showed that the risk of sinonasal cancer was significantly increased in the basic metal industry, both in the manufacture of primary iron and steel products and in the manufacture of nonferrous metal products [18]. However, these results were not confirmed by other authors.

### C.  Mining

Acheson et al. [17] found an excess of cases among miners and other workers exposed to coal and coke dust. The author did not exclude the possibility of bias due to the recording of the occupation. However, this association was confirmed by other authors [16,42].

### D.  Agricultural Work, Food Industry

Excesses of sinonasal cancer in agricultural work have been found by several authors [25,26,42]. The excess of cases was limited to squamous cell carcinoma. However, no definite conclusion could be reached about the significance of the results. Grain and hay dust might be causal agents. However, Hernberg found no excess of sinonasal cancer due to these substances.

Olsen found an excess among employees of both sexes in cocoa, chocolate, and sugar confectionery, and among females employees in canning and preserving fruits and vegetables and in farming [18]. He suggested the possibility of a common cause. Excess risks among bakers and pastry cooks were reported by Acheson et al. [17] and Luce et al. [16].

### E.  Other Occupational Exposure

An association between sinonasal cancer and the manufacture of mustard gas was found in a group of Japanese workers exposed before and during World War II [62]. However, the number of cases was small. In a cohort study in the United Kingdom, the risk of sinonasal cancer among workers of a manufacture of mustard gas was slightly elevated but not significant [57]. The manufacture of isopropyloil was associated with sinonasal cancer in several studies [63,64]. Other occupational agents have been linked to sinonasal cancer, including chemical and petroleum manufacturing and asbestos [3,5].

## VII. Current and Future Research Aspects

Most particularities of present and future research on sinonasal cancer are shared by research on occupational cancer in general. The quality of data for the retrospective evaluation of exposure is a crucial point for which much progress has been made. More emphasis is put on substances (not only on occupations). It is also increasingly frequent to use precise data on exposure, such as intensity and duration of exposure. Data are increasingly collected in a comparable manner, thus allowing comparable analysis.

Since sinonasal cancer is a rare disease, collaborative studies or common reanalysis of collected data are especially useful. In-depth comparisons between studies may also give some clues to the apparent discrepancies between countries. The use of more precise data on the type and intensity of exposure could lead to a better understanding of the reasons for differences between studies or between countries. For example, differences in the role of leather dust might be due to different levels of exposure; textile dust might have different effects according to the level of exposure and the type of textile (mainly wool or cotton). In any event, future studies will take into account the histologic type of cancer, since the role of some occupations is specific to one histologic type. Some remaining questions, such as the role of wood for squamous cell carcinomas, are limited to one histologic type.

Very strong associations exist between wood dust exposure and adenocarcinoma. It would be possible to model the probability of the occurrence of the disease in relation to the intensity, type, and duration of exposure. This would help identify which workers in the wood industry should benefit from special surveillance and which decisions might be more effective in preventing the disease. It would also help decisions to made regarding compensation.

We did not include in this chapter studies on the natural history of the disease (relations between noncancerous lesions and cancer) or relationships between exposure and noncancerous lesions. A better understanding of these relationships through prospective studies would be useful for better prevention of sinonasal cancer through early detection of histopathological changes in the nasal mucosa, or other abnormalities.

## References

1.  Muir C. Cancer incidence in five continents. IARC Scientific Publication 88. Lyon, France: IARC, 1987.
2.  Muir CS, Nectoux J. Descriptive epidemiology of malignant neoplasms of nose, nasal cavities, middle ear and accessory sinuses. Clin Otolaryngol 1980;5:195–211.

3. Roush G. Epidemiology of cancer of the nose and paranasal sinuses: current concepts. Head Neck Surg 1979;2:3–11.
4. Hayes RB, Kardaun JWPF, De Bruyn A. Tobacco use and sinonasal cancer: a case-control study. Br J Cancer 1987;56:843–46.
5. Brinton LA, Blot WJ, Becker JA, Winn DM, Browder JP, Farmer JC, Fraumeni JF. A case-control study of cancers of the nasal cavity and paranasal sinuses. Am J Epidemiol 1984;119:896–906.
6. Elwood JM. Wood exposure and smoking: association with cancer of the nasal cavity and paranasal sinuses in British Columbia. Can Med Assoc J 1981;124:1573–77.
7. Fukuda K, Shibata A, Harada K. Squamous cell cancer of the maxillary sinus in Hokkaido, Japan: a case-control study. Br J Ind Med 1987;44:263–66.
8. Moure EJ, Portmann G. Adénocarcinomes de l'ethmoïde. Rev Laryngol 1923;44:177–79.
9. Acheson ED, Cowdell RH, Hadfield E, Macbeth RG. Nasal cancer in woodworkers in the furniture industry. Br Med J 1968;2:587–96.
10. Macbeth R. Malignant disease of the paranasal sinuses. J Laryngol 1965;79:592–612.
11. IARC monograph on the evaluation of the carcinogenic risk of chemicals to humans. Vol. 25. Wood, leather and some associated industries. Lyon, France: IARC, 1981.
12. Ball MJ. Nasal cancer in woodworkers. Br Med J 1968;ii:253.
13. Mohtashamipur E, Norpoth K, Luhmann F. Cancer epidemiology of woodworking. J Cancer Res Clin Oncol 1989;115:503–15.
14. Hayes RB, Gerin M, Raatgever JW, de Bruyn A. Wood-related occupations, wood dust exposure, and sinonasal cancer. Am J Epidemiol 1986;124:569–77.
15. Battista G, Cavallucci F, Comba P, Quercia A, Vindigni C, Sartorelli E. A case-referent study on nasal cancer and exposure to wood dust in the province of Siena, Italy. Scand J Work Environ Health 1983;9:25–29.
16. Luce D, Leclerc A, Morcet JF, Casal-Lareo A, Gérin M, Brugère J, Haguenoer J, Goldberg M. Occupational risk factors for sinonasal cancer: a case-control study in France. Am J Ind Med 1992;21:163–75.
17. Acheson ED, Cowdell RH, Rang EH. Nasal cancer in England and Wales: an occupational survey. Br J Ind Med 1981;38:218–24.
18. Olsen JH. Occupational risks of sinonasal cancer in Denmark. Br J Ind Med 1988;45:329-35.
19. Malker HSR, McLaughlin JK, Blott WJ, Weiner JA, Malker BK, Ericcson JLE, Stone BJ. Nasal cancer and occupation in Sweden, 1961-1979. Am J Ind Med 1986;9:477-85.

20. Gerhardsson MR, Norell SE, Kiviranta HJ, Ahlbom A. Respiratory cancers in furniture workers. Br J Ind Med 1985;42:403–5.
21. Imbus HR, Dyson WL. A review of nasal cancer in furniture manufacturing and woodworking in North Carolina, the United States, and other countries. J Occup Med 1987;29(9):734-40.
22. Gallagher RP, Threlfall WJ, Band PR, Spinelli JJ. Cancer mortality experience of woodworkers, loggers, fishermen, farmers and miners in British Columbia. National Cancer Institute Monograph 69, Epidemiology and Cancer Registries IV. 1984.
23. Viren JR, Imbus HR. Case-control study on nasal cancer in workers employed in wood-related industries. J Occup Med 1989;31(1):35-40.
24. Finkelstein MM. Nasal cancer among North American woodworkers: another look. J Occup Med 1989;31:899–901.
25. Ng TP. A case-referent study of cancer of the nasal cavity and sinuses in Hong Kong. Int J Epidemiol 1986;15:171–75.
26. Takasaka T, Kawamoto K, Nakamura K. A case-control study of nasal cancers. An occupational survey. Acta Otolaryngol Suppl (Stockh) 1987;435:136-42.
27. Vaughan TL. Occupation and squamous cell cancers of the pharynx and sinonasal cavity. Am J Ind Med 1989;16:493–510.
28. Hernberg S, Westerholm P, Schultz-Larsen K, Degerth R, Kuosma E, Englund A, Engzell U, Hansen HS, Mutanen P. Nasal and sinonasal cancer connection with occupational exposures in Denmark, Finland and Sweden. Scand J Work Environ Health 1983;9:315–26.
29. Martinez-Cortés M. Exposition professionnelle au bois et cancer des cavités naso-sinusiennes: résultats d'une étude cas-témoin. Unpublished report. Paris: INSERM U88, 1990.
30. Vaughan TL, Davis S. Wood dust exposure and squamous cell cancers of the upper respiratory tract. Am J Epidem 1991;133(6):560-64.
31. Voss R, Stenersen T, Oppedal BR, Boysen M. Sinonasal cancer and exposure to soft wood. Acta Otolaryngol 1985;99:172–78.
32. Bolm-Audorff V, Vogel C, Woitowitz HJ. Occupation and smoking as risk factors in nasal and naso-pharyngeal cancer. In: Sakurai H, et al., eds. Occupational epidemiology. New York: Elsevier Science Publishers, 1990:71-74.
33. Acheson ED, Winter PD, Hadfield E, Macbeth RG. Is nasal adenocarcinoma in the Buckinghamshire furniture industry declining? Nature 1982;299:263-65.
34. Wills JH. Nasal carcinoma in woodworkers: a review. J Occup Med 1982;24(7):526-30.
35. Goldsmith DF, Shy CM. Respiratory health effects from occupational exposure to wood dusts. Scand J Work Environ Health 1988;14:1-15.

36.  Hardell L, Johansson BO, Axelson O. Epidemiologic study of nasal and nasopharyngeal cancer and their relation to phenoxy acid or chlorophenol exposure. Am J Ind Med 1982;3:247–57.
37.  Pippard EC, Acheson ED. The mortality of boot and shoe makers, with special reference to cancer. Scand J Work Environ Health 1985;11:249–55.
38.  Cecchi F, Buiatti E, Kriebel D, Nastasi L, Santucci M. Adenocarcinoma of the nose and paranasal sinuses in shoemakers and woodworkers in the province of Florence, Italy (1963–77). Br J Ind Med 1980;37:222–25.
39.  Merler E, Baldasseroni A, Laria R, Faravelli P, Agostini R, Pisa R, Berrino F. On the causal association between exposure to leather dust and nasal cancer: further evidence from a case-control study. Br J Ind Med 1986;43:91–95.
40.  Loi AM, Amram DL, Bramanti L, Roselli MG, Giacomini G, Simi U, Belli S, Comba P. Nasal cancer and exposure to wood and leather dust. A case-control study in Pisa area. J Exp Clin Cancer Res 1989;8(1):13–19.
41.  Brinton L, Blot WJ, Fraumeni JF. Nasal cancer in the textile and clothing industries. Br J Ind Med 1985;42:469–74.
42.  Bimbi G, Battista G, Belli S, Berrino F, Comba P. Stùdio caso contròllo sui tumóri nasali e le esposiziòni professionali. Med Lav 1988;79(4):280–87.
43.  Tola S, Hernberg S, Collan Y, Linderborg H, Korkala ML. A case-control study of the etiology of nasal cancer in Finland. Int Arch Occup Environ Health 1980;46:79–85.
44.  Magnani C, Comba P, Ferraris F, Ivaldi C, Meneghin M, Terracini B. A case-control study of carcinomas of the nose and paranasal sinuses in the woolen textile manufacturing industry. Archives of Env. Health, 1993 (in press)
45.  Albert RE, Sellakumar AR, Laskin S, Kuschner M, Nelson N, Snyder CA. Gaseous formaldehyde and hydrogen chloride induction of nasal cancer in the rat. J Natl Cancer Inst 1982;68:597–603.
46.  Swenberg JA, Kerns WD, Mitchell RI, Gralla EJ, Pavkov KL. Induction of squamous cell carcinomas of the rat nasal cavity by inhalation exposure to formaldehyde vapor. Cancer Res 1980;40:3398–3402.
47.  Kerns WD, Pavkov KL, Donofrio DJ, Gralla EJ, Swenberg JA. Carcinogenicity of formaldehyde in rats and mice after long-term inhalation exposure. Cancer Res 1983;43:4382–92.
48.  Blair A, Saracci R, Steward PA, Hayes RB, Shy C. Epidemiologic evidence of the relationship between formaldehyde exposure and cancer. Scand J Work Environ Health 1990;16:381–93.
49.  Vaughan TL, Strader C, Davis S, Daling JR. Formaldehyde and cancers of the pharynx, sinus and nasal cavity. I. Occupational exposure. Int J Cancer 1986;38:677–83.

50.  Roush GC, Walrath J, Stayner LT, Kaplan SA, Flannery JT, Blair A. Nasopharyngeal cancer, sinonasal cancer and occupations related to formaldehyde: a case-control study. J Natl Cancer Inst 1987;79(6):1221–24.

51.  Olsen JH, Asnaes S. Formaldehyde and the risk of squamous cell carcinoma of the sinonasal cavities. Br J Ind Med 1986;43:769–74.

52.  Olsen JH, Jensen SP, Hink M, Faurbo K, Breum N, Jensen OM. Occupational formaldehyde exposure and increased nasal cancer risk in man. Int J Cancer 1984;34:639–44.

53.  Hayes RB, Raatgever JW, de Bruyn A, Gerin M. Cancer of the nasal cavity and paranasal sinuses and formaldehyde exposure. Int J Cancer 1986;37:487–92.

54.  Luce D, Gerin M, Leclerc A, Morcet JF, Brugere J, Goldberg M. Sinonasal cancer and occupational exposure to formaldehyde and other substances. Int J Cancer 1993;53:1–8.

55.  Doll R, Mathews JD, Morgan LG. Cancers of the lung and nasal sinuses in nickel workers: a reassessment of the period of risk. Br J Ind Med 1977;34:102.

56.  Sunderman FW. A review of the carcinogenicities of nickel, chromium and arsenic compound in man and animals. Prev Med 1976;5:279.

57.  Easton DF, Peto J, Doll R. Cancers of the respiratory tract in mustard gas workers. Br J Ind Med 1988;45(10):652–59.

58.  Doll R, Andersen A, Cooper WC, et al. Report of the international committee on nickel carcinogenesis in man. Scand J Work Environ Health 1990;16(15):1–82.

59.  Roush GC, Meigs JW, Kelly J, Flannery JT, Burdo H. Sinonasal cancer and occupation: a case-control study. Am J Epidemiol 1980;111:183–93.

60.  Grandjean P, Andersen O, Nielsen GD. Carcinogenicity of occupational nickel exposures: an evaluation of the epidemiological evidence. Am J Ind Med 1988;13:193–209.

61.  Davies JM, Easton DF, Birdstrup PL. Mortality from respiratory cancer and other causes in United Kingdom chromate production workers. Br J Ind Med 1991;48:299–313.

62.  Wada S, Miyanishi M, Nishimoto Y, Kambe S, Miller RW. Mustard gas as a cause of neoplasia in man. Lancet 1968;1:1161–63.

63.  IARC monograph on the evaluation of the carcinogenic risk of chemicals to humans. Vol. 15. Lyon, France: IARC, 1977.

64.  Alderson MR, Rattan NS. Mortality of workers in an isopropyl alcohol plant and two MEX dewaxing plants. Br J Ind Med 1980;37:85–89.

# 6

## Occupational Asthma

JEAN-LUC MALO

Sacre-Coeur Hospital
and University of Montreal
Montreal, Quebec, Canada

## I. Introduction

Definitions can vary according to the purpose for which they are intended [1]. Epidemiological definitions will tend to be less rigid than medical or medicolegal definitions. For medical or medicolegal purposes, occupational asthma is generally defined as "reversible airways narrowing causally related to exposure in the working environment to airborne dusts, gases, vapours, or fumes" [2]. The causal relationship between exposure to an occupational agent and the onset of the disease therefore has to be proven. There are now at least 200 different agents that can cause occupational asthma [3,4]. The agents are usually classified as high- and low-molecular-weight agents, the threshold between the two classes being 1000 Da [5]. The mechanism of high-molecular-weight agents is usually IgE-mediated as with common inhalants, whereas the mechanism of asthma due to low-molecular-weight agents is generally unknown. High-molecular-weight agents generally cause immediate or dual asthmatic reactions during bronchial challenges, whereas low-molecular-weight agents more often induce late asthmatic reactions. The most frequent cause is isocyanates or polyurethanes, representing approximately 25% of cases [6,7].

Occupational asthma is now the most common occupational respiratory condition. In a national U.S. survey of 6000 respondents, Blanc found that nearly 8% identified asthma as a medical condition they suffered from and that 15% of those with asthma attributed it to the workplace [8]. Medicolegal data show that it is the most commonly reported condition, outnumbering standard pneumoconiosis (silicosis and asbestosis) [7]. Physician-based surveys have been implemented in several U.S. states [9] and in Great Britain [6,10]. In Great Britain, 554 cases were identified in 1989, making it the leading cause (26%) of occupational respiratory ailments.

The medical diagnosis of occupational asthma should be based on objective testing. A medical questionnaire is a sensitive tool, but it is not specific. It is our opinion that a history of exposure to a sensitizer previously shown to cause occupational asthma or of a work-related increase in asthma symptoms, alone or in combination with the presence of specific antibodies, or of asthma or bronchial hyperresponsiveness is insufficient to confirm a diagnosis of occupational asthma. This is based on several sources of data. In our experience, based on the prospective assessment of 162 subjects referred for possible occupational asthma on whom objective assessment (specific inhalation challenges, monitoring of PEFR and $PC_{20}$) was performed, an open questionnaire administered by chest physicians specializing in occupational asthma did not have a sufficient positive or negative predictive value to be used as a diagnostic tool. The presence or absence of typical symptoms such as improvement at weekends or during vacations was not a satisfactory index for the presence of occupational asthma [11]. Furthermore, the chest physician's impression after administering an open questionnaire did not have a sufficient predictive value either. Immunological sensitization does not mean that the subject has occupational asthma. The presence of specific antibodies is generally too sensitive in the case of an IgE-mediated condition [12]. For isocyanates, the presence or absence of specific IgG antibodies is neither sensitive nor specific enough for making a diagnosis of occupational asthma [13]. Assessing bronchial responsiveness to pharmacological agents at work or away from work merely demonstrates that a worker has bronchial responsiveness; it in no way proves that he or she has asthma or occupational asthma. However, knowing that there are changes in bronchial responsiveness between periods at work and away from work may be useful in some instances. Finally, the combination of an immediate skin reaction to an allergen and increased bronchial responsiveness does not necessarily prove that the subject will develop an asthmatic reaction when exposed to the agent. A close relationship was found for common inhalant allergens [14,15] but we have seen subjects who had skin reactivity to psyllium or guar gum and bronchial hyperresponsiveness in whom we were unable to cause significant bronchial obstruction after exposure to the specific agent [16,17].

Monitoring PEFR at work and away from work, alone or combined with assessment of nonspecific bronchial hyperresponsiveness, is an interesting tool and may be sensitive and specific enough to confirm occupational asthma [18,19]. But specific inhalation challenges are essential for confirming or excluding the diagnosis of occupational asthma and properly advising employee and employer. For these reasons we feel that the diagnosis should be based on an objective assessment, preferably specific inhalation challenges, in a laboratory if the occupational sensitizer has been identified or at work if the sensitizer is either unknown or there is more than one. These tests should be performed by specialists in centers designed for that purpose. As Burge put it, 'bronchial provocation tests are the final arbiter to prove the specific cause of occupational asthma" [20].

## II.  Natural History

Occupational asthma is a satisfactory model for asthma, from both pathophysiological and epidemiological points of view. The pathophysiology of occupational asthma due to high-molecular-weight agents can be equated to asthma due to common inhalants. Both conditions are IgE mediated. Using bronchoalveolar lavage and bronchial biopsy is now possible through fiber-optic bronchoscopy. The inflammatory reaction due to low-molecular-weight agents (plicatic acid, isocyanates) has also been described [21,22]. The model of occupational asthma can further our understanding of asthma as assessed in epidemiological and clinical studies. The natural history of occupational asthma can be illustrated as in Figure 1. This figure shows the time course of occupational asthma from onset of exposure to removal from exposure as well as its persistence.

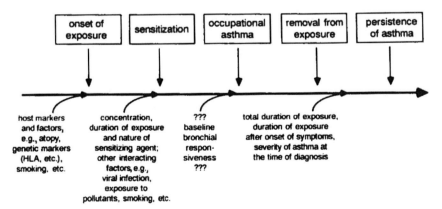

**Figure 1**  Scheme illustrating the chronological stages (in squares) of the behavior of occupational asthma before and after removal from the causal agent. The possible contributing factors at each stage are listed under the line.

### A. Host Markers and Factors Before Exposure

Atopy is a well-known predisposing factor in asthma and occupational asthma due to high-molecular-weight agents. There is an association between the presence of sensitization and occupational asthma due to high-molecular-weight agents such as detergent enzymes [23], laboratory animal–derived antigens [24], psyllium [12], guar gum [16] and snow crab [25]. However, based on the predictive values, the association is not strong. As shown in Table 1, only one-third of atopic subjects exposed to laboratory animals developed symptoms of asthma on exposure to the agent [24]. General population surveys have identified an association between smoking and total IgE production [26,27].

Smoking is not a predisposing factor in occupational asthma due to plicatic acid, the active agent in western red cedar [28] but it is a risk factor (mean relative risk of 5) in subjects exposed to platinum salts [29]. Its effect is controversial in the case of high-molecular-weight agents [30]. A higher prevalence of skin reactivity to the detergent enzyme derived from *Bacillus subtilis* was found in smokers than in nonsmokers [31]. More cases of occupational asthma due to snow crab were found among smokers than in nonsmokers [25]. Higher serum IgE antibodies were found among pharmaceutical company and coffee roastery workers who smoked than in nonsmokers [32]. However, a higher risk of developing increased specific IgE antibodies could not be demonstrated in recent surveys of nurses exposed to psyllium [17] and in carpet producers exposed to guar gum [16].

### B. Concentration, Duration, and Nature of Exposure

Anecdotal reports have suggested an association between spills of isocyanates and the likelihood of developing asthma symptoms [33]. It is doubtful, however, that these episodes could be considered as occupational asthma or reactive airways disease syndrome (RADS), a syndrome characterized by persistent asthma in subjects exposed on one or more occasions to high concentrations of an irritant [34] that has been described specifically after exposure to isocyanates [35]. Some association has been found between the concentration of exposure to colophony [36], western red cedar [37], and flour [38], on the one hand, and the presence of symptoms on exposure to the causal agent, on the other. However, this information was derived from cross-sectional studies that might be affected by the healthy survival bias. This bias can be of considerable significance in occupational asthma, as symptoms can be sufficiently troublesome or even life threatening as to force subjects to leave work. The nature of the occupational agent can also play some role in the rate of development of symptoms, as shown in Figure 2. Retrospective evidence shows that more subjects exposed to western red cedar and isocyanates develop work-related symptoms in the first two years of exposure as compared with subjects exposed to high-molecular-weight agents

**Table 1** Value of Atopy Assessed by Different Means in Predicting Asthma or Rhinitis in Laboratory Animal Workers

| | Asthma | | | Rhinitis | | | No asthma: |
|---|---|---|---|---|---|---|---|
| | *Sensitivity* | *Specificity* | *Positive predictive value* | *Sensitivity* | *Specificity* | *Positive predictive value* | *negative predictive value* |
| Personal history | 50 | 79 | 23 | 27 | 77 | 26 | 71 |
| Family history | 44 | 65 | 13 | 39 | 65 | 25 | 69 |
| Skin prick tests | 80 | 82 | 34 | 24 | 76 | 23 | 75 |

*Source:* Ref. 24.

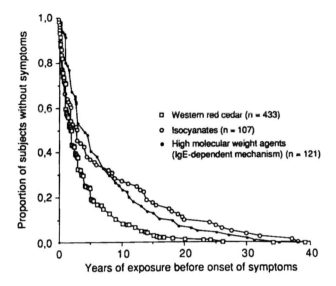

**Figure 2**   Survival analysis showing the proportion of subjects without symptoms as a function of years of exposure before onset of symptoms. Subjects exposed to western red cedar and isocyanates develop symptoms more rapidly in the first year after exposure, but the curve for isocyanates gradually joins the curve for high-molecular weight agents. All curves significantly different by log rank analysis.

(J.L. Malo and M. Chan-Yeung, work in progress). However, after five years of exposure, the rate for developing symptoms is similar for high-molecular-weight agents and isocyanates.

Once sensitization has occurred (for many low-molecular-weight agents, the mechanism of possible sensitization remains uncertain), it is unknown whether the presence of bronchial responsiveness can condition the likelihood of developing inflammatory changes in the target organ, the bronchi. It is, however, unlikely that the presence of asthma is a predisposing factor to the development of occupational asthma due to low-molecular-weight agents. Although this information is retrospective in all studies, most subjects who develop occupational asthma do not have a history of asthma before exposure to the occupational agent began. We observed workers exposed to snow crab in seasonal work. Several of them had a $PC_{20}$ value close to normal before the seasonal exposure began. After starting work, these employees progressively developed bronchial hyperresponsiveness which persisted for several months, as shown by the example in Figure 3. In a prospective study, Chan-Yeung and Desjardins found that four subjects who developed occupational asthma to western red cedar did not have bronchial hyperresponsiveness before exposure

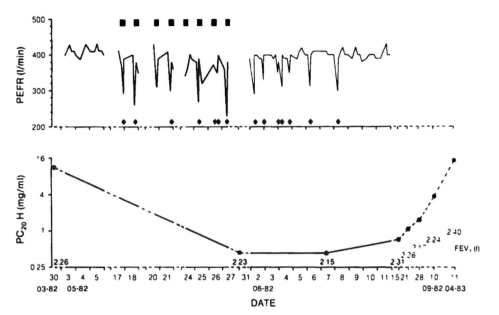

**Figure 3**  Combined monitoring of peak expiratory flow rates (upper panel) and $PC_{20}$ (lower panel) in the same subject before and after return to work in a crab processing plant. Squares represent the time spent at work; lozenges illustrate the use of inhaled salbutamol. Baseline $FEV_1$ values before each histamine inhalation tests are illustrated. After a short period of exposure at work, there are swings in PEFR and prolonged (lasting several months) changes in bronchial responsiveness to histamine. (From ref. 25.)

[39]. Although it would be interesting to investigate prospectively subjects employed in high-risk industries to see if bronchial hyperresponsiveness is a predisposing factor, the existing evidence makes this seem unlikely. It should, however, be done on subjects exposed to high- and low-molecular-weight agents as knowing the rate of development of occupational asthma after sensitization to high-molecular-weight agents, demonstrated by skin reactivity or increased specific IgE antibodies, would be useful. It would be a satisfactory model of what can occur in subjects who become sensitized to common inhalants and are at risk of developing symptoms.

### C.  Behavior of Occupational Asthma After Exposure Ends

Several retrospective studies, summarized in Table 2, have unanimously demonstrated the persistence of asthmatic symptoms, bronchial obstruction, and hyperresponsiveness in subjects with occupational asthma after they are removed

**Table 2** Retrospective Evidence for the Persistence of Symptoms and Bronchial Hyperresponsiveness After Removal from the Offending Agent

| Agent | Number of subjects | Duration of follow-up (yr) | Persistence of symptoms (%) | Persistence of hyperrespon- siveness (%) | Ref. |
|-------|-----|-----|-----|-----|-----|
| Red cedar | 38 | 0.5–4 | 29 | 38/38 (100%) | [40] |
| | 75 | 1–9 | 49 | 25/33 (76%) | [41] |
| Colophony | 20 | 1.3–3.8 | 90 | 7/20 (35%) | [42] |
| Isocyanates | 12 | 1–3 | 66 | 7/12 (58%) | [43] |
| Snow crab | 31 | 0.5–2 | 61 | 28/31 (90%) | [44] |
| | 31 | 4.8–6 | 100 | 26/31 (84%) | [48] |
| Various | 32 | 0.5–4 | 93 | 31/32 (97%) | [44] |
| Isocyanates | 50 | >4 | 82 | 12/19 (63%) | [45] |
| | 20 | 0.5–4 | 50 | 9/12 (75%) | [46] |
| | 22 | 1 | 77 | 17/22 (77%) | [47] |

from exposure. This was originally suggested by Chan-Yeung and colleagues [40] and has since been confirmed by many researchers in subjects exposed to various occupational agents [41–47]. Most studies have also shown that total duration of exposure, duration of exposure after onset of symptoms, and severity of asthma at the time of diagnosis are all determinants of the prognosis. A plateau of improvement has been shown approximately 2 years after cessation of exposure in the course of occupational asthma due to snow crab [48] (Fig. 4).

If exposure continues, there is a deterioration in the asthmatic condition, and for western red cedar asthma, wearing conventional face masks at work does not diminish the risk [49]. It is unknown, however, whether wearing tighter face masks would be more efficient in this regard.

## III. Strategies

A possible prevention scheme is illustrated in Figure 5.

### A. Primary Prevention

It would be tempting to exclude all atopic subjects from exposure to high-molecular-weight agents. Although this could be achieved ethically through direct counseling by physicians (i.e., dissuading a young atopic patient from taking specific jobs involving exposure to laboratory animals), it is not feasible for entire populations. In laboratory animal workers, the risk of developing symptoms is not sufficiently high (approximately one-third of workers) to justify

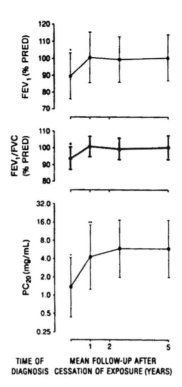

TIME OF          MEAN FOLLOW-UP AFTER
DIAGNOSIS   CESSATION OF EXPOSURE (YEARS)

**Figure 4**   Serial changes in $FEV_1$, $FEV_1/FVC$, and $PC_{20}$ in 31 subjects with occupational asthma due to snow crab after removal from exposure. A plateau of improvement in terms of $PC_{20}$ is seen approximately 2 years after exposure ends, whereas the maximum improvement in terms of $FEV_1$ and $FEV_1/FVC$ is reached earlier. (Adapted from ref. 48.)

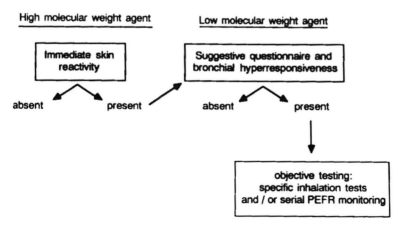

**Figure 5**   Suggested surveillance program for occupational asthma, distinguishing between high- and low-molecular-weight agents. In the first instance, skin reactivity is the cornerstone, whereas for low-molecular-weight agents, questionnaires and bronchial hyperresponsiveness are the key factors.

excluding atopic subjects [24,50]. In industries where smoking has been identified as a significant risk factor, dissuading employees from smoking appears reasonable. Keeping the concentration of the possible occupational agent low and avoiding spills also seems reasonable. But it is unrealistic to expect that replacement products will change the picture of occupational asthma over the next few years. For example, no replacement product has yet been found for isocyanate.

### B. Secondary Prevention

Routine skin testing with high-molecular-weight agents is feasible and can identify subjects who have become immunologically sensitized and should be followed more closely for development of bronchial hyperresponsiveness and asthma symptoms. For agents such as laboratory animal–derived antigens, psyllium, guar gum, and so on, skin prick testing is an easy and noninvasive means of assessing IgE-mediated sensitization. This test can easily be done every 2 years, for example. In subjects who are sensitized, regular questionnaires or assessment of bronchial responsiveness can detect subjects susceptible to developing occupational asthma at an early stage. In subjects exposed to low-molecular-weight agents, routine questionnaires, preferably coupled with assessment of bronchial responsiveness, might prove useful in identifying subjects at an early stage of the disease. In our experience, questionnaires are sensitive enough but not specific enough for this purpose. Combining both tools may be the best strategy according to preliminary results: subjects who developed occupational asthma to spiramycin were those who had both a positive question-naire and increased bronchial responsiveness [51].

### C. Tertiary Prevention

Early diagnosis of occupational asthma is important. Once the diagnosis is made, it is crucial that the subject be removed from exposure as quickly as possible. If this is done, it is less likely that the subject will be left with permanent sequelae of asthma and bronchial responsiveness requiring medication. If medicolegal compensation or private insurance does not make removal possible, efforts to diminish exposure should be undertaken. It is unknown whether taking anti-inflammatory preparations is of any help once the subject has been removed from exposure. However, retrospective evidence indicates that subjects taking anti-inflammatory preparations are left with the same level of bronchial hyperresponsiveness as those using only usual bronchodilators. It is also unknown whether the use of anti-inflammatory preparations in subjects who remain exposed can reduce the rate of functional and clinical deterioration.

## IV. Future Needs

### A. Estimating the Frequency of Occupational Asthma

The first major step in determining future needs should be to obtain figures on the frequency of occupational asthma. This has been done on a voluntary basis by physicians reporting the condition in the United Kingdom [6] and in some states in the United States [9]. But medicolegal statistics may be a poor reflection of the situation if underreporting results from unsatisfactory compensation programs.

### B. Identifying At-Risk Populations

As the number of agents that cause occupational asthma steadily increases, it is worthwhile following exposed subjects. Refining the means of identifying sensitization and occupational asthma at an early stage is important. In the same way that chest radiographs are done on subjects exposed to silica or asbestos dusts at regular intervals, it is essential to test subjects exposed to high-risk agents. The best strategy (skin testing, bronchial responsiveness) for high- and low-molecular-weight agents (see above) has to be prospectively validated. The feasibility and acceptability of this strategy also has to be tested and optimum timing established.

### C. Identifying Host Markers and Factors

Prospective studies have to be carried out on different markers and factors that can affect the likelihood of developing sensitization and occupational asthma. Atopy and smoking are the only ones to be studied so far. Other genetic markers have yet to be explored.

### D. Is There a Dose-Dependent Relationship?

As discussed above, several factors can affect the likelihood of developing occupational asthma. In this regard it would be valuable to know whether the duration of exposure or the concentration is significant. There are now means for assessing the concentration of some of the high- [52] and low-molecular-weight agents (such as isocyanates) at work. This opportunity should be taken.

## V. Conclusions

Because occupational asthma is a common occupational ailment that can cause permanent sequelae, it is essential that surveillance and prevention programs be set up to reduce the morbidity of the condition. There is much work to be done. Host and environmental predisposing factors still have to be better identified.

Strategies for surveillance programs have to be established. Assessment of the efficacy of the programs in reducing morbidity have to be done.

## Acknowledgments

We sincerely thank Katherine Tallman for reviewing the manuscript. J.L.M. is a research fellow with the Fonds de la Recherche en Santé du Québec and of the Université de Montréal School of Medicine.

## References

1. Becklake MR. Epidemiology and surveillance. Chest 1990;98:165S–72S.
2. Newman-Taylor AJ. Occupational asthma. Thorax 1980;35:241–45.
3. Chan-Yeung M, Lam S. Occupational asthma. Am Rev Respir Dis 1986;133:686–703.
4. Pauli G, Bessot JC, Dietemann-Molard A. Occupational asthma: investigations and aetiological factors. Bull Eur Physiopathol Respir 1986;22:399–425.
5. Chan-Yeung M. Occupational asthma. Chest 1990;98:148S–61S.
6. Meredith SK, Taylor VM, McDonald JC. Occupational respiratory disease in the United Kingdom 1989: a report to the British Thoracic Society and the Society of Occupational Medicine by the SWORD project group. Br J Ind Med 1991;48:292–98.
7. Lagier F, Cartier A, Malo JL. Medico-legal statistics on occupational asthma in Quebec between 1986 and 1988. Rev Mal Respir 1990;7:337–41.
8. Blanc P. Occupational asthma in a national disability survey. Chest 1987;92:613–17.
9. Matte TD, Hoffman RE, Rosenman KD, Stanbury M. Surveillance of occupational asthma under the SENSOR model. Chest 1990;98:173S–78S.
10. Carter JT. There's a lot of it about. Br J Ind Med 1991;48:289–91.
11. Malo JL, Ghezzo H, L'Archevêque J, Lagier F, Perrin B, Cartier A. Is the clinical history a satisfactory means of diagnosing occupational asthma? Am Rev Respir Dis 1991;143:528–32.
12. Bardy JD, Malo JL, Séguin P, Ghezzo H, Desjardins J, Dolovich J, Cartier A. Occupational asthma and IgE sensitization in a pharmaceutical company processing psyllium. Am Rev Respir Dis 1987;135:1033–38.
13. Cartier A, Grammer L, Malo JL, Lagier F, Ghezzo H, Harris K, Patterson R. Specific serum antibodies against isocyanates: association with occupational asthma. J Allergy Clin Immunol 1989;84:507–14.
14. Cockcroft DW, Ruffin RE, Frith PA, Cartier A, Juniper EF, Dolovich J,

Hargreave FE. Determinants of allergen-induced asthma: dose of allergen, circulating IgE antibody concentration, and bronchial responsiveness to inhaled histamine. Am Rev Respir Dis 1979;120:1053–58.

15. Cockcroft DW, Murdock KY, Kirby J, Hargreave F. Prediction of airway responsiveness to allergen from skin sensitivity to allergen and airway responsiveness to histamine. Am Rev Respir Dis 1987;135:264–67.

16. Malo JL, Cartier A, L'Archevêque J, Ghezzo H, Soucy F, Somers J, Dolovich J. Prevalence of occupational asthma and immunological sensitization to guar gum among employees at a carpet-manufacturing plant. J Allergy Clin Immunol 1990;86:562–69.

17. Malo JL, Cartier A, L'Archevêque J, Ghezzo H, Lagier F, Trudeau C, Dolovich J. Prevalence of occupational asthma and immunologic sensitization to psyllium among health personnel in chronic care hospitals. Am Rev Respir Dis 1990;142:1359–66.

18. Côté J, Kennedy S, Chan-Yeung M. Sensitivity and specificity of PC20 and peak expiratory flow rate in cedar asthma. J Allergy Clin Immunol 1990;85:592–98.

19. Perrin B, Lagier F, L'Archevêque J, Cartier A, Boulet LP, Côté J, Malo JL. Validity of investigating occupational asthma with serial monitoring of peak expiratory flow rates and bronchial responsiveness as compared to specific inhalation challenges. Eur Respir J 1992;5:40–48.

20. Burge PS. Diagnosis of occupational asthma. Clin Allergy 1989;19:649–52.

21. Lam S, LeRiche J, Phillips D, Chan-Yeung M. Cellular and protein changes in bronchial lavage fluid after late asthmatic reaction in patients with red cedar asthma. J Allergy Clin Immunol 1987;80:44–50.

22. Mapp CE, Boschetto P, Zocca E, Milani GF, Pivirotto F, Tegazzin V, Fabbri LM. Pathogenesis of late asthmatic reactions induced by exposure to isocyanates. Bull Eur Physiopathol Respir 1987;23:583–86.

23. Mitchell CA, Gandevia B. Respiratory symptoms and skin reactivity in workers exposed to proteolytic enzymes in the detergent industry. Am Rev Respir Dis 1971;104:1–12.

24. Slovak AJM, Hill RN. Does atopy have any predictive value for laboratory animal allergy? A comparison of different concepts of atopy. Br J Ind Med 1987;44:129–32.

25. Cartier A, Malo JL, Forest F, Lafrance M, Pineau L, St Aubin JJ, Dubois JY. Occupational asthma in snow crab-processing workers. J Allergy Clin Immunol 1984;74:261–69.

26. Barbee RA, Halonen M, Kaltenborn W, Lebowitz M, Burrows B. A longitudinal study of serum IgE in a community cohort: correlations with age, sex, smoking, and atopic status. J Allergy Clin Immunol 1987;79:919–27.

27.   Holt PG. Immune and inflammatory function in cigarette smokers. Thorax 1987;42:241–49.
28.   Chan-Yeung M, Vedal S, Kus J, Maclean L, Enarson D, Tse KS. Symptoms, pulmonary function, and bronchial hyperreactivity in western red cedar workers compared with those in office workers. Am Rev Respir Dis 1984;130:1038–41.
29.   Venables KM, Dally MB, Nunn AJ, Stevens JF, Stephens R, Farrer N, Hunter JY, Stewart M, Hugues EG, Newman Taylor AJ. Smoking and occupational allergy in workers in a platinum refinery. Br Med J 1989;299:939–42.
30.   Venables KM. Epidemiology and the prevention of occupational asthma (editorial). Br J Ind Med 1987;44:73–75.
31.   Greenberg M, Milne JF, Watt A. A survey of workers exposed to dusts containing derivatives of bacillus subtilis. Br Med J 1970;2:629–33.
32.   Zetterstrom O, Osterman K, Machado L, Johansson SGO. Another smoking hazard: raised serum IgE concentration and increased risk of occupational allergy. Br Med J 1981;283:1215–17.
33.   Butcher BT, Jones RN, O'Neil CE, Glindmeyer HW, Diem JE, Dharmarajan V, Weill H, Salvaggio JE. Longitudinal study of workers employed in the manufacture of toluene-diisocyanate. Am Rev Respir Dis 1977;116:411–21.
34.   Brooks SM, Weiss MA, Bernstein IL. Reactive airways dysfunction syndrome (RADS); persistent asthma syndrome after high level irritant exposures. Chest 1985;88:376–84.
35.   Luo JC, Nelsen KG, Fischbein A. Persistent reactive airway dysfunction syndrome after exposure to toluene diisocyanate. Br J Ind Med 1990;47:239–41.
36.   Burge PS, Edge G, Hawkins R, White V, Taylor AN. Occupational asthma in a factory making flux-cored solder containing colophony. Thorax 1981;36:828–34.
37.   Vedal S, Chan-Yeung M, Enarson D, Fera T, Maclean L, Tse KS, Langille R. Symptoms and pulmonary function in western red cedar workers related to duration of employment and dust exposure. Arch Environ Health 1986;41:179–83.
38.   Musk AW, Venables KM, Crook B, Nunn AJ, Hawkins R, Crook GDW, Graneek BJ, Tee RD, Farrer N, Johnson DA, Gordon DJ, Darbyshire JR, Newman Taylor AJ. Respiratory symptoms, lung function, and sensitisation to flour in a British bakery. Br J Ind Med 1989;46:636–42.
39.   Chan-Yeung M, Desjardins A. Natural history of occupational asthma due to western red cedar (thuja plicata) J Allergy Clin Immunol (in press).
40.   Chan-Yeung M. Fate of occupational asthma. A follow-up study of patients

with occupational asthma due to western red cedar (thuya plicata). Am Rev Respir Dis 1977;116:1023–29.

41. Chan-Yeung M, Lam S, Koener S. Clinical features and natural history of occupational asthma due to western red cedar (thuya plicata). Am J Med 1982;72:411–15.

42. Burge PS. Occupational asthma in electronics workers caused by colophony fumes: follow-up of affected workers. Thorax 1982;37:348–53.

43. Paggiaro PL, Loi AM, Rossi O, Ferrante B, Pardi F, Roselli MG, Baschieri L. Follow-up study of patients with respiratory disease due to toluene diisocyanate (TDI). Clin Allergy 1984;14:463–69.

44. Hudson P, Cartier A, Pineau L, Lafrance M, St Aubin JJ, Dubois JY, Malo JL. Follow-up of occupational asthma caused by crab and various agents. J Allergy Clin Immunol 1985;76:682–87.

45. Rosenberg N, Garnier R, Rousselin X, Mertz R, Gervais P. Clinical and socio-professional fate of isocyanate-induced asthma. Clin Allergy 1987;17:55–61,

46. Mapp CE, Corona PC, deMarzo N, Fabbri L. Persistent asthma due to isocyanates. A follow-up study of subjects with occupational asthma due to toluene diisocyanate. Am Rev Respir Dis 1988;137:1326–29.

47. Lozewicz S, Assoufi BK, Hawkins R, Newman-Taylor AJ. Outcome of asthma induced by isocyanates. Br J Dis Chest 1987;81:14–27.

48. Malo JL, Cartier A, Ghezzo H, Lafrance M, McCants M, Lehrer SB. Patterns of improvement on spirometry, bronchial hyperresponsiveness, and specific IgE antibody levels after cessation of exposure in occupational asthma caused by snow-crab processing. Am Rev Respir Dis 1988;138:807–12.

49. Côté J, Kennedy S, Chan-Yeung M. Outcome of patients with cedar asthma with continuous exposure. Am Rev Respir Dis 1990;141:373–76.

50. Newill CA, Evans R, Khoury MJ. Preemployment screening for allergy to laboratory animals: epidemiologic evaluation of its potential usefulness. J Occup Med 1986;28:1158–64.

51. Malo JL, Cartier A. Occupational asthma in workers of a pharmaceutical company processing spiramycin. Thorax 1988;43:371–77.

52. Reed CE, Swanson MC, Agarwal MK, Yunginger JW. Allergens that cause asthma. Identification and quantification. Chest 1985;87:40S–4S.

# 7

## Contribution of Occupational Exposures to the Occurrence of Chronic Nonspecific Lung Disease

DICK HEEDERIK

University of Wageningen
Wageningen, The Netherlands

TAEKE M. PAL

State University
Groningen, The Netherlands

## I. Introduction

Asthma, bronchitis, and emphysema, collectively called chronic nonspecific lung disease (CNSLD), form an important public health problem in the general population in many Western countries. For example, in the Netherlands, CNSLD is the fifth most common cause of death. Approximately 5.5% and 2.2%, respectively, of men and women who died in 1985 had CNSLD as the primary cause of death. For 6.6% of the men and 2.4% of the women CNSLD was mentioned on the death certificate as the secondary cause of death [1]. Morbidity statistics, however, reflect the impact of CNSLD on public health more clearly then do mortality statistics. Because of improved medical treatment techniques, CNSLD leads to death only for a minority of those with CNSLD.

Among the determinants of CNSLD, smoking is considered to be the most important. Other environmental factors, such as outdoor, indoor, and occupational air pollution, have also been studied frequently. Smoking is widespread among the general population, and it is known to be a strong determinant of CNSLD. The universality of smoking habits and the widely accepted evidence of their role in the development of airway disease have tended to overshadow the role of other environmental pollutants, such as occupational exposures [2]. In addition to this, other factors might explain the limited attention given to the role of occupational exposures in the development of CNSLD. These other reasons include [3–7]:

1. The absence of powerful longitudinal epidemiological studies of occupationally exposed workers
2. The focus on work force–based studies, which are sensitive to selection biases such as the "Healthy worker effect" instead of community-based studies
3. The complex etiology of CNSLD
4. The presence of specific lung disease such as pneumoconiosis and tuberculosis leading to increased "noise levels" in epidemiological studies of CNSLD
5. The paucity of statistical and epidemiological techniques for assessing the contribution of more than one risk factor in the development of diseases with a multifactorial etiology
6. The absence of precise and valid techniques and strategies to measure occupational pollutants

The contribution of occupational exposures to the incidence of CNSLD is not exactly known [2,8–10]. The contribution was established as being small compared to the contribution of smoking [11]. If true, strategies to prevent the development of CNSLD should aim primarily at the elimination of smoking. Others argue that specific occupational exposures can make a considerable contribution to the development of CNSLD and conclude that preventive strategies should aim at the reduction of both smoking and occupational exposures [12,13]. Specific information on the role of occupational exposures in the development of CNSLD could contribute to the development of scientifically based preventive strategies instead of sweeping generalizations on relative contributions of factors such as "smoking" and "occupational exposures" [2,11–13]. Over the last decade a number of general population studies have been performed in which the contribution of occupational exposures to the development of CNSLD has been quantified. These studies are reviewed in this chapter and used to calculate the contribution of occupational exposures to the development of CNSLD.

## II.  Definition of Chronic Nonspecific Lung Disease

Chronic obstructive lung diseases are characterized by symptoms such as chronic or recurrent episodes of cough with or without sputum production and/or chronic or intermittent episodes of shortness of breath. This group of disorders is called *chronic nonspecific lung disease* (CNSLD) if the symptoms cannot be explained by specific lung diseases, such as localized lung disease (e.g., tuberculosis), pneumoconiosis, collagen diseases, primary cardiovascular and renal diseases, diseases of the chest wall, or psychoneurosis. Within this group many distinguish asthma from chronic obstructive pulmonary disease (COPD). *Asthma* is defined as a clinical syndrome, characterized by increased responsiveness of the tracheobronchial tree to a variety of stimulants. The major symptoms are paroxysms of dyspnea, wheezing, and cough. *COPD* is a disorder characterized by abnormal tests of expiratory flow that do not change markedly over periods of several months of observation [14]. In many cases, however, the difference between asthma and COPD is unclear. Patients with COPD may have significant reversibility after treatment and patients with asthma may develop airflow obstruction with little or no reversibility [15]. These overlapping groups of patients constitute a fair percentage of the total number of patients, and categorizing COPD and asthma in one group of CNSLD patients might result in loss of information because of a poor description of the patient and incomparability of patient groups [16]. In epidemiologic studies this has been a major concern and has led to the measurement of additional information next to symptoms to specify the type of CNSLD as optimal as possible [15].

## III. Etiology of CNSLD

In 1962, Orie and co-workers postulated the *Dutch hypothesis,* which suggested that these three "diseases" were in fact expressions of one basic disease in which the combined endogenous (host) and exogenous (environmental) factors determined the patients' profile [16]. Allergic sensitization and bronchial hyperresponsiveness, two host factors that might have a genetic basis, were considered to be important mechanisms of disease [15,17]. In discussing the natural history of COPD, Fletcher et al. [18] distinguished an obstructive from a hypersecretive disorder which often occurred simultaneously. Whereas the first leads to severe disability through progressive impairment of expiratory airflow, impairment is less evident for the second. This so-called *British hypothesis* considers smoking and recurrent respiratory infections as predominant causes of both phenomena. However, a constitutional susceptibility was suggested as being important in the development of both disorders. Later, Burrows et al. [19] distinguished in their COPD patients an emphysematous subgroup and an asthma–bronchitis subgroup. The latter group had a higher survival rate and a lower rate of lung function decline than the former. They stated that the Dutch hypothesis appeared to be relevant only to their "chronic asthmatic bronchitis" group, whereas the emphysematous disorder was causally related to cigarette smoking. However, this provides no explanation of why only a minority of smokers develop this disease. The debate on splitting or lumping asthma, bronchitis, and emphysema is still going on, although there is more agreement about the importance of allergic sensitization and bronchial hyperresponsiveness (BHR) in obstructive lung disease.

## IV. Allergy and Bronchial Hyperresponsiveness

The underlying mechanism of asthma is in almost all cases immunological and characterized by the development of specific IgE antibodies. Atopic individuals tend to develop an asthmatic allergy more readily, but nonatopics can also be sensitized. Smokers have higher IgE levels than nonsmokers [20] and a increased prevalence of sensitization to some occupational agents has been demonstrated in smokers [21,22]. On the other hand, smoking appears to suppress the humoral immune response [23], which corresponds to decreased level of IgG and prevalance of positive skin tests to certain aeroallergens [24,25]. At this moment there are only a few studies that suggest a promoting effect of irritant exposure such as diesel exhaust and chlorine on allergic sensitization [26,27].

Bronchial hyperresponsiveness (BHR) is defined as an increased responsiveness of the tracheobronchial tree to a variety of stimuli in low dosages that do not cause a similar reaction in normals. In clinical and epidemiological studies BHR is usually measured as a bronchoconstrictor response to pharmacologic agents such as histamine, acetylcholine, or methacholine. Clinically, BHR may manifest itself as episodes of cough, dyspnea, or wheezing after exposure to changes in temperature (especially from warm to cold), exercise, exposure to several chemicals (e.g., sulfur dioxide), exhaust fumes, ozone, fog, smoke, and cooking smells [28]. An allergen exposure can cause a transient or persistent increase of BHR in a sensitized person [29,30]. Avoidance of allergen exposures such as house dust mite or occupational allergens may result in a decrease of symptoms and a reduction of airway obstruction, followed by a decrease of BHR [31,32]. Low-molecular-weight sensitizers, ozone, and viral infections may also induce or increase BHR [33]. Besides these inducers BHR can be provoked by inciters.

BHR is the hallmark of asthma but has also been demonstrated in patients with COPD. So there is evidence to consider BHR as a hallmark of the entire CNSLD complex [15]. The mean BHR level is significantly different between symptomatic groups; however, overlapping distributions make it impossible to distinguish individuals on the basis of BHR alone [34]. Although by now a great deal is known about BHR, its genesis is only partly understood. Inflammatory processes in the airway are now thought to play a key role in the pathway leading to BHR and airway obstruction [35–40]. One might speculate if an increased tendency to react with an inflammatory response to different types of exposure is most closely related to the underlying susceptibility, leading to CNSLD.

## V. Occupational Exposures and CNSLD

Over the years many agents have been identified as being hazardous to the respiratory organ and potentially causing CNSLD. Coal dust is known to be causally related to respiratory symptoms, accelerated lung function decline, and finally, respiratory impairment. The epidemiologic evidence is based on cross-sectional, longitudinal, and case-control studies. Becklake [2,5] applied Hill's criteria for the presence of a causal relationship between occupational exposures and CNSLD. Hill's criteria comprise requirements regarding the consistency of a relationship found, the strength of a relationship, the presence of an exposure–response relationship, the specificity of the relationship, the coherence of the relationship, and the biological plausibility of the relationship [41]. She concluded that all these criteria have been fulfilled for coal dust. For a relationship between other occupational exposures and CNSLD, the evidence is less conclusive, comprising mostly cross-sectional and some longitudinal studies among some occupational groups as well as general population studies. For example, organic dust–exposed populations show an elevated prevalence of various respiratory symptoms, and in many studies a reduced lung function has been found among those exposed. A few studies reported exposure–response relationships between dust exposure and lung function level or lung function decline. If these lung function changes eventually lead to respiratory impairment is still a matter of discussion and further study [42].

Long lists of occupational aeroallergens have been published which are known to be sensitizers and can cause occupational asthma [43]. A few occupationally exposed populations have been studied in greater detail over the last decade. For instance, high asthma prevalence rates have been found among chemical workers who are exposed to toluene diisocyanate, laboratory animal workers, and bakery workers. But the number of occupationally exposed populations for which quantitative information is absent is very high. It has been estimated that 2 to 15% of adult asthma cases may have an occupational agents as primary cause [44,45]. The quantitative evidence is limited, however, and epidemiologic studies to support further evidence are lacking.

## VI. Magnitude of the Relationship Between Occupational Exposures and CNSLD

Recent evidence on the magnitude of the relationship between occupational exposures and CNSLD consists of a series of general population studies that originate from various countries. The general population studies are in most cases morbidity studies in which respiratory symptoms and lung function were registered. Many of the general population studies started in the 1960s and 1970s. Originally, the majority of those studies was not designed to answer questions concerning the relationship between occupation or occupational exposures and lung disease. The aims were often more general; the study of the natural history of lung disease and identification of determinants of the disease or disease processes in general. In these studies the statistical analysis was often elaborate, and multivariate techniques as multiple regression analysis for lung function studies and logistic regression analysis for respiratory symptom prevalence studies were used. This made it possible to treat several independent variables simultaneously in the analysis and to adjust for confounding effects of smoking, age, and in the case of lung function studies, standing height also. The results of these population studies are summarized in Table 1. One of the first population studies presented results of a 12-year follow-up of 556 men aged 30 to 54 in 1960, who were working at that time in the surrounding industries of Paris, France [49,50]. They were mainly employed in the mechanical engineering industry, chemical industry (paint production), printing industry, and food-processing industry (flour milling). The occupational exposures were recorded after a workplace visit at the start of the study by an occupational physician or engineer. The dust exposure was estimated on a four-point scale, the exposure to gases on a two-point scale. The annual rate of decline of $FEV_1$ was calculated as the difference in lung function between 1960 and 1972. $FEV_1$ decline was significantly related to an occupational exposure to mineral dust as well as grain dust. The decline was greater for those exposed more highly. There were indications that exposure to heat had an effect on change in $FEV_1$, independent of the effect of dust exposure on lung function decline. It is noteworthy that no relationship between dust exposure and lung function was found for the 1960 cross-sectional data. After a graphical analysis of lung function level in 1960 and consecutive change, the authors concluded that a self-selection effect seems to be present among the exposed in such a way that the persons in better health remained exposed more highly. This was illustrated by an initially higher lung function with a steeper decline in the years that followed among the exposed compared to unexposed persons. Similar selection effects have also been found in other longitudinal general population studies [59].

Analyses of the Six Cities Study in the United States included 8515 white adults whose occupational history was taken by interview [52]. Based on this information, the number of years of exposure to dust, gases, or fumes was calculated per job and the total number of years of exposure for each subject. Respiratory symptoms were registered with a version of the ATS questionnaire. An index of chronic obstructive pulmonary disease (COPD) was defined as a

Tiffeneau index ($FEV_1/FVC$) smaller than 0.6. This was used as a dichotomous outcome variable in a multiple logistic regression analysis. The same statistical technique was used for analysis of the respiratory symptoms. A number of 3568 (41.9%) persons of this population had never smoked, 3028 were current smoker (35.6%), and 1919 were ex-smoker (33.5%). Of all men, 45% reported an occupational dust exposure and 47% reported an exposure to fumes or gases. Fewer females reported such exposures (19% dust, 16% fumes or gases). The adjusted odds ratios of respiratory symptoms (cough, phlegm, wheeze, and breathlessness) for subjects exposed to dust ranged from 1.3 to 1.8, respectively, for past and current exposure. For exposure to fumes or gases the odds ratios ranged from 1.3 to 1.6. There were significant positive trends for wheezing and phlegm production with increasing duration of exposure. The COPD index had a significantly elevated odds ratio of 1.5 with dust exposure. Current smokers did not appear to be more susceptible to the effect of dust or fumes on symptoms than never smokers. Those who had never smoked but had been exposed to dust had higher symptom prevalence rates than those of current smokers not exposed to dust. No significant interactions were found in this study, or in the other studies, for smoking and occupational exposure with respiratory symptoms and lung function. Gender did not modify the relationships found between occupational exposures and respiratory symptoms, but men with an occupational dust exposure had a higher COPD prevalence than women. In another study a relationship with duration of exposure was also present [46].

In most studies symptom scores were analyzed cross-sectionally. Only, one longitudinal study among 807 men with 25 years of follow-up relationships between occupational exposures and CNSLD incidence have been studied [60,61]. An average incidence density of 1.56 was found per 100 person-years of follow-up. Those with an occupational exposure to dust, fumes, or gases had an incidence density 1.4 times as high as those without such an exposure. The exposure was characterized with a job exposure matrix for the occupations held at the start of the follow-up.

Possible influences of misclassification of exposure, recall bias, or selection bias on the results of the analysis of the Six Cities Study data have been discussed extensively [52]. These comments are of general interest because designs of these general population studies are similar with respect to population sampling and characterization of the exposure. They concluded that misclassification of exposure was nondifferential because occupational status of the selected population was comparable to the total population. Such misclassification would lead to an underestimation of the magnitude of the relationship between occupational exposures and CNSLD. Recall bias (overreporting of occupational exposures among those with respiratory symptoms) was unlikely to occur because the aim of their study was not to assess effects of occupational exposure on respiratory symptoms. In addition, relationships between occupational exposures and lung

**Table 1** Overview of General Population Studies in Which Relationships Were Studied Between Occupational Exposures, Respiratory Symptoms, and Lung Function

| Country | Subjects | Health endpoint | Type of study | Exposure characterization | Exposures related to health endpoint | Quantification of results | Refs. |
|---|---|---|---|---|---|---|---|
| U.S. | 1195 men 1519 women | Symptoms, spirometry, x-ray | Cross-sectional | Interview | Specific exposure dusts, glass fibers construction industry, production industry sector | Elevated symptom prevalence with occupational exposure; no odds ratios (ORs) given, reduced FVC and $FEV_1/FVC$ | [46–48] |
| France | 556 men | FVC, $FEV_1$ | Longitudinal, 12-year follow-up | Walk through, estimation for 30 exposures | Dusts, gases, heat | Increased $FEV_1$ decline among exposed | [49,50] |
| Poland | 759 men, 1065 women | FVC, $FEV_1$, COPD incidence[a] | Longitudinal, 13-year follow-up | Interview[g] | Variable temperature (women), dusts (men) | Increased $FEV_1$ decline among exposed | [51] |
| U.S. | 8515 men | Symptoms, COPD prevalence[c] | Cross-sectional | Interviewer with questionnaire | Dusts, fumes, gases | Dust: OR = 1.3–1.6, gas or fumes: OR = 1.33–1.4 | [52] |
| Italy | 1635 working men and women | Symptoms, Lung function | Cross-sectional | Questionnaire | Dusts with fumes and chemicals | Elevated symptom prevalence with occupational exposure, no odds ratios given | [53] |

| France | 8692 men[d] | Symptoms, FVC, FEV$_1$ | Cross-sectional | Interview | Dusts, fumes, gases | Men: OR = 1.4–1.6, women: OR = 1.4–2.1 | [54,55] |
|---|---|---|---|---|---|---|---|
| Poland | 696 men, 983 women | FVC, FEV$_1$ | Longitudinal 13-year follow-up | Interview[e] | Variable temperature, dusts, chemicals | Increased FEV$_1$, decline for exposed | [56] |
| Norway | 2521 men, 2471 women | Symptoms | Cross-sectional | Questionnaire (postal) | Dusts, gases | OR = 1.8 for all symptoms | [57] |
| Netherlands | 727 men | Symptoms | Cross-sectional | Matrix[f] | Dusts, fumes, gases | OR = 1.2–2.7, OR = 0.3 for asthma | [58] |
| Netherlands | 804 men | CNSLD incidence[g] | Longitudinal 25-year follow-up | Matrix[f] | Dusts, fumes, gases | IDR = 1.4 | [59,60] |

[a]Incident cases defined as persons with a baseline FEV$_1$ ≥ 0.70 reference, and change over 13 years to < 65% of reference value.

[b]Yes/no exposure only.

[c]Prevalent cases defined as persons with a FEV$_1$/VC ratio <0.6.

[d]Manual workers not included in the analysis.

[e]Stratified by years of exposure.

[f]Occupational exposures generated with the British job exposure matrix [61].

[g]Incident cases defined on basis of symptoms or clinically confirmed morbidity.

function were also established. Selection bias toward those with a higher occupationally exposed job was unlikely because a random sample of the population was taken.

Some comments can be given. The similarity of distributions of occupational status between two populations does not necessarily mean that self-reported exposures do not show nondifferential misclassification. It seems, however, unlikely that the similarities in results between the various countries are caused by similar magnitudes of misclassification of the exposure. In almost all these studies the characterization of the occupational exposure was relatively poor. Exposures were generally self-reported and registered during an interview or based on questionnaire information. However, in one study, the occupational exposure was estimated by an occupational physician or occupational hygienist. In this study the workplace was visited and a walk-through survey was completed [50]. In the studies in the Netherlands, incidence data were used in combination with specific exposures generated with a so-called job exposure matrix [59,60]. The similarity in results of the French and Dutch studies in comparison with studies in which self-reported exposure information was used suggests that recall bias is unlikely to explain the findings.

Another factor present might be incomplete correction for confounders such as smoking and socioeconomic status resulting in so-called residual confounding bias [62]. Although this effect might be present in specific studies in which crude characterizations for smoking were used, it is unlikely that it produced the relationships found between occupational exposures and CNSLD in all studies. A strong argument against residual confounding by smoking habits is the fact that significant relationships of the same magnitude between occupational exposures and CNSLD were found for smokers as well as nonsmokers in a separate analysis [52].

## VII. Etiologic Fraction for Occupational Exposures

Although the definition of an occupational exposure varies between the studies, the presence of any occupational exposure varied between approximately 25 and 60% for all males under study and 8 to 20% for females. In all these studies relationships were found between occupational exposures and respiratory symptoms or lung function changes. Detailed analyses showed that the contribution of occupational exposures to symptoms of bronchitis can be of the same magnitude as the magnitude of the effect of moderate smoking. The magnitude of odds ratios and relative risks of the occupational exposure to dusts, fumes, and/or gases in the studies with respiratory symptoms as health endpoint are comparable between the studies and varies from 1.3 to 2.1. If we use the information from one of the longitudinal studies [59], in which approximately

30% of the males had an occupational exposure to dusts, fumes, and gases, and a comparison of those exposed with those without an occupational exposure showed an incidence density ratio of 1.4 corrected for age and smoking habits. The etiologic fraction contributable to occupational exposures is then approximately 11% (confidence limits 3 to 20%). For the Norwegian study an etiologic fraction of 11 to 19% has been calculated [57], while the etiologic fraction for smoking ranged from 28 to 54%, dependent on the symptom considered. Other studies will probably yield comparable etiologic fractions because of the comparability of results. For women the etiologic fraction will be lower because fewer women have an occupational exposure while risk ratios seem comparable.

## VIII. Concluding Remarks

It is recognized that estimates of the relative contribution of a given factor to the occurrence of disease give only a rough indication of the impact of that particular factor on the population [62,63]. Among the reasons for these difficulties are the multicausal etiology of CNSLD, uncertainties about mechanisms of disease, the role of combined exposures, and the absence of detailed qualitative as well as quantitative information about occupational exposures. One should be careful in arguing that an intervention aimed at a reduction of exposure levels to air pollution in the work environment will lead to a reduction in CNSLD equal to the etiologic fraction for occupational exposures. Not only uncertainties in the predictions but especially lack of clarity about mechanisms of disease, such as interplay of environmental and hereditary factors, could result in large deviations of estimates of the etiologic fraction from actual findings. Gaining deeper insights in the role of inflammatory responses and BHR will create new insight in possibilities for primary and also secondary prevention.

This analysis showed that the contribution of historical occupational exposures to the incidence and prevalence of CNSLD might be considerable. Because of the limitations inherent to these calculations, one should be careful to generalize the estimate of the etiological fraction to other populations and other periods. For instance, the exposure might have been changed qualitatively as well as quantitatively because of industrial developments over time. The calculations might therefore not be valid for those who are exposed at present.

This supports the need for new studies among occupationally exposed populations in order to produce estimates of the current contribution of occupation and occupational exposures to the development of CNSLD as recommended by several national and international bodies [2,8,9]. The magnitudes found in this review for the relationship between occupational exposures and CNSLD seem to be substantiated in studies among currently exposed cohorts [54,55]. This implies that preventive strategies should not only aim at a reduction in smoking habits in the general population but at the control of air contaminant levels at the workplace as well.

### References

1.  Central Bureau of Statistics. Compendium van de gezondheidsstatistiek. 's Gravenhage, The Netherlands: Staatsuitgeverij, 1985.
2.  Becklake MR. Chronic airflow limitations: its relationship to work in dusty occupations. Chest 1985;88:608–17.
3.  Smith TJ. Exposure assessment for occupational epidemiology. Am J Ind Med 1987;12:249–68.
4.  American Conference of Governmental Industrial Hygienists. International workshop on exposure assessment for epidemiology and hazard control, Woods Hole, MA, 1988.
5.  Becklake MR. Chronic airways disease: distribution and determinants, prevention and control. Report of a WHO working group, Dubrovnik, Yugoslavia, October 1988.
6.  Becklake MR. Occupational pollution. Chest 1989;96:373S–78S.
7.  Becklake MR. Occupational exposures: evidence for a causal association with chronic obstructive pulmonary disease. Am Rev Respir Dis 1989;140:S85–S91.
8.  Whittenberger JL, ed. Report on the workship on environmentally related non-oncogenic lung disease. Environ Res 1985;38:417–69.
9.  NHLBI. National Heart Lung and Blood Institute. Strategies for elucidating the relationship between occupational exposures and chronic air-flow obstruction. Am Rev Respir Dis 1987;135:268–73.
10. World Health Organization. Epidemiology of work related diseases and accidents. Technical Report 777. Geneva: WHO, 1989.
11. World Health Organization. Epidemiology of work related diseases and accidents. Technical Report 714. Geneva: WHO, 1985.
12. Jacobsen M. Smoking and disability in miners (letter to the editor). Lancet 1980;ii:740.
13. Marine WM, Gurr D, Jacobsen M. Clinically important respiratory effects of dust exposure and smoking in British coal miners. Am Rev Respir Dis 1988;137:106–12.
14. ATS statements on COPD and asthma. Am Rev Respir Dis 1987;136:225–44.
15. Sluiter HJ, Koter GH, de Monchy JGR, Postma DS, de Vries K, Orie NGM. The Dutch hypothesis (chronic non-specific lung disease) revisited. Eur Respir 1991;4:479–89.
16. Orie NGM, Sluiter HJ, de Vries K, Tammeling GJ, Witkop J. The host

factor in bronchitis. In: Orie NGM, Sluiter HJ, eds. Bronchitis. Assen, The Netherlands: Van Gorcum, 1961:43–59.

17. Meijer DA. Genetics of airway responsiveness and atopy. In: Weiss ST, Sparrow D, eds. Airway responsiveness and atopy in the development of chronic lung disease. New York: Raven Press 1989:157–80.

18. Fletcher C, Peto R, Tinker C, Speizer FE. The natural history of chronic bronchitis and emphysema. Oxford: Oxford Unversity Press, 1976.

19. Burrows B, Bloom GW, Traven GA, Cline MG. The course of different forms of chronic airways obstruction in a sample from the general population. N Engl J Med 1987;317:1309–14.

20. Burrows B, Halonen M, Barbee RA, Lebowitz MD. The relationship of serum immunoglobulin IgE to cigarette smoking. Am Rev Resp Dis 1981;124:523–28.

21. Zetterstrom O, Osterman K, Machado L, Johansson SGO. Another smoking hazard: raised serum IgE concentration and increased risk of occupational allergy. Br Med J 1981;283:1215–17.

22. Venables KM, Topping MD, Howe W, Luczynska CM, Hawkins R, Newman-Taylor AJ. Interaction of smoking and atopy in producing specific IgE antibody against a hapten protein conjugate. Br Med J 1985;290:201–4.

23. Thomas WR, Holt P, Keast O. Effect of cigarette smoking on primary and secondary humoral responses of mice. Nature 1973;243:240–41.

24. Andersen P, Pedersen OF, Bach B, Bonde GJ. Serum antibodies and immunoglobin in smokers and non-smokers. Clin Exp Immunol 1982;47:467–73.

25. Burrows B, Halonen M, Lebowitz MO, Knudson RJ, Barbee RA. The relationship of serum immunoglobin E allergy skin tests and smoking to respiratory disorders. Allergy Clin Immunol 1982;70:199–204.

26. Zwick H, Popp W, Budik G, Wanke Th, Rauscher H. Increased sensitization to aero-allergens in competitive swimmers. Lung 1990;168:111–15.

27. Muranaka M, Suzuki S, Koizumi K, Takajufi S, Miyamoto T, Ikemori R, Tokiwa H. Adjuvant activity of diesel-exhaust particulates for the production of IgE antibody in mice. J Allergy Clin Immunol 1986;77:616–23.

28. Postma DS, Koter GH, de Vries K. Clinical expression of airway hyperreactivity in adults. Clin Rev Allergy 1989;7:321–43.

29. Durham StR, Graneek BJ, Hawkins R, Newman-Taylor AJ. The temporal relationship between increases in airway responsiveness to histamine and late asthmatic responses induced by occupational agents. J Allergy Clin Immunol 1987;79:398–406.

30. Cartier A, l'Archevêque J, Malo J-L. Exposure to a sensitizing occupational agent can cause a long lasting increase in bronchial responsiveness

to histamine in the absence of significant changes in airway caliber. J Allergy Clin Immunol 1986;78:1185–89.

31.    Platts-Mills TAE, Mitchell EB, Noah P. Reduction of bronchial hyperre-activity during prolonged allergen avoidance. Lancet 1984;ii:675–77.

32.    Chan-Yeung M, MacLean L, Paggiaro PL. Follow-up of 232 patients with occupational asthma caused by western red cedar. J Allergy Clin Immunol 1987;79:792–96.

33.    Dolovich J, Hargreave FE. The asthma syndrome inciters, inducers and host characteristics. Thorax 1981;36:641–44.

34.    Rijcken B, Schouten JP, Weiss ST, Meinesz AF, de Vries K, Van der Lende R. The distribution of bronchial responsiveness to histamine in symptomatic and asymptomatic subjects: a population based analysis of various indices of responsiveness. Am Rev Respir Dis 1989;140:615–23.

35.    Barnes PJ. New concepts in the pathogenesis of bronchial hyperresponsive-ness and asthma. J Allergy Clin Immunol 1989;83:1013–26.

36.    Fine JM, Balmes JR. Airway inflammation and occupational asthma. Clin Chest Med 1988;94:577–90.

37.    Chan-Yeung M, Abboud R, Dy Buncio A, Vedal S. Peripheral leucocyte count and longitudinal decline in lung function. Thorax 1988;43:462–66.

38.    Frette L, Annesi I, Korobaeff M, Neukirch F, Dore M-F, Kauffmann F. Blood eosinophillia and $FEV_1$. Am Rev Respir Dis 1991;143:987–92.

39.    Janoff A. Elastases and emphysema. State of the art. Am Rev Respir Dis 1985;132:417–33.

40.    Postma DS, Renkema TEJ. Noordhoek JA, Faber H, Sluiter HJ, Kauffman H. Association between non-specific bronchial hyperreactivity and super-oxide anion production by polymorphonuclear leucocytes in chronic air-flow production. Am Rev Respir Dis 1988;137:57–61.

41.    Hill AB. The environment and disease: association or causation. Proc R Soc Med 1965;58:295–300.

42.    Wegman DH. Evaluation of epidemiologic approaches to the study of lung disease related to cotton dust exposures. Am J Ind Med 1987;12:661–75.

43.    Parkes WR. Occupational lung disorders. 2nd ed. London: Butterworth, 1982.

44.    Salvaggio J, ed. Occupational and environmental respiratory disease in NIAID task force report: asthma and other allergic disease. NIH Publica-tion 79-387. Washington DC: U.S. Department of Health, Education and Welfare, May 1979.

45.    Kobayashi S. Different aspects of occupational asthma in Japan. In: Frazier CA, ed. Occupational asthma. New York: Van Nostrand Reinhold, 1980:229–44.

46.    Lebowitz MD. Occupational exposures in relation to symptomalogy and lung function in a community population. Environ Res 1977;104:59–67.

47. Lebowitz MD. The relationship of socio-environmental factors to the prevalence of obstructive lung diseases and other chronic conditions. J Chron Dis 1977;30:599–611.

48. Lebowitz MD. Multivariate analysis of smoking and other risk factors for obstructive lung diseases and related symptoms. J Chron Dis 1982;35:751–58.

49. Kauffmann F, Drouet D, Lellouch J, Brille D. Occupational exposure and 12-year spirometric changes among Paris area workers. Br J Ind Med 1982;39:221–32.

50. Kauffman F, Drouet D, Lellouch J, Brille D. Occupational exposure and 12-year spirometric changes among Paris areas workers. Br J Ind Med 1982;39:221–32.

51. Krzyzanowski M, Wysocki M. The relation of thirteen-year mortality to ventilatory impairment and other respiratory symptoms: the Cracow study. Int J Epidemiol 1986;15:56–64.

52. Korn RJ, Dockery DW, Speizer FE, Ware JH, Ferris BG. Occupational exposures and chronic respiratory symptoms: a population based study. Am Rev Respir Dis 1987; 136:296–304.

53. Prediletto R, Viegi G, Paoletti P, De Pede F, Carozzi L, Carmignani G, Giuntini C. Effect of occupational exposures on respiratory symptoms and lung function in a general population (abstract). Am Rev Respir Dis 1987;135:A342.

54. Krzyzanowski M, Kauffman F. The reduction of respiratory symptoms and ventillatory function to moderate occupational exposure in a general population. Presented at the 5th International Symposium of Epidemiology in Occupational Health, University of California, Los Angeles, September 9–11, 1986.

55. Krzyzanowski M, Kauffman F. The relation of respiratory symptoms and ventilatory function to moderate occupational exposure in a general population. Results from the French PAARC study among 16,000 adults. Int J Epidemiol 1988;17:397–406.

56. Krzyzanowski M, Jedrychowski W, Wysocki M. Occupational exposures and changes in pulmonary function over 13 years among residents of Cracow. Br J Ind Med 1988;45:747–54.

57. Bakke P, Eide GE, Hanoa R, Gulsvik A. Occupational dust or gas exposure and prevalences of respiratory symptoms and asthma in a general population. Eur Respir J 1991;4:273–78.

58. Heederik D, Pouwels H, Kromhout H, Kromhout D. Chronic non-specific lung disease and occupational exposure estimated by means of a job exposure matrix: the Zutphen study. Int J Epidemiol 1989;18:382–89.

59. Heederik D, Kromhout H, Burema J, Biersteker K, Kromhout D.

Occupational exposure and 25-year incidence rate of non-specific lung disease: the Zutphen study. Int J Epidemiol 1990;19:945–52.

60. Heederik D, Kromhout H, Burema J, Biersteker K, Kromhout D. Relations between occupation, smoking, lung function, and incidence and mortality of chronic non-specific lung disease: the Zutphen study, Br J Ind Med 1992;49:299–300.

61. Pannett B, Coggon D, Acheson RED. A job exposure matrix for use in population based studies in England and Wales. Br J Ind Med 1985;42:777–83.

62. Rothman KJ. Modern epidemiology. Botson: Little, Brown, 1986.

63. Higginson J. Proportion of cancers due to occupation. Prev Med 1980;9:180–88.

# 8

# Epidemiology of Lung Cancer: Interaction Between Genetic Susceptibility and Environmental Risk Factors

ISABELLE STÜCKER,
DENIS HÉMON

INSERM U170
Villejuif, France

CATHERINE BONAITI-PELLIÉ

INSERM U155
Paris, France

## I.  Introduction

Bronchopulmonary cancer is at present the most common tumor in humans worldwide and the prime cause of death by cancer in over 35 countries. In 1980, lung cancer was estimated at about 16% of all new cases of cancer. This proportion does, however, vary by country. In Europe, lung cancer is thought to form about 23% of cancer cases. The highest annual incidences occur first in Europe (180/100,000), then in North America (91/10,000). In women, lung cancer takes sixth place among all types of cancer, and about 5% of new cancer cases are lung cancer. As with men, the highest annual incidence rates are in Europe (34/100,000) and North America (39/100,000) [1,2].

There is no doubt that tobacco presents the greatest lung cancer risk. The first evidence of the connection came from epidemiological research published in the 1950s. Many cohort studies in various countries between 1950 and 1965 showed a significantly higher risk of lung cancer in cigarette smokers, with a relative risk of around 10. In the framework of a large case-control study, Doll and Hill [3,4] showed clearly that the connection between lung cancer and the fact of smoking was causal, but added in their conclusion that this did not mean that tobacco smoke contributed to the development of all new cases of lung cancer, nor that it was the sole factor responsible for increased death rates.

In their conclusion, the multifactorial origin of lung cancer risk is clearly emphasized. It is a hypothesis that has subsequently been largely confirmed, as occupational factors do take a significant place in the etiology of lung cancers. According to population, it is thought that 5 to 35% of cases of lung cancer may be attributable to occupational exposure [5], with a estimate of 15% among males presented by Doll and Peto [6] lying approximately in the center of the wide range of estimates. Occupational factors likely to have an etiological role in lung cancer have been classified by the IARC as follows [7]:

Group 1: Agents Carcinogenic to Humans
Asbestos
Inorganic arsenic
Bis(chloromethyl) ether
Chloromethyl methyl ether
Hexavalent chromium compounds
Hematite mining
Mustard gas
Nickel refineries
Vinyl chloride
Soots, tars, and derivatives

Group 2A: Agents Probably Carcinogenic to Humans
Cadmium and certain derivatives
Nickel and certain derivatives

Group 2B: Agents Possibly Carcinogenic to Humans
Acrylonitrile
Amitrol
Beryllium and derivatives
Dimethyl sulfate

Despite the existence of certain prime risk factors in the etiology of lung cancer, it must be admitted that there is a very significant variability of risk among individuals. This variability is easily illustrated by the fact that the cumulative incidence of lung cancer in a population of smokers remains largely lower than 1. Several phenomena may be adduced to explain this variability. The first deals with the multiplicative effects, where individuals are exposed to several risk factors simultaneously. One well-known example in the literature is the risk concerning the joint exposure to tobacco and asbestos, as evaluated by Hammond et al. [8]. As shown in Table 1, the risk of lung cancer in a subject exposed simultaneously to tobacco and asbestos is approximately the product of

**Table 1** Relative Lung Cancer Risk According to Exposure to Tobacco and/or Asbestos

|  | Tobacco | |
| --- | --- | --- |
| Asbestos | No | Yes |
| No | 1 | 10.9 |
| Yes | 5.2 | 53.2 |

*Source:* Ref. 8.

risks of exposure from tobacco alone and asbestos alone. Similarly, other studies have shown the existence of multiplying effects of exposure to tobacco and radiation exposure [9,10].

In addition to the joint multiplying effects, there may also be effect modifications, which compared with the first, consist of a potentiation of the etiological factor in conjunction with another factor. In such situations the relative risk of lung cancer in subjects exposed to a first factor (P) will differ according to whether subjects are exposed (S+) or not (S–) to a second factor, S. Caporaso et al. [11] illustrate this phenomenon: In a case-control study of lung cancer risk in relation to the debrisoquine hydroxylation phenotype (S), Caporaso clearly shows that the odds ratio linked to PAH (P) or asbestos (P') exposure, are, respectively, 2.4 [95% confidence interval (CI): 0.8 to 7.4] and 2.9 (95% CI: 1.1 to 7.7) but markedly higher in S+ individuals than in S– individuals: odds ratio (OR) = 35.3 vs. 0.7 for PAH exposure and OR = 18.4 vs. 1.8 for asbestos, respectively.

It is clear that these factors, likely to bring about risk potentiation, may equally well be acquired or genetic. Among the acquired factors are age, food, life-style, and exposure to environmental agents. Genetic factors, on the other hand, may influence the metabolism of xenobiotics, skin color, or even defects in DNA repair (xeroderma pigmentosum). In this chapter we focus on genetic factors likely to have a significant influence on individual cancer risk.

## II. Biological Models of Genetic–Environment Interaction

Tobacco has various levels of influence in the process of carcinogenesis, and a person's response will depend not only on the intensity of exposure to which he or she is subjected, but also on the path taken by the carcinogen, tobacco in this case, in terms of absorption, distribution, metabolism, DNA adducts, DNA repair, and finally, of the tobacco role in the promotion and progression steps. Most of these stages are genetically controlled, which means that interactions between genotype and tobacco at each of these stages may ultimately influence individual susceptibility to cancer. Several studies have, for example, demonstrated wide individual variations in mucus production and quality, especially in its glycoprotein content, influencing the viscosity of the mucus and likely to affect the tobacco clearance rate of the lung [12]. Among all the stages listed above, the most studied is certainly that of xenobiotics metabolism. Most carcinogenic agents in the environment have to undergo metabolic activation to be carcinogenic. These substances, most of which are lipophiles, are transformed into more polar compounds before to be excreted by the organism. Most such reactions are oxidation reactions conditioned by the presence of enzymes. They lead to the formation of intermediary metabolites, some of which are carcinogens likely to react with the organism's macromolecules. These oxidation reactions are catalyzed mainly by P450 cytochrome enzymes.

Several enzymatic polymorphisms involved in the metabolism of environmental carcinogenic agents have been identified in the literature. The first polymorphism thus identified was that of the hepatic N-acetyl transferase enzyme in the 1950s. About 30 years later, discovery of the metabolism paths of arylamines, recognized carcinogens of the bladder, and in particular, the essential stage of acetylation have led several authors to look for an individual susceptibility to bladder cancer. Another polymorphism identified is that of cytochrome P4501A1 enzyme inducibility in the metabolism of polynuclear aromatic hydrocarbons. Others have subsequently been identified, in particular the glutathion S transferase polymorphism involved in detoxification of electrophile molecules, and that of the debrisoquine metabolism, which depends on cytochrome P4502D6. The relationship between these polymorphisms and susceptibility to lung cancer has been tested in several case-control studies, and we here summarize the approaches of the various authors, omitting, however, N-acetyl transferase polymorphism, which more specifically concerns bladder cancer.

### A.  Cytochrome P4501A1 Inducibility Polymorphism

Cytochromes P4501A1 and 1A2, induced by polynuclear aromatic hydrocarbons (PAH), transform these procarcinogenic substances into active carcinogens, at the same time as metabolizing a certain number of noninductive substances. Induction is under the control of the Ah locus, which encodes a cytosolic receptor capable of binding to inducers. Following translocation of the inducer–receptor complex into the nucleus, the expression of what have been called the [Ah] gene battery is augmented, including the P4501s [13–15]. Aryl hydrocarbon hydroxylase (AHH) activity probably corresponds to several isoenzymes, but essentially, to P4501A1. PAH products are capable of covalent combination with macromolecules, in particular DNA, the mechanism causing mutagenic and carcinogenic action.

On mice it has been shown that there is a polymorphism in the Ah locus connected with tumor formation [16]. After subcutaneous administration or intratracheal instillation of methylcholanthrene, mice of inducible strains locally develop a number of tumors well in excess of those of noninducible mice. For humans, Kellermann et al. [17] has shown that the distribution of AHH inducibility in the general population was trimodal and compatible with the existence of two codominant allelic forms. The study of this type of transmission from one generation to another in nuclear families has been shown to fit this model perfectly [17]. In addition, studies carried out on twins have shown a very strong correlation between monozygotic twins and a less strong one between dizygotic twins and thus prove the inheritability of the character [18]. The first case-control study to look for the existence of enhanced lung cancer risk in connection with this polymorphism was carried out by Kellermann et al. [19]. It showed a significant excess of high inducer individuals among the lung cancer group (OR = 36). Several case-control studies have subsequently been carried out. In total about 10 have been reviewed for this chapter [19–27]. To date, the results of these studies appear contradictory: Four studies have not found the risk noted by Kellermann, whereas six others have shown an excess of high inducer individuals among the cases, although still in less significant proportions than in the Kellermann study. Among these studies, Kouri [27] has shown twice as much induced activity among cases than among controls. In his study, Kouri had taken particular care to analyze all samples at the same time, to check on seasonal variations in measurement. Otherwise, it seems noteworthy that all these studies covered a relatively small number of subjects in most cases (around 50), and that most of them have taken wives of cases as controls, which could lead to confusion if the AHH activity measurement was related to sex.

### B.  Polymorphism of Glutathione S-Transferase

Glutathione S-transferase enzymes are involved in phase II metabolism. These proteins play a predominant role in the detoxification of intermediary electrophile metabolites. Thus, in general, the level of active carcinogens likely to react with DNA results from enzymatic competition between the processes of activation and detoxication. Mantel et al. (28) showed that there were in fact three GST classes relating to their "isoelectric points": GST-$\alpha$, GST-$\mu$, and GST-$\delta$. A study by Seidergard et al. [29] has shown the existence of a trimodal distribution of GST-$\mu$ activity in a population of 248 healthy individuals. A lung cancer case-control study also enabled him to show that subjects affected by lung cancer showed a significant reduction of GST mu activity compared with control subjects without cancer. This study seems to support the hypothesis that GST-$\mu$ is another factor regarding the susceptibility to PAH in the risk of lung cancer.

### C.  Polymorphism of Debrisoquine Metabolism

Debrisoquine is an antihypertension drug, the metabolism of which depends on the cytochrome P4502D6. The main metabolite is 4-hydroxydebrisoquine, and several studies have shown that there are wide variations of this metabolism among individuals. The distribution of the metabolic ratio (ratio of unchanged debrisoquine to 4-hydroxydebrisoquine) is clearly bimodal with two sub-populations: the extensive metabolizers (EMs), which represent about 90% of the population, and the poor metabolizers (PMs), 10%. Family studies have shown that this metabolism was dependent on a single autosomal locus compatible with a transmission of character on a recessive mode [30,31]. More recent studies have made it possible to locate the gene on chromosome 22 [32].

The first case-control study of the risk of lung cancer connected with this polymorphism was carried out by Ayesh et al. [33]. It showed that the EM frequency among patients affected by lung cancer was significantly higher than among controls (OR = 5.9), whereas the cases showed a significantly lower PM frequency. The case-control studies that followed showed less clear results: the EM excess in the case group compared with the control group was still not significant [34,35]. Duché et al. [36] did not find any difference in the EM frequency between the two groups. Finally, in a reanalysis of the Ayesh study, Caporaso et al. [11] have shown that relationships with the hydroxylation phenotype were even more important given that the histological type was linked to tobacco (squamous cell: OR = 7.9, small cell: OR = 12.7, adenocarcinoma: OR = 1.5) and showed a very marked increase of lung cancer risk with exposure to PAHs among EMs (OR = 35.3) compared with PMs (OR = 0.7).

The study of polymorphism of debrisoquine in relation to lung cancer, however, raises the question of the metabolic specificity of the association with regard to lung cancer. The cytochrome P4502D6 metabolizes many other drugs and chemical substances [37], and one hypothesis is that one of the constituents of tobacco has a metabolism passing via this cytochrome. A recent study by Crespi·et al. [38] seems to support this hypothesis, suggesting that 4(methyl-nitrosamino)-1-(3-pyridyl)-1-butanone (NNK), a carcinogenic tobacco deriva-tive, is activated by several P450s, including P4502D6.

### III.  Methodological Aspects

#### A.  Genotype–Environment Interaction Models

The methodology to evidence genotype–environment interaction depends partly on the underlying model. Khoury et al. [39] proposed six patterns of genotype–environment interactions which describe situations where a given genetic factor (single gene locus) may interact with an environmental agent in the occurrence of a disease (Table 2). In these models the susceptibility genotype and the

**Table 2** Disease Incidence as a Function of Exposure to Genotype G and Exposure E[a]

|        | $G^-$          | $G^+$            |
| ------ | -------------- | ---------------- |
| $E^-$  | $I$            | $R_g \times I$   |
| $E^+$  | $R_e \times I$ | $R_{ge} \times I$ |

[a] $G^-$, Subjects without the genotype; $G^+$, subjects with the genotype; $E^-$, nonexposed subjects; $E^+$, exposed subjects.

environmental exposure are both supposed to be dichotomous (present or absent). It is also assumed that the probability $f$ of exposure to the environmental agent is independent of the genotype and that among unexposed individuals without the susceptible genotype, there is a certain disease background risk $I$. The disease risk in each of the four categories, according to the presence or absence of the susceptibility genotype and the environmental agent, could be expressed in terms of relative risks in these different categories: $R_e$ the relative risk of disease for the exposure in the absence of the genotype, $R_g$ the relative risk of the genotype in the absence of exposure, and Rge the relative risk for exposed individuals with the genotype compared to unexposed people without the genotype.

In all situations, the highest risk of disease is associated with the presence of both genotype and environment ($R_{ge} > R_g$, $R_{ge} > R_e$), but no assumptions are made about the underlying statistical model of interaction. In the first pattern, individuals with the susceptibility genotype in the absence of exposure have the same risk $I$ as individuals without the genotype whatever their exposure ($R_g = R_e = 1$); only the category of individuals with both the genotype and the environment have an increased risk of the disease ($R_{ge} > 1$). In the second pattern of interaction, unexposed individuals whatever their genotype have the same risk of developing the disease ($R_g = 1$). Individuals without the genotype but exposed to the specific environmental agent have an increased risk ($R_e > 1$) with a still higher risk ($R_{ge} > R_e$) for individuals with both the genotype and the exposure. The third pattern is symmetrical to the second one: individuals without the genotype have the same risk $I$ of developing the disease, whatever their exposure ($R_e = 1$). Unexposed individuals with the genotype have a slightly higher risk ($R_g > 1$), the maximum risk being for the exposed category with the genotype ($R_{ge} > R_g$).

In the fourth pattern, both the genotype and the environment alone are associated with an increased risk of disease ($R_g > 1$, $R_e > 1$, $R_{ge} > R_g$, $R_{ge} > R_e$). The fifth and sixth patterns are somewhat different in that the smallest risk is for unexposed individuals with genotype ($R_g < 1$). In individuals without the genotype, there is no effect of exposure in pattern 5 ($R_e = 1$) and a positive effect of exposure in pattern 6 ($R_e > 1$).

There are very few examples of proven interaction of genotype and environment as shown by the particular examples given by Khoury et al. [39], where genotypes are most often rare (phenylketonuria, xeroderma pigmentosum) and environment exposure is either rare (succinylcholine administration during anesthesia) or, by contrast, universal (phenylalanine in the diet, exposure to sunlight). The example of sickle cell trait and its advantage in the case of malaria for the fifth pattern is not very convincing. However, this kind of interaction is strongly suspected in many examples with a less extreme contrast, as in the case of cytochrome P4501A1 inducibility and PAH exposure, where genotypes form around 10% of the general population and PAH (through tobacco exposure) around 70% for males. This particular model fits well with the second pattern proposed by Khoury, when $R_e$ (i.e., relative risk of smoking to lung cancer among low inducers) is $> 1$ and $R_g$ (i.e., relative risk of high inducibility among nonsmokers not exposed to environmental HPA) is 1 also and with an attempted $R_{ge}$ (relative risk for smoking and high inducers) $>> 1$. This model could also be considered an example of the fourth pattern if we assume that $R_g > 1$, considering the likely pleiotropia of the gene.

Khoury et al. [40] studied the variation in the relative risk associated with the genotype, when exposure is neglected, according to the frequency of exposure $f$ and the relative risks $R_{ge}$, $R_g$, or $R_e$ in the different patterns. He showed that the importance of genotype in disease etiology depends on the underlying model and may not be appreciated in numerous examples. As a consequence, the disease should exhibit a variable but most often low degree of familial aggregation [41], which is the usual criterion for suspecting the existence of a genetic factor not yet identified. Similar conclusions had been reached when studying the role of environmental factors and neglecting differential genetic susceptibility in disease etiology [42]. This is particularly the case when the susceptible genotype is not as rare as in most hereditary diseases, and the environmental exposure is neither universal, nor exceptional, which is probably the situation in those diseases with complex etiology that are suspected to be partly explained by an interaction between a genetic factor and a specific environmental agent.

As an illustration, let us consider a disease partly explained by the interaction between a "susceptible" allele "a" ("normal" allele A) and an environmental agent X, where allele a frequency and exposure frequency are both equal to 0.10. Suppose that alleles a and A have a codominant effect, that is, the heterozygotes Aa have an intermediate risk between homozygotes AA and aa (a model close to the model proposed by Kellermann et al. [19] for arylhydrocarbon inducibility by polynuclear aromatic hydrocarbons and its relation to lung cancer). Let us assume that unexposed individuals have a 0.001 risk of disease whatever their genotype, and that exposed individuals have risks

0.001, 0.01, and 0.1 when their genotypes are AA, Aa, and aa, respectively. Therefore, the genotypes Aa and aa confer a 10-fold and a 100-fold increased risk of the disease, respectively, as compared to the genotype AA. In the population, the frequency of AA, Aa, and aa individuals are 0.81, 0.18, and 0.01, respectively. The frequency of affected AA is 0.00081 (0.81 × 0.001) whatever their exposure. The frequency of affected Aa is 0.00018 (0.18 × 0.001) if they are unexposed and 0.0018 (0.18 × 0.01) if they are exposed to the agent X. The frequency of affected aa is 0.00001 (0.01 × 0.001) if they are unexposed and 0.001 (0.01 × 0.1) if they are exposed to the agent X. The overall frequency of the disease is thus

$$0.00081 + 0.9(0.00018 + 0.00001) + 0.1(0.0018 + 0.001) = 0.00126$$

The frequency among exposed individuals is 3.61 ‰ (0.00081 + 0.0018 + 0.001). The expected marginal relative risk associated with the agent X is thus 3.61. On the other hand, the probability of being affected for a carrier of the a allele (genotypes aa and Aa) is

$$\frac{0.18(0.9 \times 0.001 + 0.1 \times 0.01) + 0.01(0.9 \times 0.001 + 0.1 \times 0.1)}{0.19} = 0.00237$$

Thus the expected marginal relative risk associated with the "susceptible" allele is 2.37. Familial aggregation is almost absent in such a model. Indeed, the recurrence risk in siblings can be calculated using the ITO matrices of Li and Sachs [43], which provide the probability $P_{ij}$ that an individual has genotype $j$, given that his sibling has genotype $i$. Without any information on environmental exposure, the recurrence risk is 1.75‰, which leads to a relative risk of 1.4 compared to the general population. Interestingly, this risk is substantially modified when exposure is taken into account in both proband and siblings. When siblings are unexposed, their risk is simply 1.0‰, as with all unexposed individuals, whatever the exposure of the proband. If siblings are exposed to the environmental agent, their risk depends on whether the proband was exposed. If the proband was not exposed, there is no information on his genotype, and the risk for an exposed sibling is the same as for every exposed individual in the population: 3.6‰. On the other hand, when both proband and sibling are exposed, the proband, and consequently his siblings, have more chance of having genotypes aa or Aa, so that the recurrence risk in siblings becomes as high as 15.0‰ (relative risk 15), which enhances the degree of familial aggregation.

## B. Strategies to Evidence a Genotype–Environment Interaction

Such strategies must take into account the factors that have already been evidenced as possibly involved in the etiology of the disease, the possible existence of animal models, and the degree of knowledge we may have on the causal relationship between the risk factors and the disease as well as the variability of both exposure and genetic susceptibility.

If nothing at all is known about the disease, there is little chance of evidencing a genotype–environment interaction. So we will assume that at least one environmental agent has already been evidenced or suspected of playing a role in the etiology of the disease. Note that this environmental agent may have been difficult to evidence because of a low marginal relative risk, but may also have a major effect. For example, the existence of a strong relationship between tobacco and lung cancer does not imply that there is no differential susceptibility to tobacco, due to genetic factors, for developing lung cancer.

### Familial Clustering

We have seen above that familial aggregation was barely expected in the majority of models with genotype–environment interaction. This means that the absence of familial aggregation is not an argument against the role of a genetic factor. On the other hand, the existence of a high degree of familial aggregation must lead one to suspect the role of a major genetic factor (or cultural transmission mimicking genetic inheritance), with a possible minor role of environmental agents. Indeed, the presence of familial aggregation is the consequence of the correlation between relatives for a genetic trait. Even in Mendelian traits, the correlation is never more than half and decreases rapidly with the degree of relationship between relatives and the complexity of the model [44]. So this is a very indirect indicator of the existence of genetic factors.

However, we have also seen above that taking into account the exposure in both patients and relatives could improve power to detect familial clustering and could thus be a first step to investigating gene susceptibility to this agent. Such a power increase is expected only if a clear interaction (of the effect modification type) exists between the exposure and genetic characteristic and if the frequency of exposure in the general population is not very low, as for some occupational factors.

Regarding lung cancer, the existence of a family recurrence risk was shown for the first time in the study by Tokuhata and Lilienfeld [45]. More recently, the study by Ooi et al. [46] shows similarly that the risk of developing lung cancer after adjustment for tobacco, sex, and occupational exposure is 2.4 when one is a first-degree relative of an affected individual. However, this study does not identify the risks of recurrence in relatives according to whether they themselves and the proband were smokers or not.

If it is probable according to these results that there is a family component in the etiology of lung cancer, this does not seem as important as in examples such as retinoblastoma, for which numerous studies have shown the existence of a strong predisposition consistent with the effect of an autosomal dominant gene in 40% of cases.

## Evidence for a Genetic Factor

Suppose that there are sufficient arguments for suspecting the role of a genetic factor either because of successful evidencing of familial clustering or because there is a good animal model. If this genetic factor has not yet been identified, one may be tempted to use the information provided by the numerous genetic markers that have been found on the genome, using molecular biology [as restriction fragment length polymorphism (RFLP)]. These genetic markers, which are polymorphic traits segregating in a Mendelian manner, represent reference marks which can be useful to locate other genes.

### Strategy of Systematic Screening

The strategy of systematic screening of the genome has been proven to be very useful in locating genes of Mendelian diseases (e.g., cystic fibrosis [47] and neurofibromatosis [48]) through family studies using linkage analysis [49]. The principle of the method used is to test if the genetic marker segregates independently of the disease in families with at least one, and most often several, affected case(s). If independent segregation is rejected, it proves that a genetic susceptibility gene is located close to the genetic marker on the genome. However, this strategy raises some problems in the case of diseases involving several interacting risk factors.

The power of the method decreases very rapidly as the relationship between the underlying genotype and the disease becomes ambiguous. Whereas this relation is very clear for Mendelian diseases, with probabilities of phenotypes given genotypes almost always equal to 0 or 1, it is not the case for diseases with complex etiology. A way of increasing power in such a situation is to focus on multiple-case families, which, however, may be rare in the type of model we are investigating. Moreover, the true underlying disease model is usually unknown, which has several consequences on the power and robustness of the method. The power to detect genetic linkage (i.e., to evidence the existence of a susceptibility gene close to the marker) may be greatly reduced [50]. On the other hand, the method is robust to a misspecification of the genetic model for linkage conclusion but not for linkage exclusion [51,52]. In other words, there is little chance of detecting an existing susceptibility gene and a high risk of excluding the existence of a susceptibility gene in a region where it is really located.

Because of these numerous disadvantages and of the small number of informative families, one may be tempted by a case-control approach: to compare the marker allele or genotype frequencies in patients and in controls. Other kinds of problems are encountered using this approach. The rationale of this method is that under the hypothesis that a genetic factor is close to a genetic marker somewhere on the genome, one expects some degree of linkage disequilibrium (i.e., nonindependent distribution of alleles at marker and disease loci in the population). Such a disequilibrium may exist only if the genetic distance between the two loci is very small [less than 2 cM (centimorgans)]. Thus to be efficient, genetic markers should be typed at least every 2 cM. The limitation of such a strategy is that there are numerous regions of the genome, greater than 2 cM, where no genetic markers have been found. Moreover, since the length of the genome is about 3000 cM, one should investigate 1500 markers: The necessary correction for multiple tests would greatly reduce the power to detect the association. Finally, even when two genetic loci are very close to each other, the degree of linkage disequilibrium may be so small as to be undetectable [53]. For all these reasons, we think that for the study of most diseases with complex etiology, the strategy of systematic mapping of the genome will often be inefficient at the present time and that a "candidate gene" strategy should be preferred.

### Strategy of Candidate Gene

It may indeed be logical and efficient to investigate whether some genes, which may be functionally related to the disease, represent risk factors for the disease and have some chance of playing a role in interaction with the environmental factor(s) evidenced. In the example of susceptibility to PAH and lung cancer, all those genes that encode enzymes which are likely to toxify them through oxidation reactions such as enzymes of the cytochrome P450 system are candidate genes. The best candidates are, of course, the P4501A1 and 1A2, which are known to code for proteins that metabolize PAH into ultimate carcinogens, but other candidate genes may also be considered. When such candidates have been selected, the strategy depends on the possibility of measuring the expression of the gene: enzyme activity, quantity of transcript, or quantity of product. One must be sure, however, that the phenotype choosen is related as closely as possible to the genotype; in other words, this phenotype should not be too much influenced by life-long environmental exposures or constitutional factors such as age or health status. In all cases, a compromise will have to be found according to how informative the measurement is on the genotype concerned and the difficulty of measurement, which will have to be repeated on a great number of individuals. In this situation, the most efficient strategy is to investigate the degree of polymorphism and the genetic determinism through a family study in the normal population (because of the absence of selection bias) and to evaluate the relative risks given genotype and environmental exposure through a case-control study, which will have to be large enough to provide sufficient subjects according to exposure and genotype status.

In many cases the expression of the gene related to the susceptibility of the environmental agent cannot be (or is not easily) measured directly. In this situation, genetic markers located close to the candidate gene, or on the gene itself, can be used as indicators of the susceptibility genotypes. Case-control studies as well as family studies can be carried out. Because the a priori chance that a candidate gene is involved in the etiology of the disease is much greater than for a random marker gene, a lot of criticisms of the systematic screening strategy do not apply. Moreover, the information on both association and linkage may be taken into account simultaneously using the marker association segregation chi-squares (MASC) method proposed by Clerget-Darpoux et al. [54]. Compared with methods that test either association or linkage alone, this method has been shown to increase power greatly to test the involvement of a candidate gene.

Taking account of all these considerations, it seems to us that the formation of a DNA bank may be a good way of providing a return on the investment that carrying out these family studies or case controls may represent. The availability in the relatively near future of new molecular probes will actually make it possible to test new genetic–environment interaction hypotheses without having to use phenotypic expression of the gene and on already existing material.

## IV. Conclusions

At the present time a candidate gene strategy is obviously the most efficient one to evidence a possible genetic susceptibility to an environmental factor to develop a disease such as lung cancer. Study of biotransformation of potent carcinogens is one possible way of defining such candidate genes. The inducibility of cytochrome P4501A1 in the metabolism of PAHs is a good example from this point of view of an approach by candidate gene. Knowledge of the PAH toxification mechanism and its link with carcinogenesis, of the underlying genetic model suspected from the animal model and verified in humans, and the possibility of measuring its phenotypic expression, also compatible with a large number of measurements, are all elements leading to the selection of a candidate gene. This does not, however, rule out the possibility of other candidate genes in the context of genetic–environmental interaction in lung cancer (e.g., GST polymorphism or DNA repair). This is indeed both the potential interest and the difficulty of this approach, as the number of steps of the carcinogenic process that are under genetic control may be very high indeed.

In conclusion, for a factor to be likely to influence the risk of cancer, two conditions are necessary: The factor should be involved in the mechanism connecting exposure to the environmental agent to the disease (i.e., it should represent a limiting stage in the occurrence of the disease), and it should be variable among individuals. In all cases, three elements of what we could call the triangle characteristic of genotype–environment interaction must be identified: (1) a disease, (2) an environmental agent associated with the disease, and (3) a biological mechanism with some degree of polymorphism, genetically determined and susceptible to modifying the action of the environmental agent in development of the disease.

### References

1. Parkin DM. Trends in lung cancer incidence worldwide. Chest 1989;96(1):5S–8S.
2. Stanley K, Stjernswärd J. Lung cancer. A worldwide health problem. Chest 1989;96(1):1S–5S.
3. Doll R, Hill AB. Smoking and carcinoma of the lung. Br Med J 1950;2:739–48.
4. Doll R, Hill AB. A study of the aetiology of the lung. Br Med J 1952;2:1271–86.
5. Pastorino U, Berrino F, Gervasio A, Pesenti V, Riboli E, Crosignani P. Proportion of lung cancers due to occupational exposure. Int J Cancer 1984;33:231–37.
6. Doll R, Peto R. The causes of cancer: quantitative estimates of avoidable risks of cancer in the United States today. Oxford: Oxford University Press, 1981.
7. IARC monographs on the evaluation of the carcinogenic risk of chemicals to humans. Suppl. 7. Lyon, France: IARC, 1987.
8. Hammond EC, Selikoff IJ, Seidman H. Asbestos exposure, cigarette smoking and death rates. Ann NY Acad Sci 1979;330:473–90.
9. Lundin FE, Lloyd WJ, Smith EM, Archer VE, Holaday DA. Mortality of uranium miners in relation to radiation exposure, hard-rock mining and cigarette smoking: 1950 through September 1967. Health Phys 1969;16:571–79.
10. Edling C, Kling H, Axelsson O. Radon in homes. A possible cause of lung cancer. Scand J Work Environ Health 1984;10:25–34.
11. Caporaso N, Hayes RB, Dosemeci M, Hoover R, Ayesh R, Heztel M, Idle J. Lung cancer risk, occupational exposure, and the debrisoquine metabolic phenotype. Can Res 1989;49:3675–79.
12. IARC monographs on the evaluation of the carcinogenic risk of chemicals to humans. Vol. 38. Lyon, France: IARC, 1986.
13. Pelkonen O, Nebert DW. Metabolism of polycyclic aromatic hydrocarbons: etiologic role in carcinogenesis. Pharmacol Rev 1982;34:190–222.
14. Gonzales FJ, Jaiswal AK, Nebert DW. P450 genes: evolution, regulation,

and the relationship to human cancer and pharmacogenetics. Cold Spring Harbor Symp Quant Biol 1987;51:879–90.

15.    Nebert DW, Adesnick M, Coon MC, Estabrook RW, Gonzalez FJ, Guenguerich FP, Gunsalus IC, Johnson EF, Kemper B, Levin W, Phillips IR, Sato R, Waterman MR. The P450 gene superfamily: recommended nomenclature. DNA Cell Biol 1987;6:1–11.

16.    Kouri RE, Nebert DW. Genetic regulation of susceptibility to polycyclic hydrocarbon induced tumors in the mouse. In: Origins of human cancer. Cold Spring Harbor, NY: Cold Spring Harbor Laboratory, 1977:811–35.

17.    Kellermann G, Luyten-Kellermann M, Shaw CR. Genetic variation of aryl hydrocarbon hydroxylase in human lymphocytes. Am J Hum Genet 1973;25:327–31.

18.    Okuada T, Vessel ES, Plotkin E, et al. Interindividual and intraindividual variations in aryl hydrocarbons hydroxylase in monocytes from monozygoic and dizygotic twins. Cancer Res 1977;37:3904–11.

19.    Kellermann G, Shaw CR, Luyten-Kellermann M. Aryl hydrocarbon hydroxylase inducibility and bronchogenic carcinoma. N Engl J Med 1973;289:934–37.

20.    Guirgis HA, Lynch HT, Mate T, et al. Aryl hydrocarbon hydroxylase activity in lymphocytes from lung cancer patients and normal controls. Oncology 1976;33:105–9.

21.    McLemor TL, Martin RR, Busbee DL. Aryl hydrocarbon hydroxylase activity in pulmonary macrophages and lymphocytes from lung cancer and noncancer patients. Cancer Res 1977;37:1175–81.

22.    Paigen B, Gurtoo HL, Minowada J et al. Questionable relation of aryl hydrocarbon hydroxylase to lung cancer risk. N Engl J Med 1977;297:346–50.

23.    Emery AE, Anand R, Danford N, Duncan W, Paton L. Aryl hydrocarbon hydroxylase inducibility in patients with cancer. Lancet 1978;1:470–71.

24.    Ward E, Paigen B, Steenland K, et al. Aryl hydrocarbon hydroxylase in persons with lung or laryngeal cancer. Int J Cancer 1978;22:384–89.

25.    Ghamberg LG, Sekki A, Kosunen TU, Holsti LR, Makela O. Induction of aryl hydrocarbon hydroxylase activity in pulmonary carcinoma. Int J Cancer 1979;23:302–5.

26.    Prasad R, Prasad N, Harrel JE, Thornby J, Liem JH, Hudgins PT, Tsuang J. Aryl hydrocarbon hydroxylase inducibility and lymphoblast formation in lung cancer patients. Int J Cancer 1979;23:316–20.

27.    Koury RE, McKinney CE, Slomiany DR, Snodgrass, NP, Wray NP, McLemor TL. Positive correlation between high aryl hydrocarbon hydroxylase activity and primary lung cancer as analysed in cryopreserved lymphocytes. Cancer Res 1982;42:5030–37.

28.   Mantle TJ, Pickett CB, Hayes JD, eds. Gluthatione S-transferases and carcinogenesis. London: Taylor & Francis, 1987.

29.   Seidergard J, Pero R. The hereditary transmission of high gluthatione transferase activity towards silbene oxide in human mononuclear lymphocytes. Hum Genet 1985;69:66–68.

30.   Evans DA, Mahgoub A, Sloan TP, Idle JR, Smith RL. A family and population study of the genetic polymorphism of debrisoquin oxidation in a white British population. J Med Genet 1980;17:102–5.

31.   Steiner E, Iselius L, Alvan G, Lindsten J, Sjoqvist F. A family study of genetic and environmental factors determining polymorphic hydroxylation of debrisoquin. Clin Pharmacol Ther 1985;38:394–400.

32.   Eichelbaum M, Baur MP, Dengler HJ, et al. Chromosomal assignment of human chromosome P-450 (debrisoquine/sparteine type) to chromosome 22. Br J Clin Pharmacol 1987;23:455.

33.   Ayesh R, Idle JR, Ritchie JC, Crothers MJ, Hetzel MR. Metabolic oxidation phenotypes as markers for susceptibility to lung cancer. Nature 1984;312:169–70.

34.   Roots I, Drakoulis N, Ploch M, Heinemeyer G, Loddenkemper R, Minks T, Nitz M, Otte F, Koch M. Debrisoquine hydroxylation phenotype, acetylation phenotype, and ABO blood groups as genetic host factors of lung cancer risk. Klin Wochenschr 1988;66:87–97.

35.   Law MR, Hetzel MR, Idle JR. Debrisoquine metabolism and genetic predisposition to lung cancer. Br J Cancer 1989;59:686–87.

36.   Duche JC, Joanne C, Barre J, de Cremoux H, Dalphin JC, Depierre A, Brochard P, Tillement JP, Bechtel P. Lack of relationship between the polymorphism of debrisoquine oxidation and lung cancer. Br J Clin Pharmacol 1991;31:533–36.

37.   Eichelbaum M. Polymorphic drug oxydation in humans. Fed Proc 1984;43:2298.

38.   Crespi CL, Penman BW, Gelboin HV, Gonzalez FJ. A tobacco smoke-derived nitrosamine, 4-(methylnitrosamino)-1-(3-pyridyl)-1-butanone, is activated by multiple human cytochrome P450s including the polymorphic human cytochrome P4502D6. Carcinogenesis 1991;

39.   Khoury MJ, Adams MJ Jr, Flanders WD. An epidemiologic approach to ecogenetics. Am J Hum Genet 1988;42:89–95.

40.   Khoury MJ, Flanders WD, Beaty TH. Penetrance in the presence of genetic susceptibility to environmental factors. Am J Med Genet 1988;29:397–403.

41.   Khoury MJ, Beaty TH. Recurrence risks in the presence of single gene susceptibility to environmental agents. Am J Med Genet 1987;28:159–69.

42.   Khoury MJ, Stewart W, Beaty TH. The effect of genetic susceptibility on

causal inference in epidemiologic studies. Am J Epidemiol 1987;126:561–67.

43. Li C, Sacks L. The derivation of the joint distribution and correlation between relatives by the use of stochastic matrices. Biometrics 1954;10:347–60.

44. Falconer DS. The inheritance of liability to certain diseases estimated from the incidence among relatives. Am Hum Genet 1965;29:51–76.

45. Tokuata GK, Lilienfeld AM. Familial aggregation of lung cancer in humans. J Natl Cancer Inst 1963;30:289–312.

46. Ooi WL, Elston RC, Chen VW, Bailey-Wilson JE, Rotschild H. Increased familial risk for lung cancer J Natl Cancer Inst 1986;76:217–22.

47. Tsui LC, Buchwald M, Barker D, Braman JC, Knowlton R, Schumm JW, et al. Cystic fibrosis locus defined by a genetically linked polymorphic DNA marker. Science 1985;230:1054–57.

48. Barker D, Wright E, Nguyen K, Cannon L, Fain P, Goldgar D, et al. Gene for Recklinghausen neurofibromatosis is in the pericentromeric region of chromosome 17. Science 1987;236:1110–02.

49. Ott J. Analysis of human genetic linkage. Baltimore: Johns Hopkins University Press, 1985.

50. Clerget-Darpoux F, Bonaïti-Pellié C, Hochez J. Effects of misspecifying genetic parameters in load score analysis. Biometrics 1986;42:393–99.

51. Clerget-Darpoux F, Govaerts A, Feingold N. HLA and susceptibility to multiple sclerosis. Tissue Antigens 1984;24:160–69.

52. Martinez M, Goldin LR. The detection of linkage and heterogeneity in nuclear families for complex disorders; one vs. two marker loci. Am J Hum Genet 1989;44:552–59.

53. Thompson SA, Deeb S, Walker D, Motulsky AG. The detection of linkage disequilibrium between closely linked markers: RFLPs at the AI-CIII apolipoprotein genes. Am J Hum Genet 1988;42:113–24.

54. Clerget-Darpoux F, Babron M-C, Prum B, Lathrop GM, Deschamps I, Hors J. A new method to test genetic models in HLA associated diseases: the MASC method. Ann Hum Genet 1988;52:247–58.

# 9

# Measurement of Occupational Exposure and Prevention: Principal Approaches to Research

MARCEL GOLDBERG and PAQUERETTE GOLDBERG

INSERM U88
Paris, France

## I.   Measurement of Occupational Exposure: A Vast Field of Research

Occupation-related factors play an important part in both acute and chronic respiratory diseases. The impact of occupational factors is well documented, and estimates of the proportion of the principal respiratory diseases that can be attributed to them are available. Although these estimates are under constant revision, they are sometimes impressively high, as seen in certain chapters of this book. Strong scientific arguments are thus available for organizing prevention in the workplace by reducing the levels of exposure to several chemical and physical factors—even eliminating them completely if necessary and possible.

It is reasonable to suppose that the most obviously harmful substances and procedures have already been identified, and that before utilization in industry new substances undergo more thorough toxicological evaluations than in the past. However, a great many problems remain to be solved to ensure the surveillance of workers exposed to toxic substances and to identify yet unknown pathogenic factors. This involves assessing whether the occupational exposure to known toxic substances is maintained at a level at which the pathogenic risk is negligible. It also involves detecting the toxic effects of exposure to occupational factors and specifying these effects: the existence of a threshold under which no effect is detectable, the joint effect of simultaneous exposure to other factors, and modification of the effects according to various individual parameters of the exposed subjects.

Ideally, these undertakings require information concerning the internal dose of the toxic substance absorbed by the subject, the distribution and biotransformation of the substance, the fixation on critical sites of action, the biological mechanisms that induce the toxic biological effects, and the preclinical and clinical lesions. Full knowledge of such a cycle would theoretically provide all the elements for organizing the surveillance and prevention among workers exposed to toxic factors. In practice, this is far from the case. Several thousand different substances are used in industry, the conditions of exposure are often variable, and many personal parameters are involved in the toxicity. A vast field of research is thus open to various researchers, including physiologists, biologists, immunologists, geneticists, toxicologists, industrial hygienists, and epidemiologists, all of whom are concerned by the many scientific questions raised.

The one element upon which all the others depend is the dose absorbed by the individual, since it represents the initial stage of the toxic cycle. This is not as simple as it appears given the difficulty involved with human experimentation. It entails measurement of the substance actually absorbed when exposure conditions are extremely variable, the exact chemical composition of the substances to which the workers are exposed is often unknown, and in many cases the substances were absorbed several years, even decades, before a clinical or biological effect is observed.

In this chapter we present a review of the general principles and essential approaches to research involved in the work carried out on this subject, which can be entitled the "measurement of occupational exposures." Although the methods presented here refer to the study of respiratory diseases, they are not specific to studies of such diseases.

## II.   Some General Difficulties with the Measurement of Occupational Exposure

Currently, in most countries, before a new substance intended for industry is put on the market, a toxicological study must be carried out. Although the principal short-term toxic effects can be identified in this way, one can never be certain that a substance is harmless under real conditions of utilization. Neither can one be sure that there are no long-term effects. The problems discussed in this chapter thus concern the measurement of exposures in humans at work, in real situations. The practical problems are obviously different in situations in which exposure to an agent of known toxicity is monitored and in situations involving the identification of yet unknown toxic factors. In the first case, a certain amount of knowledge that may be modified (by subsequent research) is available regarding the biological mechanisms of toxicity and the permissible levels of exposure for the workers.

Efforts will be made then to define the biological indicators of exposure and/or the captors of external exposure (as described later), to check that the permissible exposure or absorption levels have not been exceeded. It is much more difficult to identify factors for which the toxicity has not yet been established and to determine whether a substance suspected of being toxic to humans is indeed toxic, and if so, under which conditions of exposure (level, duration, intensity, etc.). To understand the general principles related to research into the methods of measuring exposure adapted to these objectives (identification, confirmation, and determination of toxicity of substances used in industry), which involve mainly epidemiological methods, it is necessary to consider the pathogenic mechanisms involved, the usual exposure conditions in the workplace, and the statistical methods of analyzing exposure data in relation to clinical manifestations.

### A. Pathogenic Mechanisms

The great diversity of pathogenic mechanisms associated with the toxicity of a physical, chemical, or biological agent has a considerable effect on the measurement of occupational exposure. The principal elements that may be taken into account are the time from exposure to the manifestation of disease (especially the existence and duration of a latency period between exposure to the toxic agent and the detectable disease manifestation); the presence or absence of an age effect (variable toxicity according to the period of the life cycle during which the subject is exposed, including possible toxicity in children following exposure of a parent); the presence or absence of a threshold effect and a dose effect or dose–response relationship; the possibly different role of continuous and intermittent exposures; and the existence of a joint effect of the substance used with other exposures (potentiation or inhibition). Each of these factors will determine the methods used to measure the occupational exposure, to take into account the time (period of exposure, duration, permanent or repetitive exposure), and the intensity of exposure.

### B. Real Conditions of Exposure

In practice, conditions of exposure to toxic agents in the workplace have little in common with those reproduced in the laboratory. Many elements may modify the absorbed doses. These include the environment of the workstation (temperature, lack of space, ventilation, neighboring pollution), work conditions (e.g., the rhythm of work, which may have an effect on the physiology and modify the intensity of absorption of the toxic agent), general or individual hygiene (which may lead to cutaneous or oral absorption of toxic substances), availability and facility of use of collective or individual protective equipment (e.g., gloves, masks), and illicit working practices contrary to hygiene recommendations undertaken to work faster or more comfortably. It is important to note that exposure to a specific toxic chemical substance is very rare. Exposure usually occurs in a complex industrial environment in which substances are mixed, the exact conditions of temperature are unknown, the use of certain procedures may modify the composition or structure of the substances used, and the exact composition of the absorbed substance is not known. In addition, it should be noted that a single occupational exposure is rare. One task or successive tasks involve exposure to several substances in varying quantities. Thus simultaneous and/or sequential multiple exposures are the most usual occurrence. Finally, a particular problem encountered in epidemiological studies on the long-term effects of a toxic factor is that the exposure may have occurred long before the onset of the disease manifestation (sometimes 20 or 30 years before).

### C.  Difficulties with Statistical Analysis

An immediate and massive toxic effect is easily identifiable. The same applies when the effect is delayed but strong, especially if it results in a specific disease manifestation. However, current research involves primarily the identification of pathogenic factors with weak effects (corresponding to relative risks of little above 1) related to common diseases for which other interfering factors exist and which occur long after exposure. This leads to considerable difficulties in detecting possible toxic effects due to statistical concepts of the power and bias of the study.

The *power* of a study is defined as the ability to detect an effect if it exists in reality. If the exposure to a certain toxic substance increases the risk of developing a given disease, the power of this study will be the probability that at the end of the study an increase in risk will indeed be observed in the subjects exposed. Before carrying out the study, this probability is calculated according to several parameters, including the frequency of exposure, the number of subjects in the study, the magnitude of the expected effect, and the frequency of the disease in certain cases. The study will, of course, be carried out only if the probability of observing a real effect is considered to be sufficiently high. A *bias* is defined as an error that modifies the result of a study by producing a systematic over- or underestimate of the risk of developing the disease, compared to the reality.

A *good study* is thus a study with a strong power and no bias. However, factors related to the quality of exposure measurements may, along with others, lead to biases and a decrease in power. Two main aspects to be taken into account are the precision of the measurement itself and the misclassification of the subjects with regard to the exposure (unexposed considered as exposed, and vice versa). The poor quality of an exposure measurement (imprecision) results in a decrease in the power of the study [1,2]. Misclassification also leads to biases and/or loss of power [3–5]. These problems are not in any way theoretical, and their effects on epidemiological results can be quite spectacular [6,7]. Methods have been developed to minimize their consequences [8–11], but in most real situations they are not very effective. Although bias and loss of power may produce only a slight effect when the toxic effect is very strong, this is not the case when the toxic effect is weak and may not be detected.

The main sources of imprecision and error are related to the measuring instrument, to the investigator, and to the factors to be measured. The measuring instruments may be of poor quality. Precision, accuracy, and reproducibility are the main parameters that allow the quality of a measuring instrument to be assessed. These parameters can be assessed and the results of the assessments used to improve the quality of the instrument ("quality control").

The investigators who use the measuring instrument are themselves subject to variations, which can lead to imprecision and errors even if the instrument is excellent. A given investigator measuring the same factor at successive intervals may obtain different results ("intra-investigator" variation). Several investigators measuring a given factor might obtain different results ("inter-investigator" variation). To compensate for these imperfections, or at least to quantify them and take them into account in the analysis and interpretation of the results, procedures of follow-up and analysis of the sources of variability must be set up. Furthermore, the investigators must be given good training.

The factors studied (subjects enrolled in the studies, workstations, etc.) are subject to variation and intra- and intersubject variability are also observed. A good understanding of the factors studied and their "natural" variability is necessary to establish measurement protocols. It is often possible to overcome these difficulties either by including a sufficient number of subjects (or workstations) since the number of observations compensates for the effect of the natural variability of the factor studied, or by repeating the series of measurements with a frequency adapted to the variability over time of the factor [12], and by choosing groups of workers in such a way that intra- and intergroup variability are taken into account [2]. A detailed analysis of these aspects can be found in articles by Rappaport [13] and Kauppinen [14].

The objective of much research is thus to develop methods able to provide measurements to determine different indicators of exposure according to the pathogenic mechanisms involved. These indicators include the cumulative dose, the mean dose, and values above a threshold. For instance, the cumulative dose is often the best index of exposure for the study of long-term effects, such as cancer; it may show that intermittent exposures or peak exposures are better correlated with immunological problems [14,15]. Indicators must often take into account time variables, such as date of first exposure, time elapsed between exposure and onset of disease, total duration of exposure, and time windows of exposure [16]. The measurements must also correspond as much as possible to real exposure conditions, and they must be precise and valid. In addition, they must often be carried out on a large scale (several hundreds, even thousands, or tens of thousands of subjects, as in certain recent epidemiological studies). The measurements must therefore be easy to carry out under conditions of rigorous standardization, with the full cooperation of the workers and employers.

## III. Various Approaches to the Measurement of Occupational Exposure

The techniques used are based on extremely different methods according to whether the measurement involves the dose actually absorbed by the subject, or the levels at which the employees are exposed. In the first case, biological indicators are used, whereas in the second case measurements of the environment are undertaken. It will be seen that the term *measurement of the environment* has a wide definition, including methods by which the exposure data are indirectly assessed.

### A. Biological Indicators of Occupational Exposure

Biological indicators of occupational exposure are used to assess the internal dose absorbed by the entire organism or by a specific site of action.* The dose may have been absorbed a short time before the sampling (minutes, hours, or days before), or during the previous months for substances with a sufficiently long biological half-life, or during still longer periods for substances that accumulate in certain tissues (bone, fat tissue, etc.).

Biological measurements of exposure are theoretically the best measurements for understanding and monitoring toxic factors [18]. They are the most appropriate measurements for assessing a general or specific toxic effect, since they correspond to the dose actually absorbed. Unlike environmental measurements, they enable all exposure routes (inhalation, skin penetration, oral ingestion) to be taken into consideration. Biological measurements cover all sources of exposure, including nonoccupational exposures (household products, tobacco, environmental pollution). These measurements enable the investigator

---

*This chapter deals only with biological markers of exposure. The indicators of early effects and indicators of individual susceptibility, on which much research has been carried out [17], are not discussed here despite their great importance in understanding the toxic effects of industrial substances.

to take into account various factors related to real conditions of exposure (wearing individual protective equipment, environment of the workstation) as well as certain factors affecting penetration and absorption (ventilation, dust granulometry, individual differences in absorption and metabolism such as sex, height, and weight; physiological state; genetic variations).

However, to define reliable and appropriate biological indicators, it is necessary to have a wide knowledge of respective substances regarding the metabolism, mechanism of action, and relationships between external exposure, internal dose, and toxic effect. This is far from the case for most substances encountered in the industrial environment (for a particularly comprehensive review of available indicators, see refs. 17 to 19). The objective of most research has been to study the relationship between internal dose and external exposure [20], and to measure the substances or their metabolism in biological milieu in order to monitor very short-term exposures.

More recently, tests have been developed to measure the nontoxic biological effect correlated with the internal dose, providing an estimate (in some cases indirect) of the quantity of active substance already fixed on the critical action sites. But this approach assumes that the mechanisms of action of the incriminated substance are known, which accounts for its poor development. Most current research involves methods of estimating the quantity of active substance fixed on the critical target molecules. This approach is promising since theoretically it enables the risks to health to be assessed. This field of research is in full development given the progress in immunological techniques, which allow the detection of very slight modifications in the structure of target molecules (DNA and proteins) produced by the substances studied. Tests are gradually becoming available for some hemoglobin adducts, such as with ethylene oxide [21], and for various DNA adducts, for example with aflatoxins or benzo[a]pyrene [17,22]. Such methods must, however, be validated on groups of exposed workers before true biological indicators can be used [17,23–25].

According to Lauwerys and Bernard [18], most current approaches to research in the field of identifying biological indicators of exposure involve carrying out human studies (which are still rather infrequent), the development of tests providing more information on the interactions between active substances and target molecules or cells, the development of tests to assess the internal dose actually absorbed over a long period for substances with a short biological half-life, the development of noninvasive methods to determine the quantity of certain cumulated toxic substances in various parts of the body, and improvement in the validity of existing tests (taking into account interfering factors such as age or tobacco, using more specific analytic methods).

Biological methods are thus expected to improve greatly the assessment of occupational exposure. In the near future they will play an increasingly important role, particularly because they alone can answer the frequently posed questions on the pathogenic role of exposure at low doses of toxic substances or how to distinguish the specific role of a substance among the multitude of agents to which workers are exposed simultaneously, and how to assess the total dose of various substances from various sources absorbed by the same biological target.

However, appropriate, validated, and standardized biological indicators that would provide answers to such questions are far from available. In particular, despite the development of recent research, there are practically no indicators reflecting very old exposures, although these are necessary for studying long-term disease effects. Most markers of internal exposure either have an extremely short half-life or are biologically unstable. For instance, DNA adducts in lymphocytes represent exposures that at best took place months before. Research on these topics is developing rapidly [17,18,26–36].

Furthermore, despite all the obvious advantages of biological indicators compared to environmental measurements, the biological approach presents certain limits. The workers may refuse to provide biological specimens (particularly inconvenient in systematic and large-scale studies). The tests to measure several substances at once are unsuitable, whereas many real situations involve simultaneous and/or sequential multiple exposures. Above all, the definition of biological indicators makes the minimum assumption that a given substance is suspected of having a toxic effect. Thus since biological indicators cannot be developed for all substances used in industry, before developing adapted biological tests the substance must have been incriminated in clinical and epidemiological studies, which are based on environmental measurements.

## B.  Environmental Measurements of Exposure

Environmental measurements of exposure are classified in the following two categories: true *measurements* carried out with captors that record external exposure; and *assessments* of exposure carried out in situations for which instrument measurements are not available (no appropriate captor, study of former situations for which measurements were not made at the time) and for which the exposure can only be assessed indirectly.

### Instrument Measurements

When biological measurements of the internal dose absorbed are not available, the best measurement of external exposure is obtained by an individual captor worn by the workers exposed. If the captor is worn permanently, it should record the exposure under all the real conditions corresponding to the tasks undertaken. However, it will provide only an approximate mean value of the dose absorbed, which is all the more inexact as it does not take into account the personal characteristics of the worker or the working conditions. Moreover, the captor may be impractical to wear and may hinder workers in the execution of their tasks. The captor must often be worn far from the respiratory tract, and thus records exposures that are not related directly to the absorbed dose. Finally, it does not take in account the nonrespiratory routes (skin and mouth).

For obvious reasons of cost and facility of use, it is often preferable to carry out environmental measurements by placing captors in the workshop at sites that are presumed to be representative of the general exposure. The measurements of the general environment are, of course, even less precise than those provided by individual captors, since they do not take into account the working conditions of each subject, movements, individual protection, and other details. Due to the wide variability of exposure measurements and to the fact that underlying toxic mechanisms are to a great extent unknown, statistical analysis of exposure measurement data is often difficult. Industrial hygienists are currently trying to increase the quality of data collection and analysis. An extensive review of that domain can be found in a paper by Rappaport [13].

Instrument measurements of exposure therefore have obvious limits. In addition, they provide information on only one type of exposure at a time, and they correspond only to current exposures that are contemporaneous with the measurement. They are thus poorly adapted to the principal problems posed by the detection of unknown toxic effects, especially long-term effects. They are used essentially to monitor exposures to toxic factors already identified and especially, to check that authorized levels of any existing exposures are not exceeded. Instrument measurements are, however, important in research. They enable the relationship between external and internal doses to be studied, the importance of which has been discussed above. They are necessary for validating indirect assessments (see below). Finally, in the future, protocols of systematic measurement of the environment involving adapted sampling may advantageously replace the indirect assessment methods that are currently favored due to lack of suitable measurements. The importance of sampling must be stressed. Epidemiologic analyses of exposure data imply representativeness of the measurements regarding the real conditions of exposure. Various authors have highlighted the major biases that can occur when measurements are made for mandatory surveillance purposes, usually in the most polluted areas or among the most exposed workers [13,15,25].

### Indirect Assessment of Exposure

It is clear from the preceding pages on direct measurements of exposure (biological indicators and environmental measurements) that, on the whole, the objectives of identifying unknown toxic factors and assessing the toxicity of a substance are not reached with the current state of scientific and technical knowledge. The main exposure indicators that are useful to these objectives must be determined by other means, especially in most studies on long-term effects. Exposure assessments are therefore carried out by various procedures, but of course the precision and validity of the estimates must always be viewed with caution. Many studies are currently being carried out to improve the quality of such assessments. Traditionally, epidemiologists use two methods to study the relationship between the exposure to toxic substances and disease: job titles and ad hoc questionnaires.

### Job Titles

The use of job titles to match administrative or economic data on individuals with mortality or incidence data is a method that has been employed for a long time to detect excess mortality or incidence in certain ocupational groups [37–39]. Most well-known risk factors have been discovered in this way, due to favorable conditions such as high levels of exposure in the past, limited number of exposures for each job, large populations of exposed workers, and clear-cut correspondence between occupation and chemical exposures (e.g., shoe workers and benzene, or shipyards and asbestos). However, with this type of study, where occupation is used as a surrogate measurement of exposure, it is usually not possible to go beyond the stage of putting forth research hypotheses, since all the exposures potentially associated with an occupation cannot be distinguished. In addition, it is extremely imprecise and subject to a great many misclassifications. This is due to the fact that the codes used for occupations [International Labour Office (ILO) international code [40] or national codes] are rather approximate and give an extremely imprecise indication of the potential exposure to toxic substances. Furthermore, a given job title in fact covers different trades and working conditions, which result in different exposures. This introduces misclassification: The more general the code, the greater the number of errors. Frequently, only the occupation at the time of the studied health event is known (e.g., occupation at time of death). However, the epidemiological results that can be obtained from the occupation recorded at a given time are much less exact than if lifetime occupational histories are available [41].

Various research workers have attempted to develop questionnaires for the respective subjects or their surrogate in order to reconstitute the occupational histories and validate the information obtained in comparison with various sources, such as employers and registers [42–54]. This work is important, because despite their imperfections, studies based on job titles continue to be widely used since large data sets (death certificates, registers for cancer or other diseases) are available and enable analyses to be carried out on a large number of subjects. Studies on industrial cohorts that involve the analysis of mortality (and sometimes the incidence of certain diseases) in groups of workers within a company generally employ an approach similar to that for population-based studies using job titles. In this case the study involves a specific occupational group that is supposedly exposed to factors suspected of being pathogenic. Such a study is not usually limited to a global analysis of diseases in the company employees. It attempts to be more precise and to take into account the various jobs held by each worker. This is generally possible through the company records. Although this model does not usually include data on exposure to specific substances, it presents advantages over models using job titles alone since there is a better knowledge of the work environment of the company. Despite their limits, these studies are also in full development because they are relatively easy and allow epidemiological surveillance. Indeed, since these studies can detect new harmful substances, many people would like to see such epidemiological surveillance become systematic [55]. The systematic environmental measurements mentioned above will in the future make these surveillance studies much more effective by enabling exposure data obtained at the workstations to be incorporated.

### Ad Hoc Questionnaires

The use of specific ad hoc questionnaires is the second traditional method employed by epidemiologists to analyze the relationships between occupational exposure and disease. The objective of this type of questionnaire is to reconstitute possible exposure through detailed questions answered by the subjects included in the study. Such questionnaires are useful because being specific to a given type of exposure, it is possible to question subjects on all the circumstances under which they may have been exposed to a given factor (specific tasks, particular modes of operation, the existence and use of protective clothing, etc.). The complete exposure history can thus be reconstituted, going far back into the past. Specific questions enable the exposures to be identified even if the subjects are unaware of the exact exposures to which they were submitted. Such questionnaires have been developed for several factors, including asbestos, formaldehyde, and solvents [56–60].

Another great advantage of questionnaires is that they provide individual information on nonoccupational exposure and on possible confounding factors (e.g., tobacco). However, they have limits. The quantitative assessment of exposure can only be indirect and obviously results in inexact estimations. There are potential biases related to the mode of data collection through interviews (recall bias, objectivity of the interviewers, differences in assessment and precision according to whether the respondent is a subject in the study or a surrogate, such as a colleague or a spouse, as in certain studies). To be sufficiently precise, questionnaires are sometimes extremely long (often including several hundreds of questions and may take 1 to 2 h to complete) and require a specialized interviewer. Because of this, in practice these questionnaires are used only in population-based case-control studies on a few hundred subjects to test a hypothesis on a toxic substance, taking into account a small number of confounding factors (although some authors have tried to develop "multi-specialized" questionnaires through which several exposures are assessed [61]). Under these conditions, questionnaires are powerful epidemiological tools [62], although much remains to be done regarding the analysis of their validity. Recent publications on the study of performances and the validity of questionnaires have already been cited [42–54].

The two principal classical methods of assessing exposures (job titles and ad hoc questionnaires) indirectly have the limitations that we have mentioned. To compensate for some of these, in recent years research has been developed in two directions: to improve the use of questionnaires and to make more effective use of job titles.

### General Questionnaires with Experts

A method involving a general questionnaire with experts was introduced by Siemiatycki and Gérin in Montréal [63–65] at the beginning of the 1980s and has undergone several modifications since. The aim of this method is to extend the questionnaire technique (which is the basic tool for population-based case-control studies) to exploratory situations in which the objective is to identify unknown pathogenic factors. Ad hoc questionnaires are not adapted to this type of study, since they enable only one or a few exposures to be investigated. Thus they tend to be used when a specific hypothesis can be tested. The principle of the general questionnaire with experts is based on the dissociation of the collection of occupational history data and the actual exposure data. A general questionnaire completed with the help of a specialized interviewer aims to reconstitute the complete occupational history of a subject. It includes questions on jobs held, with the corresponding periods, and for each job relatively precise open questions provide information on the tasks undertaken and the modes of operation. The questionnaire is then translated into specific exposures by experts (specialized industrial hygienists). This method presents two very important advantages. First, the total lifetime occupational exposure (also nonoccupational exposures and the main confounding factors) of a subject can be studied without making a prior hypothesis about the role of a given factor. Second, it reduces the potential information biases since the expert works independent of the subject and is unaware of the subject's status (case or control). Thus, despite the high cost involved in using specialized interviewers to complete the questionnaires and experts to assess the exposures, this method has already been used in various studies (e.g., refs. 66 to 68) and is currently employed by several teams in different countries [69]. Certain theoretical and statistical aspects related to the use of this approach, which are common to other methods, will be discussed later in the chapter.

## Job Exposure Matrices

The principle of *job exposure matrices* was formally introduced at the beginning of the 1980s by Hoar [70]. The objective is to make more effective use of job titles, whose main inconvenience is that they do not provide information on specific exposures. The principle is simple. A job exposure matrix is a table made up of lines and columns. The lines represent occupations and the columns the toxic factors to be assessed. For the occupation of a given line, the cell of the matrix at the intersection of the line and a given column contains various indicators of average exposure to the factor corresponding to the column (Fig. 1).

There are currently two approaches regarding the field of application. There are matrices for population-based studies and matrices specific to a company or to an industrial sector. These approaches are not incompatible since they correspond to different but complementary types of epidemiological studies (studies of the general population or of specific occupational groups), with their respective advantages and disadvantages [71]. It is obvious that population-based matrices are less accurate and subject to more misclassification since they must take into account all the existing occupations (the ILO international code [40] includes no less than 1727 groups of job titles) even though the number of columns (the toxic factors) is sometimes limited. But since a large number of subjects can be included in population-based matrices, they are being developed and improved continually [72–76]. Although the matrices specific to a company or to an industry have a more specific field of application, they present the advantage of being much more precise, both in the grouping of occupations (often replaced by specific workstations) and in the estimation of exposure indicators. Thus these matrices provide better information on the work environ-

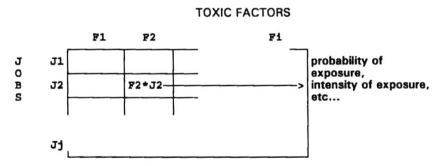

TOXIC FACTORS

Use : subject having worked for 5 years in job J1 and 10 years in job J2

Total exposure : [(F1*J1x5) + (F2*J1x5)] + [(F1*J2x10) + (F2*J2x10)]
where : Fi*Ji = level of exposure to the factor i in job j

**Figure 1**   General principle of job exposure matrices.

ment based on more data. This accounts for the increase in the number of industry-specific matrices in recent years [77–90].

In theory, the matrix method presents several advantages. Since the construction of a matrix is independent of the subjects included in epidemiological surveys, this method is economical on several accounts. The only information required for assessing all the occupational exposures of a subject is the list of all jobs held and the corresponding duration. This information is sometimes available from various administrative sources (national insurance schemes, employers, etc.) or may be collected through questionnaires at a relatively low cost. In addition, a given matrix may be used for various epidemiological surveys. Another advantage of job exposure matrices (also related to the fact that it is built independently of the subjects in the study, and that the assessment of individual exposure is "automatic") is the absence of information biases (no respondent or interviewer biases). Given all these characteristics, it follows that the job exposure matrix method is particularly useful in extremely large epidemiological studies, since there is no practical limit to the number of subjects. It has thus been used both in analyses of mortality or register data in which the data on individuals were obtained by matching records from various sources, and in large case-control studies [70,72,73,91–93]. However, the advantages provided by assessing exposures related to an occupation independent of the subjects are counterbalanced by certain disadvantages. Indeed, only mean assessments are available in a matrix. Since a given job title encompasses extremely different tasks and real work situations, the assessments will inevitably be imprecise and the attribution of exposures to a subject in a survey will always involve a certain rate of misclassification. The effect on the power of the study can be considerable [6,10,11,62,85].

Much research is under way to improve the quality of matrices and to minimize the inevitable difficulties mentioned above. The principal fields of research concern job grouping and exposure indicators. Various theoretical and methodological aspects regarding the validation of matrices and the epidemiological analysis are also being studied, but these will be discussed later since they have much in common with other approaches. The quality of a matrix is highly dependent on the definition of the *lines,* or jobs. This must be as precise as possible to minimize misclassifications. It is often necessary to use the most detailed level of job codes and even to extend existing codes for certain occupations [62]. Similarly, as indicated above, it is important for the occupational histories of the subjects to be as detailed and precise as possible since they represent the entry point of the matrix [94]. Various studies have attempted to improve and validate methods for collecting these data [42–52,64]. Another difficulty is related to the trend over time in working conditions and levels of exposure. It is important for the matrix to reflect this trend because it is often necessary to analyze extremely old exposure data, and it is essential to take time into account in epidemiological studies. It is thus usual to date assessments of exposure contained in a matrix by making as many lines as there are *job periods* for which it is appropriate to attribute different exposure values for the same job [80,95]. Recently, the notion of *task* has been introduced into the structure of matrices. Indeed, with respect to the occurrence of exposure, the differences between occupations are related essentially to the tasks undertaken. This is also true within one specific occupation. For example, the exposure among welders differs considerably according to the type of steel welded (e.g., stainless or other). Thus job-task-exposure matrices have been built with an increased number of lines [95].

Another crucial element of a matrix concerns the exposure indicators that make up the cells. These are used to determine the exposure attributed to the subjects included in epidemiological studies. This involves the choice of indicators and the way in which they are built. The very first matrices merely took into account the presence or absence of an exposure in an occupation. But it is clear that data on the average level of exposure would provide better estimates of epidemiological indices [37,92]. Various current matrices include indicators of the level (usually according to a semiquantitative mode) and even the frequency of exposure [72,73,95]. In another respect it is common knowledge that even when an exposure does occur within an occupation, all the employees working in this occupation are not subjected to it. This introduces the notion of probability of exposure to be attributed to a given worker, which corresponds to the frequency of exposure within an occupation. Recent matrices take into account such probabilities [72,73,95], which allow various strategies to be used in statistical analysis, as will be discussed later. Finally, the quality of a matrix depends essentially on the precision and validity of the estimates of the exposure levels. Such estimates are obtained through two principal approaches, the use of experts and measurements. Most current matrices are based on the use of such experts as industrial hygienists, chemists, and occupational physicians, who use existing knowledge and sometimes standardized techniques [80] to attribute values to the various exposure indices that make up the matrix. This method presents a financial advantage, but it may be considered less accurate than estimates based on environmental measurements [96]. Research is currently being undertaken to compare results obtained according to the source of information and to determine the option based on the best strategies [97].

## IV. Statistical Aspects

The many difficulties involved in the measurement of occupational exposure that have been reviewed above have obviously resulted in an abundance of statistical literature since the weaknesses and imperfections of measurement methods generate results with which it is difficult to carry out epidemiologic analyses. In parallel with research already mentioned which aims to improve the measurements of occupational exposure, current statistical research involves mainly the comparison of methods of assessing the exposure, the study of the validity of these methods, and the development of methods of analyzing complex exposure data and assessing the performance of epidemiological studies [97].

### A. Analysis of the Performance of Different Methods of Measuring Exposure

It has been seen that very different methods of measuring or assessing exposure are used (environmental measurements, questionnaires, matrices). It is of most importance to assess the performance of these approaches to determine which methods are best suited to the various situations, and to improve all these methods.

### *Evaluation of the Intrinsic Quality of a Measurement or Assessment Method*

The intrinsic quality of a measurement method is its ability to measure the true exposure correctly. For dichotomous exposure variables (presence or absence of exposure), the intrinsic quality of the measurement method is summarized by its sensitivity and specificity (respectively, the probability that the measurement will be positive when a subject is exposed, and negative when not exposed). When the prevalence of exposure in the population studied is also known, it is possible to calculate the loss of power and the bias on the relative risk, which are the most appropriate indices of epidemiological performance [5,7,9,98].

For exposure measured by quantitative or semiquantitative variables, a simple index of the intrinsic quality of a measurement does not exist, and to date, few studies have dealt with this [99]. In certain studies, a good correlation is found between environmental measurements and quantitative assessments [96], but the order of magnitude and the frequency of measurement errors are usually not quantified [20]. Finally, much theoretical work remains to be done to assess the consequences of measurement errors on the possibility of controlling confounding factors and to estimate the interactions between several risk factors [10,11,100,101].

In fact, the rigorous assessment of intrinsic performances of measurement methods requires that the "exact" measurements or measurements considered as the best be used as references. At the present time, this is possible only in a very limited number of situations, such as in studies on long-term effects, which involve measurements taken over a long period. Thus until biological research can provide indicators of former exposure, analyses of performance will continue to rely on less precise methods.

### Reproduction of Known Results

In theory, it is natural to expect that a method of assessing exposure will ultimately find known relationships between pathogenic factors and disease. It follows that such an approach could be used to assess the quality of a new method of measuring exposure, as has been done by several authors [41,102]. In fact, this method is very limited and can only be used on rare occasions since the reproducibility of epidemiological results is highly dependent on the population studied, the frequency of the exposure and the confounding factors, the sampling of the subjects, the data collected, and the methods of collection. It is thus preferable to carry out formal comparisons with exposure data obtained by different methods.

### Comparison Between Methods of Assessing Exposure

If one of the methods compared can reasonably be considered as a reference, the above-mentioned indices of intrinsic quality can be used. If not, measurements of agreement such as the kappa coefficient are generally used [103–105]. However, this type of analysis is not particularly well adapted to epidemiological studies. It is preferable, in fact, to compare estimates of relative risk and the statistical power provided by the methods studied. Several authors have made such comparisons across different populations, but as seen above, this creates numerous problems and complicates considerably the interpretation of results [106]. It is obviously better to compare methods of assessing exposure using the same data set, as has been done by several authors [93,96,98,107,108]. This type of study is very promising and in full development, since it is possible to assess the respective merits of the methods compared, to define the conditions under which they can be used and to identify the discrepancies in order to improve each method [107].

### B. Statistical Methods of Epidemiological Analysis

The epidemiological analysis of relationships between exposure and disease presents various statistical problems. Different variables can be used to determine the exposure in an epidemiological study. The total duration, average level, and cumulative dose of exposure are often taken into account. The risk associated with an exposure may also vary according to the age of the individual at first exposure and the time elapsed since this exposure [16].

As already indicated, it is particularly important to take into account the total occupational history of subjects [109]. In addition, the practically systematic presence of multiple exposures and the real conditions of exposure usually lead to a close correlation between the various parameters of exposure, and it can be very difficult to separate their respective effect on the risk [111]. The usual multivariate methods are not very effective in such situations, and certain authors have suggested using a priori models for risks [84,102], possibly combined with classical multivariate methods [112]. This is certainly a most useful approach, and much remains to be done in this field.

We have mentioned several times the problems due to misclassification regarding the exposed/nonexposed status of subjects included in epidemiologic studies. A great amount of statistical work has already been devoted to this aspect. With the increasing popularity of job-exposure matrices, controlling for misclassification is now crucial. In addition to the imprecision that is, as seen above, intrinsic to the method, the loss of power and/or the bias regarding the relative risk may be increased if misclassification is not taken into account in the statistical analysis [3,5,6,77,98,99,102–104,106,107,109,110,112]. To correct the effects of misclassification, methods of analyzing the risk are being developed specifically to take into account the probabilistic nature of exposure assessments provided by matrices. These methods can involve additional data supplied by external surveys on subgroups of subjects included in the survey analyzed [9] and/or the use of data from experts to estimate the probabilities [95]. This research is currently at a preliminary stage. For instance, few authors have studied the problems linked to misclassification when adjusting for confounding factors [10,101]. With the increase in the number of studies based on job-exposure matrices, the statistical research will lead to better knowledge and a better use of data from this type of source [7,10,11,113–115].

## V.  Trend Toward Extensive Surveillance of Occupational Exposure

The various approaches of measuring occupational exposure (biological indicators, instrument or indirect environmental measurements) all make a specific contribution and all have limits. There is not at present (and there probably never will be) a universal method enabling all types of exposure to be taken into account and able to solve all the problems posed by the surveillance of known pathogenic agents and the identification of new toxic substances. The diversity of pathogenic mechanisms and the real conditions of exposure to innumerable substances and procedures is such that progress in the knowledge required to improve the protection of workers will be achieved only through multiple approaches.

The vast field of measurement of occupational exposures is particularly multidisciplinary, involving chemists, industrial hygienists, biologists and toxicologists, epidemiologists, and statisticians. The development of research concerning the measurement of occupational exposure is a necessity in setting up extensive systems of surveillance and prevention that combine biological, environmental, and epidemiological surveillance, which are all too often dissociated.

### References

1. Armstrong BG, Oakes D. Effects of approximation in exposure assessments on estimates of exposure–response relationship. Scand J Work Environ Health 1982; 8(suppl 1):20–23.
2. Heederik D, Kromhout H, Boleij J. Variability of exposure measurements: consequences in occupational epidemiology. 5th International Symposium on Epidemiology in Occupational Health, Los Angeles, September 1986.
3. Copeland KT, Checkoway H, McMichael AJ, Holbrook RH. Bias due to misclassification in the estimation of relative risk. Am J Epidemiol 1977;105(5):488–95.
4. Flegal KM, Brownie C, Haas JD. The effects of exposure misclassification on estimates of relative risk. Am J Epidemiol 1986;123:736–51.
5. Ghozlan A, Lellouch J. L'importance des erreurs de classification en épidémiologie. Rev Epidemiol Sante Publique 1985;33:220–27.
6. Olsen J. Information bias in case-control studies in occupational health epidemiology (letter). Scand J Soc Med 1984;12(1):1–2.
7. Poole C, Trichopoulos D. Extremely low-frequency electric and magnetic fields and cancer. Cancer Causes Control 1991;2:267–76.
8. Espeland MA, Hui SL. A general approach to analyzing epidemiologic data that contain misclassification errors. Biometrics 1987;43:1001–12.
9. Greenland S. Statistical uncertainty due to misclassification: implications for validation substudies. J Clin Epidemiol 1988;41(12):1167–74.
10. Checkoway H, Savitz DA, Heyer NJ. Assessing the effects of nondifferential misclassification of exposures in occupational studies. Appl Occup Environ Hyg 1991;6:528–33.
11. Stewart WF, Correa-Villasensor A. False positive exposure errors and low exposure prevalence in community-based case-control studies. Appl Occup Environ Hyg 1991;6:534–40.
12. Heederick D, Boleij JSM, Kromhout H, Smid T. Use and analysis of exposure monitoring data in occupational epidemiology: an example of an epidemiological study in the Dutch animal food industry. Appl Occup Environ Hyg 1991;6:458–64.
13. Rappaport SM. Assessment of long-term exposures to toxic substances in air. Ann Occup Hyg 1991;35(1):61–121.
14. Kauppinen TP. Development of a classification strategy of exposure for industry-based studies. Appl Occup Environ Hyg 1991;6:482–87.
15. Rappaport SM. Selection of the measures of exposure for epidemiology studies. Appl Occup Environ Hyg 1991;6:448–57.
16. Pearce NE. Methodological problems of time related variables in occupational cohort studies. Rev Epidemiol Sante Publique 1992;40(suppl 1):43–54.

17. Vineis P. Use of biological indicators of exposure and effect in epidemiological studies of occupational cancer. Rev Epidemiol Sante Publique 1992;40(suppl 1):63–69.
18. Lauwerys R, Bernard A. Biological monitoring of exposure to industrial toxic substances. Present-day situation and prospects for development. Scand J Work Environ Health 1985;11(3 spec no):155–64.
19. CEE. Indicateurs pour l'évaluation de l'exposition aux produits chimiques génotoxiques et de leurs effets biologiques. Rapport commun. EUR 11659 FR. Luxembourg: Office des Publications Officielles des Communautés Européennes, 1989.
20. Droz PO, Berode M, Wu MM. Evaluation of concomitant biological and air monitoring results. Appl Occup Environ Hyg 1991;6:465–74.
21. Hogstedt LC. Epidemiological studies on ethylene oxide and cancer: an updating. In: Bartsch H, Hemminki K, O'Neill IK, eds. Methods for detecting DNA damaging agents in humans: applications in cancer epidemiology and prevention. IARC Scientific Publication 89. Lyon, France: IARC, 1988.
22. Hemminki K, Grzybowska E. DNA adducts in humans environmentally exposed to aromatic compounds in an industrial area in Poland. Carcinogenesis 1990;11:1229–31.
23. Brewster MA. Biomarkers of xenobiotic exposures. Ann Clin Lab Sci 1988;18(4):306–17.
24. Schulte PA. A conceptual framework for the validation and use of biologic markers. Environ Res 1989;48:129–44.
25. Vanhoorne M. A proposed framework for the assessment of exposure to (potential) carcinogens in the working environment. EEC Report EUR 11810 EN. Luxembourg: European Economic Communities, 1989.
26. Andersen I, Svenes KB. Determination of nickel in lung specimens of thirty-nine autopsied nickel workers. Int Arch Occup Environ Health 1989;61:289–95.
27. Blair A, Hoar S, Cantor KP, Stewart PA. Estimating exposure to pesticides in epidemiological studies of cancer. In: Biological monitoring of pesticide exposure. ACS Symposium Series 382. Washington, DC: American Chemical Society, 1989:38–46.
28. De Vuyst P, Dumortier P, Moulin E, Yourassowsky N, Roomans P, De Francquen P, Yernault JC. Asbestos bodies in bronchoalveolar lavage reflect lung asbestos body concentration. Eur Respir J 1988;1:362–67.
29. Hewitt PJ. Accumulation of metals in the tissues of occupationally exposed workers. Environ Geochem Health 1988;10(3/4):113–16.
30. Jarup L, Pershagen G, Wall S. Cumulative arsenic exposure and lung cancer in smelter workers: a dose–response study. Am J Ind Med 1989;15:31–41.

31. Mason HJ. Relations between liver cadmium, cumulative exposure, and renal function in cadmium alloy workers. Br J Ind Med 1988; 45:793–802.

32. Mastin JP, Stettler LE, Shelburne JD. Quantitative analysis of particulate burden in lung tissue. Scanning Microsc 1988;2(3):1613–29.

33. Raithel HJ, Schaller RH, Akslen LA. Analyses of chromium and nickel in human pulmonary tissue. Int Arch Occup Environ Health 1989;61:507–12.

34. Samuels ER, Meranger JC, Tracy BL. Lead concentrations in human bones from the Canadian population. Sci Total Environ 1989;89:261–69.

35. Somervaille LJ, Nilsson U, Chettle DR. In vivo measurements of bone lead. A comparison of two x-ray fluorescence techniques used at three different bone sites. Phys Med Biol 1989;34(12):1833–45.

36. Stern RM, Drenck K, Lyngenbo O, Dirksen H, Groth S. Thoracic magnetic dust content, occupational exposure, and respiratory status of shipyard welders. Arch Environ Health 1988;43(5):361–70.

37. Hsieh CC, Walker AM, Hoar SK. Grouping occupations according to carcinogenic potential: occupation clusters from an exposure linkage system. Am J Epidemiol 1983;117(5):575–89.

38. Magnani C, Coggon D, Osmond C, Acheson ED. Occupation and five cancers: a case-control study using death certificates. Br J Ind Med 1987;44(11):769–76.

39. Swanson GM, Schwartz AG, Burrows RW. An assessment of occupation and industry data from death certificates and hospital medical records for population-based cancer surveillance. Am J Public Health 1986;74(5):464–67.

40. Classification internationale type des professions/International standard classification of occupations. Genève: BIT, ed. rev., 1968,1991/Geneva: ILO, rev. ed., 1968, 1991.

41. Baumgarten M, Siemiatycki J, Gibbs GW. Validity of work histories obtained by interview for epidemiologic purposes. Am J Epidemiol 1983;118(4):583–91.

42. Bond GG, Bodner KM, Sobel W. Validation of work histories obtained from interviews. Am J Epidemiol 1988;128(2):343–51.

43. Bourbonnais R, Meyer F, Thériault G. Validity of self reported work history. Br J Ind Med 1988;45(1):29–32.

44. Eskenasi B, Pearson K. Validation of a self-administered questionnaire for assessing occupational and environmental exposures of pregnant women. Am J Epidemiol 1988;128(5):1117–29.

45. Goldberg JD, Siemiatycki J, Gérin M. Correspondence. Br J Ind Med 1987;44:426–28.

46. Holmberg C, Hernberg S. Congenital defects and occupational factors: a

comparison of different methodological approaches. Scand J Work Environ Health 1979;5:328–32.

47. Pershagen G, Axelson O. A validation of questionnaire information on occupational exposure and smoking. Scand J Work Environ Health 1982;8(1):24–28.

48. Rona RJ, Mosbech J. Validity and repeatability of self-reported work history in EEC countries. In: Progress in occupational epidemiology. Amsterdam: Excerpta Medica, 1988.

49. Rosenberg CR, Mulvihill MN, Fischbein A, Blum S. An analysis of the validity of self reported occupational histories using a cohort of workers exposed to PCBs. Br J Ind Med 1987;44:702–10.

50. Rosenstock L, Lofengo J, Heyer NH, Carter WB. Development and validation of a self-administered occupational health history questionnaire. J Occup Med 1984;26:50–54.

51. Stewart WF, Tonascia JA, Matanoski GM. The validity of questionnaire-reported work history in live respondents. J Occup Med 1987;29(10):795–800.

52. Turner DW, Schumacher MC, West DW. Comparison of occupational interview data to death certificate data in Utah. Am J Ind Med 1987;12:145–51.

53. Bond GG, Bodner KM, Olsen GW, Burchfiel CM, Cook RC. Validation of work histories for the purpose of epidemiological studies. Appl Occup Environ Hyg 1991;6:521–27.

54. Miligi L, Masala G. Methods of exposure assessment for community-based studies: aspects inherent to the validation of questionnaires. Appl Occup Environ Hyg 1991;6:502–7.

55. Monson RR. Editorial commentary: epidemiology and exposure to electromagnetic fields. Am J Epidemiol 1990;131:774–75.

56. Fidler AT, Baker EL, Letz RE. Estimation of long term exposure to mixed solvents from questionnaire data: a tool for epidemiological investigations. Br J Ind Med 1987;44:133–41.

57. Olsen E, Seedorf L. Exposure to organic solvents. II. An exposure epidemiologic study. Ann Occup Hyg 1990;34(4):379–89.

58. Partanen T, Kauppinen T, Nurminen M, Nickels J, Hernberg S, Hakulinen T, Pukkala E, Savonen E. Formaldehyde exposure and respiratory and related cancers. A case-referent study among Finnish woodworkers. Scand J Work Environ Health 1985;11:409–15.

59. Seedorf L, Olsen E. Exposure to organic solvents. I. A survey on the use of solvents. Ann Occup Hyg 1990;34(4):371–78.

60. Vena JE, Byers TE, Cookfair D, Swanson M. Occupation and lung cancer risk. An analysis by histologic subtypes. Cancer 1985;56:910–17.

61. Bolm-Audorff U. Experience with supplementary questionnaires in a lung case referent study. EEC Report EUR 11810 EN. Luxembourg: European Economic Communities, 1989.

62. Hémon D, Goldberg M, eds. EEC workshop: methodology of assessment of occupational exposures in the context of epidemiological detection of cancer risks. EEC Report EUR 11810 EN. Luxembourg: European Economic Communities, 1989.

63. Gérin M, Siemiatycki J, Kemper H, Begin D. Obtaining occupational exposure histories in epidemiologic case-control studies. J Occup Med 1985;27(6):420–26.

64. Goldberg JD, Siemiatycki J, Gérin M. Inter-rater agreement in assessing occupational exposure in a case-control study. Br J Ind Med 1986;43(10):667–76.

65. Siemiatycki J, Day NE, Fabry J, Cooper JA. Discovering carcinogens in the occupational environment: a novel epidemiologic approach. J Natl Cancer Inst 1981;66(2):217–25.

66. Gérin M, Siemiatycki J, Richardson L, Pellerin J, Lakhani R. Nickel and cancer associations from a multicancer occupation and case-referent study: preliminary findings. IARC Scientific Publication 53. Lyon, France: IARC, 105–15.

67. Siemiatycki J, Dewar R, Lakhani R. Cancer risks associated with 10 inorganic dusts: results from a case-control study in Montréal. Am J Ind Med 1989;16:547–67.

68. Siemiatycki J, Gérin M, Stewart P, Nadon L, Dewar R, Richardson L. Associations between several sites of cancer and ten types of exhaust and combustion products. Scand J Work Environ Health 1988;14:79–90.

69. Luce D, Leclerc A, Morcet JF, Casal Lareo A, Gérin M, Brugère J, Haguenoer JM, Goldberg M. Occupational risk factors for sinonasal cancer in a French case-control study. Am J Ind Med 1992;21:163–75.

70. Hoar S. Job exposure matrix methodology. J Toxicol Clin Toxicol 1983–84;21(1/2):9–26.

71. Checkoway H, Pearce NE, Crawford-Brown DJ. Research methods in occupational epidemiology. New York: Oxford University Press, 1989.

72. Ferrario F, Continenza D, Pisani P, Magnani C, Merletti F, Berrino F. Description of a job-exposure matrix for sixteen agents which are or may be related to respiratory cancer. In: Progress in occupational epidemiology. Amsterdam: Excerpta Medica, 1988.

73. Steineck G, Plato N, Alfredsson L, Norell SE. Industry-related urothelial carcinogens: application of a job-exposure matrix to census data. Am J Ind Med 1989;16:209–24.

74. Hoar S. Epidemiology and occupational classification system. Banbury

report 9. Quantification of occupational cancer. Peto R, Schneidermann M, eds. Cold Spring Harbor NY: Cold Spring Harbor Laboratory, 1981:455–70.

75. Pannett B, Coggon D, Acheson ED. A job-exposure matrix for use in population based studies in England and Wales. Br J Ind Med 1985;42(11):777–83.

76. Spirtas R, Fendt K. An algorithm for linking job titles with individual exposures in occupational epidemiology studies. In: Job exposure matrices. Conference report. Southampton, England: MRC, 1982;39–47.

77. Corn M, Esmen NA. Workplace exposure zones for classification of employee exposures to physical and chemical agents. Am Ind Hyg Assoc J 1979;40:47–57.

78. Froines JR, Dellenbaugh CA, Wegman DH. Occupational health surveillance: a means to identify work-related risks. Am J Public Health 1986;76(9):1089–96.

79. Gamble JF, Spirtas R, Easter P. Applications of a job classification system in occupational epidemiology. Am J Public Health 1976;66:768–72.

80. Goldberg M, Leclerc A, Chastang JF, Goldberg P, Brodeur JM, Fuhrer R, Segnan N. Evaluation rétrospective d'expositions professionnelles dans les études épidémiologiques. Utilisation de la méthode Delphi. Rev Epidemiol Sante Publique 1986;34:245–51.

81. Greenberg RA, Tamburro CH. Exposure indices for epidemiological surveillance of carcinogenic agents in an industrial chemical environment. J Occup Med 1981;23(5):353–58.

82. Guillemin MP, Madelaine P, Litzistorf G. Asbestos in buildings. Aerosol Sci Technol 1989;11:221–43.

83. Heederick D, Kromhout H, Burema J, Biersteker K, Kromhout D. Occupational exposure and 25-year incidence rate of non-specific lung disease: the Zutphen study. Int J Epidemiol 1990;19:945–52.

84. Kaldor J, Peto J, Easton D, Doll R, Hermon C, Morgan L. Models for respiratory cancer in nickel refinery workers. J Nat Cancer Inst 1986;77(4):841–48.

85. Kauppinen T, Partanen T. Use of plant- and period-specific job-exposure matrices in studies on occupational cancer. Scand J Work Environ Health 1988;14(3):161–67.

86. Miller BA, Blair A, Raynor HL, Zahm SH. Mortality among furniture workers: limitations in interpreting study findings when detailed work histories and exposure data are lacking. Scand J Work Environ Health 1987;13(2):167.

87. Ott MG, Teta Howard MJ, Greenberg L. Assessment of exposure to chemicals in a complex work environment. Am J Ind Med 1989;16:617–30.

88. Sebastien P, McDonald JC, McDonald AD. Respiratory cancer in chrysotile textile and mining industries: exposure inferences from lung cancer. Br J Ind Med 1989;46(3):180–87.

89. Vaugham TL, Strader C, Davis S, Daling JR. Formaldehyde and cancer of the pharynx sinus and nasal cavity. I. Occupational exposures. Int J Cancer 1986;38(5):677–83.

90. Wald N, Boreham J, Doll R, Bonsall J. Occupational exposure to hydrazine and subsequent risk of cancer. Br J Ind Med 1984;41:31–34.

91. Magnani C, Pannett B, Winter PD, Coggon D. Application of a job-exposure matrix to national mortality statistics for lung cancer. Br J Ind Med 1988;45(1):70–72.

92. Kjuus H. Strategies for coding data on total occupational history. Experiences from a case-referent study on lung cancer. In: Use of job exposure matrices in the Nordic countries. Copenhagen: Kraeftens Bekaempelse, Cancerregisteret, 1988.

93. Dewar R, Siemiatycki J, Gérin M. Loss of statistical power associated with the use of a job-exposure matrix in occupational case-control studies. Appl Occup Environ Hyg 1991;6:508–15.

94. Acheson ED. What are job exposures matrices? In: Job exposure matrices. Southampton, England: MRC Environmental Epidemiology Unit, University of Southampton, 1983.

95. Imbernon E, Goldberg M, Guénel P. MATEX: une matrice emplois-expositions destinée à la surveillance épidémiologique des travailleurs d'une grande entreprise (EDF-GDF). Arch Mal Prof 1991;52(8):559–66.

96. Kromhout H, Oostendorp Y, Heederik D, Boleij SM. Agreement between qualitative exposure estimates and quantitative exposure measurements. Am J Ind Med 1987;12:551–62.

97. Hémon D, Bouyer J, Berrino F, Brochard P, Glass DC, Goldberg M, Kromhout H, Lynge E, Pannett B, Segnan N, Smit HA, Retrospective evaluation of occupational exposures in cancer epidemiology: a European concerted action of research. Appl Occup Environ Hyg 1991;6:541–46.

98. Segnan N, Ronco G, Costa G, Ponti A. Marginal benefit in the assessment of the occupational exposure and validity implication. EEC Report EUR 11810 EN. Luxemburg: European Economic Communities, 1989.

99. Marshall J, Priore R, Graham S, Brasure J. On the distortion of risk estimates in multiple exposure level case-control studies. Am J Epidemiol 1981;113(4):464–73.

100. Kupper LL. Effects of the use of unreliable surrogate variables on the validity of epidemiologic research studies. Am J Epidemiol 1984;120(4):643–48.

101. Bouyer J, Hémon D. Comparison of three methods of estimating the odds-ratio with a job-exposure matrix. 8th International Symposium on Epidemiology in Occupational Health, Paris, September 1991.

102. Smith AH, Waxweiler RJ, Tyroler HA. Epidemiologic investigation of occupational carcinogenesis using a serially additive expected dose model. Am J Epidemiol 1980;112(6):787–97.
103. Fleiss JL. Statistical methods for rates and proportions. New York: Wiley, 1981.
104. Thompson WD, Walter SD. A reappraisal of the kappa coefficient. J Clin Epidemiol 1988;10:949–58.
105. Ahrens W, Pohlabeln H, Bolm-Audorff U, Jahn I, Jockel KH. Occupational exposure to cooling lubricants and lung cancer. Preliminary results from a case-control study. 8th International Symposium on Epidemiology in Occupational Health, Paris, September 1991.
106. Hémon D. Epidémiologie des risques d'origine professionnelle: quelques problémes méthodologiques. Rev Epidemiol Sante Publique 1986;34:230–36.
107. Ferrario F, Berrino F, Pisani P. Assessing occupational exposures: from job histories to structured "ad hoc" questionnaires. EEC Report EUR 11810 EN. Luxemburg: European Economic Communities, 1989.
108. Siemiatycki J, Dewar R, Richardson L. Costs and statistical power associated with five methods of collecting occupation exposure information for population-based case-control studies. Am J Epidemiol 1989;6:1236–46.
109. Illis WR, Swanson GM, Satarino ER, Schwartz AG. Summary measures of occupational history: a comparison of latest occupation and industry with usual occupation and industry. Am J Public Health 1987;77(12):1532–34.
110. Smith AH. Looking backwards from outcome to exposure to assess cancer latency. J Chron Dis 1987;40(suppl 2):113–17.
111. Doll R, Peto R. The causes of cancer. Oxford: Oxford University Press, 1981.
112. Lubin JH. A reformulation of the serially additive expected dose method for occupational cohort data. Am J Epidemiol 1983;118(4):592–98.
113. Armstrong BG, Whittemore AS, Howe GR. Analysis of case-control data with covariate measurement error: application to diet and colon cancer. Stat Med 1989;8:1151–63.
114. Rosner B, Willett WC, Spiegelman D. Correction of logistic regression relative risk estimates and confidence intervals for systematic within-person measurement error. Stat Med 1989;8:1051–69.
115. Weinkam JJ, Rosenbaum WL, Sterling TD. A practical approach to estimating the true effect of exposure despite imprecise exposure classification. Am J Ind Med 1991;19:587–601.

# Part Two

## ENVIRONMENTAL SOURCES OF RESPIRATORY DISEASES

ROLAND MASSE

The prevention of pulmonary pathologies induced by environmental factors poses a certain number of specific problems. For the clinician, the identification of environmental etiology is often difficult, apart from that of well-known allergic complaints. For health authorities, the identification and evaluation of risks are complicated by the multitude of interactions of gaseous and particulate pollutants from both indoor and outdoor environments. This particularity brings about two types of consequences: the additive or multiplicative combination of risks from toxic agents, and the interactions of pollutants leading to chemical types different from those emitted at the source, even to possible neutralizing effects such as those observed between ozone and cigarette smoke.

Numerous regulatory provisions in different countries have led to a very notable reduction in major atmospheric pollutants in urban areas and on worksites. However, new problems are appearing, such as the emergence of allergens to "compositae" and other weeds proliferating on fallow land.

Domestic exposure is much more difficult to manage and may be, in the end, one of the most worrying problems in public health. Technical and often complex solutions for prevention can be suggested for the eradication of house dust mites or for drying the air in humid dwellings; but in the case of radon, even though an important proportion of habitations exceed average exposure levels by more than one full standard measure, no realistic strategy is available to reduce this level to external environmental levels. Radical responses, such as changing residence, necessitate taking into account both individual risks, assessed by the most reliable measures, and judicious cost–benefit analysis to evaluate their real impact in the community.

# 10

## Indoor Exposure to Radon

**MARGOT TIRMARCHE**

Institut de Protection et de Sûreté Nucleaire
Fontenay-aux-Roses, France

## I. Introduction

Radon-222 is a radioactive gas occurring naturally in human environments as a decay product of radium-226, a member of the radioactive decay chain of uranium-238. Another isotope of radon is radon-220 (thoron), issued from the decay chain of thorium-232. Its contribution to the exposure of miners or the general population is relatively low, and in this chapter we focus on radon-222 and its decay products, considered as being the major component of human exposure to natural sources of ionizing radiation.

## II. Occurrence of Radon

Uranium-238 and radium-226 are present in the earth's crust in various concentrations. Radon is an inert gas, formed in soil and rocks from the decay of radium-226. It is released to the surrounding atmosphere, air, or water, but a fraction of radon can be trapped in pore spaces; it is transported in soil, over more-or-less long distances, by diffusion and by movements of air and water.

*195*

Soil porosity influences greatly the diffusion rate of radon. As soils contain various amounts of air or water as a function of their permeability, radon enters the soil gas by diffusion from soil particles. The concentration of radon in soil gas is dependent on meteorological factors: humidity, temperature, barometric pressure, wind speed, and so on. For example, heavy rain and snow reduce the exhalation rate; consequently, in winter the radon concentration in soil is increased. To a lesser extent, an increase in temperature and wind speeds may increase exhalation rates and thus decrease soil gas concentrations. As a function of these parameters, radon concentrations in soil gas may vary on a daily and seasonal basis.

Radon-222 decays with a half-life of 3.82 days into a series of radioisotopes of heavy metals (polonium, lead, bismuth) (Fig. 1). The release of radon into air is accompanied by formation of its short-lived decay products, which play a major role in its impact on health. These products occur either unattached or attached to aerosol particles of the atmosphere. The attached fraction is dependent on the concentration of dust in the air and the ventilation rate. Two of these radon daughters ($^{218}$Po and $^{214}$Po) are α-particle emitters, which, after inhalation of radon, decay in the lung and irradiate the cells of the epithelium of the respiratory tractus. The resulting effect may be carcinogenic. Uranium mining

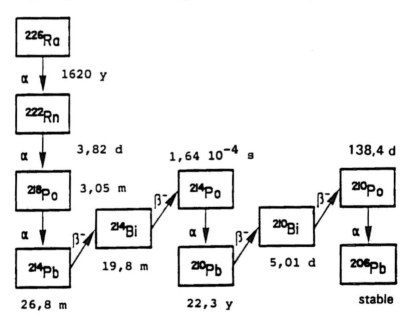

**Figure 1** Radon decay chain. Vertical arrow indicates decay by α-particle emission, diagonal arrow to decay by β-particle emission. Radioactive half-life: y = year; d = day; m = minutes; s = seconds.

is an occupational activity that results in intense exposure to radon and its decay products. Miners of other products can also be exposed to radon, but at lower concentrations in most situations.

Radon can also be detected in many houses worldwide, the concentrations in most cases being far less critical than in mining conditions. Nevertheless, in some regions the annual exposure rate for persons living in these dwellings can be relatively high. Indoor radon is a pollutant varying from one house to another depending mainly on the characteristics of the soil underneath each house. The probability of measuring high indoor levels of radon is greater in granitic than in sedimentary areas.

Sources other than soil, such as building materials, may contribute significantly to radon release inside houses. In the western United States in the 1960s, sand tailings from the processing of uranium ores were used in building construction, as bedding under foundations. In Sweden, concrete made from alum shales and naturally rich in $^{226}$Ra contributed to higher than normal levels of radon in houses. In Czechoslovakia, similar situations have been described. In most houses, the main source of domestic radon exposure is the ground underneath the house. Radon penetrates a building from numerous points: foundation points, cracks in walls or floors, and piping and electrical accessways (Fig. 2).

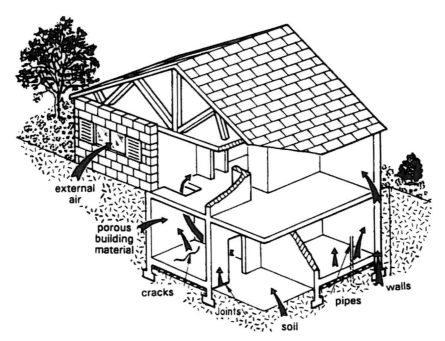

**Figure 2**   Penetration ways of radon.

### III.  Exposure to Radon in Houses and in Mines

Various techniques for measuring radon or radon decay products in mining or indoor atmosphere are presently available. They have changed over time, and when comparing quantitative values of these measurements, radon monitoring devices have to be tested in a comparable way under standard conditions. Duration of measurement is an important factor; a period of 3 to 6 months is recommended for indoor measurement to take into account the general lifestyle of the inhabitants. In some epidemiological studies where a precise quantitative value of the exposure is necessary, a 12-month measurement is used, to integrate seasonal variations. In contrast, when identifying houses with excessively high radon concentrations on a regional or national basis, short-term measurements can be realized in a period of a day to a week. The results of this technique are only indicative but have to be verified by long-term monitoring before remedial action is planned.

Because of the long latency period for lung cancer risk, most published epidemiological studies of the uranium miners are related to the exposure and working conditions during the period 1945–1970, when radon gas measurements were rare and not always realized in a systematic survey strategy. Thus the dosimetry had to be evaluated retrospectively on an individual basis for part of the period, taking in account changes in working conditions, mainly through the introduction of mechanic ventilation, which drastically reduced radon decay concentration. In past decades when radon exposure was high, dusty atmospheres were also very common. Consequently, very low values for the unattached fraction have been admitted for past mining atmospheres. When direct measurements of the $\alpha$- energy of short-lived radon decay products were rare or inexistent, estimation of the equilibrium factor has also been necessary. Indeed, in airspaces such as galleries of mines or rooms of houses, the activity concentration of the decay products does not reach radioactive equilibrium with radon, due mainly to ventilation and deposition of the decay products on surfaces. The equilibrium factor is defined as the ratio of potential $\alpha$-energy concentration of the decay product mixture to the corresponding concentration under radioactive equilibrium with radon. In mines this factor varies between 0.2 and 0.5, and even higher if the place is not ventilated. In houses it is generally admitted to be 0.4 to 0.5, and in the Unscear report of 1988 [1], values between 0.3 and 0.8 are cited.

The concentration of radon decay products in air is expressed as the total potential $\alpha$ energy concentration, being the sum of the $\alpha$ energies of the short-lived radon decay product atoms present per unit volume of air. The SI unit for the potential $\alpha$-energy concentration of radon decay products in air is joules per cubic meter ($J \cdot m^{-3}$). A special unit used in mines is the *working level* (WL), defined as being any combination of the radon progeny in 1 L of air releasing $1.3 \times 10^5$ MeV of $\alpha$- energy during the decay process. Thus 1 WL corresponds approximately to the potential $\alpha$-energy concentration of short-lived radon decay products in radioactive equilibrium with an activity concentration of $3.7 \times 10^3$ Bq radon/m$^3$ of air (100 pCi/L of air). Cumulative exposure of miners is expressed as *working level months* (WLM). Thus 1 WLM corresponds to an exposure to a concentration of 1 WL for a working period of 170 h.

For miners, a second radioactive component results from inhalation of uranium-234, thorium-230, radium-226, and polonium-210, long-lived α-particle emitters also existing in the suspended ore dusts of the mining atmosphere. At the high radon concentrations observed in the past (until 1967 in the United States), Harley et al. [2] concluded that the additional contribution to the lung dose would be less than 10% of that of the radon decay products. Measurements of these long-lived activities cited by Singh et al. [3] from autopsies of miners' lungs confirm this evaluation.

A third radioactive component present in uranium mines is the γ irradiation issued from the ore of gallery walls. This exposure has not changed drastically through time or as a function of the working conditions because it is far less affected by ventilation. Its contribution to the lung dose has not been considered when evaluating the lung cancer risk in epidemiological studies of uranium miners. Again, this contribution to the miners' exposure was considered insignificant compared with that of past radon exposure, and individual measurements of this external exposure have not always been registered in the past. To illustrate this point, it may be noted that in the French study, workers who began underground uranium mining in the years 1946–1972 have accumulated a relatively low exposure to radon and its decay products, the mean being 70 WLM. For these miners the mean cumulated γ irradiation is 100 mSv; this contribution to the lung dose leads to an additional exposure of about 1%. Depending on the types of ore in the rocks of these mines (arsenic, silica, etc.), other types of dusts and aerosols may be inhaled by miners. They can play a role as cocarcinogens or stimulate the proliferation of cells of the bronchial epithelium.

When comparing the miners' situation with domestic exposure to radon, it must be pointed out that the former is multifactorial, and that aside from radon, most of the factors differ from those observed in houses. Two other difficulties are (1) the interaction of radon with a potential carcinogenic factor such as tobacco smoking, and (2) extrapolation from a male population of low socioeconomic status such as is typical of miners, to the general population, including females and children.

The problem of indoor radon was ignored by the public in most countries until the years 1980–1985. In the United States an incident publicized in 1984 resulted in more public concern. During a routine survey, a worker in a nuclear power plant in Pennsylvania was found to be contaminated, the source of the contamination being radon in his home, located in a geological region called the Reading Prong. Since that period, indoor radon measurement has become common in the United States, and in many areas a radon test is required at the time a house is sold. In most European countries public concern for the domestic radon problem is less intense, even though in several regions (e.g., France, eastern Germany, Czechoslovakia) with past or present uranium mining industries, indoor radon concentrations may be as high as those in the United States. At present, numerous radon measurements are being carried out under the coordination of the Commission of the European Communities (CEC) to compile a radiation atlas of natural sources of ionizing radiation in Europe [4].

## IV.  Cancer Risk Estimation

Estimation of a potential risk of cancer, mainly of lung cancer, linked to inhalation of radon and its decay products in residential environment can be realized by various approaches: experimental animal research, extrapolation of the results observed on uranium miners, description of cancer incidence or mortality in regions with high or low domestic radon exposure, and finally, analyses of epidemiological studies focusing, on a large-scale national or international basis, on the risk linked to radon exposure at home, in the presence or absence of other factors of the human environment, such as tobacco use and occupational exposure.

### A.  Experimental Animal Research

Studies on animals have been conducted mainly in two centers in the United States: Pacific Northwest Laboratory (PNL) and University of Rochester, and in France (CEA–COGEMA). In most of these studies, rats, hamsters, and dogs have been exposed to high weekly exposures to radon and its decay products, varying from less than 10 to several hundreds of WLM per week. Experiments were conducted exposing rodents or dogs in inhalation chambers to radon daughters in the presence or absence of uranium dust, tobacco smoke, stable cerium hydroxide, and diesel engine exhaust.

These animal studies indicate that tumors of the respiratory tract increase with increase in cumulative exposure to radon daughters, but also, at comparable cumulative exposures, an increase is observed when the exposure rate decreases. This finding is relative to exposure rates decreasing from 300 WLM to 50 WLM per week [5]; the actual problem is to confirm if this inverse exposure-rate effect persists for low cumulative exposures, associated with low daily exposure rates. The latter situation would make the animal data more comparable to the domestic exposure rate situation, where in most situations the exposure rate is lower than 1 to 2 WLM per year.

The role of concomitant factors tested in these animal experiences [6,7] depends not only on the characteristics of the factor, but also on the sequence of administration of the various exposures. The incidence of neoplastic lesions increases if radon exposure is concomitant to uranium ore dust, diesel engine exhaust, or cigarette smoke. But the tumor incidence does not change, except for tobacco smoke. In fact, in the COGEMA experiments [7], rats exposed to cigarette smoke after exposure to radon have a higher tumor incidence, indicating that if radon acts as an initiator, tobacco smoke increases the initial risk. If tobacco smoke precedes radon exposure, the synergistic effect on tumor incidence has not been observed. On the other hand, in experiments on dogs organized at PNL, the incidence of lung tumors decreased when animals were exposed to cigarette smoke plus radon exposure.

In conclusion, we consider that the incidence of respiratory tract tumors in animals is increased linearly with cumulative radon daughter exposure, and that a decrease of exposure rate from 500 WLM to 50 WLM per week also increases this risk. An increase in the unattached fraction also increases the tumor incidence. Concomitant exposure to cigarette smoke may have a synergistic effect, depending on the sequence of exposure of these two carcinogenic factors. This last point is crucial for an understanding of the development of lung cancer in humans. More animal studies at low exposure rate and at cumulative exposures of 20 to 50 WLM are needed to determine if the inverse dose-rate effect is true at very low exposure rates. As to the incidence of cancer other than lung tumors, although higher than normal rates have been found for the kidney, bone, soft tissue, and mammary glands, a clear trend of increasing tumor incidence with exposure to radon has been demonstrated only for kidney cancer [7]. For leukemia, animal studies showed no positive trend.

### B. Epidemiology on Uranium Miners

In studies on uranium miners [8–18], the excess relative risk for lung cancer per unit of exposure that has been established is associated in most studies to a linear exposure–response relationship. Table 1 indicates that the figures on these excess coefficients are in rather good agreement, despite the various exposure conditions and uncertainties of the past. In analyzed these uranium miner studies, international committees have come to the following conclusions. The BEIR IV report [19] on the health risks of radon and other internally deposited $\alpha$ emitters concluded that after a 5-year lag time, the excess relative risk varies with time since exposure and depends on age at risk. In this model, radon exposures that occurred longer ago have less impact on the age-specific excess relative risk of lung cancer than do more recent exposures. The excess relative risk coefficient is 2.2% or 2.6% per WLM, based on internal or external analysis, with multiplicative standard errors of 1.3 and 1.2, respectively. If the combined data are fitted to a constant relative risk model, the corresponding estimates are 1.3% and 1.5% per WLM for internal and external analyses, respectively, with standard

**Table 1** Relative Risk Coefficients for Lung Cancer in Underground Miners

| Study | Excess relative risk/100 WLM |
|---|---|
| Colorado Plateau uranium miners | 0.5 |
| New Mexico uranium miners | 1.1 |
| Ontario uranium miners | 1.3 |
| Beaverlodge, Canada uranium miners | 2.6 |
| Port Radium, Canada uranium miners | 0.7 |
| Czech uranium miners | 1.9 |
| French uranium miners | 0.4 |
| Malmberget, Sweden iron miners | 1.6 |
| Newfoundland fluorspar miners | 3.0 |
| Chinese tin miners | 0.9 |

*Source:* Data from ref. 22.

errors of 1.3 and 1.2. These estimates can be compared with those in the ICRP 50 report [20], which projects an average excess relative risk coefficient of 0.01 per WLM with a probable range of 0.005 to 0.015 per WLM.

In some of the studies of miners, tobacco consumption has been reconstructed on an individual basis and is analyzed either in the cohort study or in a case-control design, but in other studies, this retrospective evaluation of tobacco consumption could not be realized in a reliable way. Most of the information on the interaction between tobacco smoke and radon exposure comes from uranium miners in Colorado and New Mexico and from iron miners in Sweden. In all these analyses a multiplicative or submultiplicative, rather than an additive, risk model is suggested to account for this interaction.

### C. Extrapolation to Low Radon Exposure

Extrapolation of these risk estimations from occupational conditions to the indoor domestic environment requires several assumptions. The models of various groups use the excess risk of lung cancer linked to past exposure to estimate the lifetime risk of the exposed public, assuming a relationship between the excess risk linked to radon decay products and the background incidence of lung cancer of this population. The 1984 model of NCRP [21] assumes for the excess risk a time-dependent exponential decline after exposure and its additivity to the background incidence. The ICRP 50 model proposes that the background rate be multiplied by the excess risk linked to radon exposure. The model of BEIR IV Committee [19], also multiplicative, incorporates a time-dependent decline in risk. With regard to the smoking effect, NCRP chooses an additive model, whereas the other two committees prefer a multiplicative model.

Comparable responsiveness to radon exposure in males and females has also been investigated. Considering the risk following exposure in childhood, the ICRP proposes a threefold increased risk of exposure before age 20. Little evidence of age effects for lung carcinogenesis after childhood radon exposure is available. The only study of miners to have included children under the age of 13 is a study of Chinese tin miners [11]. The authors conclude that exposure to arsenic or radon as a child does not increase the risk of lung cancer over that of adult exposure.

Another approach is dosimetric: Exposure to α-particles is converted into tissue dose equivalent to enable use of the cancer risk coefficients derived from epidemiological studies of survivors of atomic bombs dropped on Japan in World War II. This conversion of exposure to tissue dose equivalent requires complex transformations that consider particle size distribution and equilibrium factors, breathing rate, lung morphology, and estimation of deposition in the various regions of the lung. On the basis of this approach, the ICRP Committee projected a 20% lower risk from indoor radon exposures for the general public than the risk from mining exposures.

In conclusion, despite the discrepancies and uncertainties inherent in the data, for a typical European or American population, the various approaches conclude a lifetime risk of lung cancer of 0.3 to 0.5% for a mean annual domestic exposure to radon of 0.1 WLM (equivalent to 1mSv/yr or 20 Bq/m$^3$ of radon gas). In other words, in countries such as France and Germany, where the mean national domestic radon exposure is estimated at 40 Bq/m$^3$, 6 to 10% of lung cancer mortality may be linked to this exposure. This estimate is dependent on the percentage of smokers in a population and uncertainty about the nature of tobacco–radon interaction.

### D. Case-Control Studies

At present, various analytical epidemiological case-control studies have been organized in Europe and the United States to ascertain the potential excess risk of lung cancer in the presence or absence of other etiological factors of lung carcinogenesis, such as active and passive tobacco smoking and occupational exposure. Radon measurements have to be taken in houses occupied in the past, to retrace the exposure accumulated during the past 30 to 40 years. As the risk linked to radon is relatively low compared to other factors, such as cigarette smoking, each study may not have enough statistical power to approach the radon risk precisely. A common protocol and joint analysis are a challenge for international cooperation under the coordination of the U.S. Department of Energy and the CEC. The first results issued from these studies may be expected in the period 1993–1995. Since the 1989 report of Samet [22] on the state of descriptive geographical and case-control studies on lung cancer and domestic radon exposure, few studies have been published [23–25]. Although some of them concluded that there is increased risk, very few could demonstrate a positive trend toward greater risk with increased exposure, and they need to be confirmed by larger-scale studies.

## V. From Risk to Prevention

As verified both in animal studies and in mining atmospheres, radon is a carcinogenic substance. In studies on uranium miners, the only cancer site that shows a positive trend with regard to cumulative exposure to radon is lung cancer. A collaborative international joint analysis of these studies is necessary to determine if other cancer sites that appear in excess in isolated studies may be due to radon.

Descriptive geographical correlation studies have produced controversary results; in France, for instance, a deficit of lung cancer deaths is observed in regions where radon exposure is high. This negative result may indicate that high radon concentrations are observed predominantly in rural areas, where lung cancer incidence is relatively low compared to the rate in urban regions, and they confirm the predominant factor of smoking in lung carcinogenesis, which may mask the radon effect. Nevertheless, inhabitants of houses that have radon gas concentrations higher than 400 Bq/m$^3$ (the limit recommended by the CEC) should be informed of some of the relatively easy remedial actions, such as ventilation. Figure 3 shows the influence of ventilation on radon concentration. When indoor radon concentrations in a house exceed 800 to 1000 Bq/m$^3$, higher than the limits accepted for present mining conditions, more important remedial actions, such as transformation and isolation of the ground under the house, must be considered. It should be mentioned that in many houses, radon-220, also called thoron, a member of the decay chain of thorium-232, is considered to contribute up to 30% of the $\alpha$-particle energy measured indoors, but that this 30% corresponds to only 10% of the total lung dose. Its contribution to the lung cancer risk may be considered minor, and as the origin of this radioactive component is primarily the building material, given its short radioactive half-life (55 s), painting or some other simple wall-covering method is sufficient to isolate the inhabitants from thoron exposure.

For new houses an annual limit of exposure corresponding to 200 Bq/m$^3$ is recommended by the CEC. The U.S. Environmental Protection Agency proposes a lower limit of about 150 Bq/m$^3$. For exposures close to these limits, the cost associated with modifying the house must be compared with the potential gain in lung cancer risk of the inhabitants. Getting precise information to the public concerning the relatively low lung cancer risk due to radon compared with tobacco consumption, for example, is a rather difficult challenge, linked to the

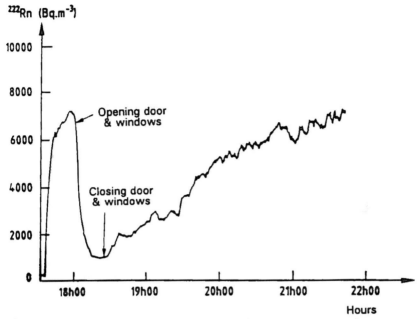

**Figure 3**   Radon concentration in a room according to ventilation conditions.

suspicious feeling of the public in front of the problem of low-level radioactivity, and to the uncertainty in the evaluation of the risk linked to the interaction of active or passive smoking and radon decay inhalation.

### References

1.  UNSCEAR report 1988. Sources, effects, and risks of ionizing radiation. Report of General Assembly, New York: United Nations Scientific Committee on the Effects of Atomic Radiation, 1988.
2.  Harley NH, Fissenne, IM. α Dose from long-lived emitters in underground uranium mine. In: Stocker H, ed. Occupational radiation safety in mining. Vol. 2. Toronto, Ontario, Canada: Canadian Nuclear Association, 1985:518–22.
3.  Singh NP, Bennett D, Saccomanno G, Wrenn ME. Concentrations of $^{210}$Pb in uranium miners' lungs and its states of equilibria with $^{238}$U, $^{234}$U, $^{230}$Th. In: Stocker H ed. Occupational radiation safety in mining. Vol. 2. Toronto, Ontario, Canada: Canadian Nuclear Association, 1985:503–6.
4.  Green BMR, Hughues JS, Lomas PR. Natural sources of ionising radiation in Europe. Radiation Atlas, 1991.

5. Chameaud J, Masse R, Morin M, Lafuma J. Lung cancer induction by radon daughters in rats, present state of the data on low dose exposures. In: Stocker H, ed. Proceedings of the International Conference on Occupational Radiation Safety in Mining. Vol. 1. Toronto, Ontario, Canada: Canadian Nuclear Association, 1985;350–53.

6. Cross FT, Palmer RF, Filipy RE, Dagle GE, Stuart BO. Carcinogenic effects of radon daughters, uranium ore dust and cigarette smoke in beagle dogs. Health Phys 1982;42:33–52.

7. Gray RG, Lafuma J, Parish SE, Peto R. Lung tumors and radon inhalation in over 2000 rats: approximate linearity across a wide range of doses and potentiation by tobacco smoke. In: Life span radiation effects studies in animals: What can they tell us? DOE Symposium Series 58. CONF-830951. 1986:592–607.

8. Hornung RW, Meinhardt TJ. Quantitative risk assessment of lung cancer in U.S. uranium miners. Health Phys 1987;52:417–30.

9. Howe GR, Nair RC, Newcombe HB, Miller AB, Burch JD, Abbat JD. Lung cancer mortality (1950–1980) in relation to radon daughter exposure in a cohort of workers at the Eldorado Port radium uranium mine: possible modification of risk by exposure rate. J Natl Cancer Inst 1987;79:1255–60.

10. Kunz E, Sevc J, Placek V, Horacek J. Lung cancer in man in relation to different time distribution of radiation exposure. Health Phys 1979;36:699–706.

11. Lubin JH, Qiao Y, Taylor PR, Yao S-X, Schatzkin A, Mao B-L, Rao J-Y, Xuan X-Z, Li J-Y. Quantitative evaluation of the radon and lung cancer association in a case control study of Chinese tin miners. Cancer Res 1990;50:174–80.

12. Muller J, Wheeler WC, Gentleman JF, Suranyi G, Kusiak R. Study of mortality of Ontario miners. In: Stocker H, ed. Proceedings of the International Conference on Occupational Radiation Safety in Mining. Vol. 1. Toronto, Ontario, Canada: Canadian Nuclear Association, 1984:335–43.

13. Morrison HI, Semenciw RM, Mao Y, Wigle DT. Cancer mortality among a group of fluorspar miners exposed to radon progeny. Am J Epidemiol 1988;128:1266–75.

14. Radford EP, St. Clair Renard KG. Lung Cancer in Swedish iron miners exposed to low doses of radon daughters. N Engl J Med 1984;310:1485–94.

15. Samet JM, Pathak DR, Morgan MV, Key CR, Valdivia AA, Lubin JH. Lung cancer mortality and exposure to Rn progeny in a cohort of New Mexico underground U miners. Health Phys 1991;61(6):745–52.

16. Sevc J, Kunz E, Tomasek L, Placek V, Horacek J. Cancer in man after exposure to Rn daughters. Health Phys 1988;54:27–46.

17. Tirmarche M, Brenot J, Piechowski J, Chameaud J, Pradel J. The present state of an epidemiological study of uranium miners in France. In: Stocker H, ed. Proceedings of the International Conference on Occupational Radiation Safety in Mining. Vol. 1. Toronto, Ontario, Canada: Canadian Nuclear Association, 1984:344–49.

18. Waxweiller RJ, Roscoe RJ, Archer VE, Thun MJ, Wagoner JK, Lundin FE. Mortality follow-up through 1977 of the white underground uranium miners cohort examined by the United States Public Health Service. In: Gomez M, ed. Radiation hazards in mining: control measurement and medical aspects. New York: Society of Mining Engineers of American Institute of Mining, Metallurgical and Petroleum Engineers, 1981:823–30.

19. BEIR IV. Health risks of radon and other internally deposited $\alpha$-mitters. Committee on the Biological Effects of Ionizing Radiations, National Research Council. Washington DC: National Academy Press, 1988.

20. ICRP 50. Lung cancer risk from indoor exposures to radon daughters. International Commission on Radiological Protection. Vol. 17. Elmsford, NY: Pergamon Press, 1987:1.

21. National Council on Radiation Protection and Measurements (NCRP). Evaluation of occupational and environmental exposure to radon and radon daughters in the United States. NCRP Report 78. Bethesda, MD: National Council on Radiation Protection and Measurements, 1984.

22. Samet JM. Radon and lung cancer. J Natl Cancer Inst 1989;81:745–57.

23. Schoenberg JB, Klotz JB, Wilcox HB, et al. Case-control study of residential radon and lung cancer among New Jersey women. Cancer Res 1990;50:6520–24.

24. Blot WJ, Xu ZY, Boice JD, et al. Indoor radon and lung cancer in China. J Natl Cancer Inst 1990;82:1025–30.

25. Roosteenoja E. Indoor radon and risk of lung cancer: an epidemiological study in Finland. STUK-A99. Helskini: Finnish Center for Radiation and Nuclear Safety. 1990.

# 11

## Pulmonary Responses to Multipollutant Airborne Particulate Matter and Other Contaminants, with Prevention Strategies

**MICHAEL D. LEBOWITZ**

University of Arizona College of Medicine
Tucson, Arizona

## I. Introduction

Humans are exposed to many particles and aerosols, both outdoors and indoors, that can affect health. There are several examples of interactions from mixed sources for given pollutants: environmental tobacco smoke (ETS) and other combustion sources produce particulate matter (PM), carbon monoxide and dioxide (CO, $CO_2$), nitrogen oxide and dioxide ($NO_2$), formaldehyde (HCHO), and organics [1–6]. More important, there are several examples of multiple pollutants from various sources having similar, possibly synergistic, effects: $NO_2$ and HCHO on irritation; PM (from ETS) and HCHO on eye and mucous membrane irritation; various PM, HCHO, and particulate allergens on "allergic" symptoms; $NO_2$, $O_3$, PM, and HCHO on pulmonary function; CO, $NO_2$, and HCHO on cognitive skills; CO, NO, $NO_2$, nitrates, and methylene chloride on carboxyhemoglobin and met-hemoglobin levels and cardiac arrhythmias; and radon and tobacco smoke on lung cancer. Several previous studies have looked at combinations of pollutants; most have looked at the combined effects of $SO_x$ and total suspended particulates (TSP) [7]. Recently, some studies have shown the interaction of allergens and bronchial irritants on bronchial responsiveness (BR) [8,9], which indicated the importance of environmental and acquired host characteristics as determinants of BR. Independent and interactive effects of indoor and outdoor pollutants, allergens, and weather variables have been shown to be related to symptoms and lung function in children and in allergic and asthmatic individuals (Table 1) [9–14].

Thus particulate pollutants, including bioaerols, may interact (additively, synergistically, or inhibitively) to produce respiratory health effects. The size of the particles or aerosols is important to potential reactions, in addition to their species (chemical and/or biological nature). Large particles (10 to 50 μm mass median aerodynamic diameter [MMAD]) affect the nose; intrathoracic airway deposition occurs with smaller particles (1 to 10 μm); and terminal airway-alreoli deposition occurs most frequently with particles under 2.5 μm. Moisture and temperature can affect the growth of viable aerosols and the size of nonviable aerosols.

To understand exposure to contaminants and the resulting effects on health, it has been suggested [3,5,15,16] that one needs to evaluate (1) the types of viable and nonviable particles, (2) the sources of contaminants and their means of dispersion, (3) the sinks for particles and the reservoirs of bioaerosols, (4) the nature and mechanisms of the morbidity effects associated with the contaminants, including the range and distribution of sensitivity in the population, and (5) the methods of evaluation (and of control). Epidemiological methods provide us with

**Table 1** Physiological Effects of Indoor–Outdoor Air Pollutants and Weather on Respiratory Symptoms and Functions in Tucson[a]

| Group | Time budget | Environmental variables[b] |
|-------|-------------|---------------------------|
| Children | Outdoors | Outdoor $O_3$, TSP, and temperature |
| Asthmatics | More indoors<br>In and out | Indoor TSP, RSP, and pollen<br>Interaction of outdoor $NO_2$ and indoor gas stoves with pollen; CO (spring), pollen, and humidity; temperature (summer) |
| Allergic subjects | Mostly outdoors | Pollen, low temp. (lag 1); humidity (spring–summer) |
| "Normals" | Both out and in | Interaction of gas stoves and outdoor $NO_2$ |

[a]Adjusted for other indoor–outdoor pollutants and meteorological variables.
[b]$O_3$, ozone; R/TSP, respiratory/total suspended particulates; $NO_2$, nitrogen dioxide; CO, carbon monoxide (a surrogate for indoor $NO_2$).

the opportunity to study the interactions of pollutants in complex environments, although most studies have not looked for interactions. Hazard assessment of respiratory effects in population is complicated by the varied biological processes that may result from exposure, separately or jointly, by irritant, infectious, and antigen challenges (NRC 1981). The health hazard assessments differ considerably with the various mechanisms (allergic, infective, or irritant/toxic).

In some diseases, such as allergy and asthma, one may see the impact of all the stimuli. Asthma (for which here we use the descriptive term *variable airways obstruction*) may be precipitated by a number of trigger factors, such as irritant pollutants (particles and/or gases), allergens and infections, exercise, and cold air. Allergy (defined as a physiological event mediated via a variety of immunological mechanisms induced and triggered by specific allergens) can be triggered by irritants as well [5,17–20]. Asthma and allergy symptoms may worsen within minutes or hours of exposure and improve after leaving the site of exposure. The late phase of dual-phase asthma may occur or reoccur 6 to 12 h after exposure to an allergic stimulus such as house dust mites [17,19,21]. Pseudoallergic reactions may be similar physiological reactions but without immunological specificity. They may be caused by direct release of mediators, complement activation, enzyme defects, or psychoneurogenic effects [22].

Responses to aeroallergens can be determined by symptoms, increased bronchial responsiveness (using allergen challenges or peak flows), increased medication use, visits to physicians or emergency rooms, and/or hospitalization [17–22]. Accuracy of the methods of detecting antibodies is very important, especially if such testing leads to probability distributions of sensitivity or immunity in populations [19,22–24]. Population models have been developed to describe attack rates and the spread of infectious diseases [23]. Each model has parameters determined by the exposure, time, and proportion of susceptibles. These compound distributions can represent the risk assessment exposure–response relationships; they can be defined for different populations.

In evaluating exposures, their type, location, and temporality are critical with respect to the various interactions related to health effects. Exposure to air pollutants is a function of pollutant concentrations in the locations or microenvironments that are "sampled" by an individual and weighted by the proportion of time spent in that location. Thus total personal exposure is highly dependent on the time–concentration component, which is attributable to spending nearly 90% of our time indoors [25–29]. This has raised questions as to whether the ambient air quality standards are appropriate, since these are based only on the health effects of outdoor exposures. It is likely that ambient monitoring data under- or overestimate actual total personal exposures and thus provide poor exposure–response estimates for use in establishing the standards and subsequent regulations for outdoor air quality.

## II.  Specific Findings of Indoor–Outdoor Multipollutant Health Effects

### A.  Indoor–Outdoor Particulates and Other Pollutants

Particulates from industrial stacks are still being characterized and studied toxicologically and epidemiologically. As mentioned, there is good evidence that PM and other combustion products released by industrial (and home) sources produce chronic respiratory disease (chronic bronchitis, ventilatory impairment) [7].

### Toxicology

In studies with *streptococuss*, Coffin [30] was able to demonstrate that $SO_x$ plus $O_3$ had a synergistic effect in increasing mortality in mice; at levels of 1 mg of $SO_x$ *(large particle) and 0.1 ppm of $O_3$*, mortality increased from 0 to between 0.5 and 3.8% when the agents were acting alone, and to 15 to 17.5% with the two together. Temperature and relative humidity were controlled. Ferrous, manganese, and nickel, as well as cadmium and zinc, showed similar results, as did zinc ammonium sulfate and ammonium sulfate. Further synergistic studies have been reviewed [1,7,31,32].

### Epidemiology

Verma et al. [33] reported that adult respiratory disease absences occurred on hot days (maximum temperature greater than 76°F) when the 24-h mean $SO_2$ levels increased. On cooler days (maximum temperature less than 50°F), when $SO_2$ and suspended sulfates were both high, respiratory illness absence rates were highest.

After accounting for temperature effects, it was found that asthma attack rates relate most closely to stepwise increases in the levels of suspended sulfates (SS) and suspended nitrates (SN) [34]. After controlling for other variables, the same team [35–37] also found differences in childhood acute respiratory disease in three different New York City communities with different levels of SS, SN, and respirable suspended particulates; there were similar findings in the Salt Lake Basin. Asthma aggravation in Los Angeles [36] was also related to variations in levels of suspended sulfates and suspended nitrates and was enhanced by the presence of elevated levels of other pollutants (e.g., ozone). In two southeastern cities, a combination of SS and SN increased asthma attacks more than either one alone [37]. Zagraniski et al. [38] saw some combined effects of sulfate particulate, ozone, and hydrogen ion concentrations in association with asthma and allergy symptoms.

Cohen et al. [39] studied attack rates in all physician-confirmed asthmatics in one town. They showed significant correlations between reported and confirmed attack rates and 24-h mean air pollution levels after the effects of temperature (a synergistic relationship) and season had been removed from the analysis. (Physician visits were used to validate attacks.) SS showed the strongest relationships; however SN, $SO_2$, and TSP individually, as well as in combination, explained a significant portion of the residual. Bates and Sizto [40] saw differential effects of sulfate and $O_3$ on hospital admissions. In Helsinki, a combination of temperature and ozone, as well as other gaseous pollutants, were associated with increased asthma admissions to hospitals [41].

Shy [42] has shown the relationship between the aggravation of asthma to elevated nitrate and sulfate levels, and the failure of respirable particle levels alone to be related to asthma. He indicates that the collinearity of nitrates and sulfates with relative humidity suggests their formation by reaction of atmospheric moisture with their precursors. Thus it is the properties of the particulates under certain climatic conditions, as well as particle size, that will determine their potential effects on health.

"Fugitive" PM exceeds the U.S. standards every year in most locations in basins in the southwest. It is primarily silica quartz, and generally averages 5 $\mu$m in size. In addition to some windblown contributions, it is often resuspended by vehicles operating over unpaved surfaces. Evidence indicates that especially with hot and dry conditions it produces both vasomotor rhinitis and regular irritant symptoms, and interacts with gases to produce symptoms and to decrease pulmonary function, especially in sensitive persons. The small PM ($>2.5$ $\mu$m) enters the indoor environment as well. The interactive effects of outdoor ozone and TSP have been shown to be synergistic [9,11]. Interestingly, passive smoking inhibits the effects of ozone [43], as active smoking does in chamber studies [32]. One could see the interactions of outdoor ozone and TSP, and of TSP–gas stove use, on peak flow (PEF), after adjustment was made for all other significant environmental variables. These interactions also demonstrate the influence of time spent indoors vs. outdoors (Table 1). The effects of TSP and gas stoves especially are either in one or the other, but not both. This type of relationship was also seen for outdoor $NO_2$ and gas stoves in asthmatics [11]. Ozone, temperature, and the use of gas stoves together were related to symptoms.

In the most recent study in Tucson, indoor PM interacted with other components of PM found in tobacco smoke (ETS) in effects on lung function; other interactions occurred between indoor and outdoor forms of PM and $NO_2$ in producing symptoms [44]. It was found that the relationship of diurnal responsiveness and $PM_{2.5}$ occurred primarily in homes independent of environmental tobacco smoke, although rates of increased diurnal responsiveness were higher in homes with more $PM_{10}$ and ETS; in the latter case, PM and ETS were collinear ($p = 0.0004$) and interactive. In children, the prevalence rate of daily bronchial responsiveness related strongly to ETS (controlling for age and sex) [45].

Adjusting for covariates, significant effects of interactions of 8-h $O_3$ with particulate matter ($PM_{10}$) and temperature on daily peak flow were found. There was some overnight effect of 8-h $O_3$, but no cumulative effect of $O_3$ in the past 4 days. These results indicate that, in general, the response of the respiratory system to low-level ambient ozone is acute, is seen more in asthmatics, and increases with its interaction with temperature and $PM_{10}$ ]12]. The interactions of outdoor pollutants and meteorological conditions on these symptoms and lung function imply greater need for total exposure assessments.

ETS interacted with indoor formaldehyde in producing symptoms and in relation to asthma and chronic bronchitis diagnoses [13]. Frigas et al. [46] showed that the HCHO particles were more important than HCHO gas alone in affecting lung function in asthmatics. Chronic respiratory symptoms and pulmonary function to current integrated levels of formaldehyde (HCHO) in homes in the sample of 298 children (6 to 15 years of age) and 613 adults in Tucson showed that significantly greater prevalence rates of asthma and chronic bronchitis were found in children from houses with current HCHO levels of 60 to 120 ppb than in those less exposed, especially in children also exposed to environmental tobacco smoke [13]. In children, levels of PEF decreased linearly with HCHO exposure, with the estimated decrease due to 60 ppb of HCHO equivalent to 22% of PEF level in nonexposed children. The effects in asthmatic children exposed to current HCHO below 50 ppb were greater than in healthy children [13]. The evidence reflects avoidance of high HCHO exposure by asthmatics; only a few were in exposure settings with levels above 50 ppb. The effects in adults were less evident: decrements in PEF related to current HCHO over 40 ppb were seen only in the morning, and mainly in smokers [13].

## B.  Bioaerosols and Other Contaminants

Biological aerosols are different from other airborne particulate matter, as they have complex, varied organic structures that do not permit simple sampling or chemical analysis [2,5]. Even in small quantities, they can have very large respiratory impacts due to infection, allergenicity, or irritation. These health effects can range from uncomfortable to disabling [2,5,17]. Only in sensitive persons would other air contaminants have such allergic or irritant effects [5,17,20,24,47]. The indoor environment is the major source of bioaerosols and has a large attributable risk for such effects. Indoors, bioaerosols contribute to overall particle mass. For instance, insects and animals can introduce by-product aerosols, which can produce a variety of allergic and irritant reactions in occupants [48,49].

Temperature and humidity contribute to the growth of some organisms that produce such particles, as well as effecting health directly [5,48,49]. Bacteria and fungi can multiply in microclimates indoors, including ventilation systems.

Viruses do not multiply indoors but may spread between humans and from a few animal sources. The airborne spread of viral disease can be facilitated by crowding of people or through the spread of airborne virus through a ventilation system [5,50]. Facilitation of pathogenicity also occurs with prior (and continued) exposure to other air contaminants [e.g., volatile organic compounds (VOCs), nitrogen dioxide ($NO_2$)] [1–6,30].

Infiltration from outdoors is responsible for most indoor pollen [51,52], the rest being from some indoor plants. Pollen, a slightly different type of suspended PM, as an allergenic has been shown to produce serious responses in those more sensitive (i.e., allergic). Indoor concentrations of fungi, insects, and animal fragments can be affected through infiltration as well [2,53]. Many of these bioaerosols end up in house dust, to be resuspended with human activity or pet activity [54,55]. Fungi, algae, and species were not related to symptoms or peak flow in Tucson after accounting for other environmental factors [11].

In Tucson, the pollutant and meteorological variables were related to respiratory symptoms and peak flow directly as well as through interactions with pollen types; specific health effects noted were rhinitis, productive cough, and attacks of wheezing dyspnea in asthmatics; and the attack and decreased peak flow in subjects with airway obstructive disease [10]. Some of the largest positive coefficients are seen in association with seasonal pollen types: specifically, rhinitis in allergics. Time-series analysis [9] showed that asthmatics had the most respiratory responses, while asymptomatics showed no significant responses. Outdoor ozone, indoor and outdoor PM and nitrogen dioxide, aeroallergens, and meteorology were significantly related, independently and interactively, with symptoms and peak flow.

The combined effect of all contaminants, especially infectious agents and those indoors, is thought to account for a substantial proportion of absenteeism in schools and workplaces and of days of restricted activity or performance; 5 to 15 days of restricted activity per year may result [5,56]. Further, a sizable proportion of the population has been or is capable of being sensitized (i.e., can develop a hypersensitivity) to these forms of bioaerosol contaminants over their lifetimes [2,20,57,58].

## III. Prevention

Strategies for prevention against the effect of airborne contaminants are of two major types, those relating to individuals and those relating to the physical environment. Prevention for the individual can occur through modification of host susceptibility (e.g., immunization for infectious agents) and avoidance of irritants or allergen pollutants. Avoidance of triggering exposures (as recommended clinically to asthmatics), including physical measures, are based predominantly on the avoidance of conditions and on the containment and removal of sources [2,5,20,59].

## A. Behavior and Socioeconomic Influences

Behavioral methods of prevention are recognized to be a major determinant, especially for contamination and exposure [3,16]. Modification of the behaviors that influence air quality and resultant exposure is often the simplest, least expensive, and most effective means of reducing adverse health effects. These factors include a range of activities: education; personal behavior, and social practices [3,5,59].

Education includes the dissemination of information to people on actions they could take to reduce or eliminate indoor bioaerosols; and the ability to recognize situations (e.g., source and source use) that might contribute to bioaerosol concentrations. Use of the information will depend upon the motivation of the individual and available resources. Individuals could use available information to reduce their exposures or remove themselves from contaminated environments in which they experience adverse health effects.

## B. Physical Methods

The goal of protecting human health is not adequately served by the application of outdoor air quality standards. Specifically, the experience gained in developing and implementing strategies for population exposure reductions in the outdoor environment is not very applicable to indoor environments, and new strategies will need to be considered, developed, tested and evaluated.

These methods of source control have been categorized by a WHO working group [5]. Because several of these controls can have the opposite effect for other contaminants, it was stated that they should be used with caution. Proper design and construction of industrial processes and buildings is the most desirable control means to avoid contamination from their system-related sources [60]. For instance, the structure of buildings should consist of nondeteriorating materials so as not to offer a substrate for microbial growth, and construction materials should be chosen to control moisture effectively, the most important factor governing microbial growth [5]. Strategies should avoid conflicts between energy conservation and effective control. Source modification offers several possibilities for control. For instance, changes in temperature or relative humidity (two interrelated parameters) can be used to control some sources but will often have an opposite effect on others; maintenance, repair, and cleaning are common control strategies [3].

Society can exert considerable pressure, or provide/promote incentives to control sources of contamination [3,60]. In addition, societal pressure can result in establishing adequate indoor ventilation standards [61]. The financial burden associated with indoor as well as outdoor controls should be estimated adequately to promote prevention measures. To protect the public, governmental guidelines for reduction of contamination have been established in some countries [3] but need further development in other countries. Strategy should be pursued as part of public policy, which should include, where necessary, the formation of standards, regulations, controls, practices, labeling requirements, recommendations, and guidelines. Governmental support of research and communication can be a primary service to encourage cooperation among participants in prevention.

## IV. Future Objectives

### A. Chronic Effects of Multipollutant Exposures

This objective includes (1) differentiation of susceptibility to chronic effects, through ongoing studies of bronchial responsiveness, immunological and physiological status, and coexisting morbidity; (2) determination of quantitative and qualitative response differences and differences in response time for susceptible and nonsusceptible individuals; (3) the study of the role of the natural history of responses to climate, biological, and nonbiological aerosols in different subpopulations as factors in subchronic and chronic responses; and (4) the study of specific pollutant interactions in chronic exposure–response relationships.

### B. Acute Effects of Multipollutant Exposures

The objectives are to relate the respiratory responses (symptoms, peak expiratory flows, spirometry, medication usage, and medical visits) and changes in activity/performance to air pollution ($O_3$, PM, $NO_2$, HCHO), to aeroallergen (pollen and mold) exposures and to meteorological conditions, as modified by host characteristics (age, sex, socioeconomic status, reactivity, or predisposition to response) and by time/activity patterns in both indoor and outdoor environments. Elevated short-term concentrations of pollutants that are related to intermittent source use, such as smoking or combustion appliances, are of special interest in assessing the health effects of these sources and pollutants on health. For example, $NO_2$ may facilitate infectious processes especially in children, and these infections may lead to more serious sequelae [62].

### C. Pollutant and Exposure Assessment

Indoors, PM generated by cigarette smoke, woodstoves and fireplaces, and other combustion is complex and contributes a major portion of the total indoor PM, so that the speciation of indoor particulate is necessary. Further, methods of evaluating adsorption or absorption of gases onto particulates are necessary, since these different combinations may have very different effects, some of which are more serious than the gas or PM alone. The size distribution of PM indoors with different combinations of sources requires further evaluation, as the indoor PM will produce major responses dependent on both its size and chemical composition. Thus characterization of the sizes and types of PM occurring both indoors and outdoors is needed to evaluate the independent effects on health of PM and the interaction of PM with other pollutants in producing effects on health.

Monitoring and time–activity diaries should directly assess levels of exposure (over time) and help to determine the major determinants of personal exposure of individuals to pollutants [2,3,63]. Quantitative assessments of total personal exposure is possible even with fixed location (microenvironmental) sampling coupled with individual time budgets [2,3,64]. Exposure classifications or models alone are probably insufficient to characterize exposure patterns of individuals. Some direct monitoring component (indoor, outdoor, and personal) is required to determine the magnitude and causes of misclassification errors, and to test the hypotheses and assumptions used.

Although peak concentrations during source use are not available directly from integrated samplers, estimates of the average concentration during source use can be derived from the reported or measured total time of source use and the measured integrated average [2,3,65,66]. This approach requires further verification with continuous monitoring data. Better models of exposure and exposure–response must be developed using real data to meet the needs of criteria for air quality standards.

### D.  Exposure–Response Studies

There are still serious limitations in our knowledge of total population exposure for each contaminant, and equally serious limitations in our knowledge of the exposure–response relationships, to both single and multiple contaminants [3–6].

The expected time interval between exposure(s) and the eventual health effect must be taken into account. Further, patterns of response [66,67] and the interaction between pollutants and other factors, such as socioeconomic characteristics, smoking, and occupational exposure, can only be shown in population studies [66].

### Acknowledgments

This work would not have been possible without the efforts of my collegues J. Quackenboss, M. K. O'Rourke, M. Krzyzanowski, P. Pfersdorf, and B. Boyer. This work was supported by NHLBI SCOR Grant HL14136 and by EPA Cooperative Agreement CR811806. Although the research described in this article has been funded in part by the U.S. Environmental Protection Agency, it has not been subjected to the agency's required peer and policy review and therefore does not necessarily reflect the views of the agency, and no official endorsement should be inferred.

### References

1. American Thoracic Society. Statement on the health effects of air pollution. New York: American Thoracic Society, 1978.
2. NRC (National Research Council). Indoor pollutants. Washington DC: National Academy of Science, 1981.
3. WHO. Indoor air quality research: Report on a WHO Meeting. EURO Reports and Studies 103. Copenhagen: WHO European Regional Office, 1986.
4. WHO. Indoor air quality: organics. EURO Reports and Studies 111. Copenhagen: World Health Organization, 1989.
5. WHO. Biological contaminants in indoor air. EURO Regional Series 31. Copenhagen: WHO, 1990.
6. WHO, Indoor air quality: combustion products. Copenhagen: WHO/EURO, 1991.
7. EPA. Air quality criteria for particulate matter and sulfur oxides. Chap. 14. Epidemiological studies of health effects. Research Triangle Park, NC: EPA, 1982.
8. O'Connor G, Sparrow D, Segal MR, Weiss ST. Smoking, atopy, and methacholine airway responsiveness among middle-aged and elderly men: the normative aging study. Am Rev Respir Dis 1989;140:1520–26.
9. Lebowitz MD, Collins L, Holberg C. Time series analysis of respiratory responses to indoor and outdoor environmental phenomena. Environ Res 1987;43:332–41.
10. Holberg CJ, O'Rourke MK, Lebowitz MD. Multivariate analysis of ambient environmental factors and respiratory effects. Int J Epidemiol 1987;16(3):399–410.
11. Lebowitz MD, Holberg CJ, Boyer B, Hayes C. Respiratory symptoms and peak flow associated with indoor and outdoor air pollutants in the Southwest. J Air Pollution Control Assoc 1985;35(11):1154–58.
12. Krzyzanowski M, Quackenboss JJ, Lebowitz MD. Sub-chronic respiratory effects from long term exposure to ozone in Tucson. Arch Environ Health 1992; 47:107–15.
13. Krzyzanowski M, Quackenboss JJ, Lebowitz MD. Chronic respiratory effects of indoor formaldehyde exposure. Environ Res 1990;52:117–25.
14. Lebowitz MD, Quackenboss JJ, Krzyzanowski M, O'Rourke MK, Hayes C. Multipollutant exposures and health responses: epidemiological aspects of particulate matter. Arch Environ Health 1992;47:71–75.

15. WHO. Guidelines on studies in environmental epidemiology. Environmental Health Criteria 27. Geneva: WHO, 1983.
16. WHO, Indoor air pollutants: exposure and health effects. WHO EURO Reports and Studies 78. Copenhagen: WHO European Regional Office, 1983.
17. Weill H, Turner-Warwick M, eds. Occupational lung diseases. New York: Marcel Dekker, 1981:143–68.
18. Rom WN, ed. Environmental and occupational medicine. Boston: Little, Brown, 1983.
19. Middleton E, Reed CE, Ellis EF. Allergy, principles and practice. 3rd ed. St. Louis: CV Mosby, 1988.
20. Lebowitz MD. Indoor bioaerosol contaminants. In: Lippmann M, ed. Environmental toxicants: human exposures and their health effects. New York: Van Nostrand Reinhold, 1992;331–59.
21. Booij-Noord H, Orie NGM, DeVries K. Immediate and late bronchial obstructive reactions to inhalation of housedust and protective effects of disodium cromoglycate and prednisolone. J Allergy Clin Immunol 1971;48:344–54.
22. Ring J. Pseudo-allergic reactions. In: Korenblat PE, Wedner HJ, eds. Allergy, theory and practice. 2nd ed. Orlando, FL: Grune & Stratton, 1989.
23. Fox JP, Hall CE, Elveback LR. Epidemiology. New York: Macmillan, 1970.
24. Turner-Warwick M. Immunology of the lung. London: Edward Arnold, 1978.
25. Dockery DW, Spengler JD, Reed MP, Ware J. Relationships among personal indoor and outdoor $NO_2$ measurements. Environ Int 1981;5:101–7.
26. Spengler JD, Treitman RD, Tosteson TD, Mage DT, Soczek ML. Personal exposures to respirable particulates and implications for air pollution epidemiology. Environ Sci Technol 1985;19:700.
27. Leaderer BP, Zagraniski RT, Berwick M, Stolwijk JAJ. Assessment of exposure to indoor air contaminants from combustion sources: methodology and application. Am J Epidemiol 1986;124:275–89.
28. Quackenboss JJ, Kanarek MS, Spengler JD, Letz R. Personal monitoring for $NO_2$ exposure: methodological considerations for a community study. Environ Int 1982;8:249.
29. Quackenboss JJ, Spengler JD, Kanarek MS, Letz R, Duffy CP. Personal exposure to nitrogen dioxide: relationship to indoor/outdoor air quality and activity patterns. Environ Sci Technol 1986;20:775.
30. Coffin DL, Gardner DE, Blommer EJ. Time/dose response for nitrogen

dioxide exposure in an infectivity model system. Environ Health Perspect 1976;13:11–15.

31. Coffin DL, Stokinger HE. Biological effects of air pollution. Vol. II. 3rd ed. Stern air pollution. New York: Academic Press, 1977:302–25.
32. EPA. Ozone criteria document. Research Triangle Park, NC: ECAO, 1984.
33. Verma MP, Schilling FJ, Becker WH. Epidemiological study of illness absences in relation to air pollution. Arch Environ Health 1969;18:536–43.
34. Finklea KF, Calafiore DC, Nelson CJ, Riggan WB, Hayes CG. Aggravation of asthma by air pollutants: 1971 Salt Lake Basin studies. In: Health consequences of sulfur oxides: a report from CHESS, 1970–71. EPA 650/1-74-004, Office of Research and Development. Washington DC: U.S. Government Printing Office, 1972:2-75-2-91.
35. Hammer DI, Miller FJ, Stead AG, Hayes CG. Air pollution and childhood lower respiratory disease. I. Exposure to sulfur oxides and particulate matter in New York 1972. In: Finkel AJ, Duel WC, eds. Clinical implications of air pollution research. Acton, MA: Publishing Sciences Group, 1976:321–37.
36. French JG. Effects of suspended sulfates on human health. Environ Health Perspect 1975;10:35–37.
37. French JG, Hasselblad V, Sharp G, Truppi L. A study of asthma in the Los Angeles basin: 1972–1973. Washington, DC: Environmental Research Council, U.S. Environmental Protection Agency, 1975.
38. Zagraniski RT, Leaderer BP, Stolwijk JAJ. Ambient sulfates, photochemical oxidants, and acute health effects: an epidemiological study. Environ Res 1979;19:306–20.
39. Cohen AA, Bromberg S, Buechley RW, Heiderscheit LT, Shy CM. Asthma and air pollution from a coal fueled power plant. Am J Public Health 1972;62:1181–88.
40. Bates DV, Sizto R. Relationship between air pollution levels and hospital admissions in Southern Ontario. Can J Public Health 1983;76:117–33.
41. Ponka A. Asthma and low level air pollution in Helsinki. Arch Environ Health 1991;46:262–70.
42. Shy, CM. Salts, gases, sulfur, nitrogen association. Photochem Oxid 1974;2:51.
43. Lebowitz MD. The effects of environmental tobacco smoke exposure and gas stoves on daily peak flow rates in asthmatic and non-asthmatic families. Eur J Respir Dis 1984;65(Suppl 133):90–97.
44. Quackenboss JJ, Krzyzanowski M, Lebowitz MD. Exposure assessment approaches to evaluate respiratory health effects of particulate matter and nitrogen dioxide. J Expos Assess Environ Epidemiol 1991;1(1):83–107.

45. Lebowitz MD, Quackenboss JJ. The effects on environmental tobacco smoke on pulmonary function. Int Arch Occup Environ Health 1989(Suppl):147–52.

46. Frigas E, Filley WV, Reed CE. Asthma induced by dust from urrea-formaldehyde foam insulating material. Chest 1981;79:706–7.

47. Lebowitz MD. The use of peak expiratory flow rate measurements in respiratory disease. Pediatr Pulmonol 1991;11:166–74.

48. RIVM. Indoor environment. In: Langeweg Ir F, ed. A national environmental survey 1985–2010, concern for tomorrow. The Netherlands: National Institute of Public Health and Environmental Protection, 1989:243–54.

49. Andersen I, Korsgaard J. Asthma and the indoor environment: assessment of the health implications of high indoor air humidity. Environ Int 1986;12:121–27.

50. Riley RL. Indoor airborne infection. Environ Int 1972;8:317–20.

51. O'Rourke MK, Lebowitz MD. A comparison of regional atmospheric pollen with pollen collected at and near homes. Grana 1984;23:55–64.

52. O'Rourke MK, Quackenboss JJ, Lebowitz MD. An epidemiologic approach investigating respiratory disease in sensitive individuals to indoor and outdoor pollen exposure in Tucson, Arizona. Aerobiologia 1989; 5:104–10.

53. Solomon WR, Burge HP. *Aspergillus fumigatus* levels in and out of doors in urban air. J Allergy Clin Immunol 1975;55:90–91.

54. Nevalainen A, Jantunen M, Pellikka M, Pitkanen E, Kalliokoski P. Airborne bacteria, fungal spores and ventilation in Finnish day-care centers. Indoor Air '87, Berlin, August 17–21, 1987:678–80.

55. Reed CE, Swanson MC. Indoor allergens: identification and quantification. Environ Int 1986;12:115–20.

56. National Center for Health Statistics (U.S.). Current estimates from the national Health Interview Survey, United States, 1987. DHHS Publication (PHS) 88-1594. Washington, DC: U.S. Government Printing Office, 1988.

57. Barbee RA, Kaltenborn W, Lebowitz MD, Burrows B. Longitudinal changes in allergen skin test reactivity in a community population sample. J Allergy Clin Immunol 1987;79:16–24.

58. Sears MR, Herbison GP, Holdaway MD, et al. The relative risks of sensitivity to grass pollen, house dust mite and cat dander in the development of childhood asthma. Clin Allergy 1989;19:419–24.

59. Samet J, ed. Environmental controls and lung disease. Am Rev Respir Dis 1990;142:915–39.

60. NRC. Policies and procedures for control of indoor air quality. Committee on Indoor Air Quality. Washington DC: National Academy Press, 1987.

61. Ventilation for acceptable air quality. ASHRAE Standard 62-1981R. Draft

for public review. Atlanta, GA: American Society of Heating, Refrigerating and Air Conditioning Engineers, 1988.

62. Burrows B, Knudson RJ, Lebowitz MD. The relationship of childhood respiratory illness to adult obstructive airway disease. Am Rev Respir Dis 1977;115:751.

63. National Academy of Sciences. Epidemiology and air pollution. Washington DC: National Academy Press, 1985.

64. Ott WR. Models of human exposure to air pollution. Technical Report 32. Stanford, CA: SIAM Institute for Mathematics and Society, Stanford University, 1990.

65. Sexton K, Letz R, Spengler JD. Estimating human exposure to nitrogen fioxide: an indoor/outdoor modeling study. Atmos Environ 1983;17:1339.

66. World Health Organization (WHO). Estimating human exposure to air pollutants. Copenhagen/Geneva: WHO, 1982.

67. Berglund B, et al. Olfactory and chemical characterization of indoor air. Towards a psychophysical model for air quality. Environ Int 1982;8(1–6):327–32.

# 12

## Prevention of Health Problems in Air-Conditioned Buildings

**CLAUDE MOLINA**

French Lung Association
and University of Clermont-Ferrand
Paris, France

## I. Introduction

Air conditioning is used in many different situations for the purposes of comfort, safety, and even noise abatement: for instance, in large blocks of fats or individual dwellings in hot countries, or in detached houses, hospitals, hotels, department stores, city office blocks, museums, and libraries containing valuable documents. It is also used in numerous industries where humidification is necessary, in printing and in such high-tech industries as electronics, data processing, and magnetic tape manufacture. Thus millions of people live or work in premises where the ventilation is regulated and where use is made of air-conditioning systems. At the same time, the problem of indoor air quality is becoming a matter of increasing concern.

Indeed, since the 1970s and the oil crisis, energy-saving measures have led to a reduction in room ventilation. Moreover, the use of synthetic materials that emit various chemical substances has led to an increase in the concentration of indoor pollutants.

In 1970, following the observations of Banaszak et al. [1], the attention of the medical profession was drawn to the development of an allergic respiratory disorder (allergic alveolitis) among employees working in air-conditioned offices (Fig. 1). This was due to contamination of air-conditioning systems by thermoactinomycetes found in air-conditioner ducts and in ambient air. The same microorganisms are found in moldy hay and provoke a hypersensitivity pneumonitis known as *farmer's lung*. So this air-conditioning disease is classified as an urban *allergic alveolitis*.

In Philadelphia in 1976 there was an outbreak of a hitherto unknown infectious disease, later called Legionnaires' disease. This serious illness, which affects primarily the lungs, was caused by a previously unidentified bacterium (later termed *Legionella*) that had probably developed in a cooling tower adjacent to the air-conditioning system of a Philadelphia hotel where the members of the American Legion were meeting. Legionnaire's disease and its more benign homolog, Pontiac fever, are now (wrongly) considered to be illnesses caused by air-conditioning systems. Several epidemics have been reported worldwide. These have been associated with a significant mortality.

Apart from these allergic and infectious disorders, doctors are confronted every day with a number of complaints related to the mucous membranes of eyes, nose, and throat, accompanied by headache and lethargy. These symptoms appear to be benign and related to the building in which the people live or work and constitute the so-called *sick-building syndrome* (SBS).

It is not surprising that health respiratory problems are common when we realize that every day we breathe more than 15,000 L of air and that most employees in air-conditioned buildings spend more than 8 h a day 5 days a week in an artificial atmosphere. An investigation carried out by Woods et al. [2] on 600 office workers in the United States showed that 20% of the employees experienced symptoms of SBS, and most of them were convinced that this reduced their working efficiency. Other estimates report that up to 30% of new and refurbished buildings throughout the world may be affected by this syndrome (WHO, 1983 and 1986). A study performed in the United Kingdom on 4373 office workers revealed that 22% of those studied experienced five or more of the characteristic symptoms of SBS [3].

## II.  Infections

### A.  Bacterial Infections

The most serious infection associated with air-conditioning systems is that caused by *Legionella pneumophila*. Subjects are infected by vapor drift containing this bacterium coming from contaminated cooling towers. This may occur in the streets in the vicinity of the cooling tower or inside buildings when water droplets are drawn into the building via the air-conditioning system. (Legionnaires'

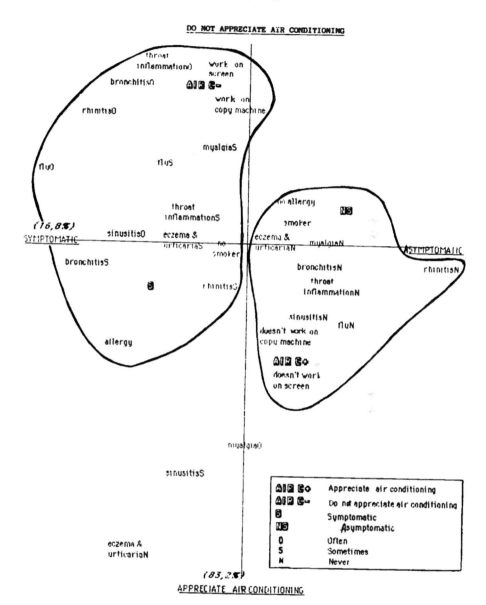

**Figure 1** Medical profiles of those who do and those who do not appreciate air-conditioning.

disease has not been described as a result of contaminated cold water spray humidifiers.)

Two clinical aspects may be observed:

1. *Legionnaires' disease.* This is a severe pneumonia with chills, fever, and lung consolidation, sometimes associated with neurologic symptoms (such as headache and drowsiness) or gastrointestinal upset. Diagnosis is made by the presence of a gram-negative bacterium, *Legionella pneumophila*, identified by direct immunofluorescence in sputum or in bronchoalveolar lavages (performed early). A few days later, diagnosis may be made by the presence of serum antibodies. Epidemics commonly break out in hotels, hospitals, or large buildings where humidification sections of heating/ventilating/air conditioning (HVAC) installations are contaminated. Some cases are fatal. Antibiotics such as erythromycine (first choice), or rifampycine associated with fluoroquinolone in severe forms, are the main efficient drugs.

2. *Pontiac fever.* This is a flulike syndrome observed among employees of the Oakland County Health Department in Pontiac (Michigan), similar to Legionnaire's disease but with benign symptoms, which can be cured in 2 to 5 days. The organism responsible for this syndrome was identified as *Legionella pneumophila*, but other serotypes of varieties of *Legionella* (*Legionella micdadei, Long-Beach, gormanee, boozemanii,* etc.) may be found as a cause of epidemics.

Other infections have been described in which the mode of spread appeared to be via air-conditioning devices, mainly in medical settings: tuberculosis [4], and infections due to *Staphylococcus aureus* (in operating rooms) [5].

### Prevention

It is well known that cooling towers located near air-conditioning systems are a source of microbial proliferation, due to water stagnation. Such towers must be built far from air-supply intakes and places where people gather (e.g., train stations, bus stops). It is necessary to take into account the dominant wind direction. The effluents of air-cooling towers must not be sucked back in by the ventilators of air-treatment casings and then blown out again inside buildings.

Good maintenance is mandatory with a check of filters for cleanliness, avoiding water stagnation and removing sludge (see Section V). Moreover, one of the best ways to reduce or eliminate microbial proliferation is the use of intermittent chlorinated compounds. Intense ultraviolet irradiation in central ventilating ducts can provide a second line of defense [6] but is very expensive.

### B. Viral Infections

An epidemic of measles has been described caused by contamination of air-conditioning systems [6]. An outbreak of influenza [7] was reported aboard a commercial airline. But buildings can also contribute to the airborne spread of viral diseases through crowding of people.

### C. Fungal Infections

Infections caused by fungal species such as *Aspergillus* as a result of contaminated incoming air have been reported, mainly in hospitals, during major building or refurbishing works [8,9]. *Aspergillus* infection affects primarily old or immunocompromized patients, or is observed after surgical procedures. The symptoms are these of *invasive* aspergillosis or atypical aspergillosis (pleural or sinusal). But other molds—*Alternaria, Aureobasidium pullulans,* and *Cladosporium*—have been isolated in the ambient air of air-conditioned rooms, even in well-supervised air-conditioning systems [10]. All these microorganisms can cause disease when airborne in sufficient number.

### D. Protozoal Infections

Motile organisms such as amoeba and ciliates grow in indoor reservoirs. A few of these protozoa can cause severe infections [11]. Most provoke hypersensitivity diseases.

## III. Allergic Diseases

Allergic indoor-related illnesses fall into four categories, as follows: rhinitis and asthma, both usually IgE-mediated, and alveolitis and humidifier fever, both usually IgG mediated.

### A. Rhinitis

Many indoor allergens induce immediate allergic responses in the upper (as well as lower) respiratory tract: house dust and mites, animal danders, chemicals (formaldehyde, TDI), and microorganisms such as *Penicillium, Aspergillus, Clados porium,* and *Bacillus subtilis.*

### B. Asthma

Cases of asthma have been described caused by a simple homemade cold water spray humidifier contaminated by microorganisms [12] or in a factory by a central cold water humidifier, especially in a poorly maintained building [13]. In these cases the features were those of occupational asthma.

### C. Alveolitis

Since the first description by Banaszak [1], a small number of cases have been reported in the literature in large air-conditioned office blocks [14], a photographic factory [15], air-conditioned homes [16], [17], and swimming pools [18]. A few hours after exposure, the main symptoms appear, including fever, malaise, and breathlessness. A sizable loss of weight is common. Late inspiratory crackles are present on ausculation, whereas chest x-rays show a micronodular infiltration. Pulmonary function tests reveal a restrictive defect with a fall in $PaO_2$ and impaired gas transfer (CO diffusion).

Serological tests show the presence of precipitating antibodies to the causative allergen. This allergen may be a thermophilic actinomycetes *(Micropolyspora faeni)*, a mold *(Aureobasidium pullulans)*, or pigeon droppings (in air intakes). We have very few data on bronchoalveolar lavages in such cases. Occasionally, lung biopsies showing characteristic features (granuloma with giant-cell and histiocytic infiltration) confirm the diagnosis.

### D.  Humidifier Fever

This condition was first described in 1959 by Pestalozzi [19]. He mentioned an outbreak of systemic and respiratory symptoms in a group of workers in a carpentry shop. Symptoms occur on the first day of the workweek. Then the symptoms improve progressively during the week, recurring after a weekend or holiday on the first day back at work. These symptoms are flulike: lethargy, myalgia, arthralgia, headache and fever, coughing, and breathlessness.

Physical examination of the patient reveals the presence of late inspiratory crackles on auscultation. Lung function tests shows a restrictive defect with impaired gas transfer, but the chest radiograph is normal. Between the attacks the lung function is normal.

Immunological investigations almost always show the presence of precipitating antibodies to antigens extracted from humidifiers. Bronchial provocation tests with water from the humidifier usually reproduce symptoms and physiological changes in affected individuals but not in control subjects. The causes of humidifier fever are not known. Outbreaks often occur when humidifiers have become heavily contaminated by microorganisms. A number of different causes have been postulated, including *Naegleria gruberi*, *Acanthamoeba polyphaga*, *Bacillus subtilis*, and endotoxins.

Recently, Polla and al. [20] suggested that there were two types of humidifier fever. The first, classical form, with precipitating antibodies, is mediated by an immune mechanism. The features of the second form include the absence of precipitins and the presence of endotoxins in large quantities in the ducts of humidifiers (their dosage being performed by biological tests, *Limulus* amoebocyte lysate) or chemical techniques.

All these hypersensitivity diseases may be due to a large variety of microorganisms. Nearly all fungi produce spores that can penetrate buildings through mechanical air intakes or cracks. However, actinomycetes are often implicated because the size of their spores are small enough (less than 1 μm) to reach alveoli. But other microorganisms may act by toxins: either bacterial endotoxins (*Pseudomonas* or *flavobacterium* species) or mycotoxins. Moreover, both toxic and immunologic mechanisms may be involved, bearing in mind that endotoxins enhance immediate or Arthus-type reactions [21,22]. Finally, many of these microorganisms produce volatile organic compounds that are mucosal irritants.

### Air Sampling

Air sampling is an expensive, time-consuming procedure, which does not always provide precise information. It is useful, however, when symptoms experienced by people living in air-conditioned buildings evoke the role of molds or bacteria or for medico-legal or research purposes.

The choice of sampler depends on the size of the bioaerosol and the time and the site of sampling (swab, liquid, dust sources). In our experience, the Cascade Impactor [23] is frequently used with culture on Sabouraud medium. Feuilhade et al. [9] confirmed the good results obtained with this device. But there is no international standard method or background data available to indicate what is "safe and normal." The relationship between reported symptoms and organisms found in air samplers may rarely be assessed.

A comparison between outdoor and indoor levels of microorganism concentration has been suggested by Burge and may be useful [24]. However, two precise studies showed the most frequent variety of microorganisms isolated in air-conditioning devices, even those most closely supervised and kept clean.

In 43 samples examined, Austwick [10] found in air and sludge a predominance of *Aspergillus, Aureobasidium,* and *Cladosporium* and in air the frequent presence of *Penicillium* and *Rhodotorula.* In nine buildings studied, Nolard Tintignier [25] found mainly *Aspergillus* (*glaucus* and *restrictus*) in the majority of cases. However, the dose–response relationship between these findings and reported symptoms could not be proved.

## IV. Sick-Building Syndrome

Sick-building syndrome (SBS) consists of various symptoms, including upper respiratory manifestations, which are experienced by people living or working in air-conditioned or hermetically sealed buildings. The absence of objective symptoms accounts for the different designations for this syndrome: tight building syndrome (United States), indoor climatee problems (Scandinavia), maladie des tours à bureaux (Canada), and maladie des bâtiments malsains (France). It is therefore diagnosed by exclusion after eliminating all other building-related illnesses.

### A. Symptomatology

The symptomatology of this syndrome is extremely varied, but five different classes of symptoms are encountered:

1. *Respiratory manifestations.* The most frequently observed symptoms are a feeling of irritation and dryness of the nasal and pharyngeal mucosae. There may also be obstructive rhinitis with or without nasal discharge. In a study carried out in a large building in the Paris region, we showed that these manifestations in the upper respiratory tract were statistically the most frequent [26]. In other cases, there are manifestations in the form of pseudoasthmatic tightness of the chest (tight syndrome) or laryngeal symptoms such as hoarseness and irritation. These sensory irritations are the dominant complaint and one of the most important criteria of diagnosis [27].

2. *Ocular manifestations.*These include dryness and irritation of the mucous membrane of the eye.

3. *Cutaneous manifestations.* Notable here are redness of the skin, itching, skin dryness, sometimes facial erythema, seborrheic dermatitis [28], and even urticaria.

4. *Odor and taste complaints.* These take the form of fetid odors or unpleasant tastes.

5. *Neuropsychic manifestations.* These are of the asthenic type, with torpor, somnolence, impairment of memory and intellectual activity, concentration difficulty, possibly headache, and occasionally, nausea and giddiness.

Overall, there is a feeling of discomfort. Many of the manifestations may be attributable to psychological factors, particularly since there are few objective signs. Exploratory tests of respiratory function fall within normal limits with regard to spirometry, carbon monoxide diffusion, and bronchial challenge tests [23].

There are two characteristics that it is important to mention. These disorders disappear during the weekend and holidays and reappear on resumption of work or activity in the same place. Usually, these symptoms are benign.

### B. Risk Factors

SBS is nowadays regarded as a multifactorial syndrome. Four major groups of factors are to be considered: physical, chemical, biological, and psychological.

#### Physical Factors

##### Temperature

The temperature standards for maintaining a certain acceptable level of comfort and occupational activity fluctuate between 20° and 26°C, taking into account clothing and relative humidity. Wyon and Holmberg [29], Jaakola and Heinonen

[30], Valbjorn and Kousgaard [31] have found a relationship between room temperatures above 22°C and the appearance of SBS symptoms.

### Relative Humidity

It is well known that high relative humidity values (above 70%), particularly when associated with high temperature, are uncomfortable. Conversely, in some people very low relative humidity (less than 20%) can cause drying of the mucous membranes and of the skin [23] or dermatitis [32]. Indirect effects could play a role, such as the buildup of static electricity and consequent electric discharges.

### Ventilation

Insufficient ventilation due to energy-saving measures has been claimed as one of the main causes for SBS symptoms. Minimum ventilation rates do exist in many countries, but vary from country to country and of course, under smoking or nonsmoking conditions [33,34]. ASHRAE recommends a rate of 30 L/s, based on a consensus standard of 80% of satisfied people. Also, *recirculation* of air, which may introduce contaminants to working areas, should be avoided.

### Artificial Light

By varying both the quantity of ultraviolet light and the ventilation, Sterling et al. [35] noted a reduction in eye symptoms but not in other symptoms of SBS [36]. In a recent personal study, we observed a major role for lighting among ergonomic factors [37].

### Noise and Vibrations

Noise, expressed as the equivalent sound pressure A-weighted level, may be a parameter causing tiredness at levels of 70 to 80 dB. But Tempest [38] has described some cases where the workers complained of unpleasant working conditions in one factory department but not in another, although the sound levels were approximately equal [61 dB(A)]. Vibrations produced in the neighborhood of buildings (e.g., underground railways) have also been accused of contributing to SBS [39].

### Ions

Finnegan et al. [13] found that ion concentration in the atmosphere did not influence the level of SBS symptoms. Moreover, negative ionizers have been described as releasing significant amounts of ozone, a potent airway irritant [40].

### Particles and Fibers

No correlation has yet been shown between SBS and total dust concentration.

## Chemical Factors

By definition, SBS is characterized by the absence of any known contaminant at harmful concentration levels. However, chemical factors are numerous and can be grouped into major categories. It should be noted that for a large number of chemicals, threshold limit values in industrial workplaces are fixed by national or international standards. The pollutant concentrations normally observed in indoor air are much lower than such limits. However, two factors should be taken into account: (1) indoor environments are characterized by complex mixtures of pollutants in which synergistic mechanisms cannot be ruled out, and (2) workplace limits are defined for healthy adults working a 40-h week, whereas children, elderly people, and hypersensitive individuals are exposed to indoor pollution for much longer periods. Finally, the concentration of chemical substances may be reduced by an increased ventilation rate.

### Environmental Tobacco Smoke

Generally speaking, environmental tobacco smoke (ETS) is by far the most important source of chemical pollution in indoor air. Sick-building syndrome is statistically more pronounced in smokers than in nonsmokers [41,42] and there are more symptoms in nonsmokers and ex-smokers exposed to ETS than in those in the same nonexposed categories.

Tobacco smoke contains several hundred compounds with particularly toxic constituents, which also act as an allergen affecting the bronchial and alveolar immune defense mechanisms [42–44]. As a rule, smoking should be prohibited in working environments and indoor spaces open to the public, particularly in air-conditioned buildings. (It is the case in French legislation since November 1992.)

### Formaldehyde

The presence of formaldehyde may result from the use of wood-based products (such as particleboard, plywood) and urea–formaldehyde foam used in insulation and a variety of other products, mainly used for disinfection, cleaning, and painting. Although it has been suggested [45,46] that formaldehyde may be the cause of SBS, the syndrome has been described where there was no formaldehyde in the ambient atmosphere [47].

### Volatile Organic Compounds

There are many volatile organic compounds (VOCs), [48]. Whether they come from building materials, furniture, household maintenance products (waxes, detergents, insecticides), personal hygiene products (cosmetics), do-it-yourself goods (resins), office materials (photocopier ink), motor vehicle exhaust, or ETS, these compounds may affect humans in different ways and sometimes are also a source of odors. However, evidence on the role of VOCs in SBS cases has not been convincing [27,35].

### Odors

Many gases and vapors give rise to sensory discomfort caused by odor and irritation, which may be a disturbing factor leading to anxiety and stress, especially when the sources are not identified. Recently, Fanger [49] introduced two new units, the *olf* and the *decipol*, to quantify air pollution sources and levels of pollution as perceived by humans. However, at the present time, no studies have been conducted that compare olf levels with sickness levels within buildings.

### Biological Factors

Air-conditioned office buildings normally present very low concentrations of mites because they do not provide appropriate conditions for the growth of such microorganisms. However, recent studies [31,50] demonstrated a correlation between the organic dust content of carpets (predominantly skin scales, bacteria, and molds) and the symptoms of SBS. Gravesen et al. [51] demonstrated a correlation between the potential immunologic components of dust in large buildings in Copenhagen and the symptoms of SBS. However, unlike chemical factors, these biological factors cannot be eliminated by an increase in ventilation rate.

### Psychosociological Factors

The initial reaction of a number of professionals confronted with repeated complaints of ill-defined discomfort has been to blame psychological factors, and all the more so since these symptoms appear to have no organic basis and women are the most frequently affected. Various studies have been carried out testing these patients either with a set of performance tests (memory, vigilance, reaction time) [52] or in the form of a psychological survey evaluating how these complainants viewed their working conditions in air-conditioned environments [53]. The performance tests showed no significant difference between symptomatic and control groups. However, in Western countries, air-conditioning is often regarded as artificial, unnecessary, and unhealthy.

In a recent personal study performed in three air-conditioned sick buildings (two in Paris and one in Clermont-Ferrand), where 250 persons were questioned and examined, we could observe the role of *ergonomic factors* and the importance of *atopic status* [37]. Our questionnaire included questions on overall environment, site and type of work, job relations (with superiors or colleagues) life-style, air-conditioning appreciation, medical history, and psychological tests (thematic aperception and Rorschach tests). This enables us to record a standard portrait of people who complain about air-conditioning (factorial analysis, Table 1): (1) two-thirds were women, (2) most were nonsmokers, (3) most worked regularly with computer screens and copy machines and (4) lighting seemed to play an important role in complaints. External environment is also a major factor since most complaints were recorded in a skyscraper in the neighborhood of Paris, with difficult access and without such facilities as food services, shopping, or transportation.

From a medical point of view, we confirm the findings of a previous survey, because in 30% of symptomatic persons we observed a past history of allergy. So as air-conditioning can be helpful to atopic patients by removing outdoor airborne allergens or indoor small particles and by decreasing humidity, which favors the growth of mites, atopy is a risk factor for the occurrence of SBS.

Finally, psychosocial factors may be taken into consideration: For example, job dissatisfaction results in complaints focusing on indoor air quality, although they may be rooted in other factors, such as stress or mood. Communicating with occupants through systematic surveys or questionnaires can often do a better job than by taking expensive and time-consuming measurements.

## V. Prevention

Health problems in relation to indoor air in general, and particularly in air-conditioned buildings, come from three main causes: (1) faulty conception of the building, with poor construction (without reliability); (2) bad adaptation to use (without flexibility); and (3) lack of maintenance of the HVAC system.

### A. How to Conduct Building-Associated Investigations: Medical and Engineering Approach

The majority of air-conditioned-building-related health problems are relatively simple to deal with. We agree with Robertson [47] when he states that 80% of problems stem from (1) inadequate ventilation, (2) inefficient filtration, and (3) poor hygiene of the air-handling system. When a significant percentage of building occupants (between 10 and 20%) complain of symptoms, the first step is to call on a trained building engineer with experience of HVAC equipment design in major buildings. This investigation should include a separate interview with the building manager, the chief engineer, and the personnel manager. It is up to the medical staff to record information or symptoms experienced by employees and potential etiologic factors.

The distribution of questionnaires (three for Samet [48]) is discussed by some authors, who believe that this is likely to exacerbate the situation, heightening employee awareness as a perceived problem and resulting in increasing stress. However, from a medical point of view, it is necessary to differentiate well-identified building-related illnesses (which deserve medical treatment and comprehensive building investigations) and SBS, which, above all, falls within the competence of building diagnosticians. The keys to these problems fall into three categories: (1) ventilation, (2) filtration, and (3) humidification.

## Ventilation

Ventilation rate should not be inferior to the minimum defined in the ASHRAE standard, which ensures a $CO_2$ level below 1000 ppm and effective dilution of other contaminants, also taking into account the quality of outdoor air, occupant density, additional thermal loads (lighting, computers), and new sources of contaminants (copy machines, printers, etc.).

## Filtration

The air-handling system must contain adequate filters, which must assure protection of the component parts themselves (against bacterial proliferation) and air quality, in keeping with the use to which the building is destined. For Rault [54] three parameters should be taken in account: (1) efficiency, (2) air blowing and resistance to airflow, and (3) air velocity. For the performance of the most common particulate filters measured by ASHRAE Standard 52.76, an efficiency of 90% (dust spot method), EU 5 to EU 9 (Eurovent 4/4), leads to removal of respirable-size particules under 3.5 $\mu$m in size. But in the case of recycling tobacco smoke or chemical pollution, it is necessary to use adsorption or gaseous removal filters (activated charcoal filters, sometimes impregnated with potassium permanganate), which are expensive.

In the case of sterile units or operation theaters in hospitals, absolute filtration is mandatory (HEPA filters, EU 13, Eurovent 4/4). This requires close to 100% efficiency (dioctyl phthalate test) at low velocity (0.45 to 0.50 m/s) without turbulence (laminar airstream). These filters must be inspected periodically to ensure continuous performance and rated efficiency ASHRAE 52.76 filters have a 6-month minimum life cycle).

## Humidification

Humidification is a source of bacterial contamination or mould proliferation. The recommendations must be stringent:

1. Use of water spray system should be avoided.
2. Whenever possible, dry-airsteam humidifiers should be used.
3. Prevent water stagnation, but if it arises, ensure easy access to the system. All sources of water associated with air-handling units (drains, coils, heat exchangers, ducts) should be examined for cleanliness.

All trained engineers have a checklist for comprehensive investigation of a building. Generally speaking, good maintenance of the air-conditioning system, with a precise checkup schedule and technical training of maintenance personnel, must be carried out. In addition, the physicians who develop a comprehensive medical history, including a physical examination of complaining employees, should discuss the recommended remedial actions and their health benefits with the building operators.

### B. Cost-Effectiveness and Medicolegal Aspects

As WHO pointed out in a publication on indoor air quality research (WHO, 1986), efforts to save energy will continue in the coming years. Unless those responsible for designing and operating buildings realize that energy economy is not the sole criterion in evaluating costs, there will be increased building problems. They point out that "energy-efficient but sick buildings often cost society far more than it gains by energy saving" and that people's confidence in the effectiveness of health and building authorities may be seriously harmed if sick buildings become a common phenomenon.

Recently, Robertson [47] made a comparative evaluation of the possible realistic cost reduction in the heating and ventilation of a large building, on the one hand, and a 1% increase in absenteeism among the employees, on the other. Under a hypotheses assumed for the calculation, the cost of the absenteeism is approximately eight times greater than the money gained through energy savings. This does not take the reduced working efficiency into account. So the public health concern is now focused not only on safety but also on the comfort of the indoor environment with an evolution in quantification risk assessment [48].

Also, the medical–legal aspect should not be forgotten. In some countries (e.g., France) allergic manifestations in employees working in air-conditioned buildings in which the air-conditioning systems are not maintained properly and/or regularly are considered occupational diseases. Finally, cooperation between air-conditioning engineers, architects, designers, and physicians may contribute to solving a large number of health problems in existing buildings and to preventing them in the conception and construction of new buildings.

### References

1. Banaszak EF, Thiede WH, Fink JN. Hypersensitivity pneumonitis due to contamination of an air conditioner. N Engl J Med 1970;283(6):271–76.
2. Woods JE, Drewry GM, Morey PR. Office workers perceptions of indoor air quality effects on discomfort and performance. Indoor Air'87, Berlin, August 17–21, 1987;464–68.
3. Wilson S, Hedge A. The office environmental survey. Building use studies, London, 1987.
4. Stead WW, Hutton MD, Bloch AB. Spread of tuberculosis from a tuberculous abscess (abstract). Am Rev Respir Dis 1987;135:A33.
5. Knudsin RC. Airborne contagion. Ann NY Acad Sci 1980;353:1.

6.  Riley RL, Nardell EA. The theory and application of ultraviolet air disinfection. Am Rev Respir Dis 1989;139:1286–94.
7.  Moser MR, Bender TR, Margolis HS, Noble GR, Kendal AP, Ritter DG. An outbreak of influenza aboard a commercial airliner. Am J Epidemiol 1979;110(1):1.
8.  Elixman JH, Jorde W, Lindsens HF. Apparition de moisissures dans les appareils d'air conditionné avant et après la mise en action. Maladie des Climatiseurs et des Humidificateurs. Colloque INSERM 1986;135:77–86.
9.  Feuilhade M, van der Meeren A, Bernaudin JF, Bignon J. Enquête d'hygiène hospitalière lors d'une épidémie nosocomiale d'aspergillose invasive en service d'hématologie. Maladie des climatiseurs. Colloque INSERM 1986;135:67–76.
10. Austwick PKC, Davies PS, Cook CP, Pickering CAC. Comparative microbiological studies in humidifier fever. Maladie des climatiseurs et des humidificateurs. Colloque INSERM 1986;135:155–64.
11. Mannis MJ, Tamaou R, Roth AM, Burns M, Thirkill C. Acanthamoeba sclerokeratitis. Arch Ophthalmol 1986;104:1313.
12. Solomon WR. Fungus aerosols arising from cold mist vaporizers. J Allergy Clin Immunol 1979;54:222–28.
13. Finnegan MJ, Pickering CAC. Prevalence of symptoms of the sick building syndrome in buildings without expressed dissatisfaction. Indoor Air '87, Proceedings of the 4th International Conference on Indoor Air Quality and Climate, Berlin, August 17–21, 1987. Vol. 2. Berlin: Institut für Wasser, Boden- und Lufthygiene, 1987:542–46.
14. Arnow PM, Fink JN, Schleuter DP. Early detection of hypersensitivity pneumonitis in office workers. Am J Med 1978;64:236–41.
15. Woodard ED, Friedlander B, Lescher RJ, Kinsey R, Hearne FT. Outbreak of hypersensitivity pneumonitis. JAMA 1988;259(13):965–69.
16. Burcke GW, Carrington CB, Strauss R, Fink JN, Gaensler EA. Allergic alveolitis caused by home humidifiers. Unusual clinical features and electron microscopy findings. JAMA 1977;238(25):2705.
17. Patterson R, Fink JN, Miles WB, Basich JE, Schleuter DB, Tinkelman DG, Roberts M. Hypersensitivity lung disease presumptively due to cephalosporium in homes contaminated by sewage flooding or by humidifier water. J Allergy Clin Immunol 68;2:129.
18. Rose CS, Newman LS, Martyny JW, Weiner D, Kreiss K, Milton DK, King TE Jr. Outbreak of hypersensitivity pneumonitis in an indoor swimming pool: clinical, physioligic, radiographic, pathologic, lavage and environmental findings. Am Rev Respir Dis 1990:A:315.
19. Pestalozzi C. Febrile Gruppenerkränkungen in einer Modellschreinerei durch Inhalation von mit Schimmelpilzen Kontaminfertem Befeuchterwasser "Befeuchterfieber". Schweiz Med Wochenschr 1959;89(27):710–13.

20. Polla BS, De Haller R, Nerbollier G, Rylander R. Humidifier disease. Role of endotoxins and precipitating antibodies. Schweiz Med Wochenschr 1988;118:1311–13.

21. Michel O, Ginanni R, Duchateau J. Endotoxin enhances the immediate skin response to house dust mite (HDM) antigen (abstract). Ann Allergy, 1990;64(January):85.

22. Caillaud D, Merrill WW, Vaerman JP, Bazin H, Molina Cl. Absence of reverse passive Arthus (RPAR) in rat lung using endotoxin-free monoclonal antibodies. Am Rev Respir Dis 1990;A:213.

23. Andersen I, Lundquist GR, Jensen PL, Proctor DF. Human response to 78 hour exposure to dry air. Arch Environ Health 1974;29:319–24.

24. Burge H. Bioaerosols: prevalence and health effects in the indoor environment. J Allergy Clin Immunol 1990;86(5):687–701.

25. Nolard Tintignier N, Beguin H, Vunckx. Mesures quantitatives et qualitatives des moisissures de l'environnement. Maladie des climatiseurs et humidificateurs. Colloque INSERM 1986;135:193–201.

26. Caillaud D, Bedu M, Brestowski D, Aiache JM, Molina Cl. Résultats d'une enquête de Médecine du Travail en atmosphère climatisée. Maladie des climatiseurs et humidificateurs. Colloque INSERM 1986;135:107–16.

27. Molhave L, Bach B, Pederson OF. Human reactions to low concentrations of volatile organic compounds. Environ Int 1986;165–67.

28. Stenberg B. Skin complaints in sick buildings. Indoor Air '87, Berlin, August 17–21, 1987:530–34.

29. Wyon DP, Holmberg I. Systematic observation of classroom behavior during moderate heat stress. Thermal comfort and moderate heat stress. Proceedings of the CIB (W 45) Symposium, Garston September 13–15, 1972. Building Establishment Report 2. London: Her Majesty's Stationery Office, 1973.

30. Jaakkola JJK, Heinonen OP. Mechanical ventilation in an office building and sick building syndrome. A short-term trial. Indoor Air '87. Proceedings of the 4th International Conference on Indoor Air Quality and Climate, Berlin August 17–21. Vol. 2. Berlin: Institut für Wasser, Boden- und Lufthygiene, 1987:454–58.

31. Valjborn O, Kousgaard N. Headache and mucous membrane irritation at home and at work. Statens Byggeforsknings Institut 175. Horsholm, Denmark, 1986.

32. Rycroft RJG. Low humidity and microtrauma. Am J Ind Med 1985;8:371–73.

33. Cain SS, Leaderer BP, Isseroff R, Berglund LG, Huer RJ, Lipsitte ED, Perlman D. Ventilation requirements in buildings. I. Control of occupancy odor and tobacco smoke odor. Atmos Environ 1983;17;1183–97.

34. Gunnarsen L, Fanger PO. Adaptation to indoor air pollution. Healthy

Buildings '88. Proceedings of a Conference, Stockholm, September 5–8, 1988, Swedish Council for Building Research, Vol. 3:157–67.

35. Sterling E, Sterling T, McIntyre D. New health hazards in sealed buildings. Am Inst Arch J 1983;72:64–67.

36. Wilkins AJ, Nimmo-Smith MI, Slater A, Bedocs L. Fluorescent lighting. Headaches and eyestrain. Proceedings of CIBSE National Lighting Conference, Cambridge, 1988:188–196.

37. Molina Cl, Aiache JM, Caillaud D, Molina N. Allergic risks due to air-conditioning. Sem Hôp Paris 1991;67(26–27):1214–17.

38. Tempest W. Infrasound and low frequency vibration. London: Academic Press, 1976.

39. Hodgson MJ, Permar E, Squire G, Cagney W., Aller A, Parkinson DK. Vibrations as a cause of "tight building syndrome" symptoms. In: Tempest W, ed. Infrasound and low frequency vibration. Vol. 2. London: Academic Press, 1976:449–53.

40. Guillemin MP, Trin Vu Duc, Bernhard CA. "Sick building syndrome" Psychose collective ou réalité? Congrés SIRMCE (EPFL-IREC). Habitat et habitations saines, Lausanne, 1987.

41. Skov P, Valbjorn O (the Danish indoor climate study group). The "sick" building syndrome" in the office environment. Indoor Air '87, Proceedings of the 4th International Conference on Indoor Air Quality and Climate, Berlin, August 17–21, 1987. Vol. 2. Berlin: Inst für Wasser, Bodenund Lufthygiene, 1987:439–443.

42. Molina Cl, Aiache JM, Viallier J, Réactions immunitaires au tabac. Nouv Presse Méd 1980;9:3171–75.

43. Warren CPW. Extrinsic allergic alveolitis: a disease common in nonsmokers. Thorax 1977;32:567–69.

44. Lehrer SB, Wilson MR, Salvaggio JE. Immunogenic properties of tobacco smoke. J Allergy Clin Immunol 1978;62;368.

45. Hendrick DJ, Lane DJ. Occupational formalin asthma. Br J Ind Med 1977;34:11–18.

46. Wanner HU, Kuhn M. Indoor air pollution by building materials. Environ Int 1986;12:311–15.

47. Robertson G. Source, nature and symptomatology of indoor air pollutants. Healthy Buildings '88. Proceedings of a Conference, Stockholm September 5–8, 1988, Swedish Council for Building Research, Vol. 3:507–16.

48. Samet J, Environmental controls and lung disease. Report of the ATS workshop on Environmental Controls and Lung Disease, Sante Fe, NM, March 24–26, 1988. Am Rev Respir Dis 1990;142:915–39.

49. Fanger PO. Introduction of the olf and the decipol unit to quantify air pollution perceived by humans indoors and outdoors. Energy Buildings 1988; 12:1–6.

50. Nexo E, Skov PG, Gravesen S. Extreme fatigue and malaise, a syndrome caused by badly cleaned wall to wall carpets. Ecol Dis 1983;2:415–18.
51. Gravesen S, Skov D. Indications for organic dusts as an etiological factor in the sick building syndrome. Allergy 1988(Suppl 7);43:1.
52. Berglund B, Berglund U, Engen T. Do sick buildings affect human performance? How should one assess them? Indoor Air '87. Proceedings of the 4th International Conference on Indoor Air Quality and Climate, Berlin, August 17–21, 1987. Vol. 2. Berlin: Institut für Wasser, Boden- und Lufthygiene, 1987:477–81.
53. Breugnon N, Clement P, Martin E, Masserand R, Molina N. Perception des conditions de travail en atmosphère climatisée. Maladie des climatiseurs et des humidificateurs. Colloque INSERM 1986;135:117–25.
54. Rault JY. Propreté particulaire des ambiances. Sem Hôp Paris 1991;67(26–27):1228–32.

# 13

## Prevention of Respiratory Diseases from Airborne Allergens

**DENIS A. CHARPIN and DANIEL VERVLOET**

Marseille School of Medicine
Marseille, France

## I. Introduction

Respiratory allergy ranks sixth among diseases of concern to the general population [1]. Reactions are especially common in young people, in whom the prevalence of atopy can reach 35% [2]. House dust mites ($HDM_2$), cat allergens, pollens, and occupational allergens account for the vast majority of sensitizations [3,4]. In this chapter we give some basic information about the aerobiology of these four major allergens, with special emphasis on prevention.

## II. House Dust Mites

A number of epidemiological studies [5] have linked exposure to house dust mites to sensitization and respiratory allergy. Two major groups of allergens have recently been distinguished in the genus *Dermatophagoides*: group I allergens (Der p I, Der f I, Der m I), excreted in feces [6], and group II allergens (Der p II, Der F II), found mainly on the body of the mite. There is no evidence for structural similarity or cross-reactivity between these two groups. More than

80% of mite allergic patients have IgE antibodies to group I and group II allergens. The relative importance of the group III allergens needs to be clarified.

The report of the Second International Workshop on dust mite allergens and asthma [5] stated that measurement of specific allergens extracted from house dust samples and expression of results as micrograms of group I mite allergen per gram of dust could still be regarded as the best validated "index of exposure." Since the proposed threshold for house dust mite sensitization is 2 μg of mite per gram of mattress dust, this is the target level for primary prevention in atopic families. Since several studies have shown that levels higher than 10 μg provoke attacks in sensitized subjects, this is the target for secondary prevention.

Platts-Mills et al. [7] showed that after disturbance of house dust, 80% of group I allergens were collected on the first stage of the impactor. This finding is in keeping with the size of these particles over 10 μg. Less than 4% of these allergens were still airborne 15 to 35 min after the disturbance. These results emphasize the fact that mite-avoidance procedures should target settled allergens.

Mite control is based on knowledge of their biological characteristics:

1.   Optimal temperature for mites ranges from 25 to 28°C. In vitro mites survive for 24 h at 45°C, 4 h at 50°C, and 1 h at 60°C [8]. At low temperature, they become inactive, but only half of a mite population die after exposure at −15°C for 6 h. Inside mattress, because of the sleeper, an optimum temperature is usually found.

2.   Mites eat scales, preferably when they have been predigested by fungi. However, there are many substitute food supplies, such as various protein material of animal or plant origin, which account for mite survival in unoccupied houses.

3.   In vitro, optimum relative humidity for mite development is around 75% at 25°C [9]. In dwellings they can survive at relative humidities of 45 to 55% at 15°C and of 55 to 65% at 25°C. In a temperate climate there is an exponential increase in house dust mite concentrations when the absolute indoor humidity exceeds 7.0 g vapor/kg dry air, corresponding to a relative humidity of 45% at an indoor air temperature of 20 to 21°C [10]. Mite development in culture [11] as well as in dwellings is mainly dependent on relative humidity, which depends on temperature, absolute humidity, and ventilation rate.

Avoidance procedures recently reviewed [12] can be classified under three headings according to the strategy used to reduce exposure to the allergen.

## A.   Elimination of Mites

The first strategy consists of reducing mite counts. This can be achieved by housekeeping to remove mites physically and by applying acaricides to kill mites. The efficacy of housekeeping in reducing mite counts is poorly documented.

Hughes and Maunsell reported [13] that vacuuming a mattress once a month in fall and winter and once or twice in spring and summer could achieve a large reduction in mite counts. Similarly, Cunnington and Gregory [14] sampled air during bedmaking and showed an eightfold reduction in mite counts following mattress vacuuming. However, both these studies involved only one mattress and did not consider a control mattress. Penaud et al. [15] reported a 30% decrease in mite counts on mattresses treated with a placebo spray. However, this study did not include unvacuumed control mattresses. Burr et al. [16] failed to find any difference in mite counts between mattresses vacuumed once a week for 8 weeks and control mattresses. Van Bronswijk [17] showed that only 5 to 10% of mites were removed after vacuum cleaning for 2 min and 20% after 40 min. Furthermore, in his study involving vacuuming of bedclothes, upholstery, furniture, and floors in addition to mattresses, Arlian et al. found no effect on mite counts [18]. In practice, patients are usually advised to vacuum mattresses once a week and to remove infested carpeting and upholstery and replace them with new furniture that has hard, smooth surfaces. Evaluation of the clinical efficacy of lowering mite counts has also provided contradictory results. Sarsfield et al. [19] reported symptomatic improvement in asthmatic children allergic to house dust mites. However, this study did not include a control group. In contrast, Burr et al.'s study [16] indicated no improvement in symptoms or peak expiratory flow in 18 asthmatic children after implementation of drastic avoidance measures, including washing pillowcases, sheets, soft toys, and blankets, using synthetic-material pillows instead of feather pillows, mattresses, or quilts, and cleaning rugs, compared to a control group of 18 asthmatic chidren who took no particular precautions. However, in a later crossover study [20] in which, in addition to the above-listed avoidance procedures, mattresses, pillows, and blankets were changed, Burr et al. demonstrated a small but significant increase in peak flow measurements. To prevent rapid reinfestation of bedding, they suggested use of sheets impregnated with benzyl benzoate [21]. Generally speaking, housekeeping alone does not seem efficient in reducing mites in mattresses and carpets or in relieving allergic reactions. Using the heat escape method, Bischoff et al. [22] showed that vacuuming withdraws only a very small percentage of mites.

    Another approach to reducing mite counts is to apply acaricides. Several substances (Table 1) kill house dust mites in laboratory cultures [23]. However, the efficacy of these chemicals in houses depends on their being brought in contact with live mites. Penetration of currently available sprays, solutions, foams, or powders into mattresses or carpets is not fully understood. Until now, only four acaricides have been evaluated in placebo-controlled studies. Dorward et al. [24] studied 21 adult asthmatic patients allergic to house dust mites, who were randomly allocated into two groups: one in which preventive measures were implemented and another in which they were not. The preventive measures included application of liquid nitrogen to mattresses and bedroom carpets, as

**Table 1**  Acaricidal Preparations Evaluated by Placebo-Controlled Studies

| Chemical name | Trade name | Mechanism of action | Form | Refs. |
|---|---|---|---|---|
| Benzylbenzoate | Acarosan | Acaricide (used for scabies) | Powder (U.S., Europe), foam (Europe only) | [26–29] |
| Pyrethroids | Actomite (Acardust) | Insecticide/acaricide | Pressurized canister (Europe only) | [25] |
| Natamycin | Tymasil | Antifungal | Powder (Europe) | [30] |
| Tannic acid (3%) | Allergy control solution | Protein denaturing | Fluid (U.S.) | [28,38] |
| Liquid nitrogen | — | Acaricide and protein denaturing agent | Fluid (Australia) | [37] |
| Mixture of surface wetting agents and solvents | Allerex | Cleaning solution used with special vacuum cleaner | Europe | [Mitchell, in preparation] |

*Source:* Data from ref. 5.

well as weekly vacuuming of mattress, cleaning of blankets, pillows, and quilts, and removing plants, soft toys, cushions, and upholstered furniture. At the end of the 8-week trial period, a significant drop in live mite counts was noted in the treated environments and a lower airway responsiveness and improved asthma symptom score were noted in the patients. These results are difficult to interpret because avoidance measures included several techniques. Furthermore, liquid nitrogen is impractical for home use. Acardust, an acaricide available in several European countries, is composed of esbiol (first-generation synthetic pyrethroid) and piperonyl butoxide. To evaluate its efficacy, 42 patients suffering from asthma and/or rhinitis with allergy to mites were included in a 3-month placebo-controlled study [25]. The antigen content, particularly for *D. pteronyssimus* antigens in dust from matresses but not the floor decreased more quickly in the Acardust group. Peak monitoring and evening flow rates improved significantly in the Acardust group, but there was little change in symptom scores. However, methodological problems hamper interpretation of these findings since the hazards of randomization led to a higher antigenic load, higher clinical score, and lower peak flow rates in the Acardust group before treatment.

Acarosan (benzyl benzoate) has been submitted to more extensive evaluation. This acaricide is available either as a foam that is sprayed on pads and spread on mattresses and upholstery or as a powder that is sprinkled on carpets and rugs. In a French study [26], levels of mite allergens and guanine were evaluated in the highly mite-infested dwellings of 20 allergic patients for 12 months. A second treatment was performed 6 to 12 months after the first. Trends in mite allergen and guanine load did not differ significantly in the treated and control dwellings. Kniest et al. [27] in the Netherlands performed a similar study in 20 houses of perennial mite-allergic rhinitic patients and found that guanine load, symptom scores, and total IgE dropped significantly in the treatment group.

An open 3-year study performed by Le Mao et al. [5] showed a significant decrease in mite Der pI allergen concentrations and in mite counts compared to baseline levels. Clinical improvement was observed 3 months after the initial treatment, but there was no significant change in daily medication requirements. In a placebo-controlled study, a German group [28] evaluated mite-antigen levels before and 10, 30, and 60 days after first treatment. A second application was carried out on day 10. There was a significant reduction in mite allergens in dust from mattresses and carpets in both Acarosan and placebo groups, but only the results on carpets in the Acarosan group were significantly different from the control group on days 30 and 60. This German group [29] also performed a placebo-controlled study using Acarosan for 12 months on the mattresses and carpets of 24 asthmatic children allergic to mites. Benzyl benzoate treatment resulted in a slight decrease in mattress allergen concentrations, but this reduction led to no change in bronchial hyperreactivity. Taken as a whole, the results of these studies indicate that time-consuming and expensive application of acaricidal preparations does not induce a clear clinical improvement. In particular, no convincing evidence has been presented that such preparations improve the symptoms of asthmatic patients. It should be mentioned that a recent placebo-controlled study using Natamycin on mattresses to kill fungi required for optimal mite growth also failed to show an improvement in the treatment group [30].

## B. Elimination of Mite Allergens

As stated above, vacuum cleaning does not reduce allergic symptoms because it leaves a large number of mites. However, although it would be difficult to prove, vacuuming might remove a fraction of the antigenic load and that could account for the drop in antigen levels observed in mattresses or carpets treated with placebo. Another interesting issue is the increase in airborne mite antigens caused by conventional vacuum cleaning [31]. This phenomenon could explain why the symptoms of mite allergic patients sometimes worsen during and following vacuum cleaning. This problem can be prevented by using high-filtration machines that retain up to 99.97% of particles over 0.3 mm in diameter (31). Vacuum cleaners that circulate warm water and cleaning solution (Allerex; see Table 1) through the pile have been designed. According to Fell and co-workers

[32], these machines can lower the antigen load by two-thirds. The lethal effects of hot water on mites were evaluated by Andersen and Roesen [33], who showed that a minimum temperature of 58°C was required. However, complete denaturation of group II allergens requires temperatures above 100°C [34]. Since dry cleaning is readily accessible, we evaluated mite-allergen levels in dust collected from five blankets by vacuuming before and after dry cleaning with perchlorethylene [35] and compared the results with five control blankets. Group I allergen levels per gram of dust were 78% lower after dry cleaning. Mean group I allergen levels per $m^2$ of dry-cleaned blankets were 98% lower. De Boer [36] compared the effects of conventional vacuum cleaning, wet cleaning, shampooing, and autoclaving on the live-mite population and mite allergen levels in rugs. Autoclaving achieved the best results but is obviously impractical for regular use. Wet cleaning appeared to be effective by removing food and/or fungi necessary for mite development, but long-term effectiveness has not been evaluated.

Since house dust is a mixture of many different allergenic proteins that can all be quickly destroyed, a promising new approach is the use of denaturing agents (Table 1). Green et al. [37] reported two studies using Allersearch DMS, a mixture of benzyl alcohol and tannic acid. In the first, they found no living mites 3 to 4 min and 50 min after treatment of dust and carpets, respectively, with DMS. In the second experiment, they observed markedly lower mite counts (–95%) and allergen levels (–100-fold) on bed blankets after spraying with DMS as compared to before spraying. Mite counts and allergen levels remained low for 6 weeks. At 16 weeks both parameters showed a slight increase. Miller et al. [38] measured mite antigens in carpets before and 24 h after spraying with a 3% tannic acid solution. Before spraying antigen levels ranged from 14.1 to 41.9 µg/g of dust, while after spraying they ranged from <0.1 (threshold of detection) to 9.7 µg/g of dust. Samples taken from one home at the end of four weekly treatments showed no detectable mite antigens. Tovey et al. [6] also demonstrated a significant decrease in Der p I concentrations on floors 2 weeks after spraying, but levels were not significantly different from baseline 4 weeks after spraying. More interestingly, Der p I concentrations on beds decreased significantly but temporarily after spraying DMS. A more sustained decrease was obtained when spraying was combined with encasing bedding in impermeable vinyl covers. Using such an approach after spraying with a 3% tannic acid solution, Ehnert et al. [29] reported a significant decrease in mite allergen in encased pillows, comforters, and mattresses. To the best of our knowledge, these authors, who also demonstrated a decrease in bronchial hyperreactivity, are the only ones to have documented in asthmatic patients a clinical benefit from an acaricidal preparation.

In addition to housekeeping and denaturing agents, a third way to decrease antigen levels is air filtration. Air-cleaning devices may be broadly divided into two groups: those that work by mechanical removal and those that use electrical attraction. Mechanical filters depend on inertial impact and Brownian motion. The best filter is the high-efficiency particulate air (HEPA) filter, which can remove 99.97% of particles over 0.3 μm in diameter. Electrical attraction devices include negative-ion generators and electronic air cleaners. All these devices were evaluated by an ad hoc committee that met in 1987 and concluded [39] that the "absence of adequate data on the clinical relevance of indoor ambient allergens levels as well as the effect of air cleaning devices on these levels, plus a general lack of health effects by these devices in published double-blind studies preclude any firm recommendations for their use." The panel stressed that because most mite allergens settle, the airborne load tends to be low in comparison to the surface load. However, a recent paper [40] showed that HEPA filters decrease particulate matter $\leq$ 0.3 μm by an average of 70%, and there was a trend toward reduction of allergic respiratory symptoms.

### C. Covering Bedding

Covers have long been used to separate the allergic sleeper from his or her contaminated bedding [19,20,41,42]. However, since plastic covers are impermeable to water vapor as well as to particulate matter, the sleeper feels uncomfortable. Recently, polyurethane backings have been applied to textiles, making them impermeable to particulate matter but permeable to water vapor. Mite allergen levels per gram of mattress dust after 12 weeks with this new covering were 1% of levels in control samples from mattresses cleaned conventionally [43]. As stated earlier, covering bedding and spraying tannic acid on carpets led to a drop in mite-antigen levels as well as in bronchial reactivity [29]. A recent international workshop recomended the use of mattresses covers made of zippered plastic or vapor-permeable fabrics as a very effective antiallergy measure. It also advised that highly infested mattresses be replaced or treated before covering [5]. It should be stressed that these covers are expensive.

### D. Environmental Control

A number of environmental measures can be taken to reduce mite infestation. A very simple measure is the use of electric blankets. Mosbech et al. [44] monitored mite counts and mite-allergen levels in 10 beds with electric blankets and in 10 beds without electric blankets for 1 year. In beds with electric blankets, mite counts dropped by 50%, and mite allergen levels fell 32% in comparison to baseline measurements made at the beginning of the study. No change was observed in control beds without electric blankets.

Another environmental approach is to control dampness (see Chapter 14). Studies aimed at grading the effects of daily activities as well as architectural features in terms of dampness are ongoing and this information could help achieve significant reductions in mite infestation. Presently available epidemiological data documents drastic differences between house dust mite antigenic levels in dry and humid areas [45]. Maintaining temperature below 20°C has an inhibiting effect. However, low temperature increases relative humidity, and it may therefore be more effective to reduce absolute humidity using a dehumidifier. Such devices are currently available on the market but have not yet been evaluated for mite control. Another approach to dehumidification is ventilation with outdoor air, which is usually drier and becomes much drier when heated. Studies evaluating these methods are in process and it has been shown that by equipping houses with a mechanical ventilation system maintaining an air exchange rate of 0.5, it is possible in areas where outdoor air is dry to reduce indoor humidity and the occurrence of house dust mites [46,47]. Another approach to lower indoor humidity could be to decrease indoor sources of water vapor, including baths and showers, steam cooking, and clothes drying indoors. Indoor air humidity could be reduced by extracting air from the dampest rooms and opening the windows in winter to allow cold air to enter the house and warm it, which decreases its relative humidity. Faulty construction could also lead to indoor humidity through seepage of groundwater.

In conclusion, epidemiological studies demonstrate that in mite allergic patients with rhinitis and/or asthma sensitized to mites, exposure to mite allergen levels greater than 10μg/g of dust [48] in bedding can provoke reactions. These epidemiological studies also suggest that in children of atopic parents, sensitization to mites occurs in early infancy [49]. High antigen levels have been measured in bedding, and six studies have reported improvement in mite allergic disease after preventive measures. As stressed by Walshaw [50], five of the six used mattress covers [19,20,41–43]. In the remaining, mattresses were soaked in liquid nitrogen [21]. Where accurate mite counts were available, posteradication levels were <50 mites/g of dust, a level considered as a threshold for inducing allergic symptoms in sensitized persons. Other avoidance procedures were able to lower mite-allergen exposure but did not lead to convincing clinical improvement. Many physicians are reluctant to involve patients in what they see as vigorous cleaning regimens. However, it is important to visit the patient at home several times to assess the situation.

## III.  Cat Allergens

The most important cat-derived protein-stimulating IgE antibodies in allergic subjects is Fel d I, a glycoprotein with a molecular weight of 37,000. First purified by Leiterman and Ohman [51]. Fel d I has been detected in fur, saliva, skin, and sebaceous gland specimens. The following facts should be kept in mind with regard to prevention of cat allergy:

1.  Unlike mite allergens, which tend to settle, small Fel d I particles remain airborne for long periods. This fact explains the distinctively rapid onset of asthma or rhinitis in allergic patients to cats and provides a basis for designing a policy to reduce airborne allergens in houses with cats [52].
2.  One study [53] has shown that even after removal of the cat from the home, Fel d I levels in mattresses remain high for a very long period. Mattresses act as an allergenic reservoir. Thus the clinical benefits of removing the animal from a cat-sensitive subject's home might may be delayed unless other measures, such as changing the mattress, are taken.
3.  A number of authors claim that saliva is the principal source of Fel dI [54] and that the pet is contaminated as a result of licking during grooming [55]. However, other findings indicate that sebaceous glands are an important extrasalivary source of Fel d I allgergen [56,57].
4.  On average, one of two households have a pet. Patients with allergic disease often keep pets [58], probably because they need love [59]. Levinson believes that pets can aid children in developing a favorable attitude toward themselves and confidence in others. It is perhaps a fortunate coincidence that the animal preferred by clinical psychologists is the dog [60], which is less allergenic than the cat [61].
5.  Desensitization may allow a cat-sensitive patient to be exposed for a longer duration without symptoms [62], Thus it is worthwhile in veterinarians. but for patients with cats at home, it is not effective.

From this evidence it is clear that atopic patients should avoid keeping cats. However, because it is often difficult for physicians to persuade patients to get rid of their cats, it is important to try to control exposure to cat allergens. Glinert et al. [63] showed that repeated washing of cats removes allergens and progressively reduces accumulated allergens. De Blay et al. [64], who measured airborne cat allergen in an experimental room, showed that airborne cat allergen can be reduced dramatically by washing the cat, reducing furnishings, vacuum cleaning, and air filtering (Table 2) and concluded that the reduction in allergen levels achieved may be sufficient to allow a cat-sensitive patient to live with a cat. A clinical study is now under way to verify the feasibility and efficacy of this approach to allergic patients.

## IV.  Pollens

Trees and weeds pollinate during different periods of the year [65,66]. The physician must know these periods to be able to attribute seasonal symptoms to a given species. Not all pollens are implicated in allergic diseases. In fact, only a few show allergenic properties.

Primary prevention (i.e., avoidance of sensitization to pollens) is not

**Table 2**  Percentage of Decrease in Total Airborne Cat Allergen (ng/m³) Measured During a 30-min Air Sampling

|  | Baseline | After air filtration for 3 hours | After vacuum cleaning and air filtration for 3 h |
|---|---|---|---|
| Uncarpeted room (n = 3) | 12.6 | 5.8 (56%) | <0.2 (98%) |
| Carpeted room (n = 2) | 11.7 | 10.9 (7%) | 3.5 (70%) |

*Source:* Data from ref. 64.

feasible. A correlation has been noted between date of birth and relative risk for sensitization to a given pollen species, but this finding is of little practical value. It might be possible to reduce exposure to some extent by not planting allergenic trees in the community.

Secondary prevention would require accurate knowledge of pollinization and the relationship between weather conditions and atmospheric pollen concentration. Temperature, relative humidity, and wind velocity are associated positively with high pollen counts. The relationship between these variables is complex and demands multiple regression analysis. Until now forecast models based on these analyses have been ineffective, and at the present time the best that can be done is to advise patients to stay indoors during pollen seasons, especially if wind blows. Thus for all practical purposes, protection of patients relies mainly on drugs and/or specific hyposensitization.

In some pollen allergies, food allergy due to allergen cross-reactivity is encountered with such a high frequency that patients should be advised to avoid offending foods. For example, food allergy has been observed in up to 53% of patients allergic to birch pollens [67], and cutaneous allergy to celery has been demonstrated in 52% of patients allergic to mugwort [68].

## V.  Occupational Allergens

### A.  Laboratory Animals

Allergy to laboratory animals is an important occupational illness that affects 15 to 30% of laboratory workers [69]. A number of substances that induce sensitization and allergic symptoms are derived from the four small mammals (i.e., the rat, mouse, guinea pig, and rabbit) commonly used for laboratory experiments [70]. Moreover, there appears to be considerable cross-reactivity between these allergens [71]. Eggleston et al. [72] demonstrated task-related variations in airborne concentrations of the major rat allergen, Rat n I, which originates from urine. Handling conscious rats or contaminated bedding exposed a worker to four- to fivefold higher concentrations. Other factors determining exposure are the number of animals and the ventilation rate in the animal room. Since atopic subjects are more prone to develop asthma than nonatopic subjects [73], the former should be discouraged from entering these occupations.

### B. Other Occupational Allergens

In addition to laboratory animals, many other products can be allergenic [73]. Occupational respiratory diseases are dealt with fully in Part One of this volume. The relationship between the symptoms and the workplace may be difficult to establish. An open medical questionnaire does not seem to be a satisfactory means of diagnosing occupational asthma [74]. Worsening of asthmatic symptoms at or after work and improvement during weekends was not conclusively linked with occupational asthma. The gold standard is still specific bronchial challenge if the interval between leaving exposure and challenge is short enough.

Understanding the route of action of the allergen is needed to implement preventive measures. This is not always straightforward. For example, rhinitis and asthma in nurses allergic to latex was first thought to be a systemic reaction to latex glove antigens, but airborne latex has been implicated in some cases [75].

Once a person has developed occupational asthma, particularly if specific IgE-mediated hypersensitivity is involved, he or she will experience symptoms after exposure to very small concentrations of the offending agent. Since it is usually impossible to reduce levels in the workplace, the only solution may be to remove the sensitive person from the workplace. In any case, even occasional exposure to low levels can increase the severity of asthma [76]. Industrial hygienists should strive to keep exposure to asthma-causing allergens as low as possible.

## VI. Conclusions

In conclusion, prevention of sensitization to airborne allergens requires knowledge of aerobiologic characteristics and the behavior of each allergen. Primary prevention would be useful for the children of atopic parents, that is, one of two children, because the prevalence of atopy in young adults is around 25%. It could include avoiding furry pets, living in a well-heated and well-ventilated house, and encasing bedding in covers. Use of an acaricide and regular washing or dry cleaning of bedding may also be valuable. However, despite prevention, medications or hyposensitization are often needed to control allergic symptoms.

## References

1.  Task force on asthma and the other allergic diseases. NIH, 1979.
2.  Vervloet D, Haddi E, Tafforeau M, Lanteaume A, Kulling G, Charpin D. Reliability of respiratory symptoms to diagnose atopy. Clin Exp Allergy 1991;21:733–37.
3.  Eriksson NE. Allergy screening in asthma and allergic rhinitis. Which allergens should be used? Allergy 1987;42:189–95.
4.  Fraisse P, Bessot JC, Kopferschmitt-Kubler MC, Dieteman-Molard A, Lenz D, Quoix E, Pauli G. Profil d'une consultation d'allergie respiratoire d'après les données informatisées de 1968 à 1984 (3962 dossiers). Rev Pneumol Clin 1987;43:282–88.
5.  Platts-Mills TAE, Thomas WR, Aalberse RC, Vervloet D, Chapman MD. Dust mite allergens and asthma. Report of the 2nd International Workshop. Minster Lovell, Oxfordshire, England, September 19–21, 1990. UCB, Brussels, Institute of Allergy, 1991.
6.  Tovey ER, Chapman MD, Platts-Mills TAE. Mite faeces are a major source of house dust allergens. Nature 1981;289:592–93.
7.  Platts-Mills TAE, Heymann PW, Longbottom JL, Wilkins SR. Airborne allergens associated with asthma: particle sizes carrying dust mite and rat allergens measured with a cascade impactor. J Allergy Clin Immunol 1986;77:850–57.
8.  Kinnaird CH. Thermal death point of Dermatophagoides Pteronyssinus (Trouessart, 1897) (Astigmata, Pyroglyphidae), the house dust mite. Acarologia 1974; 16:340–42.
9.  Wharton GW. House-dust mites. Review article. J Med Entomol 1976;12:577–621.
10. Korsgaard J. Preventive measures in house-duse allergy. Am Rev Respir Dis 1982;125:80–84.
11. Brandt RL, Arlian LG. Mortality of house dust mites, *Dermatophagoides farinae* and *Dermatophagoides pteronyssinus*, exposed to dehydrating conditions and selected pesticides. J Med Entomol 1976;13:327–31.
12. Coloff MJ, Ayres J, Carswell F, Howarth PH, et al. The control of allergens of dust mites and domestic pets: a position paper. Clin Exp Allergy 1992;22 suppl 2:1–28.
13. Hughes AM, Maunsell K. A study of a population of house dust mites in its natural environment. Clin Allergy 1973;3:127–31.
14. Cunnington AM, Gregory PH. Mites in bedroom air. Nature 1968;217:1271–72.
15. Penaud A, Nourrit J, Autran P, Timon-David P, Jacquet-Francillon M, Charpin J. Methods of destroying house-dust pyroglyphid mites. Clin Allergy 1975;5:109–14.

16. Burr ML, Dean BV, Merrett TG, Neale E, St Leger AA, Verrier-Jones ER. Effects of anti-mites measures on children with mite-sensitive asthma: a controlled trial. Thorax 1980;35:506–12.

17. Van Bronswijk JEMH. Neues zur Ökologie der Wohnungsmilben. Allergologie 1984;11:438–45.

18. Arlian LG, Bernstein IL, Gallagher JS. The prevalence of house dust mites, *Dermatophagoides* spp. and associated environmental conditions in homes in Ohio. J Allergy Clin Immunol 1982;6:527–32.

19. Sarsfield JK, Gowland G, Toy R, Norman ALE. Mite sensitive asthma of childhood: trial of avoidance measures. Arch Dis Child 1974;49:716–21.

20. Burr ML, Neale E, Dean BV, Verrier-Jones ER. Effect of a change to mite-free bedding on children with mite-sensitive asthma: a controlled trial. Thorax 1980;35:513–14.

21. Burr ML, Dean BV, Butland BK, Neale E. Prevention of mite infestation of bedding by means of an impregnated sheet. Allergy 1988;43:299–302.

22. Bischoff E, Fisher A, Schirmacher W. Assessment of mite contamination by the heat escape method and the guanine detection-test. In: Mite allergy: a world-wide problem, Bad Kreuznach, Germany, September 1–2, 1987.

23. De Saint Georges-Gridelet D, Kniest FM, Schober G, Penaud A, Van Bronswijick JEMH. Lutte chimique contre les acaciens de la poussière de maison. Note préliminaire. Rev Fr Allergol 1988;28:131–38.

24. Dorward AJ, Collof MJ, Mackay NS, McSharry C, Thomson NC. Effect of house dust mite avoidance measures on adult atopic asthma. Thorax 1988;43:98–102.

25. Charpin D, Birnbaum J, Haddi E, N'Guyen A, Fondarai J, Vervloet D. Evaluation de l'efficacité d'un acaricide, Acardust, dans le traitement de l'allergie aux acariens. Rev Fr Allergol 1990;30:149–55.

26. Pauli G, Dietemann A, Ott M, Hoyet C, Bessot JC. Levels of mite allergens and guanine after use of an acaricidal preparation or cleaning solutions in highly infested mattresses and dwellings (abstract). J Allergy Clin Immunol 1991;87:321.

27. Kniest FM, Young E, Van Praag MCG, Vos H, Kort HSM, Koers WJ, De Maat-Bleeker F, Van Bronswijk JEMH. Clinical evaluation of a double-blind dust-mite avoidance trial in mite allergic rhinitis patients. Clin Exp Allergy 1991;21:39–47.

28. Lau-Schadendorf S, Rusche AF, Weber AK, Buettner-Goetzl P, Wahn U. Short-term effect of solidified benzyl benzoate on mite-allergen concentrations in house-dust. J Allergy Clin Immunol 1991;87:41–47.

29. Ehnert B, Lau-Schadendorf S, Weber A, Buettner P, Schou C, Wahn U. Reducing domestic exposure to dust mite allergen reduces bronchial hyperreactivity in sensitive children with asthma. J Allergy Clin Immunol 1992;90:135–38.

30. Reiser J, Ingram D, Mitchell EB, Warner JO. House dust mite allergens levels and anti-mite mattress spray (natamycin) in treatment of childhood asthma. Clin Exp Allergy 1990;20:561–68.
31. Kalra S, Owen SJ, Hepworth J, Woodcock A. Airborne house dust mite antigen after vacuum cleaning. Lancet 1990;336:449.
32. Fell P, Mitchell B, Brostoff J. Wet vacuum-cleaning and housedust-mite allergen. Lancet 1992;340:788–89.
33. Andersen A, Roesen J. House dust mites, *Dermatophagoides pteronyssinus* and its allergens: effects of washing. Allergy 1989;44:396–400.
34. Lombardero M, Heymann PW, Platts-Mills TAE, Fox JW, Chapman MD. Conformational stability of B cell epitopes on Group I and Group II *Dermatophagoides* spp. allergens. Effect of thermal and chemical denaturation on the binding of murine IgG and human IgE antibodies. J Immunol 1990;144;1353–60.
35. Vandenhove T, Soler M, Birnbaum J, Charpin D, Vervloet D. Effects of dry-cleaning on mite allergens level in blankets. Allergy (in press).
36. De Boer R. The control of house dust mites allergens in rugs. J Allergy Clin Immunol 1990;86:808–14.
37. Green NF, Nicholas NR, Salome CM, Woolcock AJ. Reduction of house dust mites and mite allergens: effect of spraying carpets and blankets with Allersearch DMS, an acaricide combined with an allergen reducing agent. Clin Exp Allergy 1989;19:203–7.
38. Miller JD, Miller A, Luczynska C, Rose G, Platts-Mills TAE. Effect of tannic acid spray on dust-mite antigen levels in carpets (abstract). J Allergy Clin Immunol 1989;83:262.
39. Nelson HS, Hirsch SR, Ohman JL, Platts-Mills TAE, Reed CE, Solomon WR. Recommendations for the use of residential air-cleaning devices in the treatment of allergic respiratory diseases. J Allergy Clin Immunol 1988;82:661–69.
40. Reisman RE, Mauziello PM, Davis GB, Georgitis JW, DeMasi JM. A double-blind study of the effectiveness of a high-efficiency particulate air (HEPA) filter in the treatment of patients with perennial allergic rhinitis and asthma. J Allergy Clin Immunol 1990;85:1050–57.
41. Murray AB, Ferguson AC. Dust-free bedrooms in the treatment of asthmatic children with house dust or house dust mite allergy: a controlled trial. Pediatrics 1983;71:418–22.
42. Walshaw MJ, Evans CC. Allergen avoidance in house dust mite sensitive adult asthma. Q J Med 1986;58:199–215.
43. Owen S, Morganstern M, Hepworth J, Woodcock A. Control of house dust mite antigen in bedding. Lancet 1990;336:396–97.
44. Mosbech H, Korsgaard J, Lind P. Control of house dust mites by electrical heating blankets. J Allergy Clin Immunol 1988;81:706–10.

45. Charpin D, Birnbaum J, Haddi E, Genard G, Lanteaume A, Toumi M, Faraj F, Van der Brempt X, Vervloet D. Altitude and allergy to house-dust mites. A paradigm of the influence of environmental exposure on allergic sensitization. Am Rev Respir Dis 1991;143:983–86.

46. Korsgaard J. Mechanical ventilation and house-dust mites (abstract). ACI News 1991(Suppl 1):114.

47. Harving H, Hansen ZG, Korsgaard J, Nielsen PA, Olsen OF, Romer J, Svendsen VG, Osterballe O. House-dust mite allergy and anti-mite measures in the indoor environment. Allergy 1991;46(Suppl 11):33–38.

48. Charpin D, Vervloet D. Epidemiology of allergic diseases. Its use for clinicians. Prog Allergy Clin Immunol 1991;2:238–241.

49. Sporik R, Holgate ST, Platts-Mills TAE, Cogswell JJ. Exposure to house-dust mite allergen (Der p I) and the development of asthma in childhood. A prospective study. N Engl J Med 1990;323:502–7.

50. Walshaw MJ. Mite control: is it worthwhile? Respir Med 1990;84:257–58.

51. Leiterman K, Ohman JL. Cat allergen 1: biochemical, antigenic and allergic properties. J Allergy Clin Immunol 1984;74:147–53.

52. Luczynska CM, Chapman MD, Platts-Mills TAE. Airborne concentrations and particles size distribution of allergen derived from domestic cats *(Felis domesticus)*. Am Rev Respir Dis 1990;141:361–67.

53. Van Der Brempt X, Charpin D, Haddi E, Da Mata P, Vervloet D. Cat removal and Fel d I levels in mattresses. J Allergy Clin Immunol 1991;87:595–96.

54. Brown PR, Leiterman K, Ohman JL. Distribution of cat allergen in cat tissues and fluids. Int Arch Allergy Appl Immunol 1984;74:67–70.

55. Didierlaurent A, Fogliette MJ, Guerin B, Hewitt B, Percheron F. Comparative study on cat allergens from fur and saliva. Int Arch Allergy Appl Immunol 1984;73:27–31.

56. Dabrowsky AJ, Van Der Brempt X, Soler M, Seguret N, Lucciani P, Charpin D, Vervloet D. Cat skin as in important source of Fed d I allergen. J Allergy Clin Immunol 1990;86:462–65.

57. Charpin C, Da Mata P, Charpin D, Lavaut MN, Allasia C, Vervloet D. Fel d I allergen distribution in cat fur and skin. J Allergy Clin Immunol 1991;88:77–82.

58. Charpin D, Vervloet D, Lanteaume A, Kleisbauer JP, Kulling G, Razzouk H, Charpin J. Allergie respiratoire et animaux domestiques. A propos d'enquêtes réealisées en population générale. Rev Mal Respir 1989;6:325–28.

59. Ohman JL, Golden E. Cat attachment in allergic patients who retain cats (abstract). J Allergy Clin Immunol 1986;77:202.

60. Corson SA, Corson EO, Gwynne PH. Pet-facilitated psychotherapy in hospital setting. Curr Psychiatr Ther 1975;15:277.

61. Murray AB, Ferguson AC, Morrison BJ. The frequency and severity of

cat allergy vs. dog allergy in atopic children. J Allergy Clin Immunol 1983;72:145–49.

62. Ohman JL, Findlay SR. Leitermann KM. Immunotherapy in cat-induced asthma. Double-blind trial with evaluation of in vivo and in vitro responses. J Allergy Clin Immunol 1984;74:230–39.

63. Glinert R, Wilson P, Wedner HJ. Fel d I is markedly reduced following sequential washing of cat (abstract). J Allergy Clin Immunol 1990;85:327.

64. de Blay F, Chapman MD, Platts-Mills TAE. Airborne cat allergen (Fel d I). Environmental control with the cat in situ. Am Rev Respir Dis 1991;143:1334–39.

65. Jelks M. Allergy plants that cause wheezing and sneezing. New York: Worldwide Library, 1986.

66. Solomon W, Mathews KP. Aerobiology and inhalant allergens. In: Middleton E Jr, Reed CE, Ellis EF, eds. Allergy: principles and practice. 3rd ed. St. Louis, MO: CV Mosby, 1988.

67. Eriksson N, Formgren H, Svenonius E. Food hypersensitivity in patients with pollen allergy. Allergy 1982;37:437–43.

68. Kaupinen K, Kousa M, Reunala T. Aromatic plants. A cause of severe attacks of angio-œdema and urticaria. Contact Dermatitis 1980;6:251–54.

69. Gross NJ. Allergy to laboratory animals: epidemiologic, clinical, and physiologic aspects and a trial of cromolyn in its management. J Allergy Clin Immunol 1980;66:158–65.

70. Butcher BT, Salvaggio JE. Occupational asthma. J Allergy Clin Immunol 1986;78:547–56.

71. Ohman JL Jr, Lowell FC, Bloch KJ. Allergens of mammalian origin. II. Characterization of allergens extracted from rats, mouse, guinea pig, rabbit pelts. J Allergy Clin Immunol 1975;55:16–24.

72. Eggleston PA, Newill CA, Ansari AA, Pustelnik A, Lou SR, Evans R, Marsch D, Longbottom JL, Corn M. Task-related variation in airborne concentrations of laboratory animal allergens. Studies with rat no. 1. J Allergy Clin Immunol 1989;84:347–52.

73. Cockcroft A, Edwards J, McCarthy P, Anderson N. Allergy in laboratory animal workers. Lancet 1981; 1:827–30.

74. Malo JL, Ghezzo H, L'Archevêque J, Lagier F, Perrin B, Cartier A. Is the clinical history a satisfactory means of diagnosing occupational asthma? Am Rev Respir Dis 1991;143:528–32.

75. Lagier F, Badier M, Martigny J, Charpin D, Vervloet D. Latex as aeroallergen. Lancet 1990;336:516–17.

76. Butcher BT, O'Neil CE, Reed MA, Salvaggio JE, Weill H. Development and loss of toluene diisocyanate (TDI) reactivity: immunologic, pharmacologic and provocative inhalation challenge studies. J Allergy Clin Immunol 1982;70:231–35.

# 14

## Indoor Air Quality Problems and Patient Management

**JAMES H. DAY**

Queen's University
Kingston, Ontario, Canada

## I.  Introduction

A number of medical problems are associated with the indoor air environment. Most of these are well defined and traceable, while others are somewhat obscure, with vague symptomatology and unknown sources. Patients present with a variety of medical conditions, most of which are routinely encountered by general physicians as a part of their practices. There are, as well, distinct clinical presentations which should alert the physician as to etiology and raise suspicions as to the source. Once it is recognized that the patient presenting has a problem that may be related to the indoor environment, a methodologic approach leads on to appropriate investigation and management.

Some old players, such as formaldehyde, may not be as important in producing health effects, but concerns about them crop up from time to time. New players such as mycotoxins may well take center stage once the full implications of their role are understood. The physician, having once identified an indoor air problem or at least being suspicious of its role as the cause of symptoms, should have a plan of action that will necessarily involve collaborative

*259*

efforts with appropriate medical and building specialists. The physician must understand the importance of diagnosis and causation since any decision relative to indoor air quality could affect the well-being of the patient and have a serious economic impact, and in certain circumstances influence job security.

The health and well-being of building occupants need not be dependent on pristine air quality states but must acknowledge the considerable variability of problems arising from buildings as a consequence of changing economic and climatic conditions, age, and engineering of the building, including marked differences in the microenvironments. Any solutions to these problems must take into consideration a wide variety of factors, including the recognition that the satisfactory resolution of the problem is crucial to the safety and relative comfort of the occupants.

## II.  Recognized Medical Conditions Occurring in BRI/SDS

### A.  Allergic Rhinitis-Sinusitis, Conjunctivitis

Patients with allergic rhinitis-sinusitis present with ocular irritation, sinus fullness, headache, nasal congestion, sneezing, watery rhinorrhea, dry throat, nonproductive cough, difficulty wearing contact lenses and itching, tearing and soreness of eyes often coupled with gelatinous conjunctival discharge in the mornings, and reduced sense of well-being with irritability and fatigue [1]. Allergic rhinitis-sinusitis may be complicated by nasal polyposes and/or mucocyst development in the sinuses. Predisposing factors are personal and family history of atopic diseases.

Rhinoscopy may show pale, bluish edematous nasal turbinates coated with thin, clear secretions, and nasal membrane swelling; eye examination reveals conjunctival injection and edema [2]. Nasal washings may show prominent numbers of eosinophils [1]. Total IgE levels are frequently elevated, particularly during seasonal exacerbations, but for etiologic diagnosis, antigen-specific IgE needs to be demonstrated by skin testing, radioallergosorbent test (RAST), or by enzyme-linked immunosorbent assay (ELISA), the skin test being superior [2]. The diagnosis should be the result of the demonstration of antigen specific IgE correlated with the clinical history. Nasal challenge with suspected antigen may be necessary to establish etiology [2].

Differential diagnosis must consider nonallergic rhinitis with eosinophilia (NARES), which is featured by increased eosinophiles in nasal secretions, normal serum IgE levels, and good response to topical corticosteroid therapy minimally to antihistamines. Nonallergic rhinitis without eosinophils in the nasal secretions (vasomotor rhinitis) presents with persistent symptoms without correlation to specific allergen exposure; symptoms are usually elicited by temperature, humidity changes, or emotions and not to allergens. For rhinitis medicamentosa, repeated application of vasoconstricting nose spray leads to ischemic effects on nasal mucous membranes and is suggested by a history of chronic use of those agents. Infectious rhinitis is marked by thick, purulent nasal discharge. Many chemicals are mast cell degranulators or histamine liberators, eliciting symptoms similar to those that are allergy induced.

### B. Asthma

Asthma can be defined as reversible airway obstruction characterized by bronchial reactivity and associated airway inflammation. In allergic asthma there may be immediate or late immunological responses of the bronchi [1], whereas in nonallergic asthma, nonspecific bronchial irritability is the basis.

There are three patterns of asthmatic reaction: immediate, late, and dual (Fig. 1). The immediate reaction develops within minutes of the antigenic challenge and is of short duration. This can be prevented and readily reversed by β-adrenergic agents and cromoglycates but not by corticosteroids [3]. The late reaction develops 2 to 3 h after antigenic challenge and resolves within 24 to 36 h. The dual reaction has both early- and late-phase components. Persistent asthma is an expression of late-phase reactions that are less responsive to bronchodilators than the immediate reaction. The late-phase reaction is followed by an increase in nonspecific bronchial reactivity [3] and is modified by inhaled corticosteroids.

The hallmarks of an asthmatic reaction are dyspnea, cough, wheezing, tightness in the chest, and fatigue due to increase in respiratory effort. Physical findings depend on the severity of the asthmatic condition; a moderate attack is characterized by expiratory wheezes changing on cough and viscid mucus secretions. In a severe attack, there is use of accessory muscles, tachypnea, and pulsus paradoxus which if unchecked will lead to respiratory failure.

Laboratory tests show peripheral eosinophilia in 50% of asthmatics and normal numbers of white blood cells. The chest x-ray may be normal, reveal increased radiolucency of the lung because of hyperinflation, or complications, such as spontaneous pneumothorax and mediastinal emphysema [1,2].

In early stages, lung function tests may be normal or reveal reversible airways obstruction with reduced $FEV_1$, FVC, and MMEFR values while total lung capacity may be increased [1]. Peak expiratory flow rate (PEFR) is a convenient way of monitoring asthma and can be done by the patient at home or in suspected building environment for diagnosis and management. Total serum IgE levels are quite variable and often normal. Skin testing shows positive wheal and flare response to relevant allergen(s) in allergic subjects. Exercise test is positive in about 80% of the patients [2] and may be selective, while the methacholine/histamine challenge test, although variable in degree, is positive.

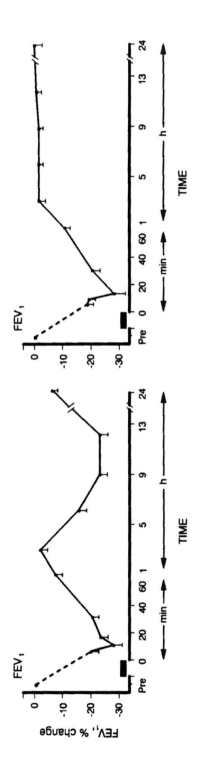

**Figure 1** Immediate and late-phase reactions to antigen challenge in the airway as represented by percent fall in FEV<sub>1</sub> <D>. The first phase is a result of mediator release, which may or may not be followed by the second inflammatory (late) phase.

Bronchial challenge tests with the appropriate allergen or irritant will reproduce symptoms.

Asthma assiciated with indoor air exposure [4] may be allergic or nonallergic (irritant) in nature. Certain allergens may also act as irritants in susceptible individuals. Causative agents of asthma occurring indoors and often associated with occupation can be divided into groups according to mechanisms of sensitization [3]. High-molecular-weight compounds cause production of specific IgE antibodies leading to a positive immediate skin test reaction. Further antigen-specific IgE antibodies can also be demonstrated by RAST or ELISA. Well-known examples include asthma induced by biologic enzymes in detergent enzyme industries; by laboratory animals among animal handlers such as in laboratory workers, farmers, veterinarians, furriers, and breeders; by psyllium and antibiotics among health professionals; and by mites among grain and flour handlers, granary workers, and bakers.

The mechanism responsible for asthmatic reaction in response to low-molecular-weight (LMW) compounds is not yet fully understood. Proposed mechanisms include the LMW compounds acting as haptens and coupling to proteins. Skin testing using the LMW compound is usually not helpful, and specific IgE antibodies directed against protein conjugates of the LMW compound are found only in a small proportion of patients. Eosinophilia is often present. Work-related asthma to LMW compounds include response to acid anhydrides such as trimellitic anhydride, isocynates, and organic dusts such as western red cedar (plicatic acid) and white cedar.

Critical to the establishment of occupational asthma and important to indoor air quality causes of asthma is the presence of methacholine/histamine responsiveness following a period of time within the suspected environment. Differential diagnosis of occupational asthma [2] includes bronchitis (acute and chronic), which is characterized by cough with expectoration. There may be a reactive component and thus some reversible changes in airflow. Chronic bronchitis is defined as productive cough on most days, for at least 3 months of the year, over two consecutive years. Eosinophilia is not typical in bronchitis. Chronic obstructive pulmonary disease (COPD), an end stage of chronic bronchitis, is a nonreversible state of airways obstruction characterized by progressive breathlessness.

### C. Hypersensitivity Pneumonitis (Extrinsic Allergic Alveolitis)

Hypersensitivity pneumonitis is an inflammatory reaction of the lungs featured by alveolar filling and interstitial reactivity resulting from intense or prolonged exposure to finely dispersed organic dusts of appropriate particle size [5]; however, clinical presentations can vary depending on the severity of disease, duration, and nature of exposure [6]. There are three forms: acute, subacute, and insidious.

The acute form is manifest as fever, headache, malaise, lethargy, chills, cough, dyspnea, sputum production, anorexia, and weight loss if exposure is chronic [1]. There may be a temporal correlation of symptoms with the building environment in which case symptoms will begin 4 to 6 h after exposure and clear 18 to 48 h after exposure ends, with the patient being asymptomatic between attacks [1].

Chest x-ray may be normal or reveal reticulonodular changes in the early stages of the disease or patchy pneumonitis. A bronchial provocation test with relevant antigens reproduces the disease. Pulmonary function tests reveal restrictive changes and diffusion defects at the end stage of the disease [6].

There may be leucocytosis as well as an elevated erythrocyte sedimentation rate. There are precipitating antibodies (IgG, IgA, IgM) in the serum to the specific organic dusts, but since these antigens are ubiquitous, their presence is not diagnostic. Total IgE levels are usually normal. The histologic appearance of pulmonary lesions is characterized by mononuclear cell interstitial and alveolar infiltrates containing mainly T suppressor cells and macrophages. Granulomata may be present particularly in chronic cases. The activity of alveolar macrophages in pulmonary lesions is increased significantly. Specific antigens within the pulmonary parenchyma can be demonstrated by immunofluorescence. There is prominent lymphokine production in symptomatic patients.

Symptoms of the subacute form appear over a period of weeks, marked by cough and dyspnea, with periods of acute illness and clinical features of tachypnea, tachycardia, fever, and bibasilar rales (1).

Laboratory findings are as for acute form, but chest x-ray may show soft reticular or patchy infiltrates with or without small, poorly defined nodules. Pulmonary function tests show a restrictive defect, decreased compliance, and at the end stages of the disease, decreased diffusion capacity.

Insidious form [1] is featured by gradual progression of symptoms with possible intermittent acute periods and progressive exertional dyspnea. It tends to occur with continuous low-level exposure to antigen. Prolonged avoidance of the offending antigen is needed in these cases for any improvement. Respiratory insufficiency may occur, usually precipitated by an acute exposure or infection.

The chest x-ray may show changes of interstitial fibrosis with prominent involvement of the peripheral lung fields and honeycombing at the end stage.

Causative agents of hypersensitivity pneumonitis indoors include the thermophilic actinomycetes, which produce acute and insidious disease as well as fungi and such as *Aurebasidium pullulans* [7], and the *Aspergillus* species [8]. Serum proteins such as avian proteins have also been reported to cause hypersensitivity pneumonitis, as do anhydrides [9].

Differential diagnosis of hypersensitivity pneumonitis should include [1] interstitial pulmonary diseases, acute pulmonary mycotoxicosis which follows massive exposure to moldy material unassociated with precipitins in the serum [1,10], collagen vascular disorders, and drug-induced lung diseases. Allergic bronchopulmonary aspergillosis should be included in the differential diagnosis, and hypersensitivity pneumonitis can occur from *Aspergillus fumigatus*.

### D. Humidifier Fever

Symptoms of humidifier fever are pyrexia and malaise, possibly cough, chest tightness, dyspnea, and weight loss [6]. There is usually a temporal correlation with building environment and onset of attacks. Episodes usually occur after absence from work for a few days, giving rise to the term "Monday sickness," with a delay of 4 to 8 h after returning to work on Mondays before symptoms occur. This is probably due to the shutting down of the air-conditioning systems over the weekend and massive exposure to accumulated endotoxins on system restart. There is usually less reactivity over the remainder of the week [6]. The disease is more frequent in the winter months, probably because during this season smaller amounts of fresh air are drawn into humidifiers than during the summer months [11]. Among the suspected causative agents of humidifier fever are bacterial endotoxins and molds. Amoebas are not the cause. A respiratory illness observed in workers in a closed swine barn has similar features and is also caused by endotoxins.

A skin prick test with humidifier antigen is often positive and is an immediate reaction; a chest x-ray is usually normal unless complicated by other conditions. Pulmonary function tests may reveal a slight restrictive defect, a reduction in gas transfer, but no permanent changes. Bronchial provocation test with humidifier material is positive, but no chronic effects are seen. Exposed workers show multiple precipitin arcs to a number of humidifier antigens, whether symptomatic or not [6]. Hypersensitivity pneumonitis may present with similar symptoms to humidifier fever, but radiographic abnormalities and permanent changes in lung function do not occur in humidifier fever.

### E. Allergic Bronchopulmonary Aspergillosis

Allergic bronchopulmonary aspergillosis is a subacute inflammatory reaction elicited by both IgE- and IgG-mediated immune response directed against *A. fumigatus* growing in the respiratory tree. *A. fumigatus* can elicit five pulmonary reactions [4], these being allergic asthma (type I hypersensitivity, IgE against mold spores, and propagules), hypersensitivity pneumonitis, fungus ball or aspergilloma, invasive aspergillosis (overwhelming diffuse pneumonia in immunocompromised host), and allergic bronchopulmonary aspergillosis.

Allergic bronchopulmonary aspergillosis presents as asthma in atopic individuals. Complaints may be nonspecific, such as anorexia, weight loss, fatigue, and flulike symptoms [1]. Generalized wheezing and localized rales are heard on physical examination.

Laboratory investigation reveal [1] marked increases in peripheral blood eosinophilia ($1000\mu L^{-1}$). Skin tests to *A. fumigatus* only produce immediate cutaneous hypersensitivity. Chest x-ray reveals recurrent migratory infiltrates and may show evidence of central bronchiectasis and pulmonary fibrosis in chronic disease. Immunological studies show a markedly elevated total serum IgE and specific anti-*A. fumigatus* IgE and IgG, as well as serum IgG precipitins to *A. fumigatus*. Inhalation challenge with antigen reproduces the symptoms; both immediate acute bronchoconstriction and late pulmonary reactions (up to 10 h after inhalation, can last 1 to 3 days) occur. The late reactions may include fever, malaise, and wheezing. Pulmonary function testing demonstrates obstructive changes, while some patients may also have a restrictive defect. The brown sputum plugs contain fungal elements.

Differential diagnosis should include allergic asthma, cystic fibrosis which may be associated with colonization of the airways by *Aspergillus*, hypersensitivity pneumonitis with infiltrates, parasitic infections with eosinophilia, and drug reactions causing pulmonary infiltrates and blood eosinophilia.

### F. Infections

Infections associated with indoor air-quality problems can be classified into two categories: those whose transmission is only facilitated by indoor air circulation and those that *live and grow* under indoor air conditions [12]. The symptoms depend on the type of infection, with the most common being bronchial infections followed by pneumonia.

The most frequent and thus important infectious diseases using HVAC systems for transmission are viruses, which include influenza, the common cold, measles, and rubella. Influenza with highest attack rate among school-aged children usually originates as epidemics in classrooms. In a study of army trainees, Brundage has linked acute respiratory infection rates to ventilation mode [13]. The transmission of measles and rubella through heating/ventilation/air conditioning (HVAC) systems is of importance mainly in pediatric settings [14].

Some infectious diseases can use HVAC systems for amplification as well as transmission. Probably the most important and best known example is Legionnaires' disease, caused by *Legionella pneumophila*. Legionnaires' disease is the pneumonic form and is a rapidly progressing respiratory illness spread from contaminated cooling towers and water systems of air-conditioning systems, hot-water systems, and showers. The illness was fatal to 29 of the 182 persons affected in Philadelphia in 1976 [15].

The symptoms are cough, which becomes productive as the illness progresses, fever, chills, rigors, weakness, and fatigue. At the end stage of the disease there may be renal failure. In the Philadelphia outbreak, shock occurred in 50% of those who died. Rales are heard on chest auscultation, the urine is positive for protein in about 20% of cases (15), and about 60% have leucocytosis $(10,000 \text{ mm}^{-3})$ and elevated sedimentation rate is found in about 30% (80 mm/h) of the cases.

*L. pneumophila* can be demonstrated from sputum cultures by direct fluorescent antibody staining using monoclonal or polyclonal antibodies. The chest x-ray typically shows pneumonia: patchy interstitial infiltrates, progressing to consolidation at later stages of the disease. Seroconversion or seropositivity is seen in immunological tests.

Pontiac fever [16] is the nonpneumonic form of *L. pneumophila* infection. The symptoms mimic mild flu and are featured by low-grade fever, headache, myalgia, and malaise. It is a self-limited disease lasting 2 to 5 days, sometimes beginning with shaking chills. The attack rate is extremely high, 95% [16]. Laboratory tests show diagnostic rises in *Legionella* antibody titers.

A less common infectious condition that can use HVAC systems to amplify is Q fever, caused by *Coxiella burnetti*, which is transmitted by laboratory animals [12]. The symptoms are flulike, but pneumonitis, hepatitis, and endocarditis may occur in some patients [6]. Twenty percent have a protracted disease for longer than 4 weeks. Complement-fixing antibody titer is elevated to phase 1 antigen.

### Fungal Infections

Fungi can become an indoor air quality problem because of universal presence indoors. The most common indoor molds are *Aspergillus, Penicillium, Cladosporium,* and *Alternaria*. There is mounting evidence that increased incidences of respiratory disease in children may have a significant mold contribution [17].

Important fungal infections known to be *tramsmitted* by air include histoplasmosis, coccidiomycosis, blastomycosis, and cryptococcus [10,12]. All cause systemic disease in unselected exposed populations. Infections are rarely building related but can occur when ventilation systems are contaminated by dust harboring the organisms mainly through bird or bat droppings. The illness usually presents as pneumonia. Lung colonization in the absence of infection can lead to allergic bronchopulmonary aspergillosis. Fungi such as *A. fumigatus* can cause invasive lung diseases in immunologically suppressed persons.

Exposure to spores and propagules of fungi may cause IgE-mediated allergy (i.e., rhinitis and asthma) and can also cause hypersensitivity pneumonitis. Massive inhalation of mycotoxins produced by fungi can lead to pulmonary mycotoxicosis, featured in some instances by severe respiratory distress [10]. Mycotoxins that are mainly secondary metabolites of molds are readily absorbed through mucous membranes since they are of low molecular weight and soluble.

Once absorbed they can exert systemic effects [10] and in high doses can be lethal. Mycotoxins may compromise the immune system, but to a large extent the effects are indirect and difficult to detect.

### G.   Dermatitis (Allergic Contact)

The signs of allergic contact dermatitis are eczematoid rash or urticaria: erythema, edema, scaling, and vesicle formation, which may leave postinflammatory hyperpigmentation. If the exposure is chronic, there may be lichenified erythematous scaling eruptions. Allergic contact dermatitic eruptions start 1 to 2 days after exposure and resolve in 1 to 2 days.

Measuring total IgE levels and blood eosinophils is of little help but can give information about the severity of the atopic disease [2]. Etiology is established by specific patch tests, but a significant incidence of false positives and negatives occur. Patch test sites should be examined 48 h and 72 h after application. Readings at 48 h only will lead to a number of false negative readings [18].

### H.   Sick-Building Syndrome

The symptoms of this relatively new condition are nonspecific, such as tiredness, lethargy, headache, and mucous membrane irritation syndromes: dryness, running or blockage of nose and eyes, dry throat, chest tightness, wheeze, and breathlessness, with no fever [19]. There is a distinct association with the building environment and symptoms may resolve once the person has left.

Various recognizable diseases must be ruled out. A detailed environmental study will not produce a causative agent, and in general, all volatile organic compounds (VOCs) and other airborne pollutants are within allowable limits. In fact, many buildings in which sick-building syndrome (SBS) occur have better indoor air quality measurements than those that do not [20].

The most important feature of SBS is its "epidemic" nature. Generally, females are more symptomatic, as are workers in lower-ranking jobs. The symptoms are less common within the first 6 months of working in a building, peak at 1 year of employment in the building, and level off after that. The problem should not be underestimated, since it has been calculated that the cost of absenteeism due to building problems is about eight times greater than the financial benefit gained through energy savings [21].

## III.   Evaluation of Patient with Health Effects Thought to Be Due to Indoor Air Pollution

### A.   The Patient

To evaluate whether the source of the problem is in the building environment, the exact history of onset of symptoms and the relationship with the building environment have to be noted, as well as the medical condition when away from the building and any other time. Personal habits that may influence symptoms should be reviewed. Finally, there must be recognition of the psychosocial component of tight building complaints and other complaints involving nonspecific symptoms; comments about unpleasant working conditions, job dissatisfaction, and other stressors should be recorded. The search for environmental and personal factors can be facilitated by questionnaires [22].

### B. The Building Environment

Once the source of a pollutant and exposure levels are established, they should be compared or correlated with the history of the problem and with observed or alleged symptoms of exposure. For a successful search of the source of an indoor air quality problem, there should be consultation and cooperation with ventilation engineers and other technical specialists.

In the case of newly suspected pollutants, there should be a systematic attempt to evaluate the health effects. These should include epidemiological studies to find susceptible groups, characterization of the patterns of the illness in question, and evaluation of predisposing factors. Controlled experiments where effects of the specific compound can be studied and at known concentrations are essential.

Finally, laboratory tests and criteria for diagnosis of particular building-related disease should be established. Commonly used laboratory tests include hematological tests to check for anemia, leucocytosis, and eosinophilia, allergen tests such as skin prick tests (type I hypersensitivity), patch tests (type IV hypersensitivity), and in vitro tests such as RAST and ELISA to detect specific IgE and IgG in the serum. In some cases special tests may be needed to confirm a diagnosis: for example, measurement of COHb, precipitating antibodies, cultures to detect possible infections/colonization or challenge tests with measurements of upper and lower airway resistance, rhinomanometry, and pulmonary function. Once the causative agent has been characterized and health effects have been established, it may be necessary to devise guidelines for exposure and standard treatment for affected persons.

### C. Management

Management of medical conditions caused by indoor air problems relate directly to the presenting complaints and causation. Clearly, removing offending sources is primary, and if necessary, affected persons may have to be restricted in some fashion within that environment (i.e., moving to an alternative place). Coincident with this may be the administration of protective equipment, medication, and other aides to provide symptomatic relief until the problem is remedied.

### Allergens Found in Homes

Allergic reactivity can be specifically managed by awareness of the circumstances under which the allergens are present in the environment. Certain allergens are well characterized; others have uncertain association. Some, such as ragweed and grass pollens, are present indoors during respective seasons; others, including molds, dust mites, and cockroaches, variably reside within the indoor environment. Allergens produced by pets constitute yet another but possibly the most important source of allergic reactivity within the household.

Pet dander, saliva, excrement, and urine can all cause allergic reactions. As well, the animal hair or feathers can collect other allergens, such as pollen, dust, and mold. Bird droppings can often be a source of bacteria, dust, and fungi. Short-haired pets can be as reactive as long-haired ones, and nonshedding animals (e.g., poodles) do not assure allergen freedom. There are considerable differences among pet species as to allergic reactivity, depending on antigen spread and antigenicity.

Cats are an especially well-known source of allergic reactivity. Over half of all homes in the United States have at least one pet, and cats are more common than dogs. Reactivity to cats and dogs affects under 5 to 10% of the general population and 15 to 40% of the allergic population, with allergy to cats being twice as common as that to dogs. Cat allergen Fel DI is derived from saliva and pelt, and for dogs Can FI is derived from pelt and saliva. Antigens from guinea pigs, rabbits, and gerbils are multiple and are derived from urine, saliva, pelt, and serum.

Allergens that consist of either dried secretions or dander become airborne with disturbance and range from less than 1 $\mu$m to greater than 20 $\mu$m with significant numbers less than 5 $\mu$m. Allergens can therefore remain airborne for long periods and will adhere to wall surfaces as opposed to house dust antigen, which is heavy, settles quickly, and is not found on walls [23,24]. The most important exposure is through respiration of airborne allergens, the level of which is the major determinant of the allergic response. Concentration of the airborne allergen is controlled by the amount of allergen in the immediate environment, degree of disturbance of the settled allergen, and ventilation of rooms or buildings. Cat sensitivity is diagnosed by history, skin tests, RAST, challenge, and a trial of avoidance.

Treatment consists of removing the animals; 4 to 6 months are required in most cases to reduce allergen levels substantially. If the animal cannot be removed, allergen reduction may be accomplished by restricting the animal's mobility, removing carpets, cleaning aggressively, increasing ventilation, using air cleaner (HEPA or electrostatic), covering mattresses, and washing cats. Pharmacotherapy is the treatment of choice, but in certain cases immunotherapy to cat and/or dog antigens may be employed, which although it has been shown to reduce sensitivity to provocation, none have demonstrated improved symptom scores for long-term exposure. Immunotherapy can therefore be quite helpful to persons with significant sensitivity and intermittent unavoidable contact, but it is less likely to confer adequate protection against daily high-dose exposure that occurs for most pet owners.

Mites flourish in warm, humidified surroundings but are present in households in temperate climates as well [25]. Since they utilize human skin scales as a food source, they are found on furniture, bedding, clothing, and carpeting. Humidity is the decisive limiting factor for mite growth [26]; higher humidity levels lead to increased mite numbers, a problem exacerbated by use of humidifiers, while air conditioning can reduce mite density if run consistently and brings humidity below 50% [27]. Agents such as tannic acid and benzyl benzoate treatment, which denatures protein antigens, helps reduce numbers, as will insecticides and natamycin [28,29]. Use of vinyl bedding and mattress encasings is a quick and simple way to reduce mattress dust samples and is especially helpful in patients with atopic dermatitis. Washing bed coverings and sheets in hot water is simple and effective. Significant reduction in symptoms cannot be expected until 3 to 4 weeks after beginning a dust mite avoidance program.

Respiratory sensitization occurs to cockroach allergens [30], a problem especially in the inner cities. These allergens include feces, skins, egg cases, and saliva. Cockroach control includes humidity reduction and pesticides.

For molds, reduced humidity and avoidance of localized water accumulation is essential. Fungicides can help, but unless underlying conditions that support fungus growth are eliminated, regrowth will occur [31]. Although pollen is mainly an outdoor allergen, it enters indoor air seasonally and may be the main constituent. Air conditioners are an effective method of reduction.

### Management Outline

In general, removing the offending agent from the subject's environment is the method of choice for treatment/management. This needs to be coupled with the education of patient, occupant, or public regarding the source and control of the problem. Although medication may be required, preventative measures are always preferable.

### *Environmental Control and Management*

The best method of control is avoidance of the offending agent by removal from the environment of the subject (e.g., tobacco smoke), reduction of periods of exposure, or other alteration of environment [32]. As the first step in creating a healthy work or home indoor air environment, attention has to be directed to proper building design and construction. This includes giving careful thought to the choice of materials of construction, the floor plan of the building, airflow patterns, and air intakes and exchanges [6]. Since newer buildings are associated with higher levels of VOCs and other pollutants, it may be useful to allow time for building bake-out and air-out time before occupation.

Once the building is occupied, modification of temperature, humidity, and ventilation settings, as well as the ratio of air recirculated versus fresh air [33] should be checked since their levels can make profound differences in indoor air quality. Continuous maintenance, repair, and cleaning of HVAC systems is essential to prevent future indoor air quality problems. Air-conditioning devices [19] may be effective in reducing indoor pollens, mold spores, and house dust mite numbers by controlling antigen intake and reducing humidity.

There are a number of filtering devices available [19] utilizing different filtering techniques. Each technique will filter out a specific range of particles. Filtering devices using inertial impaction and gravitational settling methods are best for larger particles ($>1$ $\mu g/m$). Infusion-type devices are best for smaller particles ($<0001$ $\mu g/m$ diameter). For elimination of gases and odors the method of choice is absorption to activated charcoal or chemical crystals. None of the filtering techniques are truly effective, however, if toxins or antigens produced by microorganisms too small to be trapped by normal filtration systems are the problem [31].

Mechanical filters have one or more layers of woven matting of fiber, sometimes coated with oil. Mechanical filters are effective for filtering pollen but ineffective for smoke or mold pollutants. Of the electronic air cleaners, the simplest are the negative-ion generators, which impart an electrical charge to particles, which are then attracted to surface of opposite charge. Negative-ion generators are effective for control of pollen and 89 to 90% effective for clearing environmental tobacco smoke pollutants. Their drawback is the frequent need for cleaning and ozone production.

### Infections

The most common sources of building-related infectious agents are cooling towers and water tank of humidifier systems (i.e., warm, recirculated water containing inorganic and organic solutes). For example, in perhaps the most common building-related infection and certainly the best known, Legionnaires' disease, the source of bacteria are usually cooling towers, central air-conditioning systems, and hot-water tanks.

Identified sources point to the precautions that need to be taken for the prevention of infectious diseases. One method of eliminating the solute containing warm water that supports the growth of potentially harmful microorganisms is to replace recirculating or cool mist systems with steam injection. Other meaures aim to control the growth of microorganisms; these include the use of biocides, fungicides, and anticorrosives in cooling towers and tanks, or the heating of water tanks to kill multiplying organisms. Heating or boiling of water tanks may inhibit the growth of certain microorganisms but has limited application because of its prohibitive cost. When not in use, water reservoirs shoud be drained. Sludge should be cleaned and foaming prevented. Dissolved solids should be minimized to limit bacterial growth.

For infectious agents that do not amplify in HVAC systems but merely use it for transmission, the modern building designs with tight insulation and a substantial proportion of recirculated ventilation predisposes to airborne transmission [14]. Reduction of such transmission fresh air intake versus recirculated air ratio can be adjusted ("dilution ventilation"). In susceptible subgroups of the population, such as the elderly, the immunocompromised, and the very young, vaccination is an important option.

### Other Environmental Control Measures in the Home

The aging of homes is generally associated with increased exposure to allergens due to the some breakdown of the building materials used, which can be colonized by molds or bacteria (e.g., an aging roof increases mold exposure). On the other hand, new homes are associated with increased exposure to irritants from the off-gasing of the building materials used, such as new paint and woodwork. As mentioned previously, time should be allowed for building bake-out or off-gasing before occupation. In buildings already occupied there are a number of changes that can be made in the environment to reduce the level of irritants or allergens. These include elmination of VOC-emitting items in a room, such as fireplaces, wood-burning stoves, and kerosene heaters, and replacement by electric radiant heaters. For atopic individuals, avoidance of irritants/allergens such as kapok, cotton linters, and feathers used for stuffing pillows and mattresses may be helpful.

### Behavioral Factors and Modification

There are a number of changes in behavior or habits in the building the occupants can make to minimize, primarily, the biological contaminants. These include avoiding pets, which are known reactors, elimination of environmental tobacco smoke, and avoidance of areas of known high pollution during indoor and outdoor activities.

### D. Approach to Systematic Investigation of Suspected Chemical Offenders

Although there are a number of known and established indoor air pollutants that are fairly well understood, there are still a large number that have not yet been recognized. These will probably be determined as patients present problems to health care professionals as apparent building-related complaints. If the suspected agent is not yet an established or recognized problem, an action plan must be used to investigate it. There are several steps that the physician should take beyond that of patient care. After diagnosis, the physician should establish if the problem is seen only in the patient or if it is of wider concern.

Prospective comprehensive surveillance studies correlated with exposure measurements may have to be undertaken by the scientific community with detailed criteria to document the health hazards. Although the agent in question may be innocuous to most people, there may be a subpopulation that reacts to it. In this event the pathophysiology of the health effects and those at risk should be determined. The suspected pollutant should be characterized, including its distribution and behavior in indoor and outside air in relation to health effects. Human challenge studies should be properly controlled with clear end-organ response gauges, keeping in mind that gaseous and particulate phases of the same pollutant may behave differently. This should be tested against a large data base of people of different ages, sex, and other variables.

## References

1.  Stites DP, Stobo JD, Wells JV. Basic and clinical immunology. Norwalk, CT: Appleton & Lange, 1987.
2.  Mygind, N. Essential allergy: an illustrated text for students and specialists. Oxford: Blackwell Scientific Publications, 1986.
3.  Chan-Yeung M, Malo J. Occupational asthma. Chest (Suppl) 1991;6:130–36.
4.  Kaliner M, et al. Rhinitis and asthma. JAMA 1987;258(20):2851–73.
5.  Sterling TD, Collett CW, Sterling E. Environmental tobacco smoke and indoor air quality in modern office work environments. J Occup Med 1987;29(1):57–62.
6.  Bardana EJ, et al. Building-related illness. A review of available scientific data. Clin Rev Allergy 1988;6:61–88.
7.  Woodard ED, Friedlander B, et al. Outbreak of hypersensitivity pneumonitis in an industrial setting. JAMA 1988;110(2):115–18.
8.  Jacobs RL, Andrews CP, Jacobs FO. Hypersensitivity pneumonitis treated with an electrostatic dust filter. Ann Internal Med 1989;110(2):115–18.
9.  Fink JN. Clinical features of hypersensitivity pneumonitis. 28th Annual Aspen Lung Conference, Chest 1986;89(3):193S–95S.
10. Significance of fungi in indoor air: report of a working group. Health and Welfare Canada. Working group on fungi and indoor air. Can J Public Health 1987;78:S1–S14.

11. Report of the MRC Symposium 1977. Humidifier fever. Thorax 1977;32:653–63.
12. Burge HA. Indoor air and infectious disease. State of the Art Reviews. Occupat Med 1989;4(4):713–21.
13. Brundage JF, et al. Building-associated risk of febrile acute respiratory diseases in army trainees. JAMA 1988;259(14):2108–12.
14. Bloch AB, Orenstein WA, et al. Measles outbreak in a pediatric practice: airborne transmission in an office setting. Pediatrics 1985;75(4):676–83.
15. Fraser DW, et al. Legionnaires' disease: description of an epidemic of pneumonia. N Engl J Med 1977;297(22):1189–97.
16. Glick TH, et al., Pontiac fever: an epidemic of unknown etiology in a health department. Am J Epidemiol 1978;107(2):149–60.
17. Dales RE, Zwanenburg H, Burnett R, Franklin CA. Respiratory health effects of home dampness and molds among Canadian children. AM J Epid 1991;134(2):196–203.
18. Adams RM. Recent advances in contact dermatitis. Annals of Allergy 1991;67:552–562.
19. Day JH. Investigation and management of indoor air quality problems. Indoor Air '90, 1990:309.
20. Burge PS. Building sickness: a medical approach to the causes. Indoor Air '90, 1990:3.
21. Morina Cl. Health problems in air conditioned buildings. Indoor Air '90. 1990;5:333–41.
22. Burney PGJ, et al. Validity and repeatability of the IUATLD (1984) bronchial symptoms questionnaire: an international comparison. Eur Respir J 1989;2:940–45.
23. Wood RA, Chapman MD, Adkinson NF Jr, Eggleston PA. The effect of cat removal on allergen content in household dust samples. J Allergy Clin Immunol 1989;83:730–34.
24. Wood RA, Mudd KE, Peyton AE. The distribution of cat and dust mite allergens on wall surfaces. J Allergy Clin Immunol 1992;89(1):126–30.
25. Sundell J, Wickman M, Pershagen G. Building hygiene and house dust mite infestation. Indoor Air '90. 1990;1:27–29.
26. Platts-Mills TAE, et al. Dust mite allergens and asthma: a worldwide problem. Bull WHO 1988;66(6):769–80.
27. Carpenter GB, et al. Air conditioning and house dust mite. J Allergy Clin Immunol 1985;75:121.
28. Platts-Mills TAE, Chapman MD. Dust mites: immunology, allergic disease, and environmental control. J Allergy Clin Immunol 1987;80(6):755–75.
29. Hayden ML, et al. Benzyl benzoate moist powder: investigation of acarical activity in cultures and reduction of dust mite allergens in carpets. J Allergy Clin Immunol 1992;89(2):536–45.

30. Helm RM, et al. Shared allergenic activity in Asian *(Blattella asahinai)*, German *(Blattella germanica)*, American *(Periplanta americana)*, and Oriental *(Blatta orientalis)* cockroach species. Int Arch Allergy Appl Immunol 1990;92:154–61.
31. Burge H. Bioaerosols: prevalence and health effects in the indoor environment. J Allergy Clin Immunol 1990;86(5):687–701.
32. Klein GL, Ziering RW. Environmental control of the home. Clin Rev Allergy 1988;6:3–22.
33. Nethercott JR, Holness DL. Occupational allergic contact dermatitis. Clin Rev Allergy 1989;7:399–415.

# 15

## Prevention of Respiratory Diseases from Indoor and Outdoor Air Pollution

**JONATHAN M. SAMET**

University of New Mexico School of Medicine
Albuquerque, New Mexico

**JOHN D. SPENGLER**

Harvard University School of Public Health
Boston, Massachusetts

## I. Introduction

### A. Overview

Every day adults inhale about 10,000 to 20,000 L of air. Because the volume inhaled is so large, a biologically significant dose of a potentially hazardous contaminant may be delivered to the respiratory tract even though the contaminant is present in the air at a low concentration. The ubiquitous nature of air pollution adds to the concern for adverse effects of inhaled pollutants. Exposures to air contaminants occur in many diverse indoor and outdoor locations. In the more developed countries, little time is spent in outdoor locations, an average of less than 1 h per day for adults [1], and the indoor environment, with its many sources of air pollution, is an important setting for exposure. Although outdoor locations may be the sole or predominant source of exposure to some pollutants, such as ozone for example, the exchange of indoor air with outdoor air brings pollutants from outdoor sources into buildings and vehicles.

Outdoor air pollution has long been recognized as a potential hazard to the public's health. However, until the second half of the twentieth century, there was little formal investigation into the health risks of outdoor air pollution. During the second half of the twentieth century, public health and regulatory concern with outdoor air pollution has steadily increased. During this time, new techniques for epidemiologic research have facilitated the conduct of informative community-based studies. The increasing concern for the public's health followed recognition of the substantial morbidity and mortality that can result from outdoor air pollution. From the 1930s through the 1950s, episodes of excess mortality at times of extremely high pollution levels became dramatic evidence of the danger posed by air pollution [2] (Table 1). The London fog of 1952 resulted in several thousand excess deaths [3]. In subsequent years, epidemiologic and toxicologic research on the health effects of air pollution, in addition to expanded air-quality monitoring, has provided the scientific basis for regulation of the quality of outdoor air and subsequent control of the health effects of outdoor air pollution.

Concern for the health effects of pollution in indoor air also grew during the second half of the twentieth century. Some adverse consequences of indoor air pollution, such as carbon monoxide poisoning from faulty or unvented combustion sources, had long been recognized. In the late 1960s and early 1970s, research on indoor air pollution was sparked by recognition of the contribution of the indoor environment to exposures to many pollutants, and the findings from studies that indicated the adverse health effects of such agents as environmental tobacco smoke [4] and $NO_2$ from gas cooking stoves [5]. The investigation of indoor air was subsequently stimulated by concern that modern building techniques, which have reduced building ventilation to conserve energy, would increase indoor pollutant concentrations and lead to adverse effects on health. A large body of literature is now available on diverse aspects of indoor air pollution, including the sources of pollution, concentrations, and health effects, and their control [6].

The target for prevention of respiratory diseases is large (Table 2). For example, in the United States in 1986, about 300,000 deaths were coded to

**Table 1**  Acute Air Pollution Episodes and Associated Mortality

| Location | Year | Attributed excess deaths |
|----------|------|--------------------------|
| Meuse Valley, Belgium | 1930 | 63 |
| Donora, PA, U.S. | 1948 | 20 |
| London, England | 1952 | 3500 |
| New York, NY, U.S. | 1953 | 200 |
| London, England | 1962 | 700 |
| Osaka, Japan | 1962 | 60 |

*Source:* Data from ref. 2.

**Table 2** Diseases of the Respiratory System

| Category | ICD code |
|---|---|
| Acute respiratory infections | 460–466 |
|   Acute laryngitis and tracheitis | |
|   Acute bronchitis and bronchiolitis | |
| Other diseases of the upper respiratory tract | 470–478 |
| Pneumonia and influenza | 480–487 |
| Chronic obstructive pulmonary disease and allied conditions | 480–496 |
|   Bronchitis, unspecified | |
|   Chronic bronchitis | |
|   Emphysema | |
|   Asthma | |
|   Extrinsic allergic alveolitis | |
|   Chronic airway obstruction | |
| Pneumoconioses and other lung diseases due to external agents | 500–508 |
| Other respiratory system diseases | |
|   Post inflammatory pulmonary fibrosis | |
|   Other alveolar and parietoalveolar diseases | |
|   Pneumopathy | |

disorders of the respiratory tract as the underlying cause (Table 3). The pool of persons potentially susceptible to air pollution is also large, encompassing persons with chronic lung diseases, infants, and the elderly. Through synergistic mechanisms, cigarette smokers may also be at increased risk for respiratory tract cancer from inhaled carcinogens in indoor and outdoor air.

In this chapter we address the prospects for preventing respiratory diseases by limiting exposures to indoor and outdoor air pollution. We consider the role of air pollution as a contributor to the incidence of the major respiratory diseases and as a cause of morbidity or mortality by exacerbating the status of persons with established disease (Table 2). We also consider the methods for assessing the burden of preventable respiratory diseases from air pollution and strategies for reducing this burden. We do not review the evidence linking air pollution exposure to health effects; comprehensive summaries on this topic have been published [2,6,8] and further reviews are published periodically in, for example, the criteria documents of the U.S. Environmental Protection Agency. Other chapters in this volume address specific pollutants in greater detail.

### B. Total Personal Exposure

Perhaps because of the distinct sources of pollution in outdoor and indoor air, and the separate regulatory approaches and control strategies for outdoor air, the

**Table 3** Numbers of Deaths from Respiratory Diseases in the United States, 1986

| Disease (ICD-9 No.) | Number |
|---|---|
| Diseases of newborns | |
| Respiratory distress syndrome (769) | 3,408 |
| Other respiratory conditions of newborns (770) | 3,665 |
| Nonmalignant respiratory diseases | |
| Pneumonia and influenza (480–487) | 69,812 |
| Chronic bronchitis (491) | 3,123 |
| Emphysema (492) | 14,471 |
| Asthma (493) | 3,995 |
| Chronic airways obstruction (496) | 53,513 |
| Pneumoconioses and other lung diseases due to external agents (500–508) | 8,153 |
| Interstitial lung diseases (515–516) | 5,080 |
| Pulmonary embolism (415.1) | 10,516 |
| Total (460–519) | 170,938 |
| Malignant respiratory diseases | |
| Larynx | 3,611 |
| Trachea, bronchus, lung (162) | 125,522 |

*Source:* Data from ref. 7.

workplace, home, and other indoor environments, exposures and health effects have been addressed separately for outdoor and indoor air. However, the concept of total personal exposure to air pollution is more relevant for the protection of public health (Fig. 1). Total personal exposure represents the time-weighted average of pollutant concentrations in microenvironments, physical settings that have relatively uniform concentrations of air pollutants during the time that is spent there [9]. By reflecting the exposures sustained in all environments where time is spent, estimates of total exposure provide an index of the health risk associated with a particular pollutant.

The contributions of outdoor pollutants and indoor pollutants to total personal exposure vary from pollutant to pollutant. For example, outdoor exposures to ozone are probably greater than indoor exposures in most urban areas; indoors, levels of ozone are reduced as the reactive pollutant is neutralized by surfaces [10]. However, because of the substantial proportion of time spent indoors, the home and other indoor microenvironments may contribute significantly to total personal exposure. For other pollutants (e.g., nitrogen dioxide), both indoor and in-transit exposures may make substantial contributions to total personal exposure.

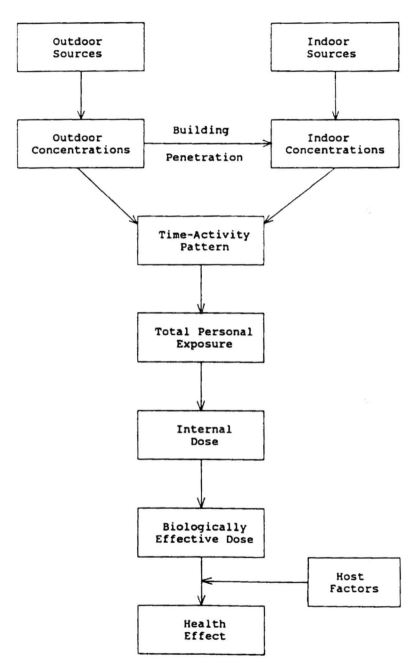

**Figure 1** Concept of total personal exposure and dose.

## II.  Trends in Air Quality

### A.  Developed Countries

In the United States, Canada, and other Western countries, standardized outdoor monitoring for several pollutants has been conducted since the 1950s. The ambient concentrations of some pollutants have decreased, and many cities that were once highly polluted by local fossil fuel-burning industries now have much cleaner air as control technologies have been put into place or factories have closed.

In the United States, there have been decreases in the ambient concentrations of total suspended particulates (TSP), sulfur dioxide, lead, and carbon monoxide [11]. Ambient levels of organic carbon compounds, such as benzo[a]pyrene, have also been reduced. These decreases probably reflect many factors, including controls on emissions from factories and vehicles, the construction of new power plants and factories in locations away from urban centers, the burning of cleaner fuels, and a decline in manufacturing-related industries.

Levels of some other pollutants have either shown no change or have increased. For example, the U.S. Environmental Protection Agency estimated that 107 communities and 135 million people live in areas that exceed the National Ambient Air Quality Standard for ozone [12]. Ozone pollution affects many regions of the United States other than southern California, where it was first identified. Most of the population east of the Mississippi experiences ozone concentrations during the spring and summer with at least 1 h above 0.10 ppm. The pervasive problem of ozone pollution reflects population growth and urban sprawl. Although newer vehicles emit lower amounts of hydrocarbons and nitrogen oxides, the precursors of photochemical pollution or smog, increasing numbers of motor vehicles and miles driven offset the lower emissions per car [12].

Even as levels of sulfur dioxide have declined, the problem of acid pollution by sulfate and nitrate species has become increasingly prominent in the United States and Canada [13]. Through complex chemical reactions, nitrogen oxides and sulfur oxides can be converted to acidic gases and particles [14]. Common acidic species include sulfuric acid, ammonia bisulfate, acidic particles, and nitrous and nitric acid gases. Concentrations of sulfate are highest in the central portion of the eastern United States, where sulfur-containing fuels, principally coal, are burned in power plants and industry. In Europe, acid pollution has been a persistent problem created by dense population, extensive industrialization, and burning of fossil fuels for power generation and space heating. Information is now becoming available on air pollution in Central and Eastern Europe, where extensive emissions of sulfur oxides and particles are now being documented [15].

We lack information on trends of indoor air quality in developed countries. In fact, survey data from population samples are available for only some of the pollutants of potential health concern: radon, nitrogen dioxide, respirable particles, and selected volatile organic compounds [14]. Reduced rates of exchange of indoor with outdoor air in buildings constructed during the 1970s and 1980s could possibly contribute to a trend of increasing indoor concentrations [6].

## B. Developing Countries

With population growth in developing countries, outdoor air pollution has become an increasingly important public health concern [16]. Uncontrolled emissions from industry, motor vehicles, and cooking and heating fuels cause the outdoor air of many of the cities of Eastern Europe, Asia, Africa, and South America to resemble the conditions found earlier in the century in London, Pittsburgh, and New York City. Since 1973 the World Health Organization through its Global Environmental Monitoring Systems (GEMS) has been documenting total suspended particulate and $SO_2$ pollution, and beginning in 1978, $NO_2$ and lead have been monitored at traffic-related stations. By 1978, about 43 countries or areas with 170 monitoring stations were participating [17]. Particulate concentrations in urban areas show a consistent negative association with gross national product per person [18]. During winter days in Beijing, particle concentrations may exceed 500 $\mu g/m^3$ [19]. Similarly, residential coal burning in the black townships of South Africa may produce particle concentrations above 1000 $\mu g/m^3$ [20,21]. In such circumstances, personal exposures can be dominated by outdoor pollution.

A recent review by Romieu and colleagues [22] provides a perspective on the increasing problem of urban air pollution in Latin America and the Caribbean. Explosive population growth and rapid economic development and industrialization have created worsening air pollution in urban areas of Central and South America. The high altitude and mountain surroundings of Mexico City, along with its population of over 20 million, large vehicle fleet, and industrial activity, have resulted in some of the highest pollution levels in the world. Romieu and colleagues estimate that about 81 million people in Latin America and the Caribbean are exposed to air pollution levels above guidelines of the World Health Organization.

Although ambient air pollution in developing countries is a problem mainly in urban areas, indoor air pollution can be quite high even in remote villages. Many of the world's poor people cook and heat their homes with biomass fuels of wood, crop residue, or dried animal dung. Some cultures use coal or briquettes made from powdered coal or charcoal. In numerous locations around the world the burning of wood, coal, charcoal, crop residue, and animal dung routinely produces indoor particle concentrations exceeding 1000 $\mu$g/m$^3$, benzo[a]pyrene concentrations exceeding 1000 $\mu$g/m$^3$, and CO concentrations exceeding 35 ppm, levels no longer encountered in developed countries with established ambient air pollution control programs [16]. Concentrations in rural village huts, whose residents burn biomass fuels, exceed by factors of 10 to 100 the concentrations of particles and organic particulate matter in homes with modern cooking and heating appliances. Data are not available on trends of indoor air pollution in developing countries.

## III.  Health Effects of Air Pollution

### A.  Outdoor Air Pollution

*Sulfur Oxides, Particulate Matter, and Acid Aerosols*

Previously, health and regulatory concerns in relation to sulfur oxides were directed primarily at the health effects of sulfur dioxide (SO$_2$), and particulate matter was considered as a separate agent. However, more recently, sulfur oxides and particulate matter have been recognized as components of a complex mixture formed as products of combustion undergo complex chemical transformations following release into the atmosphere [11,23]. Atmospheric transformations produce acidic sulfate and nitrate species; the actual causal agent for health effects associated with sulfur oxides may be hydrogen ions [23,24]. The complexity of particulate matter is also better understood. Health effects of inhaled particles depend not only on concentration but on the particles' chemistry and size distribution.

A wide array of adverse health effects has been linked to exposure to sulfur oxide and particulate pollution. Dramatic excess mortality occurred in association with the extremely high pollution occurring during the London fog of 1952 and other episodes in the United States and Europe (Table 1) [2]. However, even at today's lower levels of pollution in many developed countries, positive associations can still be demonstrated between ambient concentrations of particles and mortality [25,26].

Respiratory morbidity has also been associated with sulfur oxide and particulate pollution. Studies during the 1960s and 1970s showed that ambient air pollution with sulfur oxides and particles could increase rates of respiratory illness, increase the prevalence of respiratory symptoms, and reduce lung function in children [2]. The Harvard Six Cities Study, a large multicity study in the United States, has shown that this type of pollution is still associated with these same adverse effects, even at generally lower levels [27,28]. Other studies have provided comparable evidence for children [8].

Studies involving controlled exposures of volunteers have shown that asthmatics are particularly sensitive to sulfur dioxide [29]. Asthmatics also appear to be sensitive to acid aerosols [30]. In Canada, increased rates of admissions for respiratory diseases, including asthma, have been documented during periods of the summer when both sulfate and ozone levels are elevated [31]. A recent report by a committee of the American Thoracic Society concluded that persons with increased airways responsiveness and asthma are at risk for adverse effects from acid aerosols [32].

### Nitrogen Oxides

Like sulfur oxides, nitrogen oxides are produced by combustion processes and contribute to the formation of acid aerosols [23,33]. Outdoors, nitrogen oxides are nearly always present with other combustion pollutants. The nitrogen oxides also form nitrate species and contribute to the formation of photochemical oxidants. Thus little epidemiologic information is available on the effects of nitrogen oxides alone in ambient air. Toxicologic evidence suggests that the adverse effects in humans might include worsening of the status of asthmatics and persons with chronic obstructive pulmonary disease, increased incidence and severity of respiratory infections, and increased respiratory symptoms and reduced lung function [34].

### Ozone

The health effects of photochemical pollution, for which ozone serves as a marker compound, have received extensive investigation [35]. In animal models, long-term exposure to ozone produces airspace enlargement and damage to the small airways of the lung. Exercising volunteers exposed to ozone at levels frequently measured in urban areas experience transient reduction of lung function; markers of injury are elevated in bronchoalveolar lavage fluid obtained after such exposures [36]. While the evidence for short-term effects of ozone on lung function is convincing, uncertainty remains about the long-term effects. Together, the short-term effects of ozone and the findings of long-term effects in animal models suggest that lung function might be chronically affected by photochemical pollution. However, we still lack the needed data from prospective epidemiologic studies of sufficient size and duration. Groups with increased susceptibility to ozone have not been identified, and asthmatics have not been found to be particularly sensitive to acute exposure [35].

### Carbon Monoxide

Carbon monoxide (CO) binds to hemoglobin to form carboxyhemoglobin (COHb) and thereby reduces the capacity of the blood to deliver oxygen to tissues. At high levels, CO can cause neurologic damage and even death. Populations at potential risk from CO exposure at concentrations measured in typical indoor and outdoor environments include persons with heightened oxygen demand (e.g., vigorously exercising persons) and with compromised oxygen delivery (e.g., persons with coronary artery disease and chronic obstructive pulmonary disease). Recent evidence indicates that controlled CO exposure of patients with stable coronary artery disease can produce earlier subjective and objective evidence of myocardial ischemia at venous COHb levels as low as 2 to 4% in comparison with the level of 1% found without exposure [37]. Epidemiologic data have not readily described the adverse effects of CO exposures in the community.

### B.  Indoor Air Pollution

#### Environmental Tobacco Smoke

Environmental tobacco smoke (ETS) refers to the mixture of sidestream smoke from the smoldering cigarette with exhaled mainstream smoke. The inhalation of ETS is often referred to as "passive" or "involuntary" smoking. Studies on smoking by parents and the health of their children provided the first evidence that passive smoking has adverse effects. Maternal smoking was found to place infants at increased risk for lower respiratory infections, and smoking by household members, particularly the mother, was shown to increase the occurrence of chronic respiratory symptoms and to reduce the level of lung function in children [38,39]. Subsequently, ETS has been found to increase the risk for chronic otitis media [33].

In 1981, increased risk of lung cancer in ETS-exposed never-smokers was reported [40,41]. Since then, many studies have addressed this association; pooling of the data indicates that nonsmokers married to smokers have about a 25% increased risk of lung cancer compared to those married to never-smokers [38,42]. In 1986, reports from the International Agency for Research on Cancer [43], the U.S. Surgeon General [39], and the U.S. National Research Council concurred in concluding that involuntary smoking is a cause of lung cancer in never-smokers.

Other health effects of ETS exposure have also been investigated. Exposure to ETS adversely affects persons with asthma, although involuntary smoking has not yet been clearly linked to the onset of asthma [33]. Epidemiologic and laboratory evidence suggests that ETS may also increase mortality from ischemic heart disease [44].

#### Nitrogen Dioxide

This oxident pollutant, of concern in outdoor air, is also released indoors by combustion devices such as ranges and ovens, water heaters, and space heaters. The range of adverse effects of $NO_2$ in indoor air encompasses the same spectrum of effects as $NO_2$ in outdoor air: increased incidence and severity of respiratory infections, increased respiratory symptoms and reduced lung function, and exacerbation of asthma and chronic obstructive pulmonary disease. A number of epidemiologic investigations have addressed the effects of $NO_2$ from gas cooking stoves on children and adults; because of difficult methodologic problems, these data have been inconclusive in demonstrating adverse effects of exposure to $NO_2$ indoors [33].

### Woodsmoke

In many developed countries, wood is still burned indoors in fireplaces or stoves for space heating. The use of fireplaces and wood stoves may result in increased indoor concentrations of smoke pollutants by reentrainment of outdoor air or by direct leakage into indoor air [45]. However, limited data suggest that properly maintained and operated wood stoves and fireplaces have little effect on indoor air quality [45]. The evidence from developed countries on health effects of exposure to wood smoke indoors remains limited. By contrast, biomass fuel combustion in developing countries is associated with remarkable elevations of pollutant concentrations indoors and with excess morbidity and probably mortality from respiratory infections in childhood [16].

### Biological Agents

The biological agents, a topic covered in more detail elsewhere in this volume, represent an extremely diverse group of agents that cause disease primarily through infection and immunological mechanisms [46,47]. The potential for transmission of many infectious diseases through inhalation of indoor air has been recognized for many years. Legionnaires' disease may be transmitted by water and by mist from contaminated heating, ventilating, and air-conditioning systems. Hypersensitivity pneumonitis and humidifier fever have been linked to contaminated humidifiers and heating and cooling systems and to moisture-damaged building materials [47]. Asthma may be exacerbated by allergens in outdoor and indoor air.

### Formaldehyde and Other Volatile Organic Compounds

Although widespread exposure to formaldehyde and other volatile organic compounds has been well documented, controversy remains concerning the health effects of these indoor pollutants [48–50]. A wide array of health effects is of potential concern, including mucosal irritation, inflammation of the respiratory tract, asthma, neurobehavioral consequences, and cancer. Volatile organic compounds are also suspect causes of the sick-building syndrome.

### Radon

Exposure to radon progeny, the short-lived decay products of radon, has been causally linked to increased risk of lung cancer in uranium and other underground miners [51]. Measurements of radon in homes show that radon is present in most homes and can reach high concentrations, as high as those in underground mines with documented excess lung cancer. The hazard posed by indoor radon has been addressed primarily through risk estimation procedures [33,51]; case-control studies are in progress to estimate the risk more directly [52]. The risks for the general population are projected by extrapolating risks observed in the studies of miners. Although a number of different risk models have been developed, each of the models leads to the conclusion that radon contributes significantly to the burden of lung cancer in the population. The estimated burden of radon-related lung cancer in the general population reflects in part the synergism between radon and cigarette smoking, assumed in several of the models on the basis of the findings in underground miners [51].

## IV. Estimating the Burden of Preventable Disease

### A. Epidemiologic Approaches

Epidemiologic data can be used to estimate the burden of respiratory diseases associated with indoor and outdoor air pollution. The population attributable risk (PAR %) describes the percentage of disease in a population that would in principle be prevented if the exposure of interest were removed [53]. It is estimated as

$$\text{PAR } \% = \frac{(RR - 1) \times P}{1 + (RR - 1) \times P}$$

where RR is the relative risk of disease associated with exposure and P is the proportion of the population exposed. Thus the PAR % depends not only on the strength of a factor as a cause of disease, that is, the value of RR, but also on P, the proportion of the population exposed. A highly prevalent exposure associated with a relatively modest increase in RR may still pose a significant public health problem. For example, maternal smoking is associated with a RR of approximately 1.5 for more severe types of lower respiratory illness in early childhood [54]; the corresponding PAR %, assuming prevalence (P) of maternal smoking as 25%, is 11%. On the other hand, PAR % may be quite low for infrequent exposures that have relatively high levels of RR. For example, an occupational exposure that increased disease risk tenfold but was sustained by only 1 per 100,000 would have an associated PAR % of about one hundredth of a percent. Similarly, an exposure might be associated with a modest RR value and an unimpressive PAR % while posing unacceptable risks for susceptible individuals.

Many diseases, particularly chronic diseases, have multiple causes that may act together to increase or decrease disease risk through synergistic or antagonistic effects, respectively. For agents with interdependent effects, the PAR % includes not only the independent contribution of the agent of interest but the contribution attributable to the joint effects of the agent with other causal factors [53]. The total of PAR % estimates for a disease may exceed 100% as the joint contributions are assigned to different single agents.

Observational investigations, including cross-sectional, cohort, and case-control studies, supply the data needed to estimate PAR %. For some agents, for example, active cigarette smoking, there are abundant data on RR and exposure prevalence [55]. For most air pollutants, however, the epidemiologic evidence is neither sufficiently abundant nor certain to permit confident calculation of PAR %. Thus we cannot directly compare the PAR % for different indoor and outdoor pollutants.

### B. Risk Assessment

The technique of quantitative risk assessment is used increasingly to gauge the magnitude of risk posed by environmental pollutants, including air pollution. Quantitative risk assessment has been conceptualized as a four-step process [56]:

1. *Hazard identification:* determination of whether an agent is causally linked to the health effect of concern
2. *Dose–response assessment:* determination of the relation between level of exposure and risk of the health effect
3. *Exposure assessment:* description of the extent of human exposure
4. *Risk characterization:* description of the human risk, including uncertanties

If an agent is judged to pose a hazard and the needed information on dose–response and exposure is available, the resulting risk characterization provides an indication of the overall extent of the risk to health posed by the agent. The risk characterization serves to guide the management of risk and becomes part of the strategy for communicating risk to the public. The systematic approach inherent in conducting a quantitative risk assessment provides a framework for identifying points of uncertainty and addressing their implications for risk characterization [56].

For many indoor and outdoor air pollutants, sufficient information is still lacking for the steps of hazard identification, dose–response assessment, and exposure assessment; for others, the existence of a hazard has been adequately established, but the data on dose–response and exposure are subject to substantial uncertainty and the risk characterization is not sufficiently confident for risk management.

The problem of indoor radon and lung cancer illustrates the application of risk assessment methodology. Epidemiologic studies of underground miners, and animal and other laboratory evidence, show that radon causes lung cancer [57]. Only a few epidemiologic studies that assess the risk of indoor radon directly have been published, and estimates of PAR % from epidemiologic data have not been reported.

The extent of lung cancer attributable to indoor radon can be estimated, however, using quantitative risk analysis [51]. Surveys provide information on the population distribution of exposure, which is approximately log normal (Fig. 2), and the dose–response relation is extrapolated from the studies of miners to the indoor environment. For example, Lubin and Boice [59] estimated that approximately 14% of lung cancer deaths in the United States could be attributed to indoor radon. They further examined the attributable risk for various levels of exposure and calculated the proportions of all lung cancer deaths that would be prevented by reducing exposures above target levels to lower levels (Table 4). Reduction of the more extreme indoor exposures was projected to have little

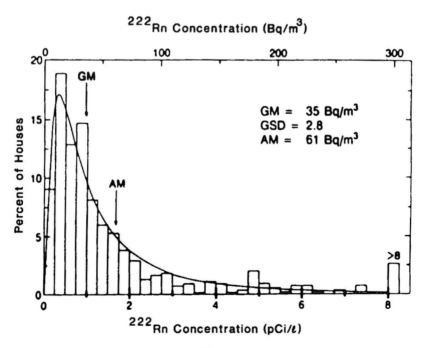

**Figure 2**  Probability distribution of $^{222}$Rn in U.S. homes. (From ref. 58.)

**Table 4** Estimated Percentages of Lung Cancer Cases Prevented in U.S. Males by Reducing Home Exposures to Radon

| Maximum exposure [Bq/m³ (pCi/L)] | Percentage of homes exceeding maximum | Attributable risk[a] (%) | | |
|---|---|---|---|---|
| | | Move to maximum | Truncate at maximum | Move to minimum |
| 2.0 (0.08) | 99 | 13.5 | 13.5 | 13.5 |
| 74.0 (2.0) | 24 | 4.5 | 7.0 | 8.6 |
| 148.0 (4.0) | 8 | 2.1 | 4.2 | 5.0 |
| 296.0 (8.0) | 2 | 0.6 | 1.6 | 1.8 |

*Source:* Based on Table 2 in ref. 59.
[a]Attributable risk estimated for three different scenarios: in "move to maximum," all exposures above the cutoff are moved to the highest value of the truncated distribution; in "truncate at maximum," the exposures above the cutoff value are assigned throughout the distribution of values below the cutoff; and in "move to minimum," values above the cutoff are moved to the lowest vale.

impact on the overall burden of lung cancer attributable to indoor radon. In fact, even the most feasible reduction at present—to approximately 2.0 pCi/L—leaves about half of the radon-related cases. For smokers, the reduction of risk following smoking cessation greatly exceeds the change in risk from lowering of radon exposure [60].

The example of indoor radon and lung cancer demonstrates the difference between the burden of disease estimated by quantitative risk assessment and the numbers of cases that are actually preventable. Because exposures to indoor radon cannot feasibly be lowered to outdoor levels, the target of preventing *all* radon-related lung cancers cannot be achieved. Reduction of exposures for the minority with unarguably high levels would have little impact on the burden of radon-related lung cancer in the population. Prevention and cessation of cigarette smoking, which has a synergistic effect with radon in causing lung cancer, is more effective for preventing radon-attributed lung cancer than is reduction of radon exposure.

Despite the limitations of quantitative risk assessment, it is used increasingly to rank the hazards posed by diverse pollutants. For example, in its Relative Risk Reduction Project, the U.S. Environmental Protection Agency used a risk-based approach to compare the relative importance of various environmental pollutants, including indoor and outdoor air pollutants [61]. The Environmental Protection Agency report acknowledges the complexity of using risk assessment to accomplish this type of ranking. Not only are needed input data lacking or highly uncertain, but a framework of societal values for combining disparate adverse effects has not yet been constructed. For example, we lack a scale for simultaneously considering mortality and morbidity or malignant and nonmalignant health outcomes.

## C. Synthesis

Although methods are available for estimating the burden of potentially preventable disease associated with indoor and outdoor air pollutants, we lack uniformly collected data for the most important agents. We also lack any framework for integrating such assessments for multiple agents. How can mortality and morbidity be compared? How are individual and population risks to be balanced? How are effects on susceptible individuals to be considered? How are feasibility and costs to be weighed against the burden of morbidity and mortality?

As an alternative to quantitative estimates of pollution-caused morbidity and mortality, assessment of the contributions of indoor and outdoor microenvironments to total personal exposures represents a complementary approach for comparing the health significance of indoor and outdoor air pollution. This approach apportions the contributions of indoor and outdoor microenvironments and may indicate the sources whose mitigation is most likely to have health benefits. Monitoring exposures in populations affords an index of potential morbidity and mortality that may be more readily applied than actually tracking patterns of disease.

## V. Strategies for Prevention

### A. Outdoor Air Pollution

Outdoor air is a community property; maintenance of acceptable air quality has required complex governmental initiatives affecting industry, transportation, and even personal life-styles. The broad goals of such initiatives include the protection of human health and the prevention of environmental degradation. The scope of programs to prevent adverse respiratory consequences of outdoor air pollution lies beyond the potential actions of individual citizens and even municipalities (Table 5). Control strategies are needed for both pollution from industries and vehicles. Transportation-related emissions of hydrocarbons and nitrogen oxides, the precursors of photochemical pollution, reflect population growth with its ever-increasing urban sprawl and motor vehicle use. Any strategy to control the rising problem of photochemical pollution in urban areas must include a reduction in motor vehicle use and implementation of effective mass transportation methods.

Regulatory strategies now in place in the United States are mandated to provide protection against adverse health effects for everyone, regardless of inherent susceptibility. Beginning in the 1950s in the United States and some

**Table 5** Prevention of Respiratory Diseases Associated with Outdoor Air Pollution

| Pollutant | Strategy |
| --- | --- |
| Sulfur oxides, particles, acidic aerosols | Source controls, concentration standards, alternative fuels |
| Ozone, photochemical oxidants | Source controls, concentration standards, reduced vehicle usage |
| Carbon monoxide | Source controls, concentration standards, reduced vehicle usage |
| Nitrogen oxides | Source controls, concentration standards, reduced vehicle usage |
| Lead | Removal of lead from gasoline |
| Hazardous pollutants | Source control |

other countries, deterioration of visibility and evidence of adverse effects on health led to research and regulatory programs. Congress enacted the first national legislation, the Air Pollution Control Act, in 1955. In passing the Clear Air Act of 1963, the federal government established its right over the states to legislate air pollution on the constitutional basis of interstate commerce. Two years later, the Motor Vehicle Air Pollution Control Act of 1965 established a process for implementing national emission standards for new motor vehicles.

The Clean Air Act Amendments of 1970 and establishment of the U.S. Environmental Protection Agency (EPA) changed the course of pollution control in the United States. Congress charged the EPA with establishing National Ambient Air Quality Standards for a number of specific pollutants and gave the agency enforcement authority. Congress imposed federal mobile source emission standards on manufacturers and ordered states to establish air pollution implementation plans to reach compliance with federal criteria. After reviewing the scientific evidence on the health and welfare effects, the EPA promulgated regulations on "criteria" pollutants, which at present are carbon monoxide, nitrogen dioxide, lead, particulate matter, sulfur dioxide, and ozone. The Clean Air Act of 1970 was amended in 1977 and again in 1990. The 1990 amendments are far-reaching and address hazardous air pollutants, acid rain, and stratospheric ozone depletion. An initial list of hazardous pollutants includes 189 compounds, primarily carcinogens, for which the EPA must set emissions standards.

By contrast, legislation in the United Kingdom has followed a strategy of smoke control [3]. The Clean Air Act of 1956 attempted to control smoke emissions from both industry and domestic sources. Smoke-control areas were established in which emissions of "black smoke" as assessed by the Ringelmann charts was prohibited. Domestic users were required to switch to fuels that burn without smoke or to electricity, and new industrial furnaces were required to be as smokeless as possible. Air quality standards were not set. However, even though smoke emissions alone were regulated, levels of sulfur dioxide declined after the institution of the regulations.

The problem of outdoor air pollution is now recognized to extend across the boundaries of individual countries. The use of tall stacks for power plants and industries sends emissions of particles and gases high into the atmosphere, thereby facilitating their long-range transport. In addition, during prolonged residence in the atmosphere, the pollutants may undergo chemical transformation. For example, sulfur oxides and nitrogen oxides may be converted into acid species. Hazardous pollutants may also be widely disseminated. The control of photochemical pollution may also need regional approaches and not simply local or national approaches. In fact, in regions like Europe, with its many geographically small but densely populated countries, control of the respiratory effects of air pollution will require an international approach.

Accidental releases of toxic pollutants also remain a persistent problem in developed and developing countries. The Bhopal incident provided a tragic reminder of the potential consequences of the release of toxic agents into inhabited areas. Such releases occur not only from industry but also from transport-related incidents involving boat, truck, or train transport.

There are some steps that people can take to reduce their exposure to outdoor air pollution. Staying indoors at times of high concentrations should reduce exposures to most pollutants, unless the building construction is open, with a high rate of exchange of indoor with outdoor air. Because exercise increases the dose of pollutants delivered to target sites in the lung, it should be avoided at such times. Public information programs designed to reduce exposures have been implemented by some governments; the public is alerted when exposures are high and individual actions should be taken to reduce exposure.

### B.  Indoor Air Pollution

In contrast to the complex regulatory strategies needed to control the health effects of outdoor air pollution, some indoor air pollution problems can be solved through the actions of the people exposed (Table 6). Prohibition of smoking in indoor spaces readily controls the contamination of homes, workplaces, and public and commercial buildings by environmental tobacco smoke. Proper use and maintenance of combustion appliances, such as ranges and heaters, reduces exposures to emissions of particles, oxides of nitrogen, and carbon monoxide. Exposures to some biological agents can be controlled by avoiding water damage and puddling of water, maintaining the proper range of humidity, and ensuring that heating, ventilating, and air-conditioning systems are properly cleaned and serviced. Effective programs have also been described for reducing exposure to house dust mite antigen [62]; measures include maintaining a sufficiently low

**Table 6** Prevention of Respiratory Diseases Associated with Indoor Air Pollution

| Pollutant | Strategy |
| --- | --- |
| Environmental tobacco smoke | Prohibition of smoking indoors, isolation of smokers from nonsmokers |
| Nitrogen oxides | Source modification, venting, proper use and maintenance |
| Carbon monoxide | Source modification, venting, proper use and maintenance |
| Volatile organic compounds | Product modification, venting and proper use, elimination of sources |
| Biological agents | Control of moisture, proper cleaning and maintenance of sources, elimination of sources |
| Radon | Measurement and mitigation, construction of low-radon housing |

relative humidity, regularly vacuuming carpets and upholstered furnishings, covering mattresses and pillows with plastic, removal of carpets, and hot washing of soft toys. Antigens from pets are of course readily controlled by not keeping animals indoors. Exposures to many volatile organic compound can be reduced by careful screening of products used in the home, storage of solvents and paints outside, and proper venting when pollution sources are used. Indoor radon concentration can readily be measured with inexpensive passive monitors that are available from retail stores. The American Thoracic Society has published a workshop report that reviews the evidence on control of the indoor environment and lung disease [63].

However, the comprehensive management of indoor air pollution requires strategies of a broader scope than can be achieved by the actions of individuals. The broad range of approaches includes the development of lower-emission products for indoor environments, building designs that reduce the potential for soil gas entry, ventilation systems that return control to the occupants with the intent of ensuring adequate comfort, more effective air cleaning systems, and elimination of smoking in indoor environments unless contamination of the air breathed by nonsmokers can be prevented. The problem of achieving comfortable indoor environments is discussed further below.

## VI. Future Challenges

### A. Safety of Current Levels of Exposure in Outdoor Air

In many developed countries, extensive regulatory systems are in place to limit pollution of outdoor air; the two principal approaches are control of emissions and standards for pollutant concentrations in ambient air. These regulatory programs are driven by the need to protect the public's health against adverse health effects. Establishing public safety poses a challenge for researchers that may not readily be met for all pollutants. Providing assurance of safety, a level of risk judged to be acceptable [64], requires precise and confident characterization of risks, and the scope of research that is needed extends beyond testing for an exposure–disease association to quantification of risk at various levels of exposure and the assessment of factors that modify the exposure–disease relationship. Epidemiologic approaches for describing the risks of lower levels of exposure require large sample sizes; even with large studies, however, the statistical power may be too limited to provide the requisite certainty. Parallel investigations, using animal models and on mechanisms of injury, should be part of the investigative program [65].

### B.  Total Exposure

Total personal exposure to pollutants is a more biologically relevant index of health risk than concentrations of pollutants in indoor and outdoor air, the indexes typically incorporated into regulatory strategies. Monitoring population patterns of exposure rather than patterns of disease may offer a more sensitive index of the benefits of preventive strategies. Assessing the contributions of indoor and outdoor environments to total personal exposure indicates the relative importance of indoor and outdoor air; microenvironments where control of sources would effectively reduce personal exposures can be identified. For example, the Total Exposure Assessment Methodology (TEAM) Study conducted by the U.S. Environmental Protection Agency examined sources of exposure to selected volatile organic compounds [50]. Surprisingly, even in areas with industrial emissions of volatile organic compounds, indoor microenvironments were the dominant location for exposure. The cancer risk associated with the compounds assessed was attributed primarily to the indoor environment. Thus in many settings, reduction of the adverse health effects of this diverse and ubiquitous group of agents would be more effectively accomplished by reducing indoor rather than outdoor emissions.

A recent National Research Council report [9] advocates reduction of personal exposures by directing controls and other interventions at the major contributing microenvironments rather than simply implementing universal controls or primarily focusing control efforts on outdoor sources. This suggestion acknowledges the greater relevance for health of considering total personal exposure. Its implementation would require more broadly based strategies for control than the present focus on outdoor air in regulatory programs.

### C.  Community Sources

In many communities, visible pollution by industry and sites of waste disposal prompt concern by residents over possible adverse health effects. The concerns are often broad and encompass a wide array of health effects, and adequate data to address these broad concerns are not routinely available. For public health officials and epidemiologic researchers, investigating the health effects of community sources of pollution poses not only a difficult methodologic challenge but requires skills in information-gathering and risk communication, often under the cloud of community suspicion and litigation. The population at risk may be small and the likelihood of detecting statistically significant effects may be correspondingly low. Publicity and community concern may increase the potential for nonparticipation in investigations and for biased responses to questionnaires. Investigating clusters of disease attributed to point sources, while often warranted by a high level of community concern, rarely identifies a specific causal agent [53].

Despite these difficulties in conducting population-based studies of community sources of air pollution, a number of investigations have been conducted and reported (see, e.g., ref. 66 and 67). The experience gained in these and comparable investigations provides some general guidance. Community involvement is needed at all phases of the investigation; an advisory group representing all parties within the community should be assembled and the advisory group should participate as the study is planned, conducted, and then reported to the community. Initially, community input needs to be openly obtained as the focus of the study is identified.

For example, following the Bhopal incident residents of the Kanawha Valley in West Virginia, site of one of the world's largest petrochemical industries, expressed fears that emissions from the plants were affecting their health adversely. The potential adverse effects of concern were wide ranging and included adverse reproductive outcomes, respiratory morbidity in children and adults, and cancer. An organization representing a coalition of the community's industries used funding from the Environmental Protection Agency to support population-based research on exposures and health effects. As the project was planned, open workshops involving researchers and the community were conducted and the study design evolved with guidance from external scientists and community representatives. In addition to limited indoor and outdoor monitoring, the project included a survey of respiratory morbidity in school-children and short-term studies of the status of children with respiratory symptoms and diseases and of control children in relation to levels of volatile organic compounds.

## D. New Sources

As technologies evolve, we are likely to be faced with new sources emitting pollutants that may have adverse health effects. New industries, changing vehicle technologies and fuels, and waste incineration are evident examples. While toxicologic studies may raise concern for adverse effects, such as the release of formaldehyde from combustion of methanol-containing fuels, characterizing the consequences for the population requires an understanding of the patterns of exposure and, possibly, direct epidemiologic evidence of adverse health effects. The number of new agents that may be released into indoor and outdoor air precludes a systematic assessment, and risk assessment represents the most appropriate basis for assigning priorities.

### E.  Indoor Air

Although control strategies have been widely implemented for outdoor air, we lack a comprehensive legal, regulatory, administrative, and technical framework for approaching the problem of indoor air pollution. Indoor air quality problems may result from natural sources, poor building design, inadequate building maintenance, structural components and furnishings, consumer products, and occupant activities. The control of these diverse sources of pollution in the air of public and private buildings poses an unprecedented challenge. Development of standards or guidelines for indoor concentrations is made difficult by the diversity of pollutants and the wide range of health effects of concern. Simply transferring standards developed for occupational settings to indoor settings or for outdoor air to indoor air is not appropriate in light of the time spent indoors and the wide range of potential susceptibility. Adopting safety factors into such concentration limits does not adequately redress their limitations. Similarly, specifying a minimum rate of exchange between indoor and outdoor air does not ensure either a comfortable or a healthy indoor environment.

Providing comfortable indoor air for all occupants of indoor environments may prove to be one of the most challenging aspects of indoor air pollution. In addition to the level of air pollutants that have adverse and detectable effects, the elements of comfort include temperature, temperature gradients, draftiness, humidity, noise, odors, and lighting. Subjective components also influence an occupant's perception of the environment. We do not yet have comprehensive data on the bounds that should be set for these factors to achieve acceptable indoor environmental quality. We also lack a definition of comfort that is universally accepted and can be readily applied in approaching indoor air quality problems.

### References

1.   Ott W. Human activity patterns: a review of the literature for estimating time spent indoors, outdoors, and in transit. In: Stark TH, ed. Proceedings of the Research Planning Conference on Human Activity Patterns, U.S. Environmental Protection Agency, Las Vegas, NV. EPA/600/4-89/004.

2. Shy CM, Goldsmith JR, Hackney JD, Lebowitz MD, Menzel DB. Health effects of air pollution. ATS News 1978;6:1–63.
3. Brimblecombe P. The big smoke. London: Routledge, Chapman & Hall, 1987.
4. Harlap S, Davies AM. Infant admissions to hospital and maternal smoking. Lancet 1974;1:529–32.
5. Melia RJ, Florey CV, Altman DG, Swan AV. Association between gas cooking and respiratory disease in children. Br Med J 1977;2:149–52.
6. Samet JM, Spengler JD, eds. Indoor air pollution: a health perspective. Baltimore: Johns Hopkins University Press, 1991.
7. National Center for Health Statistics. Vital statistics of the United States, 1985. Vol. II. DHHS Publication (PHS) 890-1101 (Mortality; Part A). Washington, DC: U.S. Government Printing Office, 1988.
8. Lambert WE, Samet JM, Dockery DW. Community air pollution. In: Rom W, ed. Environmental and occupational medicine. Second edition. Boston: Little, Brown, 1992:1223–42.
9. National Research Council, Committee on Advances in Assessing Human Exposure to Airborne Pollutants. Human exposure assessment for airborne pollutants: advances and opportunities. Washington, DC: National Academy Press, 1991.
10. Weschler CJ, Shields HC, Naik DV. Indoor ozone exposures. J Air Pollut Control Assoc 1989;39:1562–68.
11. U.S. Environmental Protection Agency, Office of Air Quality Planning and Standards, Monitoring and Reports Branch. National air quality and emission trends report, March 1989. Publication EPA-450/4-89-001. Research Triangle Park, NC: U.S. Government Printing Office, 1989.
12. Office of Technology Assessment. Catching our Breath: next steps to reducing urban ozone. OTA-0-412. Washington, DC: U.S. Government Printing Office, 1989.
13. U.S. Environmental Protection Agency. An acid aerosols issue paper. Health effects and aerometrics. Publication EPA-600/8-88/005F. Washington, DC: Office of Health and Environmental Assessment, U.S. EPA, 1989.
14. Spengler JD. Sources and concentrations of indoor air pollution. In: Samet JM, Spengler JD, eds. Indoor air pollution: a health perspective. Baltimore: Johns Hopkins University Press, 1991:33–67.
15. Levy BS. Air pollution in central and eastern Europe. Health and public policy. In: Levy BS, ed. Proceedings of the 2nd Annual Symposium on Environmental and Occupational Health During Societal Transition in Central and Eastern Europe, Czechoslovakia (CSFR), June 14–19, 1991. Boston: Management Sciences for Health, 1991.
16. Smith KR. Biofuels, air pollution, and health: a global review. New York: Plenum Press, 1987.

17.  World Health Organization. Air quality in selected urban areas, 1975–
     1976. Offset Publication 41. Geneva: WHO, 1978.
18.  Smith KR. Air pollution, assessing total exposure in developing countries.
     Environment 1988;30:16.
19.  World Health Organization. Urban air pollution in the People's Republic of
     China, 1981–1984. EHE/EFP/85.5. (Not a formal publication, prepared to
     assist with implementation of WHO/UNEP Global Air Monitoring Project.)
20.  Kemeny E, Ellerback RH, Briggs AB. An assessment of smoke pollution
     in Soweto: residential air pollution. Proceedings of the National Associa-
     tion for Clean Air, Pretoria, South Africa, November 10–11, 1988:152–63.
     Available through NACA, P.O. Box 5777, Johannesburg 2000, South
     Africa.
21.  Tshangwe HT, Kgamphe JS, Annegarn HJ. Indoor–outdoor air particulate
     study in a Soweto home: residential air pollution. Proceedings of the
     National Association for Clean Air, Pretoria, South Africa, November
     10–11, 1988:164–75. Available through NACA, P.O. Box 5777, Johan-
     nesburg 2000, South Africa.
22.  Romieu I, Weitzenfeld H, Finkleman J. Urban air pollution in Latin
     America and the Caribbean. J Air Waste Manage Assoc 1991;41:1166–71.
23.  Spengler JD, Brauer M, Koutrakis P. Acid air and health. Environ Sci
     Technol 1990;24:946–56.
24.  Amdur MO, Chen LC. Furnace-generated acid aerosols: specification and
     pulmonary effects. Environ Health Perspect 1989;79:147–50.
25.  Schwartz J, Dockery DW. Particulate air pollution and daily mortality in
     Steubenville, Ohio. Am J Epidemiol 1992;135:12–19.
26.  Dockery DW, Schwartz J. Authors' response to Waller and Swan
     commentary (pages 20–23) on their article published on pages 12–19. Am
     J Epidemiol 1992;135:23–25.
27.  Dockery DW, Ware JH, Ferris BG Jr, Speizer FE, Cook NR, Herman
     SM. Change in pulmonary function associated with air pollution episodes.
     J Air Pollut Control Assoc 1982;32:937–42.
28.  Dockery DW, Speizer FE, Stram DO, Ware JH, Spengler JD. Effects of
     inhalable particles in respiratory health of children. Am Rev Respir Dis
     1989;139:587–94.
29.  Bromberg PA. Asthma and automotive emissions. In: Waston AY, Bates
     RR, eds. Air pollution: the automobile and public health. Washington,
     DC: National Academy Press, 1988:465–98.
30.  Utell MJ, Morrow PE, Speers DM, Daring J, Hyde RW. Airway responses
     to sulfate and sulfuric acid aerosols in asthmatics. Am Rev Respir Dis
     1983;128:444–50.
31.  Bates DV, Sizto R. Air pollution and hospital admissions in southern
     Ontario: the acid summer haze effect. Environ Res 1987;43:317–31.

32. American Thoracic Society. Report of the ATS workshop on the health effects of atmospheric acids and their precursors. Am Rev Respir Dis 1991;144:464–67.

33. Samet JM. Nitrogen dioxide. In: Samet JM, Spengler JD, eds. Indoor air pollution: a health perspective. Baltimore: Johns Hopkins University Press, 1991:170–86.

34. Samet JM, Utell JM. The risk of nitrogen dioxide: what have we learned from epidemiological and clinical studies? Toxicol Ind Health 1990;6:247–62.

35. Lippman M. Ozone. In: Lippmann M, ed. Environmental toxicants: human exposures and their health effects. New York: Van Nostrand Reinhold, 1992.

36. Devlin RB, McDonnell WF, Mann R, Becker S, House DE, Schreinemachers D, Koren HS. Exposure of humans to ambient levels of ozone for 6.6 hours causes cellular and biochemical changes in the lung. Am J Respir Cell Mol Biol 1991;4:72–81.

37. Allred EN, Bleecker ER, Chaitman BR, Dahms TE, Gottlieb SO, Hackney JD, Pagano M, Selvester RH, Walden SM, Warren J. Short-term effects of carbon monoxide exposure on the exercise performance of subjects with coronary artery disease. N Engl J Med 1989;321:1426–32.

38. National Research Council, Committee on Passive Smoking. Environmental tobacco smoke: measuring exposures and assessing health effects. Washington, DC: National Academy Press, 1986.

39. U.S. Department of Health and Human Services. The health consequences of involuntary smoking. A report of the Surgeon General. DHHS Publication (CDC) 87-8398. Rockville, MD: U.S. Government Printing Office, 1986.

40. Hirayama T. Nonsmoking wives of heavy smokers have a higher risk of lung cancer: a study from Japan. Br Med J 1981;282:183–5.

41. Trichopoulos D, Kalandidi A, Sparros L, MacMahon B. Lung cancer and passive smoking. Int J Cancer 1981;27:1–4.

42. Wald NJ, Nanchakal K, Thompson SG, Cuckle HS. Does breathing other people's tobacco smoke cause lung cancer? Br Med J 1986;293:1217–22.

43. IARC monographs on the evaluation of the carcinogenic risk of chemicals to humans. Vol. 38. Tobacco smoking. Lyon, France: IARC, 1986.

44. Glantz SA, Parmley WW. Passive smoking and heart disease: epidemiology, physiology, and biochemistry. Circulation 1991;83:1–12.

45. Marbury MC. Wood smoke. In: Samet JM, Spengler JD, eds. Indoor air pollution: a health perspective. Baltimore: Johns Hopkins University Press, 1991:209–22.

46. Burge HA, Feeley JC. Indoor air pollution and infectious diseases. In: Samet JM, Spengler JD, eds. Indoor air pollution: a health perspective. Baltimore: Johns Hopkins University Press, 1991:273–84.

47.   Weissman DN, Schuyler MR. Biological agents and allergic diseases. In: Samet JM, Spengler JD, eds. Indoor air pollution: a health perspective. Baltimore: Johns Hopkins University Press, 1991:285–305.
48.   Leikauf GD. Formaldehydes and other aldehydes. In: Lippmann M, ed. Critical reviews of environmental toxicants: human exposures and their health effects. New York: Van Nostrand Reinhold, 1991.
49.   Marbury MC, Krieger RA. Formaldehyde. In: Samet JM, Spengler JD, eds. Indoor air pollution: a health perspective. Baltimore: Johns Hopkins University Press, 1991:223–52.
50.   Wallace LA. Volatile organic compounds. In: Samet JM, Spengler JD, eds. Indoor air pollution: a health perspective. Baltimore: Johns Hopkins University Press, 1991:252–72.
51.   Samet JM. Radon and lung cancer. J Natl Cancer Inst 1989;81:745–57.
52.   Samet JM, Stolwijk J, Rose SL. Summary: international workshop on residential radon epidemiology. Health Phys 1991;60:223–27.
53.   Rothman KJ. A sobering start for the cluster busters conference. Am J Epidemiol 1990;132:S6–S13.
54.   Wu AH, Samet JM. Environmental tobacco smoke: exposure–response relationships in epidemiological studies. Risk Anal 1990;10:39–48.
55.   U.S. Department of Health and Human Services. Reducing the health consequences of smoking: 25 years of progress. A report of the surgeon general. DHHS (CDC) Publication 89-8411. Washington DC: U.S. Government Printing Office, 1989.
56.   National Research Council. Committee on the Institutional Means for Assessment of Risks to Public Health. Risk assessment in the federal government: managing the means. Washington DC: National Academy Press, 1983.
57.   National Research Council, Committee on the Biological Effects of Ionizing Radiation. Health risks of radon and other internally deposited α-emitters: BEIR IV. Washington, DC: National Academy Press, 1988.
58.   Nero AV Jr. Radon and its decay products in indoor air: an overview. In: Nazaroff WW, Nero AV Jr, eds. Radon and its decay products in indoor air. New York: Wiley, 1988:1–53.
59.   Lubin JH, Boice JD. Estimating radon-induced lung cancer in the U.S. Health Phys 1989;57:417–27.
60.   Ennever FK. Predicted reduction in lung cancer risk following cessation of smoking and radon exposure. Epidemiology 1990;1:134–40.
61.   U.S. Environmental Protection Agency, Office of Air and Radiation. Implementation strategy for the clean air act amendments of 1990. Seattle, WA: U.S. EPA, 1991.
62.   Platts-Mills TAE, Chapman MD. Dust mites: immunology, allergic disease, and environmental control. J Allergy Clin Immunol 1987;80:755–75.

63. American Thoracic Society. Environmental controls and lung disease. Am Rev Respir Dis 1990;142:915–39.
64. Lowrance WW. Of acceptable risk: science and the determination of safety. Los Altos, CA: William Kaufmann, 1976.
65. Mauderly JL, Samet JM. General environment. In: Crystal RG, West JB, eds. The lung: scientific foundations. New York: Raven Press, 1991:1947–60.
66. Dales RE, Spitzer WO, Suissa S, Schechter MC, Tousignant P, Steinmetz N. Respiratory health of a population living downwind from natural gas refineries. Am Rev Respir Dis 1989;139:595–600.
67. Ware JH, Spengler J, Samet J, Wagner G, Neas L, Coultas D, Ozkaynak H, Schwab M. Respiratory and irritant health effects of emissions from chemical manufacturing: the Kanawha County Health Study (submitted for publication).

# Part Three

## BIOLOGICAL MARKERS

JEAN-PIERRE MARTIN

Several factors play a determining role in the appearance and evolution of respiratory diseases. Tobacco use, occupational factors, environmental sources, and genetic or individual factors combine, and several mechanisms lead to such diseases as asthma, cancer, bronchitis, and emphysema. Prevention of respiratory diseases can be aided with knowledge of the biological markers that determine the appearance or nonappearance of a disease and its possible evolution.

In most complex diseases such as pulmonary diseases, the genetic determination has to be proven and its place among other factors assessed, as discussed in Chapter 16. Molecular biology has made great progress in determining the linkage between markers and diseases, leading to the identification, for example, of candidate genes and DNA polymorphism. Studies of the genetics of diseases have used familial aggregation of a disease (including twin studies) and familial segregation analysis to identify the role of the main gene responsible. Studies using genetic markers have been employed in families (lod score, linkage) and in populations (HLA and diseases), but this method is not really adapted to multifactorial diseases. Risk estimations can include information concerning a marker and the estimated risks for an affected subject. The choice of a marker for a monogenic disease such as cystic fibrosis permits screening for the genome with all available markers, but for multifactorial diseases, the power to detect linkage with a marker is very weak. This is illustrated in the case of asthma, where familial and genetic markers associated with environmental aspects and a strong allergic component could lead to a better understanding of the disease. In multifactorial diseases such as asthma and emphysema, the effect of genetic factors that may interact among themselves and with environmental factors needs further investigation. Such epidemiological and genetic studies could lead to preventing the development of a disease.

The protease inhibitor (PI) phenotype is a typical biological marker that has been assessed to be associated with emphysema, as discussed in Chapter 17. The protease inhibitor (PI system) and its main marker for panlobular emphysema, PI Z, are of great interest in the theory of a balance between the proteolytic activity (which destroys elastic tissue of the lung) and its inhibitors. The determination of PI phenotypes is important in families or in populations and can be considered as a marker for the risk of emphysema. This genetic deficiency shown by the determination of the PI phenotypes is nevertheless very rare, and affects only one subject among 3000 within Caucasian population. The genetic deficiency affecting $\alpha_1$-antitrypsin (the main protease inhibitor in human plasma) sometimes leads to the appearance of a panlobular emphysema, especially in smokers. PI phenotypes are therefore good markers to evaluate emphysema.

Collagen and elastin are the two major structural proteins of the lung extracellular matrix. Fibrillar cross-linking of collagen and lung elastin are distributed between the various microarchitectures of the alveolar wall. Collagen and elastin degradation by various proteinases (metalloproteases, elastases), resulting primarily in plasma and urinary peptides release, is believed to be an important component of such physiological processes as morphogenesis and remodeling of the lung, wound healing, and embryogenesis. In addition to the maintenance of normal pulmonary function, the process of uncontrolled matrix destruction has received attention in the study of pathological states, including lung fibrosis, emphysema, and tumor metastasis. The environmental conditions are shown particularly in the mechanism of tobacco smoke–induced lung emphysema, discussed in Chapter 18.

Two principal types of markers can be used to evaluate lung degradation and to prevent it. (see Chapter 19):

1. *Collagen peptides*. Collagen molecules are the major constituents of the extracellular matrix of most organs. Fourteen collagen types have been described so far; collagen synthesis is a multiple process, and each of these steps may be deregulated and lead to pathological situations. The main studies on the physiopathological significance of collagen peptides assays in pulmonary disease deal with type III procollagen, which is often synthesized during the initial phase of the fibroproliferative response. This is interesting for the monitoring of antifibrotic treatment.

2. *Elastin peptides and desmosine*. The alteration observed during emphysema is the fragmentation of elastic fibers. Two types of assays have been developed to measure elastin degradation: desmosine in urine and elastin peptides in all fluids. In chronic obstructive pulmonary disease, the level of circulating or excreted elastin peptides is increased. Urinary desmosine is a more specific marker of elastin degradation and elastin reconstruction. Nevertheless, the ability of desmosine tests to measure the increase of elastin degradation in emphysema and in smokers needs to be demonstrated in further studies.

The genetic aspects of lung cancer can be related to cytochrome, as discussed in Chapter 20. The genetic polymorphisms of cytochrome P450 are important in the discovery of genes that predispose to lung cancer. Expression of cytochrome P450 in the lung tissue has focused interest on the localized metabolism of xenobiotic. For example, restriction fragment length polymorphism (RFLP) on cytochrome P4501A1 shows that benzo[a]pyrene metabolites produced by this enzyme are 10 to 100 times more mutagenic than those produced by other cytochromes. The carcinogenicity of these compounds can be modulated through bioactivation or through detoxication. Polymease chain reaction (PCR) allowed identification of more than 95% of the various mutated allees. The results raise the possibility that inheritance might play an important role in individual susceptibility to lung cancer.

# 16

## Genetic Markers in Complex Diseases

**MARIE-HÉLÈNE DIZIER and JOSUÉ FEINGOLD**

INSERM U155
Paris, France

## I. Introduction

The aim of genetic epidemiology is to study the genetic determinism of diseases. The pattern of such determinism may be simple, as for Mendelian diseases, which depend on the effect of one gene, or more complex, as for some common multifactorial diseases, which depend on several genetic and environmental factors. For Mendelian diseases the pattern of genetic inheritance is determined easily by studying the familial distribution of the disease. For multifactorial diseases, such studies lead to detecting a genetic component rather than to determining the exact pattern of inheritance.

One result of genetic studies is to localize and identify the gene (or genes) involved in a disease and eventually to determine its (or their) product function(s). This could lead to better understanding of the nature of the underlying biological mechanisms involved, which for the majority of diseases is unknown. To evidence the effect of genes and to localize them will again be easier for Mendelian diseases, which depend on a rare defective allele, than for multifactorial diseases, which depend on several common genes that could each independently have a minor effect.

However, for both types of diseases, important advances have been made by the use of information on genetic markers to seek linkage between markers and diseases. The first markers studied were the blood groups; subsequently, progress in molecular biology has led to identification of a large number of DNA polymorphisms, which can be used in genetic studies of disease. Different strategies exist according to the choice of marker. The marker may be a candidate gene for the disease, because it is a known genetic function that could itself be involved in the disease. It may also be a DNA polymorphism located in the region of a known genetic function. When the candidate gene is not sufficiently polymorphic, it can be more efficient to study DNA polymorphisms close or adjacent to the candidate gene. Another possibility is that the marker is an arbitrary DNA polymorphism. In this case the strategy of walking on the chromosome toward the disease gene could be applied, although this represents a large amount of work. The disease gene may be then identified and cloned, and its protein function determined.

A recently developed approach is to study well-defined animal models for a disease and to look for linkage with many genetic markers. When evidence of linkage with markers is obtained in animal studies, homologeous loci are sought in the human and can then be studied to confirm linkage. If the marker is a candidate gene, evidence for linkage between a marker and a disease may make it possible to conclude involvement of the candidate gene in the disease; in other cases it may lead to identification of the gene involved in the disease by walking on the chromosome. On the other hand, a linkage between a marker and a disease also directly provides other interesting information, such as the predictive risk to be affected for a person given the marker genes that he or she possesses. For multifactorial diseases, risks may be low when considering only one genetic factor, but may become high when considering several genetic and environmental factors interacting between them.

We present here the various approaches for studying diseases and genetic markers as well as the choice of markers used to study multifactorial diseases. Finally, the genetics of asthma is presented as an interesting example of genetic study of a multifactorial disease.

## II.  Study of Genetics of Diseases

The effect of a genetic component may first be suggested by familial aggregation of a disease. Twin studies comparing concordance for the disease between dizygous and monozygous twins, assuming they share the same environment, may show a genetic component in a disease if there is a greater concordance level in monozygous twins. However, this type of study gives no indication as to the genetic inheritance pattern of the disease. For this purpose familial segregation analysis [1] can be performed. It allows us to determine the most simple model that best explains the distribution of the disease in a family sample by the maximum likelihood approach. More commonly studied genetic hypotheses are the effect of a major gene and/or of a polygenic component. When the effect of a major gene is shown, its frequency and penetrance values are estimated and its transmission mode, dominant or recessive, is precised. Then localization of the major gene will be assessed by studies with genetic markers or DNA polymorphism. However, for multifactorial diseases, which depend on the effects of several genetic and/or environmental factors, familial aggregation can be explained by the effect of either genetic factors or a shared familial environment; segregation analysis is therefore often inconclusive as to the inheritance pattern of the disease. Recently, familial segregation analysis has been developed for studying simultaneously the effect of a major gene and/or of a polygenic component and environmental factors [2]. It has not as yet been extended to the study of the effect of more than one major gene. In fact, according to whether the genetic inheritance pattern of the disease is known, the methods for seeking linkage with genetic markers are appropriated differently.

## III. Studies Using Genetic Markers

Two types of studies using genetic markers can be distinguished: familial and population.

### A. Familial Analysis

One type of familial analysis is the lod-score method [3]. This method is based on the principle of the maximum likelihood approach and uses information on the joint segregation of a marker and the disease in families. The purpose is to test the absence against the presence of linkage between the marker and the disease gene. The recombination fraction between the marker and the disease gene, 0.5 under the absence of linkage and <0.5 if there is linkage, is estimated by maximization of the likelihood under the hypothesis of linkage. Likelihood calculation also depends on gene frequency, penetrance values, and transmission mode (recessive or dominant), which are estimated by segregation analysis. An error in these parameters will strongly affect estimation of the recombination fraction and the conclusion regarding linkage. Thus this approach is not really adaptable to multifactorial diseases with an obscure genetic inheritance pattern. However, the lod score test is robust, and the use of arbitrary parameters cannot lead to a false conclusion regarding linkage but will decrease the power to detect true linkage [4]. This is true as long as different sets of parameters are not used for the lod-score test; in the case of multiple tests, false conclusions of linkage may arise [5].

Because of all these problems, other approaches are preferred for diseases for which segregation analysis has been inconclusive, particularly methods for which no assumptions as to the inheritance pattern are needed to look for linkage. One of these approaches is the sib-pair method [6–8]. This approach uses information on affected sibpairs, which are classified according to the number of IBD (identify by descent) of parental genes of the marker they share. The variable IBD could then take a value of 2, 1, or 0. Under the hypothesis of no linkage or independent segregation between the marker and the disease, 25% of sib pairs are expected to share two genes, 50% to share one gene, and 25% to share zero genes. Under the hypothesis of linkage, an excess of sib pairs sharing two genes is expected. Absence of linkage can be tested by comparing the IBD distribution observed in a sib-pair sample and that expected under independence (0.25, 0.5, 0.25). This method was developed for the HLA marker and widely used for such HLA-associated diseases as insulin-dependent diabetes, rheumatoid arthritis, and coeliac diseases [9]. IBD distribution expected under the hypothesis of linkage is a function of the frequency of the gene of susceptibility, penetrance values, and recombination fraction. However, information given by IBD distribution in affected sib pairs is not always sufficient to give an estimate of all parameters simultaneously. The approach was then extended to use information on IBS (identity by state) among all affected relatives in a pedigree [10], which also makes it possible to test absence of linkage without making an inference as to the inheritance pattern of the disease.

## B. Population Studies

Differences in allele frequencies of a marker between affected and healthy individuals show an association between the marker and the disease. Such an association could be explained by linkage between the marker and the susceptibility gene of the disease, but also by stratification between the two populations of cases and controls. However, population association due to linkage can be detected only for very close linkage, in contrast with familial analyses, which can detect linkage of about 10% of recombination. Thus if linkage has been evidenced by a nonindependent familial segregation of the disease and the marker, and association has been evidenced on the population level, it will give strong support for very close linkage. For example, linkage between HLA and a gene of susceptibility to some diseases evidenced by nonindependent familial segregation of HLA and the disease was strongly assumed to be very close because of association of the population level between HLA genes and the diseases. This was also supported by involvement of the HLA genes in the immune response.

## IV. Risk Estimation

Given the information available on a linked genetic marker, risks may be estimated using information on either population or familial data. When association has been evidenced between marker genes and the disease, we may estimate the risk to be affected according to whether or not associated genes are present in a person. When nonindependence of segregation has been evidenced between a marker and the disease in sib pairs, we can estimate the risk to be affected by a sib of affected index, according to whether they share zero, one, or two parental marker genes. A new approach, the marker association segregation chi-square (MASC) method [11], has recently been proposed that allows us to use information simultaneously on the segregation and association of the marker with the disease, to estimate risk that a person will be affected.

## V. Choice of Markers

One strategy is to use arbitrary DNA polymorphisms and to screen the genome by studying all available markers. When linkage is obtained with a marker, we can walk on the chromosome to the gene involved in the disease. This strategy has been applied successfully to such monogenic diseases as cystic fibrosis. However, for multifactorial diseases, which depend on several factors each with a small effect, the power to detect linkage with a marker will be weak if the marker is not very close to the gene involved in the disease. For these diseases it would be more efficient to study candidate genes rather than arbitrary DNA polymorphisms [12], since if such genes are really involved in the disease, very close linkage is expected.

## VI. Genetics of Asthma

The genetic inheritance of asthma still remains unclear, probably because of its complexity. Familial studies have shown familial aggregation of the disease [13], and twin studies have confirmed a genetic component [14]. However, it is known that there is also strong participation by the environment, including smoking (active and passive), conditions of life, occupational exposure, and other factors. In addition, the strong association of asthma with bronchic hyperreactivity and allergy, for which a genetic component has also been shown, leads us to assume the effect of more than one gene in this disease. We can hope, however, that use of genetic markers will be helpful in advancing study of the genetics of this disease.

Studies on genetic markers have so far been performed essentially with the HLA system. Some studies have shown an association with antigens HLA-A1 and B8 [15–16], but these results were not confirmed by other studies [17,18]. Thus there is no clear evidence of association between HLA antigens and asthma. In contrast, two studies on affected sib pairs have shown nonindependence of segregation of allergic asthma and HLA [19,20]. If the involvement of HLA is confirmed by further studies, it would be interesting to understand the exact biological implication of HLA in allergic asthma—more specifically, in asthma and allergy.

Because of the strong allergic component of asthma, studies on allergy could also lead to better understanding of the genetics of asthma. Interesting results have already been obtained with allergy and genetic markers. First, an association has been evidenced between some specific allergic responses to particular allergens and HLA antigens [21]. A study of allergic families has suggested a linkage between allergy and a polymorphism located on the short arm of chromosome 11 [22]. This result has to be confirmed by other studies. If linkage is confirmed, it will be possible to walk on the chromosome to a disease gene, identify it and the corresponding protein, and understand its function in the development of the disease. Another alternative is to study some candidate genes on chromosome 11 known to be involved in the synthesis of T-cell receptors. In the future it will also be possible to study other candidate genes, known to be involved in IgE synthesis, such as genes coding for interleukin-4 or interferon-α.

On the other hand, bronchic hyperreactivity is a syndrome well identified in animals such as the rat and mouse. Genetic studies on rats and mice have already shown a genetic component, and linkage studies with markers lead to the identification of loci linked to bronchic hyperreactivity [23]. It would then be possible to look for homologeous loci in humans and to confirm linkage.

## VII.  Conclusions

The aim of genetic studies in common multifactorial diseases such as asthma and emphysema is to evidence the effect of genetic factors, which may interact among themselves and with environmental factors. The complexicity of these diseases makes such genetic studies difficult. However, the study of genetic markers and preferentially, candidate genes by looking for linkage with disease may provide important progress in the study of diseases. Evidence of linkage may allow us to show the involvement of a candidate gene in the disease and could then be a way to better understand the biological mechanisms of the disease by studying the exact implications of the function of the gene in development of the disease. However, such a strategy requires a sizable amount of work and may not lead to a specific treatment for a long time. Another interesting result of evidence of linkage with a marker, which could lead to more direct application, is to define a person's risk of being affected according to the information available on the marker. When an interactive effect of several factors (other candidate genes or environmental factors) has been evidenced, such information could be used for better estimating a person's risk of being affected. It would then be possible in the high-risk population to propose prevention or management of the disease much earlier in its evolution. To apply such a strategy, however, we first have to know how to prevent development of the disease.

## References

1. Morton NE, Maclean CJ. Analysis of family resemblance. III. Complex segregation analysis of quantitative traits. Am J Hum Genet 1974;26:489–503.
2. Bonney GE. On the statistical determination of major gene mechanisms in continuous human traits: regressive models. Am J Med Genet 1984;18:731–49.
3. Morton NE. The detection and estimation of linkage between the genes for elliptocytosis and the Rh blood type. Am J Hum Genet 1956;8:80–96.
4. Clerget-Darpoux F, Bonaïti-Pellié C, Hochez J. Effects of misspecifying genetic parameters in lod score analysis. Biometrics 1986;42:393–99.
5. Clerget-Darpoux F, Bonaïti-Pellié C, Babron MC. Assessing the effect of multiple linkage test in complex diseases. Genet Epidemiol 1990;7:245–53.
6. Day NE, Simons MJ. Disease susceptibility genes: their identification by multiple case family studies. Tissue Antigens 1976;8:109–19.
7. Thomson G, Bodmer WF. The genetic analysis of HLA and disease associations. In: Dausset J, Svejgaard A, eds. HLA and disease. Vol. 8. Copenhagen: Munksgaard, 1977:84–93.
8. Suarez BK. The affected sib pair IBD distribution for HLA-linked disease susceptibility genes. Tissue Antigens 1978;12:87–93.
9. Svejgaard A, Platz P, Ryder LP. HLA and disease 1982: a survey. Immunol Rev 1983;70:193–218.
10. Weeks DE, Lange K. The affected-pedigree-member method of linkage analysis. Am J Hum Genet 1988;42:315–26.
11. Clerget-Darpoux F, Babron MC, Prum B, Lathrop GM, Deschamps I, Hors J. A new method to test genetic models in HLA associated diseases: the MASC method. Ann Hum Genet 19 ;52:247–258.
12. Clerget-Darpoux F, Bonaïti-Pellié C. Strategies based on marker information for the study of human diseases. Ann Hum Genet (submitted for publication).

13. Schwartz M. Heredity in bronchial asthma. Acta Allergol 1952;5(Suppl 11).
14. Edfors-Lubs ML. Allergy in 7000 twin pairs. Acta Allergol 1971;26:249–85.
15. Thorsby E, Engset A, Lie SO. HLA antigens and susceptibility to diseases. A study of patients with acute lymphoblastic leukemia, Hodgkin's disease and childhood asthma. Tissue Antigens 1971;1:147–52.
16. Soothill JF, Stokes CR, Turner MW, Norman AP, Taylor B. Predisposing factors and the development of reaginic allergy in infancy. Clin Allergy 1976;6:305.
17. Turton CMG, Morris L, Buckingham JA, Lawler SD, Turner-Warwick M. Histocompatibility antigens in asthma: population and family studies. Thorax 1979;34(5):670–76.
18. Morris MJ, Faux JA, Ting A, Morris PJ, Land DJ. HLA-A, B and C and DR antigens in intrinsic and allergic asthma. Clin Allergy 1980;10:173–79.
19. Hafez M, Zedan M, El-Shennawy FA, Abd El-Hafez SA, El-Khayat H. HLA antigens and extrinsic bronchial asthma. Asthma 1984;21(4):259–63.
20. Caraballo LR, Hernandez M. HLA haplotype segregation in families with allergic asthma. Tissue Antigens 1990;35:182–86.
21. Marsh DG, Zwollo P, Ansari AA. Toward a total human immune response finger print: the allergy model. In: Said EL, Sami A, Merrett TG, eds. Allergy and molecular biology. Elmsford, NY: Pergamon Press, 1989;65–82.
22. Cookson WOCM, Faux JA, Sharp PA, Hopkin JM. Linkage between immunoglobulin E responses underlying asthma and rhinitis and chromosome 11q. Lancet 1989;1:1292–94.
23. Levitt RC, Mitzner W. Autosomal recessive inheritance of airway reactivity to 5-hydroxytryptamine. Appl Physiol 1989;67:1125–32.

# 17

## Protease–Antiprotease System

**RICHARD SESBOÜÉ and JEAN-PIERRE MARTIN**

INSERM U295
Rouen, France

## I. Introduction

Many protease inhibitors regulate the cascade of proteolytic events occurring both at the tissular (pulmonary alveolus) and humoral (coagulation) levels. The proteins that inhibit the proteolytic enzymes whose active site is a serine (elastase, trypsin, chymotrypsin, thrombin, etc.) are called serine protease inhibitors, or serpins [1]. The most representative protein in this family is $\alpha_1$-antitrypsin (A1AT), whose main role consists of inactivating human leukocyte elastase. Laurell and Eriksson's observation in 1963 of the association between A1AT deficiency and early pulmonary emphysema [2] gradually led to the concept of a protease–antiprotease balance. Thus the integrity of the normal lung structure would be dependent on a system opposing the destructive activity of human leukocyte elastase and the protective effect of the serpins, especially A1AT. There is great clinical variability in the development of emphysema in subjects with a genetic A1AT deficiency, but the preponderant role of tobacco should be noted, as the disease appears 15 to 20 years earlier in smokers.

The recent availability of purified human A1AT has made it possible to initiate replacement therapy by means of weekly injections in order to generate a sufficient concentration in the plasma, and especially the lung, to protect the alveolus; however, while the biologic efficacy of this method has been demonstrated, the same is not true of its clinical efficacy.

## II.  Structure, Function, and Synthesis of A1AT

A1AT is a glycoprotein of 394 amino acids to which three carbohydrate chains are attached through asparagine residues. These saccharide chains are double or triple branched and terminate in a neuraminic acid. Functionally, the most important residue is methionine 358, the key amino acid of the elastase inhibitory site exposed on the outside of the native molecule [3]. However, this amino acid is particularly sensitive to oxidizing agents, which cause inactivation of the molecule [4]. Like the other serpins, A1AT forms a stable stoichiometric complex (1:1 ratio) with its target enzyme, elastase, and is hydrolyzed between the 358 (methionine) and 359 (serine) residues.

A1AT is produced mainly by the liver, but also by macrophages. It circulates in plasma with a half-life of 5 days, and diffuses into many organs, especially the lung, where it is found in the alveolus. Its synthesis is controlled by a gene localized on chromosome 14, at position q31–32.3 [5].

## III.  Genetics of A1AT: the PI system

The genetic variants of A1AT constitute the protease inhibitor (PI) system. The alleles of the PI system, described originally in relation to their electrophoretic mobility [6] as anodal or fast (F), cathodal or slow (S), and medium (M), are inherited according to the autosomal codominant mode. The most common variant, PI*M, occurs in 90% of Caucasians. The characteristic allele of A1AT deficiency, PI*Z, results from a single nucleotide substitution, leading to the replacement of glutamic acid with lysine at position 342 on the protein. This gene is very rare, if not absent, in Negroid and Mongoloid populations. The PI*S allele, found more frequently in populations of Hispanic origin, also results from a point mutation whereby glutamic acid is replaced with valine at position 246 [7].

## IV.  Clinical Evolution of Subjects with a Genetic Deficiency in A1AT

In the typical form [8], these subjects are male smokers (ratio of two men to one woman). The disease appears insidiously as progressive dyspnea before age 40.

Antecedents include childhood respiratory infections, atopic asthma, recurrent pneumonias with cough, and sputum. Physiopathologically, the important point is the reduction in the $FEV_1$ value; the often rapid progression of emphysema is accompanied by bronchitis with hypersecretion and bronchospasm. Gas exchanges deteriorate rapidly, as reflected by the reduction in the DLCO value; conventional x-ray pictures reveal a predominant hyperlucency at the bases. Diagnosis and evolution are essentially assessed by high-resolution computerized axial tomography. Tobacco smoke is the principal agent responsible for the early onset of emphysema and the appearance of clinical signs, notably dyspnea. Death results from complications of emphysema, with a considerably shortened rate of survival (by 10 to 20 years) among smokers [9]. Therefore, it is essential to arrive at an early diagnosis of A1AT deficiency in order to limit and, if possible, exclude the use of tobacco among deficient homozygotes.

The A1AT deficiency is seldom recognized in the child, where it may express itself in the form of neonatal cholestasis. Clinical and biological signs of liver disorders exist in half the cases at about 1 year of age, but a genuine hepatopathy appears in only 15% of the cases [10]. In children, liver disease is rarely serious, and death by cirrhosis is exceptional. In adults, on the other hand, liver cirrhosis is reportedly present in 30% of the cases; based on anatomical data, half these subjects also have liver cancer. The reasons for the liver disease are still unclear, although there exists a strong correlation with the presence of A1AT globules blocked inside the endoplasmic reticulum of the hepatocytes [11].

## V. Diagnosis and PI Phenotype

A diagnosis of A1AT deficiency must be considered when the $\alpha_1$ zone of the serum protein electrophoresis is reduced or absent. This diagnosis can be corroborated by measuring the concentration of A1AT in plasma or serum by an immunochemical method [2]. However, since A1AT is part of the proteins of the acute inflammatory phase, its plasma concentration rises considerably, doubling and even tripling during many illnesses, as well as during pregnancy or contraceptive treatment. This is why the precise determination of the variants of A1AT requires more elaborate techniques. The PI phenotype is currently being investigated by isoelectric focusing in polyacrylamide gels with a low pH gradient (pH 4 to 5). In such a medium, A1AT presents itself as many bands, whose intensity and position vary with the person. This microheterogeneity has to do on the one hand, with amino acid changes (genetic variants) and on the other hand, with the number and structure of the carbohydrate chains in a given type of protein. Molecular biology techniques, involving synthetic oligonucleotide probes specific to the different alleles (PI*M, PI*S, and especially PI*Z), can also be used; they are ordinarily reserved for antenatal diagnoses [12].

## VI.  Genetic Variants

More than 70 alleles of the PI system have been described, but the frequency of
occurrence of rare variants is not known precisely because the studies have been
conducted on limited population samples. The frequency of PI*M is well
established among Caucasians (0.95): 90% of northern Europeans have the PI
MM phenotype. The frequency of PI*Z has been especially well investigated in
Sweden, thanks to a prospective study of 200,000 infants, according to which
one subject out of 1700 has the PI*ZZ phenotype [10]. The A1AT observed in
PI Z homozygotes is linked to a reduction in the production of protein by the
liver. The synthesis of the protein begins normally, but a major portion of it
remains blocked in the endoplasmic reticulum, which results in a plasma level
on the order of 15% of normal. The A1AT isolated from hepatocyte inclusions
has a pronounced tendency to aggregate and is not readily soluble [11].

Other, extremely rare variants correspond to a virtually complete absence
of A1AT [7]: these are the "weak" PI*M and especially the PI*Q0 (or PI*Nil)
variants, which were able to be brought to light only in special cases (in
homozygotes, or when associated with another deficient allele), and correspond
to major anomalies in the gene (deletion, appearance of a stop codon, unstable
mRNA) or the protein (instability, intrahepatocyte deterioration). Pulmonary
emphysema appears at an extremely early stage in such subjects. Other alleles,
such as PI*S and PI*P, also cause a slight decrease in A1AT concentration,
although usually without pathological consequences.

Deficient heterozygous subjects have depressed theoretical concentrations
of A1AT in plasma—60% of normal in persons with the PI MZ phenotype and
35% in PI SZ subjects. They do not usually exhibit any lung disease, although
a minor risk may exist in the latter [13]. Based on these data, it has been possible
to conclude empirically that the threshold of the A1AT plasma concentration for
protection against the proteases is about 35% of normal.

## VII.  Protease–Antiprotease Balance in the Pulmonary Alveolus

During the initial investigations of A1AT deficiency [8], Eriksson suggested that
$\alpha_1$-antitrypsin played a role in protecting the connective tissue of the lung against
the proteolytic enzymes synthesized by the polymorphonuclear neutrophil.
Moreover, experimental emphysema was produced in the rat by the intratracheal
instillation of papain, an enzyme capable of digesting elastin.

The concept gradually developed that maintenance of the integrity of the
lung structure is due to the existence of a balance between, on the one hand, the
rate of leukocyte elastase and, on the other hand, protection of the lung tissue
by protease inhibitors. The existence of a methionine residue at the level of the
A1AT active site and the demonstration that tobacco smoke extracts are

responsible for the degradation of A1AT's inhibitory powers have helped explain the role of tobacco in emphysema [14]. In fact, tobacco causes inflammation in the lung parenchyma while oxidizing and inactivating A1AT, which results in a functional A1AT deficiency in the smoker.

The A1AT level in the bronchoalveolar lavage fluid is naturally lower in PI Z subjects than in PI M subjects [15]. In smokers, the ponderal (immunochemical) level of A1AT is normal, but its functional level (elastase inhibition) is depressed. Only a fraction of the A1AT found in plasma exists, in an active (free) or inactive (oxidized or fragmented) form, in the alveolar liquid. Obviously, any event resulting in an increase in the number of neutrophils in the lung, or favoring the release of elastase, upsets the balance toward destruction by the proteases and the constitution of emphysema. Thus the lung defense system rests essentially on A1AT.

## VIII. Replacement Therapy

None of the currently known data proves that replacement therapy can prevent the development of emphysema due to A1AT deficiency, although theoretically, this should be the case. Ideally, A1AT should be administered before the lung structure is affected, but this replacement therapy is not recommended for asymptomatic subjects, as a significant number of them do not present any deterioration of lung function. Following the diagnosis (determination of the PI phenotype), these subjects must be followed up periodically, especially by spirometry, at least every 4 months during the first year, and annually thereafter if there are no symptoms. Replacement therapy cannot be recommended in deficient homozygous subjects who continue to smoke. The goal of the treatment is to slow down the progression of the destruction of the emphysematous lung by raising the level of active inhibitor in the lung. The scheme offering the best guarantee of efficacy at this time is weekly intravenous administration of 60 mg/kg of active inhibitor, as such treatment results in a doubling of the level of alveolar A1AT [16]. At this time it is not possible to determine if other methods (identical doses, higher but less frequent doses, administration only during aggressive manifestations of pulmonary illness) could prevent or delay the appearance of emphysema.

Modern cell and molecular biology techniques make it possible to contemplate other therapeutic possibilities in the future [17]. Human A1AT has been produced in bacteria and yeast; it retains its immunologic and functional activity without glycosylation. Such a protein has a very short plasma half-life and is probably not suitable for intravenous administration. However, animal experiments show that aerosol administration leads to the presence of a significant quantity of inhibitor at the level of the alveolar fluid. The protein also diffuses into the lung. Products in which methionine 358 has been replaced with valine are also available; these proteins are capable of inhibiting leukocyte elastase without being sensitive to oxidants.

Finally, gene therapy experiments have been conducted with animals. Mouse embryos in which the gene of human A1AT has been injected or transfected produce large quantities of human A1AT at the adult stage [18]. Gene therapy thus seems to be a reasonable future goal, but many obstacles remain.

### References

1.  Carrell RW, Boswell DR. Serpins: the superfamily of plasma serine proteinase inhibitors. In: Barrett AJ, Salvesen G, eds. Research monographs in cell and tissue physiology: proteinase inhibitors. Vol. 12. Amsterdam: Elsevier, 1986:403–20.
2.  Laurell CB, Eriksson S. The electrophoretic $\alpha$-1-globulin pattern of serum in $\alpha$-1-antitrypsin deficiency. Scand J Clin Lab Invest 1963;15:132–40.
3.  Loebermann H, Tokuoka R, Deisenhofer J, Huber R. Human $\alpha$-1-proteinase inhibitor. Crystal structure analysis of two crystal modifications, molecular model and preliminary analysis of the implications for function. J Mol Biol 1984;177:531–56.
4.  Carp H, Janoff A. In vitro suppression of serum elastase-inhibitory capacity by reactive oxygen species generated by phagocytosing polymorphonuclear leukocytes. J Clin Invest 1979;63:793–97.
5.  Cox DW, Markovic VC, Teshima IE. Genes for immunoglobulin heavy chains and for $\alpha$-1-antitrypsin are localized to specific regions of chromosome 14q. Nature 1982;297:428–30.
6.  Fagerhol MK, Laurell CB. The polymorphism of "prealbumins" and $\alpha$-1-antitrypsin in human sera. Clin Chim Acta 1967;16:199–203.
7.  Crystal RG. $\alpha$-1-antitrypsin deficiency, emphysema, and liver disease. Genetic basis and strategies for therapy. J Clin Invest 1990;85:1343–52.
8.  Eriksson S. Studies in $\alpha$-1-antitrypsin deficiency. Acta Med Scand 1965;177(Suppl 432):1–85.
9.  Larsson C. Natural history and life expectancy in severe $\alpha$-1-antitrypsin deficiency, Pi Z. Acta Med Scand 1978;204:345–51.
10. Sveger T. Liver disease in $\alpha$-1-antitrypsin deficiency detected by screening of 200,000 infants. N Engl J Med 1976;294:1316–21.
11. Perlmutter DH. The cellular basis for liver injury in $\alpha$-1-antitrypsin deficiency. Hepatology 1991;13:172–85.
12. Kidd VJ, Golbus MS, Wallace RB, Itakura K, Woo SLC. Prenatal diagnosis of $\alpha$-1-antitrypsin deficiency by direct analysis of the mutation site in the gene. N Engl J Med 1984;310:639–42.

13. Tobin MJ, Hutchinson DCS. An overview of the pulmonary features of α-1-antitrypsin deficiency. Ann Intern Med 1982;142:1342–48.

14. Janoff A. Biochemical links between cigarette smoking and pulmonary emphysema. J Appl Physiol 1983;55:285–93.

15. Gadek JE, Fells GA, Zimmerman RL, Rennard SI, Crystal RG. Anti-elastases of the human alveolar structures. Implications for the protease-antiprotease theory of emphysema. J Clin Invest 1981;68:889–98.

16. Wewers MD, Casolaro MA, Sellers SE, Swayze SC, McPhaul KM, Wittes JT, Crystal RG. Replacement therapy for α-1-antitrypsin deficiency associated with emphysema. N Engl J Med 1987;316:1055–62.

17. Courtney M. Novel serine protease inhibitors obtained by protein engineering. Bull Inst Pasteur 1988;86:85–94.

18. Sifers RN, Carlson JA, Clift SM, DeMayo JL, Bullock DW, Woo SLC. Tissue specific expression of the human α-1-antitrypsin gene in transgenic mice. Nucleic Acids Res 1987;15:1459–75.

# 18

## Mechanisms of Tobacco Smoke-Induced Lung Emphysema

JOSEPH G. BIETH

INSERM U237
Illkirch, France

## I. Introduction

Lung emphysema is characterized by an enlargement of the airspaces distal to the terminal nonrespiratory bronchioles accompanied by destructive changes in the alveolar walls. A major improvement in understanding of the pathogenesis of this disease came from the observation of an association between inherited $\alpha_1$-proteinase inhibitor ($\alpha_1$PI) deficiency and early panlobular emphysema. The $\alpha_1$PI is present in the lower respiratory tract and is the major physiological inhibitor of neutrophil elastase (NE), an enzyme capable of digesting elastin and other lung matrix proteins. This key observation, together with the ability of NE to induce emphysematous-like lesions in the animal, led to a proposal called the elastase–antielastase hypothesis of emphysema. This theory holds that alveolar structures are normally protected against NE released accidentally from activated neutrophils by $\alpha_1$PI present in the lung interstitium. Emphysema occurs as a result of a more-or-less complete lack of antielastase protection of the lower respiratory tract. This hypothesis rationalizes the familial disease where $\alpha_1$PI is either absent (Pi NulNul individuals) or occurs in very low amounts in the lung

(Pi ZZ patients). In such patients NE may attack elastin fibers in an almost unimpaired way [1,2].

Emphysema due to $\alpha_1$PI deficiency is, however, relatively rare. The most frequent form of the disease is centrilobular emphysema (destruction of bronchioles), which occurs in $\alpha_1$PI-sufficient persons as a result of cigarette smoking. It was difficult using the elastase–antielastase theory to account for smokers' emphysema until it was discovered that oxidants present in cigarette smoke or secreted in situ by activated phagocytes may transform methionine 358, the $P_1$ residue of the active center of $\alpha_1$PI into methionine sulfoxide, with a resulting 2000-fold decrease in $k_{ass}$, the second-order rate constant for the association of the inhibitor with NE. As a consequence, the oxidized inhibitor reacts too slowly with NE to prevent the latter's proteolytic action. On the other hand, smoking recruits neutrophils and macrophages in the lung and causes these cells to release oxidants. A biochemical link between smokers' emphysema and tobacco consumption was thus established. This led to the oxidant theory of smokers' emphysema, which holds that $\alpha_1$PI-sufficient individuals who smoke may get an acquired decrease in $\alpha_1$PI activity whose magnitude is comparable to that of the genetic defect of the $\alpha_1$PI protein. A number of observations strongly suggest that expressed in those terms, the oxidation hypothesis is not valid. For example, healthy smokers and nonsmokers have similar levels of active $\alpha_1$PI in their bronchoalveolar lavage fluids [1,3]. Moreover, acute smoking does not decrease the activity of $\alpha_1$PI in healthy persons [3]. Even heavy smokers with emphysema have high amounts of active $\alpha_1$PI in their lower respiratory tract [4,5]. Furthermore, smokers and nonsmokers have similar levels of oxidized $\alpha_1$PI in lung secretions, and these levels are exceedingly small ($<0.1\%$ of total $\alpha_1$PI). The foregoing observations do not rule out the role of oxidants in the pathogenesis of smokers' emphysema (see below). They simply rule out the possibility that oxidants may oxidatively inactivate the bulk of lung $\alpha_1$PI and depress the antielastase protection of $\alpha_1$PI-sufficient smokers to an extent similar to that experienced by $\alpha_1$PI-deficient nonsmokers. Smokers' emphysema can therefore not be viewed as a monomolecular disease like familial emphysema. In this chapter we list a number of pathogenic factors and mechanisms that might explain why a number of $\alpha_1$PI-sufficient smokers develop emphysema.

## II. Neutrophil Elastase-Mediated Proteolysis in the Presence of $\alpha_1$-Proteinase Inhibitor

If one assumes that NE induces emphysematous lesions in $\alpha_1$PI-sufficient persons, one must also assume that NE cleaves elastin and other extracellular matrix proteins despite the presence of $\alpha_1$PI. This is possible under certain circumstances, as shown below.

### A. Proteolysis as a Consequence of Competitive Inhibition

If NE (E) is released from neutrophils in a milieu that contains both substrate (S) and $\alpha_1$PI (I), there will be competition between S and I for the binding of E as shown in the following scheme:

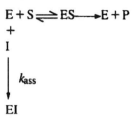

Thus whatever $[I_0]$, the in vivo $\alpha_1$PI concentration or $k_{ass}$, the second-order association rate constant, there will invariably be some substrate breakdown during the irreversible inhibition of NE by $\alpha_1$PI. The concentration of product at the end of the inhibition process $[P\infty]$ is given by [6]:

$$[P_\infty] = \frac{k_{cat} \, [E_0] \, [S_0]}{K_m} \, \frac{1}{k_{ass} \, [I_0]}$$

This equation shows that the amount of substrate broken down during the inhibition of NE by $\alpha_1$PI is proportional to the amount of NE released from neutrophils. Smokers have more lung neutrophils than do nonsmokers. In addition, the smokers' neutrophils are activated and may release NE. Smokers may therefore have significant NE-mediated proteolysis just because of the competitive nature of the $\alpha_1$PI-mediated inhibition process.

### B. Proteolysis as a Consequence of Uneven Distribution of Elastase and Elastin

The neutrophil distribution within the lung interstitium is probably highly heterogeneous since these cells accumulate at sites of phagocytosis while being present in lower amounts in other parts of the interstitium. On the other hand, elastin, and to a lesser extent the other NE substrates of the extracellular matrix [1], are also heterogeneously distributed within the interstitium. This uneven distribution of enzyme and substrate may favor proteolysis, for reasons given below.

### Effect of High Local Concentration of Elastase

The NE concentration in the azurophil granules is thought to be as high as 25 mM [7]. Thus, in the immediate vicinity of a degranulating neutrophil there has been, for some time, a local NE concentration that is much higher than the $\alpha_1$PI concentration. In this local area, proteolysis will therefore occur in a totally unimpaired way.

### Effect of High Local Concentration of Elastin

Equation (1) shows that the extent of substrate breakdown is proportional to the concentration of substrate. If neutrophils degranulate in the immediate vicinity of an elastin fiber, elastin may therefore strongly compete with $\alpha_1$PI for the binding of NE. Hence a substantial part of NE may escape inhibition and bind to elastin. In vitro experiments clearly demonstrate this behavior [8]. On the other hand, several investigators have shown that about 30% of the elastin-bound NE resists inhibition by $\alpha_1$PI (ref. 9 and references therein). In conclusion, neutrophil degranulation in the close vicinity of an elastin fiber may result in NE-mediated elastolysis despite the presence of $\alpha_1$PI. It must be noted, however, that the low-molecular-weight mucus proteinase inhibitor ($Mr = 11.7$ kDa), whose concentration is about tenfold lower than that of $\alpha_1$PI in the lower respiratory tract [4], readily inhibits elastin-bound elastase [9].

### C. Proteolysis as a Consequence of Local Inactivation of $\alpha_1$-Proteinase Inhibitor

#### Oxidation of $\alpha_1$PI

The activated neutrophil secretes not only proteinases but also superoxide anions ($O_2^{\cdot -}$) and myeloperoxidase. As shown below, the latter generate hypochlorite (HOCl), which readily oxidizes methionine 358 of $\alpha_1$PI into methionine sulfoxide. Since the $k_{ass}$ of oxidized $\alpha_1$PI is about 2000-fold lower than that of native $\alpha_1$PI [10 and references therein], there will be 2000-fold more substrate broken down during the inhibition of NE by oxidized $\alpha_1$PI than during the inhibition of NE by native $\alpha_1$PI.

Macrophages of smokers but not of nonsmokers have also been shown to oxidatively inactivate $\alpha_1$PI in vitro [11] by a process that requires the presence of myeloperoxidase [12]. It is therefore likely that $\alpha_1$PI is oxidized in the areas of the smokers' lung interstitium where macrophages accumulate. If NE is released in such areas, it may cleave elastin and other proteins in an almost fully unimpaired way. The amount of $\alpha_1$PI oxidized by neutrophils or macrophages may be very low compared to the total amount of inhibitor collected by bronchoalveolar lavage. This may explain why very low levels of oxidized $\alpha_1$PI have been found in lung lavage fluids [13].

#### Proteolytic Inactivation of $\alpha_1$PI

$\alpha_1$PI is inactivated by metalloproteinases from neutrophils [14–15], cathepsin L from macrophages [16], and proteinases from bacteria such as *Serratia marcescens* [17], *Pseudomonas aeruginosa* [18], *Staphylococcus aureas* [19], and *Legionella pneumophila* [20]. The inactivation occurs as a result of proteolytic cleavage of the inhibitor at or near its active center. Thus activated neutrophils and macrophages impair the activity of $\alpha_1$PI through the combined action of oxidants and proteinases. On the other hand, lung infections may promote elastolysis through the direct action of bacterial proteinases (e.g., *P. aeruginosa* elastase [21]) and through indirect mechanisms: increased neutrophil counts and inactivation of $\alpha_1$PI.

### D.  Proteolysis as a Consequence of Close Cell–Matrix Contact

When neutrophils are in close contact with insoluble matrix proteins, they exclude molecules having molecular weights larger than 25 kDa. This allows pericellular matrix degradation despite the presence of $\alpha_1$PI ($M_r$ = 53 kDa) [7,22,23]. The low-molecular-weight mucus proteinase inhibitor ($M_r$ = 11.7 kDa) is, however, able to inhibit NE-mediated proteolysis at the cell–matrix interface [23].

### E.  Proteolysis as a Consequence of Impaired Rate of Inhibition of Elastase by $\alpha_1$-Proteinase Inhibitor

NE forms a tight complex with heparin. This complex is enzymatically less active than free NE but reacts with $\alpha_1$PI with a 300-fold lower $k_{ass}$ value than that of the free enzyme [24]. NE and other positively charged enzymes are stored in the azurophil granules together with negatively charged proteoglycans [25]. Neutrophil degranulation is therefore likely to release NE in complex with these ligands. This might lower the $k_{ass}$ value in the immediate vicinity of the neutrophil. Moreover, heparin is abundant in the lung since this organ is a commercial source of this compound [26]. Lung mast cells, which secrete heparin [26], are found in large quantities in the alveolar walls [2]. If NE binds heparin faster than $\alpha_1$PI in vivo, as it does in vitro [24], it may be suggested that the $k_{ass}$ value for the NE + $\alpha_1$PI association in the lung is much lower than that measured in vitro (i.e., there is more proteolysis in the presence of $\alpha_1$PI than expected). On the other hand, heparin combines with the mucus proteinase inhibitor and strongly enhances its rate of inhibition of NE [27]. This inhibitor might therefore play a more significant function than expected from its concentration in the lower respiratory tract.

Ogushi et al. [28] recently showed that $\alpha_1$PI isolated from smokers' lung lavage fluids has a lower $k_{ass}$ value for NE ($6.5 \times 10^6 \, M^{-1} \, s^{-1}$) than $\alpha_1$PI isolated from nonsmokers' fluids ($8.1 \times 10^6 \, M^{-1} \, s^{-1}$). These authors also measured the $\alpha_1$PI concentration in the epithelial lining fluid of the two groups of subjects and calculated the delay time of inhibition ($d(t)$ [i.e., the time required to get almost full inhibition of NE in vivo; $d(t) = 5/k_{ass} \, [I_0]$ where $[I_0]$ is the in vivo inhibitor concentration (see refs. 6 and 29)]. They found that $d(t) = 0.34$ s for smokers and $(d(t) = 0.17$ s for nonsmokers and suggested that this increased $d(t)$ is part of the risk factors for the development of emphysema.

## III.  Lung Elastases Different From Neutrophil Elastase

### A.  Elastases from Neutrophils

The azurophil granules of neutrophils contain two additional elastolytic serine proteinases: cathepsin G and proteinase-3. (Table 1). The former occurs in about the same amount as NE and shares 36% sequence identify with it [30]. Its elastolytic activity is about 10% that of NE. In addition, cathepsin G enhances the elastolytic activity of NE [31–33]. Its physiological inhibitor, $\alpha_1$-antichymotrypsin ($k_{ass} = 3 \times 10^7 M^{-1} s^{-1}$, ref. 1) occurs in very low amounts in the lung and has been found to be inactive in lung secretions [34]. Cathepsin G is also inhibited by $\alpha_1$PI with a $k_{ass}$ value of $4 \times 10^5 M^{-1}s^{-1}$ [1]. Taking into account the $\alpha_1$PI concentration in the epithelial lining fluid ($4.6 \times 10^{-6} M$ [35]), one gets a delay time of inhibition of 2.7 s, a value 16-fold higher than that calculated for NE [35]. Thus $\alpha_1$PI is a poor inhibitor of cathepsin G in vivo. Cathepsin G is also inhibited by the low-molecular-weight mucus proteinase inhibitor.

Proteinase-3 solubilizes elastin and induces emphysema in the hamster [36]. Its elastolytic activity is about one-half that of NE at pH 7.4 but 40% higher than that of NE at pH 6.5. The quantity of proteinase-3 purified for neutrophil granules is about one-third that of NE. Proteinase-3 is inhibited by $\alpha_1$PI with a $k_{ass}$ value of $3 \times 10^6 M^{-1} s^{-1}$, from which a delay time of inhibition of 0.17 s

**Table 1**  Lung Elastolytic Proteinases and Their Inhibitors

| Name | Source[a] | Proteinase Class | Inhibitors[b] |
|------|-----------|------------------|---------------|
| Elastase | PMN, MAC | Serine | $\alpha_1$PI, MPI |
| Cathepsin G | PMN | Serine | $\alpha_1$ACHY, $\alpha_1$PI, MPI |
| Proteinase-3 | PMN | Serine | $\alpha_1$PI |
| 92-kDa collagenase (MMP-9)[c] | MAC | Metallo | TIMP |
| Cathepsin L | MAC | Cysteine | Cystatin |
| Smoke-induced cysteine-proteinase | MAC | Cysteine | Cystatin |

[a]PMN, polymorphonuclear leukocytes; MAC, alveolar macrophages.
[b]$\alpha_1$PI, $\alpha_1$-proteinase inhibitor; MPI, mucus proteinase inhibitor; $\alpha_1$ACHY, $\alpha_1$-antichymotrypsin; TIMP, tissue inhibitor of metalloproteinases.
[c]MMP, matrix metalloproteinase.

may be calculated using the foregoing $\alpha_1$PI concentration in the epithelial lining fluid [37]. This figure is identical to that calculated for NE [35], indicating that proteinase-3 and NE are inhibited with the same efficiency in the lower respiratory tract. Unlike NE, proteinase-3 is not inhibited by the mucus proteinase inhibitor [23,37]. As discussed above, this inhibitor readily inhibits elastin-bound NE, a property not shared by $\alpha_1$PI. If elastin-bound proteinase-3 is also resistant to inhibition by $\alpha_1$PI, elastolysis may occur despite the presence of $\alpha_1$PI.

### B. Elastases from Alveolar Macrophages

Smokers have many more macrophages in their lower respiratory tract than do nonsmokers. In addition, a markedly increased number of these cells are found in the vicinity of those small airways, where destructive changes are most prominent [38]. Smoking rapidly alters the cell surface protein composition [39] and the plasma membrane fluidity of alveolar macrophages [40]. These changes persist for a long time after smoking cessation.

Human alveolar macrophages have been shown to internalize human NE in vitro and in vivo and to release this enzyme in an active form [1]. By this mechanism NE may escape the action of endogenous elastase inhibitors and may be liberated at sites where the antielastase protection is weak. Senior et al. [41] recently observed that elastin degradation by human alveolar macrophages was largely inhibited by tissue inhibitor of metalloproteinases (TIMP), suggesting that it is due, at least in part, to one or more metalloproteinases. Later, these authors found that the activity was due to the 92-kDa type IV collage-nase/gelatinase, also called matrix metalloproteinase-9 (MMP-9). On a molar basis MMP-9 was 30% as active as NE, an important finding [42]. Macrophages also synthesize TIMP [43].

Human alveolar macrophages also degrade elastin by a process that involves acidic cysteine proteinases [1]. Liver lysosomal cathepsin L, a cysteine proteinase, solubilizes elastin at a slightly acidic pH. An immunologically and functionally related enzyme has been partially purified from human alveolar macrophages. The participation of macrophage cathepsin L in the degradation of elastin is possible because macrophages are able to generate a local acidic environment (ref. 44 and references therein). Cigarette smoking induces a further elastolytic cysteine proteinase different from cathepsin L [45]. Plasma-derived cysteine proteinase inhibitors might control this activity [46]. The macrophage itself synthesizes cystatin C [47].

### IV. Stimulation of Elastolysis by Nonelastolytic Proteinases

Nonelastolytic proteinases may stimulate the elastolytic activity of neutrophil and macrophage elastases by cleaving extracellular matrix proteins other than elastin.

This unmasks elastin fibers and therefore eases their elastase-catalyzed break-down. In addition, these nonelastolytic proteinases may inactivate proteinase inhibitors and therefore enable unimpaired proteolysis.

## A. Cleavage of Extracellular Matrix Proteins

Lung elastic fibers are embedded in a complex mix of structural proteins (collagen, proteoglycans) and nonstructural glycoproteins (fibronectin, laminin). Degradation of these matrix components probably facilitates the action of elastases on elastin as suggested by experiments with in vitro–prepared extracel-lular matrices [1]. NE and cathepsin G themselves are able to cleave interstitial collagen (i.e., collagen I, II, III), proteoglycans, and fibronectin [1].

Neutrophils and macrophages synthesize latent collagenases named ma-trix metalloproteinase-8 (neutrophils) and matrix metalloproteinase-9 (macro-phages). These enzymes are active on lung interstitial collagens. The neutro-phils' collagenase is stored in the specific granules of these cells. The sequence of its 467 amino acids has recently been deduced from the nucleotide sequence of a cDNA clone [48]. Macrophages also secrete matrix metalloproteinases-3 (stromelysin), which also acts on matrix components. All these matrix me-talloproteinases are secreted as latent enzymes. They are activated in vivo by plasmin, NE, and cathepsin G [49] or by oxidants [50]. The main physiologic inhibitor of these proteinases is the tissue inhibitor of metalloproteinases (TIMP) [51].

The specific granules of neutrophils contain plasminogen activator, a trypsin-like proteinase that is also associated with the cell membrane of macrophages. This enzyme generates plasmin from plasminogen, a proenzyme present in the lung interstitium [52]. Plasmin activates latent matrix metallopro-teinases and cleaves fibronectin, laminin, and other interstitial glycoproteins. Its activity is regulated primarily by $\alpha_2$-antiplasmin. The physiologic inhibitor of plasminogen activator is plasminogen activator inhibitor 1. Chapman et al. [52] cultured macrophages on an elastin-rich extracellular matrix and showed that the rate of elastin solubilization increased markedly upon addition of plasminogen, thus providing in vitro evidence for plasminogen activator–induced stimulation of elastolysis.

## B. Inactivation of Proteinase Inhibitors

The proteolytic inactivation of $\alpha_1$PI has been dealt with in Section II.C. NE is able to inactivate $\alpha_1$-antichymotrypsin [53], $\alpha_2$-antiplasmin [54], TIMP [55], and cystatin C [56]. This will facilitate the proteolytic degradation of lung matrix proteins other than elastin (see Fig. 1).

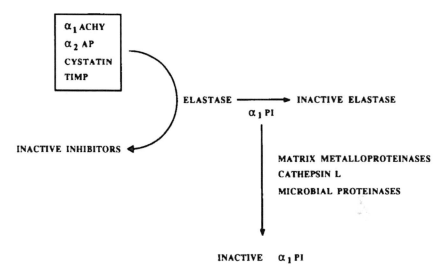

**Figure 1** Proteolytic inactivation of proteinase inhibitors. $\alpha_1$ACHY, $\alpha_1$-antichymotrypsin; $\alpha_2$AP, $\alpha_2$-antiplasmin; TIMP, tissue inhibitor of metalloproteinases; $\alpha_1$PI, $\alpha_1$-proteinase inhibitor.

## V. Stimulation of Elastolysis by Oxidants

### A. Source and Nature of Oxidants

Air may contain oxidants such as ozone ($O_3$) and nitrogene dioxide ($NO_2$). Welding fumes contain large amounts of these species. The gas phase of cigarette smoke contains free radicals (R·), which may generate the superoxide anion ($O_2^{·-}$), hydrogen peroxide ($H_2O_2$), and the hydroxyl radical (·OH). One puff of cigarette is thought to contain $5 \times 10^{14}$ free radicals. Because these radicals are long-lived (>5 min), they may still be deleterious in sidestream smoke. Cigarette tar also contains free radicals [57]. The generation of oxidants by phagocytes is illustrated in Figure 2. Hydrochlorite (HOCl), the major product of the neutrophil's respiratory burst, is an extremely potent and stable oxidant responsible for most of the oxidation reactions [50].

### B. Biological Effects of Oxidants

The oxidation of $\alpha_1$PI discussed in Section II.C is not the only mechanism by which oxidants may stimulate elastolysis. Mucus proteinase inhibitor, the inhibitor of elastin-bound NE, also undergoes oxidant-mediated inactivation [1,58]. Oxidants may increase elastolysis by at least two other mechanisms (see

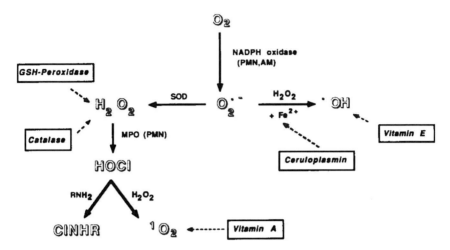

**Figure 2** Oxidants and antioxidants secreted by lung phagocytes. PMN, polymorphonuclear leukocyte; AM, alveolar macrophage; SOD, superoxide dismutase; GSH, glutathion; MPO, myeloperoxidase. The boxed compounds are antioxidants. During the
respiratory burst, latent membrane-bound NADPH oxidase from PMN and AM is activated
and transforms molecular oxygen ($O_2$) into the superoxide anion ($O_2^{.-}$), a short-lived and
poor oxidant (better qualified as a reducing agent), which is nevertheless dramatically
harmful because it generates potent oxidants. The Haber–Weiss reaction, which leads to
the strongly oxidant hydroxyl radical ($^.OH$), is probably of little importance in vivo because
(1) lactoferrin, present in the extracellular milieu, scavenges $Fe^{2+}$, and (2) $H_2O_2$ is rapidly
transformed by MPO into hypochlorite (HOCl), a very potent and stable oxidant. This
species may react with amines to yield the less potent but very stable chloramines ClNHR.
Hypochlorite may also decay into singlet oxygen ($^1O_2$).

Fig. 3). First, activation of latent metalloproteinases [50] may lead to enhanced
$\alpha_1$PI inactivation, increased cleavage of extracellular matrix proteins, or even
macrophage MMP-9-mediated elastolysis (see Section III.B). Second, inactivation of plasminogen activator inhibitor [59] leads to an overproduction of plasmin
with resultant cleavage of matrix glycoproteins and activation of latent matrix
metalloproteinases (see Section IV).

Oxidants may also impair the resynthesis of elastin by decreasing the
activity of lysyloxidase, the enzyme that cross-links tropoelastin [2]. Elastase-
induced emphysema in rats is enhanced by cigarette smoke [60] as a result of
an impairment of elastin resynthesis [61]. Finally, it should be mentioned that
oxidants may injure epithelial cells, collagen, hyaluronic acid, and elastin directly
[2,62].

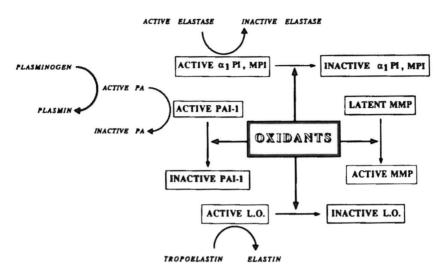

**Figure 3**   Some effects of oxidants on the proteinase–antiproteinase–elastin system. $\alpha_1$PI, $\alpha_1$-proteinase inhibitor; MPI, mucus proteinase inhibitor; PA, plasminogen activator; PAI-1, plasminogen activator inhibitor-1; MMP, matrix metalloproteinase; L.O., lysyloxidase.

### C.   Antioxidants

Oxidants are buffered to some extent by endogenous antioxidants some of which are shown in Figure 2. Although it generates $H_2O_2$, superoxide dismutase is considered as the major antioxidant of the lung because it prevents the transformation of $O_2^{\cdot-}$ into the highly toxic radical $^{\cdot}OH$. The glutathion (GSH), glutathion peroxidase, and glutathion reductase system is also a very important antioxidant:

$$2GSH + H_2O_2 \; \underset{\substack{\text{GSSG-reductase} \\ + \text{ NADPH}}}{\overset{\text{GSH-peroxidase}}{\rightleftharpoons}} \; GSSG + 2H_2O$$

This system also reduces cell membrane lipid peroxides. Glutathion is synthesized by most mammalian cells and occurs in high concentration in the epithelial lining fluid [50,63]. The spontaneous dismutation of $H_2O_2$ into $H_2O + O_2$ is enhanced considerably by catalase, the third antioxidant enzyme. Catalase is present in the alveolar epithelial lining fluid [64].

Methionine peptide sulfoxide reductase may be considered as an antioxidant since it catalyzes the reduction of methionine sulfoxide into methionine in proteins. This enzyme is able to reduce and reactivate oxidized $\alpha_1$PI [1], oxidized mucus proteinase inhibitor [58], and oxidized plasminogen activator inhibitor I [59]. This reductase is present in neutrophils and type II pneumocytes. Its in vivo function is, however, unclear [65].

Ceruloplasmin oxidizes $Fe^{2+}$ into $Fe^{3+}$ and therefore prevents the formation of $\cdot OH$ (see Fig. 1). This 134-kDa plasma protein occurs, however, in low amounts in the epithelial lining fluid. Vitamin A, C, and E are further antioxidants. These oxidant scavengers appear to play a minor role compared to that of the antioxidant enzymes [50]. Chronic smoking results in an increase in the activity of superoxide dismutase and catalase in macrophages as a possible response to the oxidant burden [66].

## VI.  Summary and Discussion

Smoking is undoubtedly a major risk factor for the development of emphysema in $\alpha_1$PI-sufficient individuals. It induces chronic lung inflammation characterized by an important recruitment and activation of phagocytes with a resultant proteinase and oxidant burden. Oxidation considerably reduces the activity of $\alpha_1$PI but does not lead to an acquired deficiency in $\alpha_1$PI activity in smokers' lungs since high amounts of active $\alpha_1$PI are present in lung lavage fluids of heavy smokers with emphysema. Oxidative inactivation of $\alpha_1$PI with resultant NE-mediated proteolysis, may, however occur in the immediate surroundings of the activated neutrophil. These local phenomena cannot be detected by lung lavage. There are several other mechanisms by which NE may exert proteolysis in the presence of $\alpha_1$PI: (1) partial proteolysis is the unavoidable consequence of in vivo competitive inhibition; (2) the inhibitory activity of $\alpha_1$PI may be overcome or strongly impaired by proteolytic inactivation in the immediate vicinity of a neutrophil; (3) if a neutrophil contacts an extracellular matrix protein, $\alpha_1$PI is excluded from the pericellular environment; and (4) a significant part of elastin-bound NE resists inhibition by $\alpha_1$PI.

Neutrophils secrete cathepsin G and proteinase-3, two additional elastolytic serine proteinases inhibited by $\alpha_1$PI. These enzymes may mediate proteolysis in the presence of $\alpha_1$PI for reasons similar to those given for NE. On the other hand, alveolar macrophages have three $\alpha_1$PI-resistant elastases: matrix metalloproteinase-9, cathepsin L, and a smoking-induced cysteine proteinase. Elastolysis may be potentiated by nonelastolytic proteinases such as collagenases and plasminogen activator. These enzymes are able to cleave matrix proteins and may inactivate proteinase inhibitors.

Oxidants are potent cofactors of the proteolytic systems described above. They strongly impair the inhibitory potential of $\alpha_1$PI, mucus proteinase inhibitor, and plasminogen activator inhibitor I. They also activate latent metalloproteinases, injure lung proteins and cells directly, and impair the resynthesis of elastin. The importance of the mucus proteinase inhibitor in the lower respiratory tract is commonly overlooked. This protein is fully able to inhibit elastin-bound NE and to prevent NE-mediated proteolysis at the cell–matrix interface, two properties not shared by $\alpha_1$PI. In addition, its activity is enhanced by glycosaminoglycans.

The pathogenic functions of the numerous factors listed above have been deduced from in vitro experiments. What is the in vivo mechanism for the development of emphysema in $\alpha_1$PI-sufficient individuals? There is no answer to that question as yet. A number of reasonable guesses may be made, however. There are reasons to believe that NE is a very important pathogenic factor. This enzyme occurs in very large quantities: 75 mg are present in 5 L of human blood. Also, NE has the highest specific elastolytic activity among all lung elastases. Further, patients with emphysema have elevated levels of NE–$\alpha_1$PI complex in their epithelial lining fluid and these levels increase with the severity of the disease, indicating that in emphysema there is a marked increase in the rate of neutrophil degranulation [4]. On the other hand, NE has been found to be associated with elastin fibers in emphysematous lung tissue [67]. It should also be restated that NE not only solubilizes elastin but also cleaves interstitial collagen, proteoglycans, and fibronectin and inactivates $\alpha_1$-antichymotrypsin, $\alpha_2$-antiplasmin, tissue inhibitor of metalloproteinases, and cystatin. Thus NE may mediate general proteolysis of lung matrix proteins either directly or indirectly through proteinase inhibitor inactivation.

There is, however, no reason to believe that other elastolytic enzymes do not play a significant role in the pathogenesis of emphysema. For instance, proteinase-3, which is not inhibited by mucus proteinase inhibitor, may exert proteolysis at the neutrophil–matrix interface. On the other hand, cathepsin G might also play a role since it occurs in high amounts in neutrophils, stimulates the activity of NE, and is poorly regulated in the lower respiratory tract. The increased prevalence of abnormal residual lung volume and total lung capacity in persons with heterozygous $\alpha_1$-antichymotrypsin deficiency [68] favors this hypothesis.

The macrophage internalizes NE and may excrete it at sites where the anti-NE protection is weak. Moreover, the smoker's activated macrophage has three additional elastases, one metalloproteinase and two cysteine proteinases. These enzymes are resistant to the inhibitory action of $\alpha_1$PI and mucus proteinase inhibitor. Moreover, a close cell/matrix contact also prevents the action of the metallo- and the cysteine proteinase inhibitors that normally block the action of these enzymes. Macrophages-mediated elastolysis might therefore also play an important role in emphysema. It is worth restating that a markedly increased number of macrophages is found in the vicinity of those small airways where tissue destruction is most prominent and that the smoke-induced changes in the membrane properties of these cells persist long after smoking cessation.

Synthetic or natural NE inhibitors may soon be used in humans to stop the progression of emphysema. These drugs will tell us a great deal about the pathogenetic importance of NE in emphysema.

### References

1. Bieth JG. Elastases: catalytic and biological properties. In: Mecham RP, ed. Regulation of matrix accumulation. New York: Academic Press, 1986:217–320.
2. Janoff A. Emphysema: proteinase–antiproteinase imbalance. In: Gallin JI, Goldstein IM, Snyderman R, eds. Inflammation: basic principles and clinical correlates. New York: Raven Press, 1988:803–14.
3. Abboud RT, Fera T, Richter A, Tabona MZ, Johal S. Acute effect of smoking on the functional activity of $\alpha_1$-proteinase inhibitor in broncho-alveolar lavage fluid. Am Rev Respir Dis 1985;131:79–85.
4. Gast A, Dietemann-Molard A, Pelletier A, Pauli G, Bieth JG. The antielastase screen of the lower respiratory tract of $\alpha_1$-proteinase inhibitor-sufficient patients with emphysema or pneumothorax. Am Rev Respir Dis 1990;141:880–3.
5. Fujita J, Nelson NL, Daughton DM, Dobry CA, Spurzem JR, Irino S, Rennard SI. Evaluation of elastase and antielastase balance in patients with chronic bronchitis and pulmonary emphysema. Am Rev Respir Dis 1990;142:57–62.
6. Bieth JG. In vivo significance of kinetic constants of protein proteinase inhibitors. Biochem Med 1984;32:387–97.
7. Campbell EJ. Preventative therapy of emphysema. Lessons from the elastase model. Am Rev Respir Dis 1986;134:435–37.
8. Padrines M, Bieth JG. Elastin decreases the efficiency of neutrophil elastase inhibitors. Am J Respir Cell Mol Biol 1991;4:187–93.
9. Bruch M, Bieth JG. Influence of elastin on the inhibition of leucocyte elastase by a 1-proteinase inhibitor and bronchial inhibitor. Potent inhibition of elastin-bound elastase by bronchial inhibitor. Biochem J 1986:269–73.
10. Padrines M, Schneider-Pozzer M, Bieth JG. Inhibition of neutrophil elastase by a1-proteinase inhibitor oxidized by activated neutrophils. Am Rev Respir Dis 1989;139:783–90.
11. Hubbard RC, Ogushi F, Fells GA, Cantin AM, Jallat S, Courtney M, Crystal RG. Oxidants spontaneously released by alveolar macrophages of cigarette smokers can inactivate the active site of $\alpha_1$-antitrypsin, rendering it

ineffective as an inhibitor of neutrophil elastase. J Clin Invest 1987;80:1289–95.

12. Wallaert B, Gressier B, Aerts C, Mizon C, Voisin, C, Mizon J. Oxidative inactivation of $\alpha_1$-proteinase inhibitor by alveolar macrophages from healthy smokers requires the presence of myeloperoxidase. Am J Respir Cell Mol Biol 1991;5:437–44.

13. Campbell EJ, Endicott SK, Rios-Mollineda RA. Assessment of oxidation of $\alpha_1$-proteinase inhibitor in bronchoalveolar lining fluid by monoclonal immunoassay: comparison of smokers and non-smokers. Am Rev Respir Dis 1987;135:A156.

14. Desrochers PE, Weiss S. Proteolytic inactivation of $\alpha_1$-proteinase inhibitor by a neutrophil metalloproteinase. J Clin Invest 1988;81:1646–50.

15. Vissers MCM, George PM, Bathurt IC, Brennan OS, Winterbourn CC. Cleavage and inactivation of $\alpha_1$-antitrypsin by metalloproteinases released from neutrophils. J Clin Invest 1888;82:706–11.

16. Johnson DA, Barrett AJ, Mason RW. Cathepsin L inactivates $\alpha_1$-proteinase inhibitor by cleavage in the reactive site region. J Biol Chem 1986;261:14748–51.

17. Virca GD, Lyerly D, Kreger A, Travis J. Inactivation of $\alpha_1$-proteinase inhibitor by *Serratia marcescens* metalloproteinase. Biochim Biophys Acta 1982;704:267–71.

18. Morihara K, Tsuzuki H, Harada M, Iwata T. Purification of human plasma $\alpha_1$-proteinase inhibitor and its inactivation by *Pseudomonas* elastase. J Biochem 1984;95:795–804.

19. Potempa J, Watorek W, Travis J. Inactivation of human $\alpha_1$-proteinase inhibitor by *Staphylococcus aureus* proteinases. J Biol Chem 1986; 261:14330–4.

20. Conlan JW, Williams A, Ashworth LAE. Inactivation of human $\alpha_1$-antitrypsin by a tissue-destructive protease of *Legionella pneumophila*. J Gen Microbiol 1988;134:481–87.

21. Hamdaoui A, Wund-Bisseret F, Bieth JG. Fast solubilization of human lung elastin by *Pseudomonas aeruginosa* elastase. Am Rev Respir Dis 1987;135:860–36.

22. Campbell EJ, Campbell MA. Pericellular proteolysis by neutrophils in the presence of proteinase inhibitors: effects of substrate opsonisation. J Cell Biol 1988;106:667–76.

23. Rice WG, Weiss SJ. Regulation of proteolysis at the neutrophil–substrate interface by secretory leukoprotease inhibitor. Science 1990;249:178–81.

24. Frommherz KJ, Faller B, Bieth JG. Heparin strongly decreases the rate of inhibition of neutrophil elastase by $a_1$-proteinase inhibitor. J Biol Chem 1991;266:15356–62.

25. Navia MA, McKeever BM, Springer JP, Lin TY, Williams HR, Fluder

EM, Dorn CP, Hoogsteen K. Structure of human neutrophil elastase in complex with a peptide chloromethyl ketone inhibitor at 1.84-Å resolution. Proc Natl Acad Sci USA 1989;86:7–11.

26. Clark JG, Kuhn C, McDonald JA, Mecham RP. Lung connective tissue. In: Hall DA, Jackson DS, eds. International review of connective tissue research. Vol. 10. New York: Academic Press, 1983:249–331.

27. Faller B, Bieth JG. Heparin increases the rate of inhibition of neutrophil elastase by mucus proteinase inhibitor. Am Rev Respir Dis 1991; 143(Suppl):A328.

28. Ogushi F, Hubbard RC, Vogelmeier C, Fells GA, Crystal RG. Risk factors for emphysema. Cigarette smoking is associated with a reduction in the association rate constant of lung $\alpha_1$-antitrypsin for neutrophil elastase. J Clin Invest 1991;87:1060–65.

29. Bieth JG. Pathophysiological interpretation of kinetic constants of protease inhibitors. Bull Eur Physiopathol Respir 1980;16(Suppl):183–95.

30. Salvesen G, Farley D, Shuman J, Przybyla A, Reilly C, Travis J. Molecular cloning of human cathepsin G: structural similarity to mast cell and cytotoxic T lymphocyte proteinase. Biochemistry 1987;26:2289–93.

31. Boudier C, Holle C, Bieth JG. Stimulation of the elastolytic activity of leukocyte elastase by leukocyte cathepsin G. J Biol Chem 1981;256:10256–58.

32. Lucey EC, Stone JP, Breuer R, Christensen TG, Calore JD, Cantanese A, Franzblau C, Snider GL. Effects of combined human neutrophil cathepsin G and elastase on induction of secretory cell metaplasia and emphysema in hamster with in vitro observations on elastolysis by these enzymes. Am Rev Respir Dis 1985;132:362–66.

33. Boudier C, Godeau G, Hornebeck W, Robert L. Bieth JG. The elastolytic activity of cathepsin G. An ex vivo study with dermal elastin. Am J Respir Cell Mol Biol 1991;4:497–503.

34. Berman G, Afford SC, Burnett D, Stockley SA. $\alpha_1$-Antichymotrypsin in lung secretions is not an effective proteinase inhibitor. J Biol Chem 1986;261:14095–99.

35. Ogushi F, Hubbard RC, Fells GA, Casolaro MA, Curiel DT, Brandy ML, Crystal RG. Evaluation of the S-type of $\alpha_1$-antitrypsin as an in vivo and in vitro inhibitor of neutrophil elastase. Am Rev Respir Dis 1988;137:364–70.

36. Kao RC, Wehner NG, Skubitz KM, Gray BH, Hoidal JR. Proteinase 3. A distinct human polymorphonuclear leukocyte proteinase that produces emphysema in hamsters. J Clin Invest 1988;82:1963–73.

37. Rao, NV, Wehner NG, Marshall BC, Gray WR, Gray BH, Hoidal JR. Characterization of proteinase-3 (PR-3), a neutrophil serine proteinase. Structural and functional properties. J Biol Chem 1991;266:9540–48.

38. Niewoehner DE, Kleinerman J, Rice DB, Pathologic changes in the peripheral airways of young cigarette smokers. N Engl J Med 1974;291:755–58.
39. Skubitz KM, Northfelt DW, McGowan SE, Hoidal JR. Changes in the cell surface protein composition of human alveolar macrophages induced by smoking. Cancer Res 1987;47:3072–82.
40. Hannan SE, Harris JO, Sheridan NP, Patel JM. Cigarette smoke alters plasma membrane fluidity of rat alveolar macrophages. Am Rev Respir Dis 1989;140:168–73.
41. Senior RM, Connoly NL, Cury JD, Welgus HG, Campbell EJ. Elastin degradation by human alveolar macrophages. Am Rev Respir Dis 1989;139:1251–56.
42. Senior RM, Griffin GL, Fliszar CJ, Shapiro SD, Goldberg GI, Welgus HG. Human 92– and 72-kilodalton type IV collagenases are elastases. J Biol Chem 1991;266:7870–75.
43. Albin RJ, Senior RM, Welgus HG, Connoly NL, Campbell EJ. Human alveolar macrophages secrete an inhibitor of metalloproteinase elastase. Am Rev Respir Dis 1987;135:1281–85.
44. Reilly JJ Jr, Mason RW, Chen P, Joseph LJ, Sukhatme VP, Yee R, Chapmann HA Jr. Synthesis and processing of cathepsin L, an elastase by human alveolar macrophages. Biochem J 1989;257:493–98.
45. Reilly JJ Jr, Chen P, Sailor LZ, Wilcox D, Mason RW, Chapman RA Jr. Cigarette smoking induces an elastolytic cysteine proteinase in macrophages distinct from cathepsin L. Am J Physiol 1991;261:L41–L48.
46. Barrett AJ, Rawlings D, Davies ME, Machleidt W, Salvesen G, Turk V. Cysteine proteinase inhibitors of the cystatin superfamily. In: Barrett AJ, Salvesen G, eds. Proteinase inhibitors. New York: Elsevier, 1986:515–69.
47. Chapman HA, Reilly JJ Jr, Yee R, Grubb A. Identification of cystatin C, a cysteine proteinase inhibitor, as a major secretory product of human alveolar macrophages in vitro. Am Rev Respir Dis 1990;141:698–705.
48. Hasty KA, Pourmotabbed TF, Goldberg GI, Thompson JP, Spinella DG, Stevens RM, Mainardi CL. Human neutrophil collagenase. A distinct gene product with homology to other matrix metalloproteinases. J Biol Chem 1990;265:11421–24.
49. Okada Y, Nakanishi I. Inactivation of matrix metalloproteinase 3 (stromelysin) and matrix metalloproteinase 2 ("gelatinase") by human elastase and cathepsin G. FEBS Lett 1989;249;353–56.
50. Weiss SJ. Mechanisms of disease. Tissue destruction by neutrophils. N Engl J Med 1989;320:365–76.
51. Sibille Y, Reynolds HY. Macrophages and polymorphonuclear neutrophils in lung defense and injury. Am Rev Respir Dis 1990;141:471–501.
52. Chapman HA Jr, Reilly JJ Jr, Kobzik L. Role of plasminogen activator

in degradation of extracellular matrix protein by live human alveolar macrophages. Am Rev Respir Dis 1988;137:412–19.

53. Morii M, Travis J. Amino acid sequence at the reactive site of human a₁-antichymotrypsin. J Biol Chem 1983;258:12749–52.

54. Brower MS, Harpel PC. Proteolytic cleavage and inactivation of a₂-plasmin inhibitor and C1 inactivator by human polymorphonuclear leukocyte elastase. J Biol Chem 1982;257:9849–54.

55. Okada Y, Watanabe S, Nakanishi I, Kishi JI, Hayakawa T, Warorek W, Travis J, Nagase I. Inactivation of tissue inhibitor of metalloproteinase by neutrophil elastase and other proteinases. FEBS Lett 1988;229:157–60.

56. Abrahamson M, Mason RW, Hansson H, Buttle DJ, Grubb A, Ohlsson K. Human cystatin C. Role of the N-terminal segment in the inhibition of human cysteine proteinases and in its inactivation by leucocyte elastase. Biochem J 1991;273:621–26.

57. Pryor WA, Prier DG, Church DF. Electron-spin resonance study of mainstream and sidestream cigarette smoke: nature of the free radicals in gas-phase smoke and in cigarette tar. Environ Health Perspect 1983;47:345–55.

58. Kramps JA, van Twisk C, Appelhans H, Meckelein B, Nikiforov T, Dijkman JH. Proteinase inhibitory activities of antileukoprotease are represented by its second COOH-terminal domain. Biochim Biophys Acta 1990;1038:178–85.

59. Lawrence DA, Loskutoff DJ. Inactivation of plasminogen activator inhibitor by oxidants. Biochemistry 1986;25:6351–55.

60. Kimmel EC, Winsett DW, Diamond L. Augmentation of elastase-induced emphysema by cigarette smoke. Description of a model and a review of possible mechanisms. Am Rev Respir Dis 1985;132:885–93.

61. Osman M, Kaldany RRJ, Cantor JO, Turino GM, Mandl I. Stimulation of lung lysyl oxidase activity in hamsters with elastase-induced emphysema. Am Rev Respir Dis 1985;131:169–70.

62. Rao NV, Hoidal JR. Oxidized halogens degrade elastin: a potential mechanism for smoking-induced emphysema. In: Mittman C. Taylor JC, eds. 2nd International Symposium on Pulmonary Emphysema and Proteolysis. New York: Academic Press, 1986.

63. Janoff A. Biochemical links between cigarette smoking and pulmonary emphysema. J Appl Physiol Respir Environ Exercise Physiol 1983;55:285–93.

64. Cantin AM, Fells GA, Hubbard RC, Crystal RG. Antioxidant macromolecules in the epithelial lining fluid of the normal human lower respiratory tract. J Clin Invest 1990;86:962–71.

65. Swaim MW, Pizzo SV. Methionine sulfoxide and the oxidative regulation of plasma proteinase inhibitors. J Leukocyte Biol 1988;43:365–79.

66. McCusker K, Hoidal J. Selective increase of antioxidant enzyme activity in the alveolar macrophages from cigarette smokers and smoke-exposed hamsters. J Clin Invest 1990;86:962–71.

67. Damiano VV, Tsang A, Kucich U, Abrams WR, Rosenbloom J, Kimbel P, Fallahnejad M, Weinbaum G. Immunolocalization of elastase in human emphysematous lungs. J Clin Invest 1986;78:482–83.

68. Lindmark BEM, Arborelius M Jr, Erikson SG. Pulmonary function in middle-aged women with heterozygous deficiency of the serine proteinase inhibitor $a_1$-antichymotrypsin. Am Rev Respir Dis 1990;141:884–88.

# 19

## Serum and Urinary Markers for Lung Elastin and Collagen Degradation

**D. J. HARTMANN**

Institut Pasteur de Lyon
Lyon, France

**P. A. LAURENT**

INSERM U139
Créteil, France

**M. P. JACOB and C. LAFUMA**

CNRS (UA CNRS 1460)
Créteil, France

## I. Introduction

Collagen and elastin are the two major structural proteins of the lung extracellular matrix. Fibrillar cross-linked types I, III, and V collagen, beaded filaments of type VI collagen, sheets of type IV collagen, and anchoring fibrils of type VII collagen [1] are variously distributed among the microarchitectures of the alveolar wall. Also, lung elastin is secreted as its proform, tropoelastin, which is deposited onto microfibrils [2] and cross-linked extracellularly to form mature fibers. So the elastic fiber network in the lung contributes to its resilience. Collagen and elastin degradation by various proteinases, mostly resulting in plasma and urinary peptides release, is believed to be an important component of physiologic processes such as morphogenesis and remodeling of the lung, wound healing, and embryogenesis. In addition to the maintenance of normal pulmonary function, the process of uncontrolled matrix destruction has received attention in the study of pathologic states including lung fibrosis, emphysema, and tumor metastasis.

Several classes of metalloproteinases secreted by resident lung cells are involved in the extracellular degradation of collagen. As the enzyme responsible for initiating the degradation of interstitial fibrillar collagens [3], the collagenase (matrix metalloproteinase-1) constitutes one of the pivotal control points for collagen metabolism; it can cleave the native tripe helical region into characteristic ¾ and ¼ collagen degradation fragments that may be degraded further by other matrix metalloendoproteinases. Matrix metalloproteinase-5 [4] degrades native 3/4 collagen fragments, whereas matrix metalloproteinase-2, also designated type IV collagenase or gelatinase, cleaves denatured α chains of collagen, as well as native full-length type IV collagen [5]. Both 72- and 92-kDa type IV collagenases have been reported to be identical to gelatinases secreted by connective tissue cells, leucocytes, and tumor cells, whereas macrophage 92 kDa would be able to degrade type V collagen [6]. On the other hand, stromelysin, also designated proteoglycanase (matrix metalloproteinase-3), secreted from the connective tissue cells, is also able to degrade type IV collagen as well as gelatin and removes the $NH_2$-terminal propeptides of type I procollagen [3,7,8]; it is also thought to be the mediator necessary for assumption of full collagenolytic activity [9]. Stromelysin itself, as well as gelatinases, may be activated by human neutrophil elastase and cathepsin G [10]. Furthermore, telopeptidase (matrix metalloproteinase-4) may facilitate collagenolysis by the cleavage of the carboxy-terminal telopeptide region of collagen [11]. Regulation of all these matrix metalloproteinases expression by growth factors, oncogenes, or mediators of inflammation and tumor promoters can occur either at the level of gene expression, including transcription and translation, at the level of activation, or at the level of inhibition by tissue inhibitor of metalloproteinases (TIMP) and $\alpha_2$-macroglobuline [12]. Also, a role for lysosomal collagenolytic lung cysteine proteinases (cathepsins B, L, N, and T) may be considered because of their ability to degrade native collagen at acid pH in the pericellular microenvironment [14]. Finally, lysosomal serine proteinase, such as leucocyte elastase, exhibits broad specificity toward collagen types II and III as well as collagen type IV or types IX, X, and XI (for a review, see ref. 14). Moreover, changes in degradation of newly synthesized lung collagen [15] would probably occur intracellularly and may be relevant in various pathological states, such as pulmonary fibrosis, where excessive collagen deposition occurs.

Elastin degradation and imperfect repair are held to be pivotal in the pathogenesis of pulmonary emphysema [16]. Elastin degradation may be effected by proteinases, designated "elastases," with variable specificities and mechanisms of action. It is well known that (1) elastinolysis may lead to peptide bond cleavage with or without generation of soluble peptides, and (2) elastases are not "specific" for elastin, since they hydrolyze other extracellular matrix components as well [17]. The catalytic sites and mechanisms of peptide bond hydrolysis by serine, cysteine, or metalloelastases have been reviewed [16]. Three serine elastinolytic enzymes—human leucocyte elastase, cathepsin G, and proteinase-3—are able to degrade elastin and so to induce or potentialize lung emphysema [18,19]. Human alveolar macrophages contain cathepsin L, a cysteine proteinase exhibiting elastinolytic activity [20]; and a second elastino-lytic cysteine proteinase with optimal activity at pH 5.5 has been identified in human alveolar macrophages [21] and was proposed to increase the potential of these cells to participate in the connective lung matrix destruction that is the hallmark of emphysema. Furthermore, macrophage metalloelastase has been described extensively (for a review, see ref. 22) and more recently, matrix metalloproteinases such as 92- and 72-kDa type IV collagenases, both present in alveolar cells or septa, were found to possess elastase activity [23] and are thought to be involved in the pathogenesis of chronic disorders such as pulmonary emphysema. Finally, metalloelastase of *Pseudomonas aeruginosa* causing serine pulmonary infection is also well known to actively degrade elastin into small peptides [24,25] as well as to inactivate human leucocyte inhibitors, so favorizing the destruction of lung tissue.

We propose here a synthesis review about the evaluation of plasma or urinary collagen, elastin peptides, and desmosine, as well as their possible use as biological markers of lung collagen and elastin degradation, more particularly during lung disorders.

## II. Collagen Peptides

It is well known that collagen molecules are major constituents of the extracellular matrix of most organs; they function primarily as supporting elements, but they also have other roles through their interaction with cells. They include in their structure one or several domains with a characteristic triple helical conformation formed of three $\alpha$ chains, the primary sequence of which is composed of repetition of the triplet Gly-Xaa-Yaa, Pro and OH-Pro often in the Xaa and Yaa positions, respectively. Fourteen collagen types have been described so far (for a review, see Van der Rest and Garrone [1]), formed of at least 28 polypeptide chains representing unique gene products. They could be divided into [1]:

1. Collagens forming homo- and heterofibrils: types I, II, III, V, and XI
2. Collagens forming nonfibrillar networks: types IV (in basement membranes), VI forming thin-beaded filaments, VIII (in Descemet's membrane), and probably X (in the hypertrophic cartilage)
3. Other collagens playing a connective role between tissue components, including the fibril-associated collagens with interrupted triple helices (FACITs) (types IX, XII, and XIV) and the type VII (anchoring fibrils) (Table 1)

In the mammalian lung, the region bounded by the basement membranes of the alveolar epithelium and the capillary endothelium contains fibrillar

**Table 1** Collagen Types

| Collagen type | Molecule | Tissular distribution | Characteristics |
|---|---|---|---|
| I | $[\alpha1(I)]_2\, \alpha2(I)$ | Skin, tendon, bone, lung, and many connective tissues | Thick, well-organized fibrils, low level of Hyl and carbohydrates |
| I trimer | $[\alpha1(I)]_3$ | Embryonic or pathological tissues, low amount in tissues (skin, dentin) | More Hyl than in type I, different peptide pattern after V8 protease action |
| II | $[\alpha1(II)]_3$ | Hyaline cartilage, intervertebral disk, vitreous body | Fine fibrils; rich in Hyl, Gal-Hyl, and Glc-Gal-Hyl |
| III | $[\alpha1(III)]_3$ | Skin, vessels, liver, placenta, lung, embryonic tissues (often associated with type I) | Presence of Cys and intramolecular disulfide bonds |
| IV | $[\alpha1(IV)]_2\, \alpha2(IV)$ $\alpha3(IV),\, \alpha4(IV),\, \alpha5(IV)$ (?) | Basement membranes Glomerular basement membrane | Rich in Hyp-Hyl, low level of Ala, Arg; several residues of 3-Hyp; highly glycosylated |
| V | $[\alpha1(V)]_2\, \alpha2(V)$ $\alpha1(V)\alpha2(V)\alpha3(V)$ $[\alpha1(V)]_3$ | Fetal membranes, bone, skin, lung Placenta Hamster lung cells cultures (associated with type I fibrils) | Rich in basic amino acids, low level of Ala, no Cys |
| VI | $[\alpha1(VI)\alpha2(VI)\alpha3(VI)]$ | Aorta intima, placenta, skin, cartilage, intervertebral disk, lung, liver, vessels | High-molecular-weight aggregates; many noncollagenic domains; rich in Cys, Tyr, Hyl, and glycosylated Hyl; low levels in Ala and Hyp; presence of glucosamine |
| VII | $[\alpha1(VII)]_3$ | Dermal-epidermal junction (anchoring fibrils) | Large triple helical domain, rich in Cys |
| VIII | $\alpha1(VIII),\, \alpha2(VIII)$ (?) | Descemet membrane, endothelial cells cultures | Rich in 3-Hyp and glycosylated Hyl, absence of disulfide bonds despite a high concentration in Cys, highly sensitive to proteases, many homologies with type X |
| IX | $[\alpha1(IX)\alpha2(IX)\alpha3(IX)]$ | Hyaline cartilage, intervertebral disk, vitreous humour | FACIT, rich in Cys, presence of a GAG chain, located at the surface of type II fibrils |
| X | $[\alpha1(X)]_3$ | Growth plate | Rich in Tyr, Met, and imino acids |
| XI | $[\alpha1(XI)\alpha2(XI)\alpha3(XI)]$ | Hyaline cartilage, chondrosarcoma (associated with type II fibrils) | $\alpha3(XI)$ identical to $\alpha1(II)$ but hyperglycosylated |
| XII | $[\alpha1(XII)]_3$ | Embryonic tendon and skin, periodontal ligament (associated with type I fibrils) | FACIT, many noncollagenous domains |
| XIII | $\alpha1(XIII)(?)$ | Endothelial cell cultures | Described from ADNc studies, presence of 4 ARNm |
| XIV | $[\alpha1(XIV)]_3$ | Fetal tendon and skin | FACIT, similar structure with type XII |

collagens types I, III, and V [26]. As in other tissues, they are of crucial importance for structural and mechanical properties of the lung; they account for about 20% of the dry weight of normal lung in a ratio of 18:3:1 for types I, III, and V, respectively. The cross-banded fibers and smaller fibrils are composed of these collagens, mixed or not. Lung also contains type VI collagen, forming independent filaments and perhaps type XII. Moreover, type IV collagen is also present but only in the basement membranes [26]. The collagens are synthesized and secreted as high-molecular-weight precursors, the procollagens, composed of the collagen molecule and two extension peptides (the amino- and carboxy-terminal propeptides) at both ends that can be cleaved enzymatically following a not completely known process during fibrillogenesis [27].

Lung cells, including fibroblasts, endothelial cells, or alveolar epithelial cells, produce different types of collagen molecules. Many collagen genes have been isolated and found to be very large with a size of 25,000 to 50,000 base pairs divided into many coding exons (44 for triple helix coding, many of them of 54 bp or multiples of 54 bp) and long interrupting introns. After the transcription step and the processing of premRNA into mature mRNA in the nuclei, the latter is translated into the procollagen chains by the membrane-bound polysomes of the rough endoplasmic reticulum. Then occurs the hydroxylation of proline and lysine residues under the control of prolyl-4 hydroxylase and lysyl hydroxylase, respectively, and some of the hydroxylysine residues are glyco-sylated. Prolyl-4 hydroxylase is a key enzyme because without hydroxylation of the proline, the collagen chains do not fold into stable triple helices and are either intracellularly degraded or secreted as nonfunctional protein [27]. Thus specific inhibition of this enzyme is a pharmacological target for fibrotic diseases. Then the chains can aggregate to form the specific triple helical structure. Later, the procollagen molecule is secreted. At the extracellular level, fibrillogenesis, which is a complex phenomenon, can occur with or without cleavage of propeptides by specific enzymes and leading to a supramolecular structure; finally, intra- and intermolecular reducible and mature cross-links are generated and catalyzed by lysyl oxidase. Thus collagen biosynthesis is a multistep process (Tables 2 and 3); each of these steps may be deregulating and leading to pathological situations.

## A. Methods for Assessing Collagen Peptides

The remodeling of extracellular matrix is often a slow process involving both synthesis and degradation. As a matter of fact, fibrosis is the result of fibrogenesis and fibrolysis. With the exception of assays for specific enzymes (which are outside the scope of this chapter), analytical methods often measure the resultant of the two [28]. Several collagen products have been detected in human body fluids; however, little is known about the normal phases and regulation of collagen in the human body, particularly the lung. As type III procollagen is

**Table 2**  Biosynthesis of Collagen

Transcription and translation
  Biosynthesis and processing of pre-mRNA
  Translation

Intracellular modifications
  Removal of prepeptide sequences
  4-Hydroxylation of peptidyl proline
  3-Hydroxylation of peptidyl proline
  Hydroxylation of peptidyl lysine
  Glycosylation of peptidyl hydroxylysine
  Glycosylation of propeptides
  Chain association and disulfide bonding
  Triple helix formation
  Translocation and secretion of procollagen

Extracellular modifications (not for all collagen types)
  Conversion of procollagen to collagen
  Ordered aggregation
  Cross-link formation

**Table 3**  Co- and Post-Translational Modifications of Collagen

| Enzyme | Substrate | Cofactors | Inhibitors | Effect on collagen |
|---|---|---|---|---|
| Prolyl 4-hydroxylase | Proline | 2-Oxoglutarate ascorbate, $Fe^{2+}$, $O_2$ | $\alpha\alpha'$-Dipyridyl, $N_2$ atmosphere | Stability of triple helix |
| Lysyl hydroxylase | Lysine | Ascorbate, $Fe^{2+}$, $O_2$ | $\alpha\alpha'$-Dipyridyl, $N_2$ atmosphere | Stabilization of covalent cross-links, attachment site for sugar moieties |
| Glucosyltransferase | Procollagen | — | — | Linkage to oligosaccharides |
| Gal-Glc-transferase | Procollagen | — | — | Linkage to oligosaccharides |
| N-/C-Propeptidase | Procollagen | — | — | Cleavage of propeptides |
| Lysyl oxidase | Collagen | $Cu^{2+}$ (pyridoxal 5'-phosphate or pyrroloquinoline quinone) | $\beta$-Aminopropionitrile, D-penicillamine | Intermolecular cross-links |

often synthesized during the initial phase of the fibroproliferative response, assays for its metabolic products are of clinical interest and have been developed. Additional assays for type I and IV collagens have been proposed. An assay for type VI collagen was described several years ago but never applied to lung diseases [29].

## Type III Procollagen-Derived Antigens

In human biological fluids, the antigens recognized in the various assays for type III procollagen–derived molecules were found to be heterogeneous: Indeed, there are at least four immunoreactive forms (termed A to D) [28], which differ in their molecular size and can be separated by gel filtration. Aminoterminal propeptide of type III procollagen (form C) is the intact trimeric propeptide (Col 1–3) with a molecular mass of $M_r = 45,000$. Its degradation product, Col-1 $(M_r = 10,000)$ is eluted as form D. Also, larger forms are recognized by the antibodies directed to type III procollagen: One (form A) may represent entire type III procollagen or p-N-III collagen; the other (form B), somewhat larger than the propeptide itself, may be aggregated amino-terminal propeptide or a degradation product of type III procollagen. Form A is also recognized by an antibody to fully processed type III collagen (unpublished results). These circulating antigens do not express the same affinity for the antibodies as do purified molecules, so leading to various apparent proportions of the various forms in any serum sample, according to the antisera and the assay conditions used. Two types of assays have already been developed.

### Amino-terminal Propeptide of Type III Procollagen (PIIINP)

The first radioimmunoassay for amino-terminal propeptide of type III procollagen was described by Rohde et al. in 1979 [30]; it is available from Behring in Germany. Since the curve slope was less steep than that for the bovine reference peptide, the following improvements were proposed. To quantitate mainly the low-molecular-weight forms, Pierard et al. [31] reported a modified radioimmunoassay using, as standard, the antigen generated by cleavage of bovine aminoterminal propeptide of type III procollagen with bacterial collagenase (Col-1 plus Col-2). Rohde et al. [32] introduced an assay using pepsin-cleaved antibody ($F_{ab}$ fragments), the affinity of the intact propeptide and its degradation product (Col-1) to these $F_{ab}$ being nearly identical. Niemelä purified human Col-1 and developed the corresponding assay [33]. By contrast, Risteli et al. [34] using highly purified human PIIINP and precise assay conditions proposed an assay, now commercially available from Farmos in Finland, which did not detect Col-1 and showed satisfactory dilution tests. A two-sites immunoradiometric assay with monoclonal antibodies has been developed (available from Behring in Germany). In our studies we used a modified assay from Pierard et al. [31] with Col 1–3 as standard. Under the reaction conditions chosen [35] the reactivity of the small degradation products was reduced and the displacement curves obtained with the antigen and serially diluted human sera or BALF [99] were parallel.

An increased serum PIIINP might reflect a de novo synthesis of type III procollagen in the lung, since the aminopropeptide is partly liberated during conversion of procollagen into collagen in stoichiometric amounts, but it may also reflect either the degradation of tissue type III collagen still containing the amino-terminal propeptide, or impaired elimination [28]. In BALF, PIIINP is a marker of synthesis since high-molecular-weight antigens and Col 1–3 are predominant [36,99].

### Type III Collagen (CIII)

Using human type III collagen extracted with pepsin from placenta, we developed a liquid-phase radioimmunoassay for fully processed type III collagen. Only high-molecular-weight components (form A) are recognized. Thus this assay probably reflects fibrogenesis.

## *Type I Procollagen-Derived Antigens*

Less is known regarding type I procollagen antigens in human fluids. The circulating immunoreactive forms seem less numerous than for type III procollagen. As for type III procollagen, two kinds of assays have been reported.

### Carboxyterminal Propeptide of Type I Procollagen (PICP)

Although described in 1974, this radioimmunoassay was less popular than that of PIIINP [28]. As the assay [37] is now commercially available (from Farmos, Finland), several studies have been undertaken but not, to date, on lung diseases. In biological fluids, after gel filtration, the antigen recognized in the assay has the same molecular size as standard PICP; thus PICP can be considered as a synthesis marker.

### Type I Collagen (CI)

Using human acid-soluble type I collagen extracted from skin, we developed a liquid-phase radioimmunoassay for fully processed type I collagen [38]. After gel filtration, two peaks can be separated in serum or BALF: One may represent entire type I collagen, and the other, whose nature is unknown, a degradation product. PICP appeared at another elution position. Denatured type I collagen is not recognized in the assay. In liver diseases, serum CI is correlated with already established cirrhosis and reflects degradation (fibrolysis) [38]. This assay has been applied in serum and BALF from patients with pneumonia and ARDS; in that situation, CI was shown to represent mainly fibrogenesis [99].

### Type IV Collagen-Derived Antigens

The type IV collagen molecule is composed of a large triple-helical domain with a pepsin-resistant amino-terminal domain, named 7S, and a globular carboxy-terminal domain $NC_1$. In contrast with type I or III procollagens, no peptides are cleaved prior to tissue deposition. Assays have been set up against both $NC_1$ and 7S antigens and also against pepsinized type IV collagen lacking $NC_1$ (CIV) [28], $NC_1$ being a marker of degradation, and 7S or CIV, markers of both synthesis and degradation.

### B. Application and Physiopathological Significance of Collagen Peptide Assays in Pulmonary Diseases

Some of the assays described previously, notably the PIIINP assay, have been applied to serum from patients with pulmonary diseases. As bronchoalveolar lavage may contribute to a better understanding of what happens locally, measurements of connective tissue components in BALF have received increasing attention; to our knowledge and in contrast with other pathologies, nothing has been reported in urine. Several studies have focused on PIIINP, in serum and/or BALF (rarely both together), alone or in conjunction with other extracellular matrix molecules, such as hyaluronic acid, fibronectin, laminin, or enzymes (galactosylhydroxylysyl glucosyltransferase). Only our group has also measured fully processed type I and III collagens (CI and CIII). The major findings are summarized in Table 4.

In humans, lung fibrosis is a heterogeneous group of diseases; however, some general comments can be drawn up from the various studies (Table 4). As for liver diseases, the tissue changes leading to lung fibrosis seem to be reflected in the serum concentrations of extracellular matrix components. Slightly increased levels of PIIINP were reported in studies with patients having idiopathic pulmonary fibrosis [39], sarcoidosis [40], systemic sclerosis [41], chronic bronchitis [40], or farmer's lung [42], or in a model of bleomycin-induced pulmonary fibrosis in rabbit [43]. In other studies, no significant changes were observed [43–45]. Only in ARDS was a dramatic increase in serum PIIINP [46–48,99] CI, or CIII [99] noted. As these changes are likely to be due to overproduction of collagen in lung tissues, the increases in collagen peptide concentration occur earlier and are of greater magnitude in BALF than in serum; this has been demonstrated in sarcoidosis [36,44,45,49,50], idiopathic pulmonary fibrosis [36,45,51–53], systemic sclerosis [41], farmer's lung [54], asbestosis [55], and ARDS [99]. No clear association between serum or BALF PIIINP and pulmonary function was noted [40,41,45,47,50], nor between PIIINP and the acute stage of a disease (e.g., farmer's lung) [42]. However, PIIINP levels were increased with inflammation [41] or alveolitis [49].

In conclusion, circulating collagen antigens, markers of fibroblast activa-

**Table 4** Application of Collagen Assays to Pulmonary Diseases

| Pathology | Collagen marker (other ECM marker tested) | Assay[a] | Biological fluid | Number | Concentration range (mean) pathological/normal | Ref. |
|---|---|---|---|---|---|---|
| Sarcoidosis | PIIINP | 1 | BALF serum | 9 | 1.76–66.0 (18.2)/0.29–2.50 (0.91) ng/mL 10.1–21.4 (12.1)/9.7–11.9 (11.0) ng/mL | [45] |
| Idiopathic pulmonary fibrosis | PIIINP | 1 | BALF serum | 11 | 0.32–66.0 (22.2)/0.29–2.50 (0.91) ng/mL 10.2–13.1 (11.7)/9.7–11.9 (11.0) ng/mL | [45] |
| Sarcoidosis | PIIINP | 1 | Serum | 4 | 3–20 (12)/5–14 (9) ng/mL | [43] |
| Idiopathic pulmonary fibrosis | PIIINP | 1 | Serum | 14 | 3–17 (9)/5–14 (9) ng/mL | [43] |
| Chronic bronchitis | PIIINP | 1 | Serum | 13 | 3–35 (14)/5–14 (9) ng/mL | [43] |
| Bronchial asthma | PIIINP | 1 | Serum | 18 | 2–19 (10)/5–14 (9) ng/mL | [43] |
| Pulmonary tuberculosis | PIIINP | 1 | Serum | 27 | 4–27 (13)/5–14 (9) ng/mL | [43] |
| Primary lung cancer | PIIINP | 1 | Serum | 22 | 4–42 (19)/5–14 (9) ng/mL | [43] |
| Sarcoidosis | PIIINP | 1 | BALF serum | 110 | <0.2–19.5 (0.6)/<0.2 ng/mL (16.2)/(15.4) ng/mL | [44] |
| Sarcoidosis | PIIINP (FN) | 1 | BALF | 84 | <0.2–80/<0.2–0.8 ng/mg protein | [50] |
| Sarcoidosis | PIIINP (FN,HA) | 1 | BALF | 74 | <0.2–50 (0.77)/<0.2 ng/mL | [49] |
| Sarcoidosis | PIIINP | 1 | Serum | 38 | 4–25 (18 in type I progressive)/5–13 (9.5) ng/mL | [40] |
| Chronic bronchitis | PIIINP | 1 | Serum | 15 | 3–25 (11)/5–13 (9.5) ng/mL | [40] |
| Farmer's lung | PIIINP (GGT) | 1 | Serum | 40 | (7.6) treated (8.1) nontreated/(7.0) ng/mL | [42] |
| Farmer's lung | PIIINP (HA) | 1 | BALF | 10 | 2.8–19.4 (7.3)/<0.2 ng/mL | [54] |
| Asbestosis | PIIINP (FN) | 1 | BALF | 34 | (2.0)/1.2 ng/mg albumin | [55] |
| Systemic sclerosis | PIIINP | 3 | BALF serum | 34 | <0.1–2.0/<0.1 ng/mL 40–120/35–65 ng/mL | [41] |

| Disease | Marker | Method | Sample | n | Values | Ref. |
|---|---|---|---|---|---|---|
| Idiopathic pulmonary fibrosis and other diseases | PIIINP | 1 | BALF/serum | 12 | 0.6–6.8 (3.1)/(0.25) ng/dL, 10.8–24.5 (14.3)/(9.3) ng/dL | [51] |
| Idiopathic pulmonary fibrosis | PIIINP | 1 | BALF | 31 | 0.05–8.0 (1.2)/0.05–0.3(0.1) ng/mL | [36] |
| Idiopathic pulmonary fibrosis | PIIINP (HA) | 1 | BALF | 22 | <0.2–12.2 (0.4)/<0.2 ng/mL | [53] |
| Cryptogenic fibrosing alveolitis | PIIINP | 1 | Serum | 23 | 8–18 (13)/5–15(9) ng/mL | [39] |
| Diffuse fibrosing alveolitis | PIIINP | 1 | BALF | 42 | (1.72) in group with Met(O) > 6%/<0.2 ng/mL | [52] |
| ARDS | PIIINP (LN) | 1 | Serum | 10 | 62–113/2–12 (8) ng/mL | [48] |
| ARDS | PIIINP | 4 | Serum | 8 | 9–20 (13)/(0.5) U/mL | [46] |
| ARDS | PIIINP (HA,LN) | 1 | Serum | 16 | 50–180 (90)/(12) ng/mL | [47] |
| ARDS | PIIINP (GGT) | 2 | BALF/serum | 19 | 1.5–92 (53)/<0.2–1.5 (1) ng/mL; 8–49 (35)/5–14 (9) ng/mL | [99] |
| | CI | 5 | BALF/serum | | 0.5–123 (86)/<0.2–15 (9) ng/mL; 140–315 (240)/140–192 (161) ng/mL | |
| | CIII | 5 | BALF/serum | | 0.8–45 (34)/<0.2–15 (11) ng/mL, 15–78 (51)/<10–30 (13) ng/mL | |
| Pneumonia (infectious and other) | PIIINP (GGT) | 2 | BALF/serum | 29 | 0.5–51 (20)/<0.2–1.5 (1) ng/mL, 8–49 (35)/5–14 (9) ng/mL | [99] |
| | CI | 5 | BALF/serum | | 0.8–69 (41)/<0.2–15 (1) ng/mL, 140–275 (230)/140–192 (161) ng/mL | |
| | CIII | 5 | BALF/serum | | <0.2–21 (13)/<0.2–15 (11) ng/mL; 12–61 (35)/<10–30 (13) ng/mL | |

*1, RIA derived from the method described in ref. 30; 2, RIA modified from the method described in refs. 31 and 35; 3, RIA derived from the method described in ref. 32; 4, coated tubes IRMA; 5, in-house RIA [38].

tion, would more likely be representative, primarily in BALF, of ongoing fibrogenesis in lung diseases. The determination of serum of BALF collagen peptides levels:

1. May be useful for distinguishing active disease from inactive disease, as in sarcoidosis [40], idiopathic pulmonary fibrosis [53], or farmer's lung [54].
2. May be useful for assessing the response to therapy: for example, to the glucocorticoid treatment in sarcoidosis [40] and cryptogenic alveolitis [39] or to extracorporeal $CO_2$ removal in ARDS [47,48];however, no relationship with treatment was noted in farmer's lung, where the collagen peptides levels decreased during recovery and returned to normal during clinical remission [54].
3. May provide prognostic information in sarcoidosis (PIIINP levels were increased with deterioration [40] or in ARDS when the nonsurvivors have the highest PIIINP, CI, and CIII levels [99].

However, long-term longitudinal studies are still needed to assess more clearly the clinical usefulness of the different collagen assays in lung diseases, particularly for the monitoring of antifibrotic treatment.

### III.  Elastin Peptides and Desmosine as Biological Markers of Lung Elastin

Elastin can be considered as a polymer of linear polypeptide chains (tropoelastin) stabilized by lysine-derived cross-links, such as desmosine, isodesmosine, dehydrolysylnorleucine, or lysylnorleucine. Desmosine (MW = 526 Da) and isodesmosine are the major cross-linking amino acids in elastin and are synthesized by condensation of three residues of α-aminoadipic-δ-semialdehyde (allysine) with one lysine residue lying in close proximity to another within and between adjacent polypeptide chains of tropoelastin. Allysine, in turn, is formed extracellularly by the oxidative deamination of the amino group of lysine, a reaction catalyzed by the copper-dependent enzyme lysyl oxidase. Elastin is characterized by the presence of large areas with β-spiral structure and regions having a helix structure in which cross-links are located. Elastin resistance to enzymatic degradation is related to the presence of cross-links. The synthesis of desmosine cross-links occurs in extracellular space and is dependent on lysyl oxidase enzyme.

Lysine-derived cross-links are not necessary for elastin fiber formation. Tropoelastin monomer coacervates as fiber by hydrophobic interactions. Penicillamine, which prevents the formation of desmosine cross-links, induces the production of new elastin fibers which appear normal from the ultrastructural point of view [56]. However, inhibition of desmosine cross-link formation by penicillamine or by inhibition of lysyl oxidase (vitamin $B_6$ and copper deficiency, β-aminopropionitrile) leads to formation of parenchymal lesions very close to those observed in lung emphysema.

The desmosine content of elastin fibers is considered constant and is estimated as 4 desmosines per 1000 amino acids in purified elastin [57]. However, the desmosine content of the isolated elastin may vary in abnormal or neosynthesized connective tissue. Elastin synthesized in the uterus during pregnancy has been shown to be poorly cross-linked [58]. Furthermore, in the aortic media of patients with Marfan's syndrome, desmosine content was reduced by approximately 50% [59]. This less-cross-linked elastin is probably quicker to degrade by proteases or during a purification procedure using sodium hydroxide or proteases. Richmond demonstrates that 11% of lung elastin was degraded by trypsin and chymotrypsin, enzymes devoided of elastinolytic capacities. However, the material solubilized by these enzymes contained lysynonorleucine, whereas desmosine cross-links were present only in the elastase digest [60]. Considerable differences were found in the content of desmosine cross-links between the results obtained by means of a cyanogen bromide method and those determined in the sample after alkaline hydrolysis [61].

Elastin turnover in tissue declines very rapidly from birth to the age of 20, after which, in normal tissues, almost no synthesis occurs [62]. The total body elastin degradation per day can be estimated at 2.5 mg/day, this representing only about 1% of the total body elastin pool turnover per year [63]. However, this apparent stability of elastin tissue in adults is no longer true in the case of tissue aggression. Moreover, elevated levels (eightfold) of urinary desmosine are found during pregnancy in rats and are probably due to elastin remodeling in the uterus [64]. In the lung, one of the most striking alterations observed during emphysema is the fragmentation of elastic fibers. To measure elastin degradation by noninvasive methods, two types of assays were developed: assays for desmosine in urine and assays for elastin peptides in serum, plasma, or urine. All these assays are based on specific immunological recognition by antibodies.

### A. Elastin Peptide Assays

Several studies used elastin peptide antibodies to determine elastin peptide concentration in serum, plasma, or urine by ELISA assay or solid-phase RIA (Table 5). These assays measure peptides derived from tropoelastin, the soluble precursor of elastin, as well as peptides derived from degradation of matrix cross-linked elastin. The studies reported agreed on the fact that, in chronic obstructive pulmonary disease, the level of circulating or excreted elastin peptides is increased [65–70]. However, great discrepancies exist in the reported average elastin peptide concentrations of normal nonsmoker blood samples, varying from

**Table 5**   Elastin Peptide Assays in Serum, Plasma, or Urine

| Sample | Healthy non-smokers | Healthy smokers | Chronic obstructive lung disease (COPD) | Ref. |
|---|---|---|---|---|
| Serum | 11.9 ng/mL | 53.5 ng/mL | 81.1 ng/mL | [65] |
| | 19.9 ± 10.5 μg/mL | 17.6 ± 8.5 μg/mL | 53.4 ± 22.5 μg/mL | [66] |
| | 2.48 ± 0.21 μg/mL | | | [68] |
| Plasma | 58 ± 15 ng/mL (<40 years) | 59 ± 15 ng/mL (low EDP[a] group) | 127 ± 46 ng/mL | [67] |
| | 60 ± 22 ng/mL (>40 years) | 135 ± 54 ng/mL (high EDP group) | | [67] |
| | 22.6 ± 8.2 ng/mL | 36.0 ± 6.8 ng/mL | 66.8 ± 5.8 ng/mL | [69] |
| Urine | 215 ± 28 ng/mg creatinine | 362 ± 116 ng/mg creatinine | 911 ± 106 ng/mg creatinine | [69] |
| | 88 ± 60 ng/mg creatinine | 87 ± 57 ng/mg creatinine | 252 ± 162 ng/mg creatinine | [70] |

[a]EDP, elastin-derived peptides.

11.9 ng/mL to 2.5 or 19.9 μg/mL [65,66,68], and may be related to the various methods used to obtain elastin peptides and antibodies.

To elucidate more precisely the above-mentioned discrepancies, we hydrolyzed elastin from human aorta using either chemical or enzymatic procedures, and we produced monoclonal or polyclonal antibodies with each elastin peptide preparation; these elastin peptide preparations and corresponding antibodies were then used in ELISA assays to quantitate elastin peptides in human sera. Competitive ELISA assays were developed as described by Rennard et al. [71]. Wells of microtiter plates were coated with elastin peptides (0.4 μg or 1.11 μg/mL PBS, 100 μL/well), incubated at 37°C for 2 h, and stored at 4°C. Simultaneously, in other microtiter plate wells, 60 μL of elastin peptide solution [0.5 ng to 10 μg per 50 μL PBST (PBS + Tween 20 0.05%), BSA 70 mg/mL] or sample (undiluted serum) was mixed with 60 μL of antisera or monoclonal antibodies (diluted in PBST) and incubated overnight at 4°C. Before use, elastin peptide–coated plates were washed three times with PBST; 100 μL of elastin peptides or sample and antibody mixtures was then transferred on this plate and incubated at 37°C for 30 min. After three washings, 100 μL of peroxidase-labeled goat antirabbit IgG antibodies (dilution: 1/4000) or rat antimice IgG1 antibodies (dilution: 1/5000) were added and incubated for 1 h at 37°C. Wells were washed with PBST and 100 μL of o-phenylenediamine (0.5 mg/mL), $H_2O_2$ 0.06% in sodium phosphate–citrate buffer (pH 5.0) were added. After 15 min at 37°C, the enzymatic reaction was stopped with 50 μL of 2 N HCl. Absorbance values were determined at 490 nm using an ELISA reader. Using this method and the various elastin peptide and antibody preparations, we measured the elastin peptide concentration in human sera and observed that its value varied greatly with the nature of the elastin peptide and antibody preparations used for the ELISA assay (Tables 6 and 7) [72]. These variations might be explained by several factors:

1. The heterogeneity of elastin peptide preparations with regard to their molecular weight and their amino acid sequence. The same amino acid sequence of insoluble elastin may exhibit different conformations resulting in different immunological recognition, depending on whether it is contained in a small (molecular weight $\approx$ 10 kDa) or a large (molecular weight $\approx$ 100 kDa) peptide. Furthermore, human serum elastin peptides appear somewhat different from elastin peptides produced in vitro. Our recent experimental data indicated that the major fraction ($\approx$ 80%) of elastin peptides in human sera had molecular weight lower than 5 kDa, whereas a minor fraction (20%) would be associated with HDL [75]. In their recent study, Kucich and al. [73] also detected, but to a lesser extent, the presence of small elastin peptides (molecular weight < 20 kDa) in the plasma of some normal smokers and of patients with chronic obstructive pulmonary diseases, but surprisingly not in the plasma of normal nonsmokers.

**Table 6** Elastin Peptide Concentration in Human Serum[a]

| Antigen/immune serum used for the competitive ELISA assay[b] | Elastin peptide concentration (mean ± SD, $n$ = 14) | $r^c$ |
|---|---|---|
| κ-EP/κ-EP immune serum | 1.28 ± 0.97 μg κ-EP equivalents /mL | |
| P95% EP/P95% EP immune serum | 6.90 ± 3.80 μg P95% EP equivalents /mL | 0.93 |
| L25% EP/L25% EP immune serum | 4.49 ± 3.27 μg L25% EP equivalents /mL | 0.94 |
| L85% EP/L85% EP immune serum | 0.56 ± 0.50 μg L85% EP equivalents /mL | 0.82 |

*Source:* Ref. 72.

[a]Meaurements were carried out by competitive ELISA assay using four human aorta EP preparations and polyclonal antibodies raised against them.

[b] κ-EP, elastin peptides obtained during hydrolysis of elastin with KOH 1 $M$ in ethanol 80%; P95% EP, elastin peptides obtained during hydrolysis of elastin with porcine pancreatic elastase until 95% of elastin is solubilized; L25% EP, elastin peptides obtained during hydrolysis of elastin with rat leucocyte elastase until 25% of elastin is solubilized; L85% EP, elastin peptides obtained during hydrolysis of elastin with rat leucocyte elastase until 85% of elastin is solubilized.

[c]Correlation coefficient between elastin peptide concentrations (measured by using an elastin peptide preparation and corresponding antibodies) and elastin peptide concentrations (measured by using κ-elastin and κ-elastin peptide antibodies).

**Table 7**  Elastin Peptide Concentration in Human Serum[a]

| Antigen/antibody used for the competitive ELISA assay[b] | Elastin peptide concentration (mean ± SD, n = 23) | r[c] |
|---|---|---|
| κ-EP/κ-EP immune serum | 1.40 ± 1.00 μg κ-EP equivalents /mL | |
| κ-EP/κ-EP mAb A2,1 | 1.04 ± 0.32 μg κ-EP equivalents /mL | 0.80 |
| κ-EP/κEP mAb A6,1 | 39.0 ± 18.0 μg κ-EP equivalents /mL | 0.87 |
| κ-EP/α-EP mAb A7,1 | 0.76 ± 0.36 μg κ-EP equivalents /mL | 0.76 |
| κ-EP/κ-EP mAb G8,1 | 19.4 ± 9.0 ng κ-EP equivalents /mL | 0.80 |

*Source:* Ref. 72.
[a]Measurements were carried out by competitive ELISA assay using κ-elastin peptides and polyclonal or monoclonal antibodies (mAb) raised against them.
[b]κ-EP, elastin peptides obtained during hydrolysis of elastin with KOH 1 $M$ in ethanol 80%.
[c]Correlation coefficient between elastin peptide concentrations (measured by using κ-elastin and a monoclonal antibody) and elastin peptide concentrations (measured by using κ-elastin and κ-elastin immune serum).

2.  The differences in elastin peptide preparations obtained when using either chemical reagent (KOH) or enzymes (pancreatic or leucocyte elastase). KOH hydrolyzes insoluble elastin with less specificity than do enzymes; during the enzymatic reaction, the P1 amino acid specificity is alanine (240 per 1000 amino acids in elastin) for porcine pancreatic elastase, and more probably valine (140 per 1000 amino acids in elastin) for rat leukocyte elastase [74]. Therefore, elastin peptide preparation obtained with pancreatic elastase contains epitopes liable to be themselves cleaved by leucocyte elastase. Thus antibodies raised against the various elastin peptide preparations may recognize different epitopes, so leading to different immunological recognition of elastin peptides in human sera as a function of antibody preparation specificities. Also, elastin peptide concentration measured in human sera varies when different monoclonal antibodies are used in the ELISA assay, although all these monoclonal antibodies are produced against κ-elastin.

3.  Chemical treatment may induce conformational change in elastin peptides and consequently modify their reactivity against antibodies. For example, we have shown [75] that treatment of human serum with 4 $M$ urea caused a fivefold decrease in elastin peptide concentration, whereas treatment with ethanol (final concentration of 80%) induced a 70-fold increase.

All these data clearly indicate that serum evaluation of elastin peptide concentration by ELISA assays provides relative values as a function of the nature of elastin peptides or antibody preparations. However, it is of interest to note that a significant correlation was observed between the various measurements of elastin peptides, thus indicating their value in comparative studies. Our recent clinical and epidemiological studies were effected by using κ-elastin peptides and corresponding antibodies in the ELISA assay, to avoid the possible presence of antielastase antibodies in immunized animals. A first study carried out on the serum of 54 control subjects did not allow us to detect any significant change with age. Nevertheless, in another study, including a larger group of 310 normal subjects, we evidenced a significant decrease in elastin peptide level with age (2.18 ± 1.14 μg/mL in men older than 50 years vs. 2.92 ± 1.54 μg/mL in men younger than 30 years) [76]. We also found a lower elastin peptide level in serum of non-$\alpha_1$Pi MM healthy patients, but we did not evidence any difference related to smoking habits or FEV$_1$. Cohen et al. [77] recently reported a significant inverse relation of plasma elastin peptide concentration to FEV$_1$ (expressed in liters) among 46 patients with chronic obstructive pulmonary disease (COPD); nevertheless, no correlation was observed when FEV$_1$ was expressed as a percent of predicted value.

In conclusion, actual data are in agreement on the elevated plasma elastin–derived values in COPD compared with nonsmoking adults. Although the absolute concentration differed, the relative differences between groups were similar, patients with COPD having mean values approximately 300% higher than those of nonsmokers (Table 5). Such results highly suggest that blood elastin peptide levels may serve as markers of elastin breakdown and turnover during COPD and would be useful in diagnosis or in therapeutic monitoring of this disease. Tissues other than lung, such as vascular wall and skin, contain significant amounts of elastic fibers in their matrices, the turnover of which could contribute to plasma elastin concentration. Nevertheless, lung appears to be the privileged organ of origin, since the estimated elastin peptide concentration in bronchoalveolar lavage fluid is very elevated in COPD patients with high urine values [69]. Little information is available about elastin peptide level in urine, and little is known about the renal clearance of elastin degradation products. However, recent studies [69] reported that elastin peptides (1) can be rapidly cleared into the urine, making urine a more sensitive assay than plasma, and (2) were higher in the urine of subjects with COPD than in healthy patients.

Concerning the plasma level of elastin peptide in healthy smokers, it appears unchanged in most reported work, although moderately increased in a few reports (Table 5). This variation in elastin peptide level probably reflects the severity of smoking habits or individual risk of developing pulmonary elastin degradation in response to cigarette smoke.

Finally, our studies [76] related to the diminution with age of serum elastin peptide level in a large population of middle-aged, predominantly healthy, men cast some doubt on the use of elastin peptide level as a marker of elastin degradation or lung destruction. We suggested that several factors (e.g., age, alcohol consumption, and non $\alpha_1$Pi MM phenotype) may, rather, be associated with decreased elastin neosynthesis. Further studies conducted with various age classes, including estimates of the degree of lung destruction, are needed to unravel the mechanisms underlying lysis and resynthesis of lung elastin.

### B.  Urinary Desmosine Assays

The specificity of desmosine as a marker of elastin brought the development of various techniques for its quantitation. In addition, it should be noted that desmosine is a structure common to all vertebrate elastin, thus making it possible to use the test in different species. Antibodies obtained with desmosine-haptenized macromolecules allowed the development of specific radioimmuno-assays and later of ELISAs [63,78–80]. These assays quantitate desmosine in the range 1 to 100 p$M$ (0.5 to 50 ng) in tissue and urinary samples. The low cross-reactivity observed with other lysine-derived cross-links (7% w/w with isodesmosine <0.1% with lysinonorleucine) and with amino acids (0.001% w/w) is the main factor limiting the sensitivity and specificity of these assays. In one of these assays, a cross reaction was found with pyridinoline, a nonreducible collagen cross-link [79]. Desmosine can always be measured if the desmosine/protein ratio of the sample exceeds 0.001% w/w. So far, elastin quantitation is feasible in elastin-rich tissue (aorta, skin, lung) but not in serum unless elastin peptides are partially purified first. Urinary desmosine excretion has been evaluated at $\approx$ 100 to 200 nmol per 24 h; a good correlation had been shown between daily urinary desmosine excretion and desmosine/creatine ratio ($\approx$ 74 pm/mg). Despite its low level (2.9 pmol per 100 $\mu$L BALF, CI 1.9 to 4.7), desmosine was measurable in bronchoalveolar lavage fluid [81].

Several high-performance liquid chromatographic (HPLC) methods for desmosine measure have been developed [82–86]. These assays are sensitive in the range 100 pmol to 10 nmol. The assay developed by Lunte et al. seems to be the most sensitive since it can detect 0.1 pmol [87]. These assays allow complete separation and quantification of desmosine and separately, of its isomer isodesmosine. Stone et al. reported a desmosine excretion of 25 nmol per 24 h when HPLC analysis was preceded by Sephadex G15 chromatography to remove contaminants. This value is less by a factor of 5 than the values reported in the literature. These authors indicate that results obtained with HPLC techniques or amino acid analysis could have been overestimated because of interfering peaks from contaminants. On the other hand, interference with components present in urine samples has been reported with ELISA techniques. However, these interferences are negligible if the concentration of urine in the reaction mixture in the assay is not too high [79]. Gunja-Smith [80] showed that a known amount of desmosine added to urine was quantified perfectly by the ELISA method.

Several studies have been done to evaluate the usefulness of desmosine cross-links for monitoring lung elastolysis. We will separate studies on chronic diseases such as emphysema from acute inflammatory pulmonary diseases [pneumonia, adult respiratory distress syndrome (ARDS)]. Alveolar tissue destruction and distension observed in emphysematous lung have been demonstrated to be related to elastic fiber destruction. Only enzymes that hydrolyze fibrous elastin in vitro are able to induce emphysematous lesions when injected intratracheally in animals. The pathogeny of lung emphysema is thought to be related to an increase in elastolytic forces. Since human alveolar macrophages can degrade elastin by a cell contact–dependent process, it is interesting to point out that cells binding to elastin require an intact cross-linked molecule [88]. The apparent discrepancy between this theory and the normal content in elastin of lung of emphysematous patients demonstrates the ability of lung cells to resynthesize elastin fibers and eventually to keep up with elastin destruction. Lung emphysema could result from a lack of synergy between elastin degradation and elastin reconstruction [89].

Several studies have been undertaken to evaluate the hypothesis that lung elastin degradation is accelerated in emphysema. Pehlam et al. studied 17 homozygous $\alpha_1$-antitrypsin-deficient persons with emphysema. Urine desmosine was not significantly elevated in either group compared with the age-matched control subjects [90]. These results explain that urine excretion did not change following $\alpha_1$-antitrypsin infusion in PI Z patients [91]. Davies et al. [92] were unable to detect any association between desmosine and current smoking status, total lifetime cigarette consumption, or spirometric functions in 157 men. In a study including 46 patients with chronic obstructive pulmonary disease (mean $FEV_1$ % $\approx$ 58% $\pm$ 8), Cohen et al. found a desmosine/creatinine ratio of 77 pmol/mg, very close to the normal value [69]. In a limited number of patients with COPD, Harel et al. showed that desmosine excretion was larger than that of unaffected control subjects [63]. These data suggest that pathologic lung elastolysis in patients with emphysema may constitute too small a fraction of total elastin turnover to be detected. Indeed, since the adult human lung contains 30 mg of desmosine, if all lung elastin was degraded at a constant rate over a 20-yr span, average daily excretion would be only about 7 n$M$ [92]. Alternatively, degradation of elastin may be episodic, occurring during lung infection, rather than continuous.

In opposition to emphysema, cross-linked elastin has been shown to be increased in animal models of lung fibrosis. This has been documented in lung tissue with bleomycin and amiodarone-induced fibrosis [93]. Desmosine in BAL fluid was elevated in bleomycin-treated marmosets. However, no consistent clinical studies have been published on desmosine excretion in human lung fibrosis.

The release of large quantities of neutral proteases (human leucocyte elastase) by neutrophils during inflammation suggests that elastinolysis occurs during acute inflammatory injuries. This risk for proteolysis of lung connective tissue was evaluated in patients with cystic fibrosis. Urinary cross-link excretion was significantly higher than in controls. There was a significant correlation between urinary desmosine excretion and the severity of lung disease as indicated by chest roentgenogram score [94]. Elevated urinary desmosine have also been found in newborns whose respiratory insufficiency required ventilation with high concentrations of $O_2$. In this study desmosine excretion was significantly greater in infants who later developed bronchopulmonary dysplasia. However, if elevated desmosine excretion through day 9 was shown to reflect lung injury, decreased desmosine excretion beyond that time suggested that elastin synthesis and turnover were impaired [95].

We observed a three- to tenfold augmentation of urinary desmosine above the normal level in patients with bacterial pneumonias (unpublished data). Such an increase was also observed by McCarren et al. in 10 patients with a variety of bacterial pneumonia [96]. Increased activity of neutrophil elastase in bronchoalveolar lavage suggests a major role for this enzyme in lung damage occurring in patients who have an ARDS [97]. Urinary desmosine was shown to increase markedly (tenfold) in patients with ARDS as well as in patients with pneumonias. However, the total amount of desmosine excreted distinguished patients with ARDS from patients with pneumonia without pulmonary edema. Patients with cardiogenic pulmonary edema has a normal level of urinary desmosine. No prospective study has been made to evaluate if the measure of desmosine excretion could be a marker of lung injury or repair in ARDS patients.

In conclusion, although numerous methods have been developed to measure elastin cross-links, very few studies have been done in the field of lung pathology. If desmosine assays seem sensitive enough to evaluate elastin degradation in acute diseases (ARDS, pneumonias), we cannot make a determination regarding its predictive capability concerning the onset of these diseases. The ability of the desmosine test to measure an increase in elastin degradation in emphysema or in smokers is not actually demonstrated. Clinical studies on desmosine excretion in a larger series of patients with serial follow-up should be made. Comparative studies evaluating desmosine and elastin peptide excretion concomitantly should be worth performing to shed light on the discrepancy observed between these two types of tests, especially in emphysema patients. Only one study [69] related the concomitant measurement of plasma elastin peptide concentration and urinary desmosine excretion during chronic obstructive pulmonary disease, and no correlation was observed between these two specific parameters of elastin peptide quantitation. This discrepancy might be due to the inability of elastin peptides quantitation tests to distinguish mature elastin fibers and tropoelastin products of degradation. Indeed, elastin cross-links are specific to mature elastin fibers, and this dictates against the use of elastin peptide quantitation tests, which measure indistinctly mature elastin fibers and tropoelastin products of degradation.

Moreover, since dietary desmosine is not absorbed from the intestine, we can postulate that urinary desmosine reflects elastin degradation quantitatively [98]. However, even if tropoelastin does not seem to be degraded directly in vivo before cross-linking, there are no data indicating that this condition remains unchanged during elastin resynthesis occurring following injury to the lung.

### References

1. Van der Rest M, Garrone R. Collagen family of proteins. FASEB J 1991;5:2814–23.
2. Cleary EG, Gibson MA. Elastin associated microfibrils and microfibrillar proteins. Int Rev Connect Tissue Res 1983;10:97–209.
3. Okada Y, Nagase N, Harris ED. A metalloproteinase from human rheumatoid synovial fibroblasts that digests connective tissue components. J Biol Chem 1986;261:14245–55.
4. Murphy G, McAlpine C, Poll CG, Reynolds JJ. Biochem Biophys Acta 1985;831:49–58.
5. Mackay AR, Hartzler JL, Pelina MD, Thorgeirsson UP. Studies on the ability of 65 kDa and 92 kDa tumor cell gelatinases to degrade Type IV collagen. J Biol Chem 1990;265(35):2129–21934.
6. Hibbs M, Hoidal JR, Kang AH. Expression of a metalloproteinase that degrades native type V collagen and denatures collagens by cultured human alveolar macrophages. J Clin Invest 1987;80:1644–50.
7. Galloway WA, Murphy G, Sandy JD, Gavrilovitch J, Cawston TE, Reynolds JJ. Stromelysin, a connective tissue degrading metalloendopeptidase secreted by stimulated rabbit synovial fibroblasts in parallel with collagenase. Biochem J 1983;209:741–52.
8. Chin JR, Murphy G, Werb ZJ. Purification and characterization of a rabbit bone metalloproteinase that degrade proteoglycan and other connective tissue components. J Biol Chem 1985;260:12367–76.
9. Unemori EN, Bair MJ, Bauer EA, Amento EP. Stromelysin expression regulates collagenase activation in human fibroblasts. J Biol Chem 1991;266(34):23477–82.
10. Okada Y, Nakatishi I. Activation of matrix metalloproteinase-3 (Stromelysin) and matrix metalloproteinase-2 (gelatinase) by human neutrophil elastase and cathepsin G. FEBS 1989;249(2):353–56.
11. Goldberg HA, Scott PG. Connect Tissue Res 1986;15:209–19.
12. Matrisian LM. Metalloproteinases and their inhibitors in matrix remodelling. TIG 1990;6:121–125.
13. Delaissé JM, Ledent P, Vaes G. Collagenolytic cysteine proteinases of bone tissue. Biochem J 1991;279:167–74.

14. Lafuma C. Elastases et pathologies pulmonaires. In: Sebastien P, ed. Mechanisms in occupational lung diseases. Colloque INSERM Ed. P. Sebastien. Paris. 1991;203:49–69.

15. Macnulty RJ, Laurent JG. Collagen synthesis and degradation in vivo. Evidence for rapid rates of collagen turnover with entensive degradation of newly synthesized collagen in tissues of the adult rat. Collagen Relat Res 1987;7:93–104.

16. Janoff A. Elastases and emphysema. Current assessment of the protease antiprotease hypothesis. Am Rev Respir Dis 1985;132:417–33.

17. Bieth JG. Mechanisms of action of elastases. In: Robert L, Hornebeck W, eds. Elastin and elastases. Vol. 2. Boca Raton, FL: CRC Press, 1989:13–20

18. Lucey EC, Stone PJ, Breuer R, Christensen TG, Calore JD, Catanese A, Franzblau C, Snider GL. Effect of combined human neutrophil cathepsin G and elastase on induction of secretory cell metaplasia and emphysema with in vitro elastolysis by these enzymes. Am Rev Respir Dis 1985;132:362–66.

19. Kao R, Wehner NG, Skulitz KM, Gray BH, Hoidal JR. A distinct human polymorphonuclear leucocyte proteinase that produces emphysema in hamsters. J Clin Invest 1988;82:1963–73.

20. Reilly JJ, Mason RN, Chen P, Joseph LJ, Sukhatme VP, Yee R, Chapman HA. Biochem J 1989;257:493–98.

21. Reilly JJ, Chen P, Sailor LZ, Wilcose D, Mason JW, Chapman HA. Cigarette smoking induces an elastolytic cysteine proteinase in macrophages distinct from cathepsin L. Lung Cell Mol Physiol 1991;5:L41–L48.

22. Lafuma C, Hornebeck W. Macrophage elastase. In: Robert L, Hornebeck W, eds. Elastin and elastases. Vol. 2. Boca Raton, FL: CRC Press, 1989:39–48.

23. Senior RM, Griffin GL, Fliszar CJ, Shapiro S, Goldberg GI, Welgus HG. Human 92 and 72 kilodalton type IV collagenases are elastases. J Biol Chem 1991;266(12):7870–75.

24. Saulnier JM, Curtil FM, Duclos MC, Wallach JM. Elastolytic activity of *Pseudomonas aeruginosa* elastase. Biochem Biophys Acta 1989;995:285–90.

25. Morihara K. *Pseudomonas aeruginosa* elastase. In: Robert L, Hornebeck W, eds. Elastin and elastases. Vol. 2. Boca Raton, FL: CRC Press, 1989:73–84.

26. Bienkowski RS. Interstitial collagens. In: Crystal RG, West JB, et al. eds. The lung. New York: Raven Press, 1991:381–88.

27. Nerlich AG, Pöschl E, Voss T, Müller PK. Biosynthesis of collagen and its control. Rheumatology 1986;10:70–90.

28. Risteli L, Risteli J. Noninvasive methods for detection of organ fibrosis.

In: Rojkind M, ed. Focus on connective tissue in health and disease. Vol. 1. New York: CRC Press, 1990:61–98.

29. Schuppan D, Rühlmann T, Hahn EG. Radioimmunoassay for human type VI collagen and its application to tissue and body fluids. Anal Biochem 1985;149:238–47.

30. Rohde H, Vargas L, Hahn E, Kalbfleisch H, Bruguera M, Timpl R. Radioimmunoassay for type III procollagen peptide and its application to human liver disease. Eur J Clin Invest 1979;9:451–59.

31. Pierard D, Nusgens BV, Lapiere CM. Radioimmunoassay for the amino-terminal sequences of type III procollagen in human body fluids measuring fragmented precursor sequences. Anal Biochem 1984;141:127–36.

32. Rohde H, Langer I, Krieg T, Timpl R. Serum and urine analysis of the amino-terminal procollagen peptide type III by radioimmunoassay with antibody Fab fragments. Collagen Relat Res 1983;3:371–79.

33. Niemelä O. Radioimmunoassays for type III procollagen amino-terminal peptides in humans. Clin Chem 1985;31:1301–5.

34. Risteli J, Niemi S, Trivedi P, Mäentausta O, Mowat AP, Risteli L. Rapid equilibrium radioimmunoassay for the amino-terminal propeptide of human type III procollagen. Clin Chem 1988;34:715–8.

35. Fayol V, Hassanein HI, El-Badrawy N, Ville G, Hartmann DJ. Amino-terminal propeptide of type III procollagen: a marker of disease activity in schistosomal patients. Eur J Clin Chem Clin Biochem 1991;29:737–41.

36. Cantin AM, Boileau R, Bégin R, Increased procollagen III aminoterminal peptide-related antigens and fibroblast growth signals in the lungs of patients with idiopathic pulmonary fibrosis. Am Rev Respir Dis 1988;137:572–78.

37. Melkko J, Niemi S, Risteli L, Risteli J. Radioimmunoassay of the carboxyterminal propeptide of human type I procollagen. Clin Chem 1990;36:1328–32.

38. Hartmann DJ, Trinchet JC, Ricard-Blum S, Beaugrand M, Callard M, Ville G. Radioimmunoassay of type I collagen that mainly detects degradation products in serum: application to patients with liver diseases. Clin Chem 1990;36:421–26.

39. Kirk JME, Bateman ED, Haslam PL, Laurent GJ, Turner-Warwick M. Serum type III procollagen peptide concentration in cryptogenic fibrosing alveolitis and its clinical relevance. Thorax 1984;39:726–32.

40. Pohl WR, Thompson AB, Köhn H, Losch S, Umek H, Legenstein E, Kummer F, Rennard SI, Klech H. Serum procollagen III peptide levels in subjects with sarcoidosis. A 5-year follow-up study. Am Rev Respir Dis 1992;145:412–17.

41. Harrison NK, McAnulty RJ, Haslam PL, Black CM, Laurent GJ. Evidence for protein oedema, neutrophil influx and enhanced collagen production in lungs of patients with systemic sclerosis. Thorax 1990;45:606–10.

42. Anttinen H, Terho EO, Myllylä R, Savolainen E-R. Two serum markers of collagen biosynthesis as possible indicators of irreversible pulmonary impairment in farmer's lung. Am Rev Respir Dis 1986;133:88–93.

43. Watanabe Y, Yamaki K, Yamakawa I, Takagi K, Satake T. Type III procollagen N-terminal peptides in experimental pulmonary fibrosis and human respiratory diseases. Eur J Respir Dis 1985;67:10–16.

44. Bjermer L, Thunell M, Hällgren R. Procollagen III peptide in bronchoalveolar lavage fluid. A potential marker of altered collagen synthesis reflecting pulmonary disease in sarcoidosis. Lab Invest 1986;55:654–56.

45. Low RB, Cutroneo KR, Davis GS, Giancola MS. Lavage type III procollagen N-terminal peptides in human pulmonary fibrosis and sarcoidosis. Lab Invest 1983;48:755–59.

46. Entzian P, Hückstädt A, Kreipe H, Barth J. Determination of serum concentrations of type III procollagen peptide in mechanically ventilated patients. Am Rev Respir Dis 1990;142:1079–82.

47. Kropf J, Grobe E, Knoch M, Lammers M, Gressner AM, Lennartz H. The prognostic value of extracellular matrix component concentrations in serum during treatment of adult respiratory distress syndrome with extracorporeal $CO_2$ removal. Eur J Clin Chem Clin Biochem 1991;29:805–12.

48. Lammers M, Grobe E, Knoch M, Gressner AM, Lennartz H. Serum laminin and procollagen type III propeptide in patients with respiratory distress syndrome: potentially useful markers of therapy success. Fresenius Z Anal Chem 1988;330:443–44.

49. Blaschke E, Eklund A, Hernbrand R. Extracellular matrix components in bronchoalveolar lavage fluid in sarcoidosis and their relationship to signs of alveolitis. Am Rev Respir Dis 1990;141:1020–25.

50. O'Connor C, Ward K, Van Breda A, McIlgorm A, Fitzgerald MX. Type 3 procollagen peptide in bronchoalveolar lavage fluid. Poor indicator of course and prognosis in sarcoidosis. Chest 1989;96:339–44.

51. Aresu G, Pascalis L, Pia G, Rosetti L, Giglio S. Procollagen III peptide in the blood and in the fluid of bronchoalveolar lavage of subjects affected by pulmonary fibrosis. IRCS Med Sci 1986;14:871–72.

52. Behr J, Maier K, Krombach F, Adelmann-Grill BC. Pathogenic significance of reactive oxygen species in diffuse fibrosing alveolitis. Am Rev Respir Dis 1991;144:146–50.

53. Bjermer L, Lundgren R, Hällgren R. Hyaluronan and type III procollagen peptide concentrations in bronchoalveolar lavage fluid in idiopathic pulmonary fibrosis. Thorax 1989;44:126–31.

54. Bjermer L, Engström-Laurent A, Lundgren R, Rosenhall L, Hällgren R. Hyaluronate and type III procollagen peptide concentrations in bronchoalveolar lavage fluid as markers of disease activity in farmer's lung. Br Med J 1987;295:803–6.

55. Bégin R, Martel M, Desmarais Y, Drapeau G, Boileau R, Rola-Pleszczynski M, Massé S. Fibronectin and procollagen-3 levels in bronchoalveolar lavage of asbestos-exposed human subjects and sheep. Chest 1986;89:237–43.

56. Pasquali-Ronchetti I, Contri MB, Fornieri C, Quaglino D Jr, Mori G. Alteration of elastin fibrogenesis by inhibition of the formation of desmosine crosslinks. Comparison between the effect of β-aminopropionitrile and penicillamine. Connect Tissue Res 1985;14:159–67.

57. Sandberg LB, Soskel NT, Leslie JG. Elastin structure, biosynthesis and relation to disease state. N Engl J Med 1981;304:566–79.

58. Gunja-Smith Z, Lin J, Woessner JF Jr. Changes in desmosine and pyridinoline cross links during rapid synthesis and degradation of elastin and collagen in the rat uterus. Matrix 1989;9:21–27.

59. Peredja AJ, Abraham PA, Carnes WH, Coulson WF, Uitto J. Marfan's syndrome: structural, biochemical, and mechanical studies of the aortic media. J Lab Clin Med 1985;106:376–83.

60. Richmond VL. Elastin and elastin-associated protein of porcine aorta and lung. Connect Tissue Res 1990;25:131–37.

61. Wimmerova J, Benesova J, Kosar K, Ledvina M. Changes of insoluble elastin in the rat aorta depending on isolation method. Sb Ved Pr Lek Fak Kralove 1989;32:149–56.

62. Gunja-Smith Z, Boucek RJ. Desmosine in human urine. Biochem J 1981; 193:915–18.

63. Harel S, Janoff A, Yu SH, Hurewitz A, Bergofsky. Desmosine radioimmunoassay for measuring elastin degradation in vivo. Am Rev Respir Dis 1980;122:769–75.

64. Starcher B, Percival S. Elastin turnover in the rat uterus. Connect Tissue Res 1985;13:207–15.

65. Kucich U, Christner P, Lippmann M, Fein A, Goldberg A, Kimbel P, Weinbaum G, Rosenbloom J. Immunologic measurement of elastin-derived peptides in human serum. Am Rev Respir Dis 1983;127:S28–S30.

66. Darnule TV, McKee M, Darnule AT, Turino GM, Mandl I. Solid-phase radioimmunoassay for estimation of elastin peptides in human sera. Anal Biochem 1982;122:302–7.

67. Kucich U, Christner P, Lippmann M, Kimbel P, Williams G, Rosenbloom J, Weinbaum G. Utilization of a peroxidase antiperoxidase complex in an enzyme linked immunosorbent assay of elastin derived peptides in human plasma. Am Rev Respir Dis 1985;131:709–13.

68. Fülöp T Jr, Wei SM, Robert L, Jacob MP. Determination of elastin peptides in normal and arteriosclerotic human sera by ELISA. Clin Physiol Biochem 1990;8:273–82.

69. Schriver EE, Davidson JM, Sutcliffe MC, Swindell BB, Bernard GR.

Comparison of elastin peptide concentrations in body fluids from healthy volunteers, smokers and patients with chronic obstructive pulmonary disease. Am Rev Respir Dis 1991;145:762–66

70. Kucich U, Hamilton J, Akers S, Kimbel P, Rosenbloom J, Weinbaum G. Urine from emphysema patients contains elevated levels of elastin-derived peptides. Am Rev Respir Dis 1990;A232.

71. Rennard SI, Martin GR, Crystal RG. Enzyme-linked immunoassay (ELISA) for connective tissue proteins: type I collagen. In: Furthmayr H, ed. Immunochemistry of the extracellular matrix. Vol. 1. Boca Raton, FL: CRC Press, 1982:237–52.

72. Wei SM, Robert L, Jacob MP. Elastin peptide concentration in human serum: variations with antibody and elastin peptide preparation used for the enzyme-linked immunosorbent assay (submitted for publication).

73. Kucich U, Rosenbloom J, Kimbel P, Weinbaum G, Abrams WR. Size distribution of human lung elastin-derived peptide antigens generated in vitro and in vivo. Am Rev Respir Dis 1991;143:279–83.

74. Hornebeck W, Soleilhac JM, Tixier JM, Moczar E, Robert L. Inhibition by elastase inhibitors of the formyl-met-leu-phe-induced chemotaxis of rat polymorphonuclear leukocytes. Cell Biochem Funct 1987;5:113–22.

75. Wei SM, Robert L, Jacob MP. Characterization of elastin peptides from human serum (manuscript in preparation).

76. Frette C, Wei SM, Neukirch F, Sesboüé R, Martin JP, Jacob MP, Kauffmann F. Relation of serum elastin peptide concentration to age, FEV(1), smoking habits, alcohol consumption, and protease inhibitor phenotype. An epidemiological study in working men. Thorax 1992; 47:937–942.

77. Cohen AB, Girard W, McLarty J, Starcher B, Stevens M, Fair DS, Davis D, James H, Rosenbloom J, Kucich U. A controlled trial of colchicine to reduce the elastase load in the lungs of cigarette smokers with chronic obstructive pulmonary disease. Am Rev Respir Dis 1990;142:63–72.

78. King GS, Mohan VS, Starcher BC. Radioimmunoassay for desmosine. Connect Tissue Res 1980;7:263–68.

79. Laurent P, Magne L, DePalmas J, Bigon J, Jaurand M-C. Quantitation of elastin in human urine and rat pleural mesothelial cell matrix by a sensitive avidin-biotin ELISA for desmosine. J Immunol Methods 1988;107:1–11.

80. Gunja-Smith Z. An enzyme linked immunosorbent assay to quantitate the elastin crosslink desmosine in tissue and urine samples. Anal Biochem 1985;147:258–64.

81. Idell S, Thrall RS, Maunder R, Martin TR, McLarty J, Scott M, Starcher BC. Bronchoalveolar lavage desmosine in bleomycin-induced lung injury in marmoset and patients with adults respiratory distress syndrome. Exp Lung Res 1989;15:739–53.

82. Zarkadas CG, Zardakas GC, Karatzas CN, Khalili AD, Nguyen Q. Rapid method for determining desmosine, isodesmosine, 5-hydroxylysine tryptophan, lysinoalaline and the amino sugars in proteins and tissues. J Chromatogr 1986;378:67–76.

83. Zarkadas CG, Rochemont JA, Zarkadas GC, Khalili AD. Determination of methylated basic, 5-hydroxylysine, elastine crosslinks, other amino acids, and the amino sugars in proteins and tissues. Anal Biochem 1987;160:251–66.

84. Yamaguchi Y, Haginaka J, Kunimoto M, Bando Y. High-performance liquid chromatographic determination of desmosine and isodesmosine in tissues and its application to studies of alteration of elastin induced by atherosclerosis. J Chromatogr 1987;422:53–59.

85. Soskel NT. High-performance liquid chromatographic quantitation of desmosine plus isodesmosine in elastin and whole tissue hydrolysate. Anal Biochem 1987;160:98–104.

86. Stone PJ, Bryan-Rhadfi J, Lucey EC, Ciccolella DE, Crombie G, Faris B, Snider GL, Franzblau C. Measurement of urinary desmosine by isotope dilution and high performance chromatography. Correlation between elastase-induced air space enlargement in the hamster and elevation of urinary desmosine. Am Rev Respir Dis 1991;144:284–90.

87. Lunte SM, Mohabat T, Wong OS, Kuwana T. Determination of desmosine, isodesmosine, and other amino acids by liquid chromotography with electrochemical detection following precolumn derivatization with naphtalenedialdehyde/cyanide. Anal Biochem 1989;178:202–7.

88. Tobias JW, Bern MM, Zetter BR. Monocyte adhesion to subendothelial components. Blood 1987;69:1265–68.

89. Laurent P, Janoff A, Kagan HM. Cigarette smoke block cross linking of elastin in vitro. Am Rev Respir Dis 1983;127:189–92.

90. Pelham F, Wewers M, Crystal R, Buist AS, Janoff A. Urinary excretion of desmosine (elastin cross-links) in subjects with PiZZ alpha-1-antitrypsin deficiency, a phenotype associated with hereditary predisposition to pulmonary emphysema. Am Rev Respir Dis 1985;132:821–23.

91. Moser KM, Smith RM, Spragg RG, Tisi GM. Intravenous administration of α-1-antiproteinase inhibitor in patients of PiZ and PiM phenotype. Preliminary report. Am J Med 1988;84(6A):70–74.

92. Davies SF, Offord KP, Brown MG, Campe H, Niewoehner D. Urine desmosine is unrelated to cigarette smoking or to spirometric function. Am Rev Respir Dis 1983;128:473–75.

93. Cantor JO, Keller S, Mandl I, Turino GM. Increased synthesis of elastin in amiodarone-induced pulmonary fibrosis. J Lab Clin Med 1987;109:480–85.

94. Bruce MC, Poncz L, Klinger JD, Stern RC, Tomashefski JF, Dearborn

DG. Biochemical and pathologic evidence for proteolytic destruction of lung connective tissue in cystic fibrosis. Am Rev Respir Dis 1985;132:529–35.

95. Bruce MC, Wedig KE, Jentoft N, Martin RJ, Cheng PW, Boat TF, Fanaroff AA. Altered urinary excretion of elastin cross-links in premature infants who develop bronchopulmonary dysplasia. Am Rev Respir Dis 1985;131:586–72.

96. McCarren JP, Bergeron-Lynn G. Urinary excretion of desmosine from patients with bacterial pneumonias. Am Rev Respir Dis 1985;131:A384.

97. Tenholder MR, Rajagopal KR, Phillip YY, Dillard TA, Bennett LL, Mundie TG, Tellie CJ. Urinary desmosine excretion as a marker of lung injury in the adult respiratory distress syndrome. Chest 1991;100:1385–90.

98. Starcher BC, Goldstein RA. Studies on the absorption of desmosine and isodesmosine. J Lab Clin Med 1979;94:848–52.

99. Farjanel J, Hartmann DJ, Guidet B, Luquel L, Offenstadt G. Four markers of collagen metabolism as possible indicators of disease in the adult respiratory distress syndrome (submitted).

# 20

## Cytochrome P450 Polymorphisms as Markers of Genetic Risk for Lung Cancer

**P. A. LAURENT, J. COSME**
**and J. C. PAIRON**

INSERM U139
Créteil, France

### I. Introduction

Cigarette smoking is widely recognized as the major cause of lung cancer, the risk increasing with the number of cigarettes smoked and the duration of smoking. Yet the lower incidence of lung cancer in people exposed to the same dose of tobacco suggests a population subgroup that has a different susceptibility to the disease [1,2].

Several lines of evidence suggest that human primary lung carcinoma in smokers arises from gene mutation induced by the chemicals in tobacco smoke. Cigarette smoke is the major source of human exposure to polycyclic aromatic hydrocarbons (PAHs), nitrosamines, and aromatic amines. Paradoxically, most of these chemicals are inert procarcinogens that require metabolic activation to exert their carcinogenic effects (Table 1) [3]. Xenobiotic metabolism leads to the formation of highly reactive metabolites that can form DNA adducts, so most studies focus on bioactivation enzymes, specifically the cytochrome P450-dependent monooxygenase system. Expression of cytochromes P450 in the lung tissue, although lower than that of the liver, has focused interest on localized metabolic activation of xenobiotics [4,5]. Studies with experimental animals have clearly shown that some differences in cancer susceptibility between different strains were related to differences in xenobiotic metabolism. On the other hand, striking differences in cytochrome P450 activities among human subpopulations are related to allelic differences in a single gene. Thus it is hypothesized that lung cancer is a disease resulting from interaction between a susceptibility gene and an environmental risk factor. In this model both the genotype and the environmental risk factors are required to raise risk. As we know, many forms of cytochrome P450 exist and the level of expression is influenced by xenobiotics themselves. Several reviews deal with the characteristics of P450 enzymes and the reader is directed to these [6,7].

Cytochrome P450 enzymes are a multigenic superfamily; investigations have shown that 10 to 20 P450 proteins are expressed in rat, rabbit, and humans. In this chapter we use the nomenclature of the gene superfamily based on the structural homology of P450 protein sequences [8]. Among those genes, *CYP1A1, 1A2, 2E1,* and *3A1/3A4* are of particular interest because of their capacities to bioactivate cigarette smoke components. Yet attention has been focused primarily on polymorphic cytochromes P450 1A1/1A2 and 2D6. These enzymes, including CYP2D6, bioactivate procarcinogens [9].

Among the various components of cigarette smoke, some were recognized to be potent carcinogens (Table 1). The attention has been focused particularly on polycyclic aromatic hydrocarbons (i.e., benzo[*a*]pyrene, 3-methylcholanthrene), aromatic amines (*N*-dimethylnitrosamine), and chemicals derived from tryptophan pyrolysis [trp-p-1 (3-amino-1,4-dimethyl-5*H*-pyrido[4,5-*f* ]quinoline)].

## II.  Expression of Lung Cytochromes P450

In contrast with the liver, rodent lung cytochromes P450 are located in only three of the 42 different specific cell types contained in this organ. They are found

**Table 1**  Activation of Procarcinogens by Human Cytochromes P450

| | |
|---|---|
| P4501A1 | Polycyclic aromatic hydrocarbons: benzo[*a*]pyrene, 3-methylcholanthrene, benzo[*a*]fluorene, etc. |
| P4501A2 | Aromatic amines: 2-(acetylamino)fluorene, 2-aminofluorene, 2-aminoanthracene, tryptophane and glutamic pyrolysis product: 2-amino-6-methyldi-pyrydol[1,2-a3',2']imidazole (Glu P-1), 3-amino-1-methyl-5*H*-pyrydo[4,3-*b*]indole (Trp P-2) |
| P4502A6 | *N*-Nitrosodiethylamine |
| P4502D6 | 4-(Methylnitrosamino)-1-(3-pyridyl)-1-butanone |
| P4502E1 | *N*-Nitrosodimethylamine, benzene |
| P4503A4 | 7,8-Dihydroxy-7,8-dihydrobenzo[*a*]pyrene,3,4-dihydroxy-3,4-dihydro-7-12-dimethylbenz[*a*]anthracene, 1-nitropyrene |

mainly in epithelial cells (Clara cells, alveolar type II cells) and to a lesser degree in endothelial cells. Given their location in the small airways and alveoli at the air–blood interface, the epithelial cells can be expected to play a major role in biometabolization of airborne xenobiotics. Most of the reactive metabolites generated by cytochrome P450 metabolism of xenobiotic react with DNA within the cells where they have been formed. Against this hypothesis, studies involving transplants of rat livers argue that the liver is the main source of benzo[a]pyrene metabolites for extrahepatic adducts [10]. The strong correlation between the cell localization of P450 enzymes and the type of cell transformed by procarcinogens as well as the observed influence of the route of administration of these compounds on the localization of the tumors or DNA adducts formation are good arguments for in situ bioactivation [11,12]. Intratracheal injection to rodents of PAH diluted in solvent provokes the formation of bronchoalveolar tumor derived from Clara cells and alveolar type II cells. Normal lung tissues from smokers with lung cancer showed higher levels of PAH–DNA adducts than did lung tissue from control smokers [13–15]. PAHs are three times as likely to form adducts in lung tissue as in the liver [16]. The selective expression of CYP1A1 enzyme in extrahepatic tissue may explain why PAH adducts are preferentially found in those tissues (i.e., lung, placenta). It should be noted that minor expression of cytochromes P450 has recently been shown in ciliated cells [17]. Even if this expression is low, it could play an important role in transformation of bronchial cells. When PAHs were intratracheally injected as particles, most of the tumors were of epidermoid type and occurred in the bronchi where particles were deposited [18].

The observation of an increased incidence of the disease in some families suggests a genetic predisposition, although lung cancer may affect only a minority of people (see ref. 19). This "reduced penetrance" suggests that expression of a dominant susceptibility allele is influenced by environmental factors.

## III.  *Ah* Receptor-Dependent Induction of Cytochrome P4501A1

Genes of CYP1A subfamily are of considerable interest regarding lung cancer pathogenesis because of their capabilities to bioactivate PAHs and their expression in lung tissue. The mechanism by which PAHs contained in cigarette smoke exert their deleterious biological effects on pulmonary tissue has been studied extensively in rodents and humans [20]. PAHs, and especially benzo[a]pyrene, are prevalent tobacco smoke carcinogens [21]. The metabolism of PAHs such as benzo[a]pyrene (see ref. 3) is carried out by several P450 enzymes but mostly by CYP1A enzymes [22]. The main and ultimate mutagenic metabolite of benzo[a]pyrene, the *trans*-7,8-diol9,10-epoxide, is dependent primarily on CYP1A1 enzyme activity and not on other cytochromes P450 that produce the

4,5 diols. In recent years, benzo[a]pyrene diol-epoxide adducts were found to bind selectively to specific DNA sites [23,24].

### A. Induction of CYP1A1 Activity (Aryl Hydrocarbon Hydroxylase) and Lung Cancer Risk

The cytochrome P4501A gene family has two members, 1A1 and 1A2 [25]. Many studies have shown that these two genes have very different tissue-specific expression patterns. While 1A2 is found only in liver tissue, 1A1 is expressed in extrahepatic tissues except in rodents, where it is also found in the liver. CYP1A1 is expressed at the mRNA and protein levels in the lung of rodents [26] and humans [27–31]. CYP1A1 enzyme, which supports the aryl hydrocarbon hydroxylase activity (AHH), was shown to produce 10 to 100 times more mutagenic metabolites than non-CYP1A1 enzyme. The induction of *CYP1A1* gene is an important characteristic of this enzyme. It occurs in response to PAH substrates or polychlorinated dibenzo-*p*-dioxin compounds such as 2, 3, 7, 8-tetrachloro-*p*-dioxin (TCDD) [32]. While the basal level of CYP1A1 protein is negligible, its expression is 50- to greater than 100-fold in tissues of induced animals. Microsomes from 3-methylcholanthrene-treated rats contain approximately 70% of their total cytochromes P450 as cytochrome P4501A1. Cigarette smoke induces CYP1A1 activity predominantly in extrahepatic tissue, particularly in the lung [40, 41] and the placenta [33]. The positive relationship between mutagenicity, initiation of tumors, and the induction of this enzyme was shown clearly in different organs [34]. In lung, pulmonary carcinogenesis occurred in mice that had received PAHs intratracheally [35].

Studies of the induction mechanism at a molecular level have been documented extensively in recent review articles [36,37]. High inducibility of CYP1A1 activity was shown to be genetically determined in mice [35]. Unresponsive mice are at a decreased risk for subcutaneous sarcoma compared with the responsive (inducible) mice receiving subcutaneously the same dose of benzo[a]pyrene. Studies of induction in cell culture provided a large body of evidence suggesting that this induction is not the result of the direct effect of PAHs on CYP1A but is mediated through a specific protein known as the *Ah* (Aryl hydrocarbon) receptor [38]. The gene that determines responsiveness to PAHs is designated the *Ah* locus and encodes a protein receptor. Binding experiments with TCDD, which is 30,000 times more potent than methylcholanthrene as an inducer of CYP1A1, has led to a better understanding of *Ah* receptor function. This receptor, which belongs to the estrogen and retinoic receptor family, has not yet been purified or cloned. The receptor binds PAHs (or TCDD) in the cytosolic space. The receptor-ligand complex translocates into the nucleus and binds a DNA recognition site located about 1000 base pairs upstream of the *CYP1A1* transcriptional promoter. This xenobiotic responsive element (XRE) has the properties of a cis-acting transcriptional enhancer (see refs. 36 and 39). The Ah locus polymorphism in responsive and unresponsive mice was shown to be due to the presence of a low affinity *Ah* receptor for PAHs (except TCDD). In smokers, several reports have shown induction of CYP1A1 enzyme activity or mRNA [40,41]. On the other hand, contents in DNA adducts in human lung were shown to correlate with cigarette smoke exposure [15,16,42] and AHH activity in parenchymal tissue [43].

In humans, lung P4501A cannot easily be measured in vivo. Aryl hydrocarbon hydroxylase activity (AHH) in lymphocytes treated with PAH was taken as a surrogate marker of CYP1A1 enzyme induction. The interindividual variations of AHH in cultured lymphocytes using twins were shown to be under genetic control [44]. The enzymatic induction observed in lymphocytes was well correlated with mRNA induction [45]. A polymorphic distribution of the inducible AHH was shown to be present with a trimodal distribution of high, low, and intermediate enzyme induction, consistent with an autosomal codominant transmission [46]. A similar study performed in 2000 male smokers confirms this three-model phenotype distribution [47]. In this study the degree of induction was ≥3.6, 2.6 to 3.6, and ≤2.5, respectively, for high, intermediate, and low inducibility. It should be noted that other studies reported a unimodal distribution [44,48]. In Kellerman's study, a higher level of inducible AHH was associated with bronchogenic carcinoma [46]. This observation suggests that in humans, genetic difference in cancer risk is associated with the *Ah* locus and that altered receptor gene would be suspected rather than an altered *CYP1A1* gene. Since this report, contradictory reports have appeared concerning the relationship between AHH inducibility and human lung cancer [40,49–51]. Kouri et al. developed a standardized assay in which lymphocytes are cryopreserved, allowing the simultaneous culture and enzymatic assay of all lymphocyte samples. In this assay lymphocytes are cultivated for 96 to 120 h in the presence of mitogen phytohemagglutinin, benzo[*a*]anthracene as inducer, and human AB serum, fetal calf serum resulting in some AHH-inducing activity [52]. AHH activity is measured by fluorescence associated with the formation of 3-hydroxybenzo[*a*]pyrene. This enzyme activity, shared by several cytochromes P450, was shown to be due only to CYP1A1 enzyme in lymphocytes but not in monocytes [53]. The half-life of AHH in culture is 5 to 6 h and is thus very low in control lymphocytes after the 96 to 120 h of culture. Thus environmental induction was not considered [52,54]. Using this technique, Kouri et al. reported that the ratio AHH activity/NADH-dependent cytochrome *C* reductase activity was higher in patients with lung cancer [52]. NADH-dependent cytochrome *C* reductase activity is a method of quantitation of endoplasmic reticulum; this enzyme activity is not induced by PAHs. In cancer patients the frequency of the highly inducible allele was estimated twice that of control population and the risk for lung cancer was estimated to be approximately 30-fold greater in highly inducible individuals than in the low-inducible group. The relationship between higher AHH inducibility in lymphocytes and the occurrence of lung cancer was shown in previous studies by some authors [49,55] but not by others [56]. No subsequent studies using the technique developed by Kouri et al. have been performed.

It remains to be determined whether the genetic regulation of CYP1A1 enzyme in lymphocytes reflects the regulation in the lung. There could be some tissue specificity of induction as described for P4502B1 in rat. CYP2B1 is not expressed in the liver unless animals are treated with phenobarbital, whereas this enzyme is constitutively expressed in lung tissue. Such a tissue expression specificity has also been described for CYP1A2 in humans (as discussed below). Abnormal responsiveness to phytohemagglutinine was suggested to occur in lymphocytes of lung cancer patients [57,58]. Some intraindividual variations in AHH activity were observed, suggesting that a variety of epigenetic stimuli (environmental, physiological, and pathological) may occur. Paigen et al. reported a tenfold higher induced AHH activity during late summer versus the values observed in spring [59]. However, the addition of hormones to culture medium did not affect induced AHH activity.

AHH activity in lymphocytes remains difficult to test and cannot be used easily in clinical or epidemiological study. Some more specific or sensitive enzyme assays, such as ethoxyresorufin $O$-deethylase activity (EROD) or ethoxyfluorescein ethyl esterose, might be proposed for AHH activity [38]. EROD activity that is detectable in intact cells may be used for quick screening of many samples [60]. Other sensitive assays based on DNA technology have been developed. In this regard mRNA is now quantified in induced or noninduced peripheral lymphocytes [31,61]. The level of induced P4501A1 mRNA was shown to reflect accurately AHH activities. This technique should bring interesting results if performed on lymphocytes and monocytes obtained by bronchoalveolar lavage, since those cells were shown to express higher CYP1A1 activities in smokers [62].

### B.  Caffeine as a Drug Marker of Liver CYP1A2 Activity

Cigarette smoke contains PAHs and many arylamines. 4-aminobiphenyl, 2-naph-tylamine, or $o$-toluidine are present in mainstream and sidestream cigarette smoke. N-oxidation of primary arylamines, which leads to the formation of carcinogenic metabolites, is catalyzed mainly through P4501A2 and to a lesser degree by cytochrome P4501A1 [63].

Although, in humans CYP1A2 is not found in the lung, it appears that its in vivo assessment would be worthy of study in patients with primary lung carcinoma. Both the CYP1A1 and CYP1A2 enzymes are inducible by polycyclic aromatic hydrocarbons. An increase in the rate of rat *CYP1A2* gene transcription through the binding of *Ah* receptor to an XRE element has been found following inducer treatment, although a post-transcriptional regulatory element appears to be involved [38,64,65]. Taken together these data suggest that the phenotyping of this cytochrome should be a potential indirect probe for the study of *Ah*-dependent inducibility [66].

The study of caffeine metabolism in vivo in human subjects has been shown to yield estimates of the activities of CYP1A2 and of *N*-acetyl transferase and xanthine oxidase. Caffeine in 1,3,7-trimethylxanthine (137X) is mostly metabolized by CYP1A2 in humans by 3-demethylation to form 1,7-dimethylxanthine (17X). 1,7-dimethylurate (17U), 1-methylxanthine (1X), 5-acetylamino-6-amino-3-methyluracil (AAMU), and 1-methylurate (1U) metabolites are formed by *N*-acetyl transferase, xanthine oxidase, and other unknown cytochrome P450 enzymes.

The measure of urinary caffeine metabolites by a high-performance liquid chromatographic (HPLC) technique has been proposed as an indicator of CYP1A2 activity in humans [67]. This test is more convenient than the caffeine breath test, which requires the use of isotopically labeled caffeine. A caffeine metabolite ratio has been defined to be a CYP1A2 index. It is defined as follows: CYP1A2 index = (AAMU + 1X + 1U)/17U [67,68]. The protocol for assessment of this ratio includes an overnight urine collection after absorption of 75 mg of caffeine. Since the demethylation rate of caffeine is saturable, the daily intake of caffeine should be restricted on the test day. Moreover, this test is often not feasible because of interferences of coadministered drugs [69]; the metabolic ratio is decreased in women taking contraceptives [68,70]. Circadian variations in caffeine metabolism seem important and have to be considered. Nevertheless, this widely used compound may be employed to measure the CYP1A2 phenotype and to evaluate its role in human susceptibility to chemical-induced cancer.

In a population study the caffeine index showed a log-normal distribution, with the values of most subjects covering a 6.3-fold range [70]. This distribution could indicate that the enzyme is not polymorphically variable. These results contrast with variations in the amounts of immunoreactive CYP1A2 observed in human liver microsomes. On the other hand, wide variations (57-fold) in the ability to catalyze the 3-demethylation of caffeine were found in vitro in 22 liver biopsies [71]. There was a substantial increase in the caffeine CYP1A2 index in smokers [69,72]. Epidemiological studies with the caffeine test should be made to determine whether interindividual variations due to environmental and genetic factors may contribute to susceptibility to primary lung carcinoma.

## IV. Restriction Fragment Length Polymorphism Studies on CYP1A1 and CYP2E1

Polymorphic changes in the DNA sequence of cytochromes P450 could result in altered functional proteins. This altered enzymatic activity may constitute a risk factor for lung cancer. In humans the wide variation of cytochrome P450 content described for several cytochromes may be the result of both genetic and environmental influences (see ref. 73). *CYP2D6* genetic polymorphism has been studied most intensively (discussed below). There are few data concerning the genetic origin of polymorphism of other P450s. A genetic polymorphism has been reported but not confirmed for CYP2C10, which supports the hydroxylation of tolbutamide [74]. Restriction fragment length polymorphism (RFLP) is often found in these P450 genes, but few of them are correlated with functional deficiency of the protein.

Lung cancer risk was correlated with *MspI* polymorphism of CYP1A1 in 64 Japanese patients [75]. Genotype frequencies in the healthy population were 0.49 for the predominant heterozygote, 0.40 for the heterozygote, and 0.11 for the homozygous rare allele. Among lung cancer patients the homozygous rare allele was found to be threefold higher than among healthy people. This polymorphism was shown to segregate concordantly with CYP1A1 inducibility phenotype (AHH) [76]. A study of 221 Norwegian lung cancer individuals and 212 controls did not find an association between the *MspI* polymorphism and an increased risk of lung cancer [77]. Linkage disequilibrium of this polymorphism with a gene regulating *CYP1A1* inducibility or its activity could explain why these two characters cosegregate in the Japanese population but not in the Norwegian population. In this perspective it is worth noting that *MspI* polymorphism is associated with a point mutation in the region of gene coding for the heme binding region [78]. Phenotypic expression of this mutant has not yet been characterized. Other RFLPs on CYP1A1 were found but are not related to lung cancer risk [79].

CYP2E1 is the only member of this P450 family in rat and humans. This enzyme bioactivates procarcinogens, especially $N,N$-dimethylnitrosamine, $N$-nitrosamine, and benzene [80]. It is readily inducible by the administration of various chemicals, especially by ethanol via a post-transcriptional mechanism. Expression of this enzyme in human lung has not been described, whereas it is expressed in rabbit lung [81]. Large interindividual differences have been found in the CYP2E1 content in human liver, but it is not known if this polymorphism is of genetic origin or results from environmental factors [82]. These data suggest that CYP2E1 may be responsible for variations in individual susceptibility to cancers induced by nitrosamines. This underlines the interest of a noninvasive probe to assess its in vivo level and function. The 6-hydroxylation of chlorzoxazone, a therapeutic muscle relaxant, that was shown to be specifically catalyzed by CYP2E1 constitutes a noninvasive probe in humans. It should prove useful to assess in vivo level and function of CYP2E1 in clinical studies [83]. An association between a *DraI* RFLP of the human CYP2E1 gene and susceptibility to lung cancer was observed recently in 47 Japanese individuals [84]. A genetic polymorphism of CYP2E1 was composed of several point mutations in the distal

5'-flanking region of the gene [85]. This difference induced a change in the expression level of P450 mRNA. The mutated DNA fragment placed upstream of SV40 promoter and the chloramphenicol acetyltransferase gene enhanced about 10 times the expression of the gene. Results of DNase footprinting experiments suggest that this polymorphism affects the binding of trans-acting factor to CYP2E1 and changes its transcriptional regulation. This mutation could be responsible of interindividual differences jn CYP2E1 activity. Its relation to lung cancer susceptibility has not yet been studied.

## V. CYP2D6 Polymorphism as Marker of Lung Cancer Risk

### A. Debrisoquine Hydroxylase Polymorphism

Individual differences in the drug response in patients treated with debrisoquine, an antihypertensive agent, and the occurrence of adverse reactions to the drug were shown to occur because of a defective oxidative drug metabolism. This defective drug metabolism is due to the absence of specific cytochrome, P4502D6. Deficiency in the 4-hydroxylation of debrisoquine was the first genetic polymorphism to be recognized among the hepatic microsomal P450s and has been studied intensively. Two distinct phenotypes can be defined, the extensive metabolizer (EM) and the poor metabolizer (PM). They differ in their ability to perform the oxidation of debrisoquine, sparteine, and other drugs.

Determination of the phenotype required the administration of a probe drug (debrisoquine, sparteine, or dextrometorphan [86]) followed by collection of urine for several hours. The determination of the drug and of its chief metabolites is performed through HPLC procedure [87]. With debrisoquine the metabolic phenotype is determined by calculating the ratio, which is the percent dose excreted of unchanged drug divided by the percent dose excreted as 4-hydroxydebrisoquine.

Population and family studies performed with debrisoquine demonstrated that the level of enzyme activity segregated within families in a Mendelian fashion. This defective oxidative drug phenotype is inherited as an autosomal recessive trait [88,89], but other studies found data consistent with an autosomal codominant transmission [90]. The human *CYP2D6* cDNA has been cloned and the gene fully sequenced, and its locus is on the long arm of chromosome 22 (22q11.2-qter) [91–93]. A subgroup of approximately 5 to 10% of subjects with PM phenotype is found in Caucasian populations [88,90].

In a case-control study, where lung cancer patients were compared to a chronic bronchitis population, extensive metabolizers of debrisoquine were at increased risk for developing bronchial carcinoma compared to poor metabolizers [94]. Other studies considering this association have produced conflicting results or were criticized for their epidemiologic methods [95–98]. In a recent case-control study the debrisoquine phenotype was determined in 42 black and 42 white lung cancer patients [90]. Those with chronic obstructive pulmonary diseases or a variety of other cancers formed two groups of controls. Both black and white lung cancer patients EM were at significantly greater risk of lung cancer than were those who were poor metabolizer and intermediate metabolizers. The odd ratio was 4.5 and 10.2 for black and white patients, respectively, and was close to that calculated from the data of Ayesh et al. [91,94]. This increased risk was also found when the two control groups were considered separately; distributions of the debrisoquine phenotype were identical in both control groups. EM phenotype is associated with the risk of lung cancer, but whether this phenotype is cause or effect of the tumor is not known.

Discrepancies between the different clinical studies may be explained partly by some technical difficulties. The protocol for testing the CYP2D6 phenotype with drugs suffers from some drawbacks. The debrisoquine phenotype does not sort well into trimodal groups with heterozygotes clearly distinguished from other groups; thus misclassification of intermediate phenotypes may occur. This test is often not feasible because of interference by coadministered drugs, potential medical adverse effects of the drugs, or inability to schedule protocol requirements [99]. More than 40% of eligible subjects for debrisoquine study were excluded in the Caporaso study because of these limitations of the phenotyping procedure [90].

### B. CYP2D6 Polymorphism

A polymerase chain reaction assay associated with a RFLP procedure allowing identification of more than 95% of the different mutated alleles has been developed. This assay should shed light on the existence and significance of a link between CYP2D6 and lung cancer. Subsequent to the cloning of the CYP2D6 gene, several mutated alleles were described. A pseudogene, not transcribed because of interruption by stop codons CYP2D8P, and a related gene CYP2D7 occur in tandem with the CYP2D6 gene [94]. Analysis of poor metabolizer-genomic DNA by restriction fragment length polymorphism analysis using XbaI enzyme allowed detection of three mutant alleles of the CYP2D6 gene [100,101]. These mutants are characterized by 44- and 11.5-kb fragments and a pair of fragments of 16 and 9 kb. The 44-kb fragment has an insertion gene due to nonhomologous recombination between CYP2D6 and CYP2D7 genes. The 11.5-kb allele represents deletion of the entire CYP2D6 gene [102]. Cloning and sequencing genes from poor metabolizers permitted the characterization of three-point mutated alleles. The allele termed 29A has a single base deletion in exon 5 that causes a shift in the reading frame. The 29B contains four point mutations, one of which is at the splice site consensus sequence between intron 3 and exon 4 [103]. The 29C is characterized by a single 3-bp deletion of the fifth exon [104]. Identification of about 95% of mutant alleles is allowed by the combined use of oligonucleotide primers specific for mutations and the normal sequence and of amplification of genomic DNA by polymerase chain reaction (allele-specific PCR) [105].

The mechanism responsible for the relation between the EM phenotype and lung cancer is discussed. For CYP1A1, animal, molecular, and clinical studies suggest that this susceptibility factor modifies the effect of tobacco smoke. In contrast, the CYP2D6 phenotype appears to be an independent risk factor for lung cancer [91]. The normal allele and mutated alleles may be in linkage disequilibrium, respectively, with a gene that induces transformation or protects against cancer. Another hypothesis has been proposed based on the observation of similar binding affinities of some dopamine uptake blockers for both brain CYP2D6 and the dopamine transporter [106]. Thus it was envisioned that CYP2D6 activity may be of importance to the regulation of one effector of cell growth. In this perspective the development of a molecular biology procedure allowing identification of more than 95% of the different mutated alleles should lead to a better understanding of the relationship existing between CYP2D6 function and enhanced risk of lung cancer. However, it is possible that genetic "phenotyping" may not resolve this question completely. If the mutation explains almost all the cases of poor metabolizer phenotype, the variation within the extensive metabolizer phenotype is still considerable (about 100-fold) [107]. It is possible that even if there is not clear evidence for induction of CYP2D6, these variations may involve some cis- or trans-acting regulatory elements.

It remains to be determined whether CYP2D6 is expressed in the lung tissue, and if not, whether variations in the enzyme activity in the liver are causal in lung cancer occurrence or if the CYP2D6 gene is in linkage disequilibrium with another gene important in the carcinogenic process.

## VI. Role of Other Human Lung Cytochromes P450 in Cancer

CYP3A4 is involved in the bioactivation of 7,8-dihydroxy-7,8-dihydro-benzo[a]pyrene and of other dihydrodiol derivatives of polycyclic aromatic hydrocarbons. This enzyme expressed in rat lung (CYP3A1) was shown to be expressed in human lung by immunoinhibition or induction ($\alpha$-naphtoflavone) of the microsomal enzymatic activity. It is not known if the large variations observed in the enzyme liver content are related to genetic factors. An evaluation of the increase in the 6$\beta$-hydroxycortisol/free cortisol urinary ratio after administration of drug inducer of CYP3A has been proposed to figure out whether or not P4503A inducibility is genetically controlled [108].

The question of participation of other cytochromes P450 in bioactivation of PAH should be raised. Benzo[a]pyrene metabolites produced by CYP1A1 enzyme are 10 to 100 times more mutagenic than those produced by other cytochromes, such as enzymes encoded by the 2C gene subfamily [109]. It should be kept in mind that if these enzymes are expressed at a high level, they could, through bioactivation or detoxication processes of PAHs, modulate the carcinogenicity of these compounds. Some cytochrome P450 have been shown to be specifically expressed in human lung [110,111]. However, there are critically few data about their efficacy in the procarcinogen bioactivation processes, and no polymorphism (phenotypic or genetic) has been described yet.

## VII.  Conclusions

Studies involving the polymorphism of cytochromes P450 are important in the discovery of genes that predispose to lung cancer. Although we have amassed a lot of information, our data are not complete for any form of cytochrome P450. These results do raise the possibility that inheritance might play an important role in individual susceptibility to lung cancer, but to date, there is no definite evidence that a true cytochrome P450 polymorphism is an etiological factor. There is much controversy concerning the observations describing relationships between polymorphism of CYP1A1 and 2D6, and enhanced risk for lung cancer.

Identification of a genetic risk for lung cancer is of major interest in an understanding of cancer. The ultimate validity of a biologic marker is the extent to which it can predict disease occurrence. In this perspective, in vivo cytochrome P450 phenotyping or genotyping does not yet seem to meet the standard. However, these tests should strengthen epidemiologic researches and help us in advancing knowledge concerning exposure–disease relationships and identification of susceptibility genes for environmentally related diseases. Investigation of the genetic mutations for a polymorphic cytochrome could be of some interest in the occupational environment. Screening might prove efficacious if focused on small high-risk groups, which is not the case of cigarette smokers with regard to the CYP2D6 polymorphism. Developments in molecular genetics together with the development of in vivo tests specific to one cytochrome P450 and easy to perform would enable comprehensive studies to be executed.

## References

1. Frank AL. Epidemiology of lung cancer. In: Roth JA, Ruckdeschel JC, Weisenberger TH, eds. Thoracic oncology. Philadelphia: WB Saunders, 1989:6–15.
2. Loeb LA, Ernster VL, Warner KE, et al. Smoking and lung cancer: an overview. Cancer Res 1984;44:5940–58.
3. Thakker DR, Yagi H, Levin W, Wood AW, Conney AH, Jerina DM. Polycyclic aromatic hydrocarbons: metabolic activation to ultimate carcin-

ogens. In: MW Anders, ed. Bioactivation of foreign compounds. New York: Academic Press, 1985:177–242.

4. Philpot RM, Smith BR. Role of cytochrome P-450 and related enzymes in the pulmonary metabolism of xenobiotics. Environ Health Perspect 1984;55:359–67.

5. Baron J, Voigt JM. Localization, distribution, and induction of xenobiotic-metabolizing enzymes and aryl hydrocarbon hydroxylase within lung. Pharmacol Ther 1990;47:419–45.

6. Guengerich FP. Enzymatic oxidation of xenobiotic chemicals. Biochem Mol Biol 1990;25:97–153.

7. Gonzalez FJ. Molecular genetics of the P-450 superfamily. Pharmacol Ther 1990;45:1–38.

8. Nebert DW, Nelson DR, Coon MJ, Estabrook RW, Gonzalez FJ, Feyereisen R, Fujiikuriyama Y, Guengerich FP, Gunsalus IC, Johnson EF, Lopper JC, Phillips IR, Sato R, Waterman MR, Waxman DJ. The P450 superfamily: update on new sequences, gene mapping, and recommended nomenclature. DNA Cell Biol 1991;10:1–14.

9. Crespi CL, Penman BW, Gelboin HV, Gonzalez FJA. Tobacco smoke-derived nitrosamine, 4-(methylnitrosamino)-1-(3-pyridyl)-1-butanone, is activated by multiple human cytochrome P450s including the polymorphic human cytochrome P450 IID6. Carcinogenesis 1991;12:1197–1201.

10. Wall KL, Gao W, Koepple JM, Kwei GY, Kauffman FC, Thurman RG. The liver plays a central role in the mechanism of chemical carcinogenesis due to polycyclic aromatic hydrocarbons. Carcinogenesis (Lond) 1991;11:783–86.

11. Kouri RE, Billups L, Rude TH, Whitmire CE, Sass B, Henry CJ. Correlation of inducibility of arylhydrocarbon hydroxylase activity with susceptibility to 3-methylcholanthrene-induced lung cancer. Cancer Lett 1980;9:277–84.

12. Lu L-JW, Harvey RG, Lee H, Baxter JR, Anderson LM. Age-, tissue-, and *Ah* genotype-dependent difference in the binding of 3-methyl-cholanthrene and its metabolite(s) to mouse DNA. Cancer Res 1990;20:4239–47.

13. Perera F, Mayer J, Jretzji A, et al. Comparison of DNA adducts and sister chromatid exchange in lung cancer cases and controls. Cancer Res 1989;49:4456–61.

14. Phillips DH, Hewer A, Martin CN, Garner RC, King MM. Correlation of DNA adduct levels in human lung and cigarette smoking. Nature 1988;36:790–92.

15. Randerath E, Miller RH, Mittal D, Avitts TA, Weinstein IB, Randerath K. Covalent DNA damage in tissues of cigarette smokers as determined by $^{32}$P-postlabelling assay. J Natl Cancer Inst 1989;81:341–47.

16. Cuzick J, Routledge MN, Jenkins D, et al. DNA adducts in different tissue of smokers and nonsmokers. Int J Cancer 1990;45:673–78.
17. Voigt JM, Kwabata TT, Burke JP, Martin MV, Guengerich FP, Baron J. In situ localization and distribution of xenobiotic-activating enzymes and aryl hydrocarbon hydroxylase activity in lungs of untreated rats. Mol Pharmacol 1990;37:182–91.
18. Rehm S, Kellof GJ. Histologic characterization of mouse bronchiolar cell hyperplasia, metaplasia and neoplasia induced intratracheally by 3-methylcholanthrene. Exp Lung Res 1991;17:229–44.
19. Law MR. Genetic predisposition to lung cancer. Br J Cancer 1990;6:195–206.
20. Nebert DW. The *Ah* locus: genetic differences in toxicity, cancer, mutation, and birth defect. Crit Rev Toxicol 1989;20:137–52.
21. Whitehead JK, Rothwell K. The mouse skin carcinogenicity of cigarette smoke condensate fractionated by solvent partition methods. Br J Cancer 1969;23:840–57.
22. Yun C-H, Shimada T, Guengerich FP. Role of human liver cytochrome P4502C and 3A enzymes in the 3-hydroxylation of benzo(*a*)pyrene. Cancer Res 1992;52:1868–74.
23. Boles TC, Hogan ME. Site specific binding to DNA. Proc Natl Acad Sci USA 1984;81:5623–27.
24. Dittrich KA, Krugh TR. Analysis of site-specific binding of (+/–)-anti-benzo<*a*>pyrene diol epoxide to restriction fragments of pBR322 DNA via photochemical mapping. Chem Res Toxicol 1991;4:270–76.
25. Jaiswal AK, Gonzalez FJ, Nebert DW. Human dioxin-inducible cyto-chrome $P_1$-450 complementary DNA and amino acid sequence. Science 1985;228:80–83.
26. Domin BA, Devereux TR, Philpot RM. The cytochrome P-450 monooxy-genase system of the rabbit lung: enzyme components, activities, and induction in the nonciliated epithelial (Clara) cell, alveolar type II, and alveolar macrophage. Mol Pharmacol 1986;30:296–303.
27. Prough AR, Patrizi VW, Okita RT, Masters BS, Jakobson SW. Charac-teristic of benzo(a)pyrene metabolism by kidney, liver, and lung micro-somal fractions from rodents and humans. Cancer Res 1979;390:1199–1206.
28. Wheeler CW, Park SS, Guenthner TM. Immunochemical analysis of a cytochrome P-450IA1 homologue in human lung microsomes. Mol Pharmacol 1990;38:634–43.
29. McLemore TL, Adelberg S, Czerwinski M, Hubbard WC, Yu SJ, Storeng R, Wood TG, Hines RN, Boyd MR. Altered regulation of the cytochrome P4501A1-gene: novel inducer-independent gene expression in pulmonary carcinoma cell lines. J Natl Cancer Inst 1989;81:1787–94.

30. Wheeler CW, Guenthner TM. Cytochrome P-450-dependent metabolism of xenobiotics in human lung. J Biochem Toxicol 1991;3:163–69.
31. Omiecinski CJ, Redlich CA, Costa P. Induction and developmental expression of cytochrome P450IA1 messenger RNA in rat and human tissue by the polymerase chain reaction. Cancer Res 1990;50:4315–21.
32. Poland AP, Glover E. 2,3,7,8-Tetrachlorodibenzo-*p*-dioxin: segregation of toxicity with the *Ah* locus. Mol Pharmacol 1980;17:86–90.
33. Pelkonen O, Kärki NT, Korhonnen P, Koisvisto M, Tuimala R, Kauppila A. Human placental aryl hydrocarbon hydroxylase: genetics and environmental influences. In: Jones PW, Lebers P, eds. Polynuclear aromatic hydrocarbons. Ann Arbor, MI: Ann Arbor Science Publishers 1979:765–77.
34. Nebert DW, Janssen NM. The *Ah* locus genetic regulation of the metabolism of carcinogens, drugs, and other environmental chemicals by cytochrome P-450-mediated monooxygenases. CRC Crit Rev Biochem 1979;6:401–37.
35. Nebert DW, Benedict WF, Kouri RE. Aromatic hydrocarbon-produced tumorigenesis and the genetic differences in aryl hydrocarbon hydroxylase induction. In: Ts'o POP, DiPaolo JA, eds. Chemical carcinogenesis. New York: Marcel Dekker, 1974;271–88.
36. Nebert DW, Jones JE. Regulation of the mammalian cytochrome $P_1450$ *(CYPIAI)* gene. Int J Biochem 1989;21:243–52.
37. Okey AB, Denison MS, Prokipcak RD, Roberts EA, Harper PA. Receptors of polycyclic aromatic hydrocarbons. In: Galteau MM, Siest G, Henny J, eds. Biologie prospective. Paris: John Libbey Eurotext, 1989;605–10.
38. Puga A, Raychaudhuri B, Salata K, Zhang Y-H, Nebert DW. Stable expression of mouse *Cyp1a1* and human CYP1A2 cDNAs transfected into mouse hepatoma cells lacking P-450 enzyme activity. DNA Cell Biol 1990;9:425–36.
39. Landers JP, Bunce NJ. The *Ah* receptor and the mechanism of dioxin toxicity. Biochem J 1991;276:273–87.
40. McLemore TL, Martin RR, Pickard LR, Springer RK, Wray NP, Toppell KL, Mattox KL, Guin GA, Cantrell ET, Busbee DL. Analysis of aryl hydrocarbon hydroxylase activity in human lung tissue, pulmonary macrophages and blood monocytes. Cancer (Phila) 1978;41:2292–2300.
41. McLemore TL, Adelberg S, Liu MC, McMahon NA, Yu SJ, Hubard WC, Czerwinski M, Wood TG, Storeng R, Lubet RA, Eggleston JC, Boyd MR, Hines MR. Expression of CYP1A1 gene in patients with lung cancer: evidence for cigarette smoke-induced gene expression in normal lung tissue and for altered gene regulation in primary pulmonary carcinomas. J Natl Cancer Inst 1990;82:1333–39.
42. Randerath E, Avitts TA, Reddy MV, Miller RH, Everson RB, Randerath

K. Comparative $^{32}$P-analysis of cigarette smoke-induced DNA damage in human tissues and mouse skin. Cancer Res 1986;46:5869–77.

43. Geneste O, Camus A-M, Castegnero M, Petruzelli S, Macchiarini P, Angeletti CA, Giuntini C, Bartsch H. Comparison of pulmonary DNA adduct levels measured by $^{32}$P-postlabelling and aryl hydrocarbon hydroxylase activity in lung parenchyma of smokers and ex-smokers. Carcinogenesis 1991;12:1301–5.

44. Atlas SA, Vessel ES, Nebert DW. Genetic control of interindividual variations in the inducibility of aryl hydrocarbon hydroxylase in cultured human lymphocytes. Cancer Res 1976;36:4619–30.

45. Jaiswal AK, Gonzalez FJ, Nebert DW. Human $P_1$-450 gene sequence and correlation of mRNA with genetic differences in benzo[a]pyrene metabolism. Nucleic Acids Res 1985;13:4503–20.

46. Kellerman G, Shaw CR, Luyten-Kellerman M. Aryl hydrocarbon hydroxylase inducibility and bronchogenic carcinoma. N Engl J Med 1973;289:934–37.

47. Trell L, Korsgaard R, Janzon L, Trell E. Distribution and reproducibility of aryl hydrocarbon hydroxylase inducibility in a prospective population study of middle-aged male smokers and nonsmokers. Cancer 1985;56:1988–94.

48. Okuda T, Vessell ES, Plotkin E, Tarone R, Bast RC, Gelboin HV. Interindividual and intraindividual variations in aryl hydrocarbon hydroxylase in monocytes from monozygotic and dizygotic twins. Cancer Res 1977;37:3904–7.

49. Guirgis H, Lynch HT, Mate T, Harris RE, Wells I, Caha L, Anderson J, Maloney K, Rankin L. Aryl hydrocarbon hydroxylase activity in lymphocytes from lung cancer patients and normal controls. Oncology (Basel) 1976;3:105–9.

50. Jett JR, Moses HL, Branum EL, Taylor WF, Fontana RS. Benzo(a)pyrene metabolism and blast transformation in peripheral blood mononuclear cells from smoking and nonsmoking populations and lung cancer patients. Cancer (Phila) 1970;40:191–200.

51. Paigen B, Gurtoo HL, Minowada J, Houten L, Vincent R, Paigen K, Parker NB, Ward E, Hayner NT. Questionable relation of aryl hydrocarbon hydroxylase to lung cancer risk. N Engl J Med 1977;297:346–50.

52. Kouri RE, Imblum RL, Sosnowski RG, Slomiany J, McKinney CE. Parameters influencing quantitation of 3-methylcholanthrene-induced aryl hydrocarbon hydroxylase activity in cultured human lymphocytes. J Environ Pathol Toxicol 1979;2:1079–98.

53. Robie-Suh K, Robinson R, Gelboin HV, Guengerich FP. Aryl hydrocarbon hydroxylase is inhibited by antibody to rat liver cytochrome P-450. Science; 1980;208:1031–33.

54. Bast RC, Okuda T, Plotkin E, Tarone R, Rapp HJ, Gelboin HV. Development of an assay for aryl hydrocarbon [benzo(a)pyrene] hydroxylase in human peripheral blood monocytes. Cancer Res 1976;36:1967–74.

55. Emery AEM, Danford M, Anan R, Duncan W, Paton L. Aryl hydrocarbon hydroxylase inducibility in patients with lung cancer. Lancet 1978;3:470–71.

56. Karki NT, Pokela R, Nuutinene L, Pelkonen O. Aryl hydrocarbon hydroxylase in lymphocytes and lung tissue from lung cancer patients and controls. Int J Cancer 1987;39:565–68.

57. Ducos J, Migueres J, Colombies P, Kessous A, Poujoulet N. Lymphocyte response to phytohemagglutin in patients with lung cancer. Lancet 1970;1:1111–12.

58. Rao LGS. AHH inducibility and lung cancer. Lancet 1974;1:1228.

59. Paigen B, Ward E, Reilly A, Houten L, Gurtoo HL, Minowada J, Steenland K, Havens MB, Sartori P. Seasonal variations of aryl hydrocarbon hydroxylase activity in human lymphocytes. Cancer Res 1981;41:2757–61.

60. Hammond DK, Strobel HW. Ethoxyresorufin O-deethylase activity in intact human cells. Toxicol in Vitro 1992;1:41–46.

61. Cosma GN, Toniolo P, Currie D, Pasternack BS, Garte SJ. Expression of the CYP1A1 gene in peripheral lymphocytes as a marker of exposure to creosote in railroad workers. Cancer Epidemiol Biomed Prev 1992;1:137–42.

62. Harris CC, Hsu IC, Stoner GD, Trump BF, Selkirk JK. Human pulmonary alveolar macrophages metabolize benzo(a)pyrene to proximate and ultimate mutagens. Nature (London) 1978;272:633–34.

63. Aoyama T, Gonzalez F, Gelboin HV. Human cDNA expressed cytochrome P450 1A2: mutagen activation and substrate specificity. Mol Carcinog 1989;2:192–98.

64. Quattrochi LC, Tukey RH. The human cytochrome CYP1A2 gene contains regulatory elements responsive to 3-methylcholanthrene. Mol Pharmacol 1989;36:66–71.

65. Voorman R, Aust SD. Inducer of cytochrome P-450d: influence on microsomal catalytic activities and differential regulation by enzyme stabilization. Arch Biochem Biophys 1988;262:76–84.

66. Sesardic D, Pasanen M, Palkonen O, Boobis AR. Differential expression and regulation of members of the cytochrome-P450IA gene subfamily in human tissues. Carcinogenesis 1990;12:1183–88.

67. Campbell ME, Spielberg SP, Kalow W. A urinary metabolite ratio that reflects systemic caffeine clearance. Clin Pharmacol Ther 1987;42:157–65.

68. Kalow W, Tang B-K. Use of caffeine metabolite ratios to explore CYP1A2 and xanthine oxidase activities. Clin Pharmacol Ther 1991;50:508–19.

69. Tarrus E, Cami J, Roberts DJ, Spickett RGW, Celdran E, Segura J. Accumulation of caffeine in healthy volunteers treated with furafylline. Br J Clin Pharmacol 1987;23:9–18.

70. Callahan MM, Robertson RS, Arnaud MJ, Branfman AR, McCormish MF, Yesair DW. Human metabolism of [1-methyl-$^{14}$C] and [2-$^{14}$C]caffeine after oral administration. Drug Metab Dispos 1982;10:417–23.

71. Butler MA, Iwasaki M, Guengerich FP, Kadlubar FF. Human cytochrome P-450$_{PA}$ (P-450IA2), the phenacetin $O$-deethylase, is primarily responsible for the hepatic 3-demethylation of caffeine and N-oxidation of carcinogenic arylamines. Proc Natl Acad Sci USA 1989;86:7696–7700.

72. Kalow W, Tang B-K. Caffeine as a metabolic probe: exploration of the enzyme-inducing effect of cigarette smoking. Clin Pharmacol Ther 1991;49:44–48.

73. Guengerich FP. Polymorphism of cytochrome P-450 in humans. Trends Pharmacol Sci 1989;10:107–9.

74. Shimada T, Misono KS, Guengerich FP. Human liver cytochrome P-450 mephenytoin 4-hydroxylase, a prototype of genetic polymorphism in oxidative drug metabolism. J Biol Chem 1986;261:909–21.

75. Kawajiri K, Nakachi K, Imai K, Yoshii A, Shinoda N, Watanabe J. Identification of genetically high risk individuals to lung cancer by DNA polymorphism of the cytochrome P450IA1 gene. FEBS Lett 1990;263:131–33.

76. Petersen DD, McKinney CE, Ikeeya K, Smith HH, Bale AE, McBride OW, Nebert DW. Human CYP1A1 gene: cosegregation of the enzyme inducibility phenotype and an RFLP. Am J Hum Genet 1991;48:720–25.

77. Tefre T, Rydberg D, Haugen A, Nebert DW, Skuag V, Brgger A, Brresen A-L. Human $CYP1A1$ (cytochrome P$_1$450) gene: lack of association between the $Msp$ I restriction length polymorphism and incidence of lung cancer in a Norwegian population. Pharmacogenetics 1991;1:20–25.

78. Hayashi S-I, Watanabe J, Nakachi K, Kawajiri K. Genetic linkage of lung cancer associated $Msp$I polymorphisms with aminoacid replacement in the heme binding region of the human cytochrome P450IA1 gene. J Biochem 1991;110:407–11.

79. Haugen A, Willey J, Brressen A-L, Tefre T. PstI polymorphism at the human P$_1$450 gene on chromosome 15. Nucleic Acids Res 1990;18:3114.

80. Guengerich FP, Kim DH, Iwasaki M. Role of human cytochrome-P-450-IIE1 in the oxidation of many low molecular weight cancer suspects. Chem Res Toxicol 1991;4:168–79.

81. Porter T, Khani SC, Coon MJ. Induction and tissue-specific expression of rabbit cytochrome P450IIE1 and IIE2 gene. Mol Pharmacol 1989;36:61–65.
82. Perrot N, Nalpas B, Yang CS, Beaune Ph. Modulation of cytochrome P450 isozymes in human liver by ethanol and drug intake. Eur J Clin Invest 1989;19:549–55.
83. Peter R, Böcker R, Beaune Ph, Iwasaki M, Guengerich FP, Yang CS. Hydroxylation of chlorzoxazone as a specific probe for human liver cytochrome P-450IIE1. Chem Res Toxicol 1990;3:566–73.
84. Uematsu F, Kikuchi H, Motomiya M, Abe T, Sagami I, Ohmachi T, Wakui A, Kanamaru R, Watanabe M. Association between restriction fragment length polymorphism of the human cytochrome P450IIE1 gene and susceptibility to lung cancer. Jpn J Cancer Res 1991;82:254–56.
85. Hayashi S-I, Watanabe J, Kawajiri K. Genetic polymorphism in the 5'-flanking region change transcriptional regulation of the human cytochrome P45OIIE1 gene. J Biochem 1991;110:559–65.
86. Schmid B, Bircher MD, Preisig R, Küpfer A. Polymorphic dextrometorphan metabolism: co-segregation of oxidative O-demethylation with debrisoquine hydroxylation. Clin Pharmacol Ther 1985;38:618–24.
87. Idle JR, Mahgoub A, Angelo MM, Dring LG, Lancaster R, Smith RL. The metabolism of [14C]debrisoquine in man. Br J Clin Pharmacol 1979;7:257–66.
88. Price-Evans DAP, Maghoub A, Sloan TP, Idle JR, Smith RL. A family and population study of the genetic polymorphism of debrisoquine oxidation in a white British population. J Med Genet 1980;17:102–5.
89. Alvan G, Bechtel P, Iselius L, Gundert-Remy U. Hydroxylation polymorphism of debrisoquin and mephenytoin in European populations. Eur J Clin Pharmacol 1990;39:533–37.
90. Caporaso NE, Tucker MA, Hoover RN, Hayes RB, Pickle LW, Isaaq HJ, Muschik GM, Green-Gallo L., Buivys D, Aisner S, Resau JH, Trum BF, Tollerud D, Weston A, Harris CC. Lung cancer and the debrisoquine metabolic phenotype. J Natl Cancer Inst 1990;82:1264–72.
91. Eichelbaum M, Baur MP, Osikowa-Evers BO, Tieves G, Zekorn C, Rittner C. Chromosomal assignment of human cytochrome P450 debrisoquine/sparteine type to chromosome 22. Br J Clin Pharmacol 1987;23:455–58.
92. Gonzalez FJ, Skoda RC, Kimura S, Umeno M, Zanger UM, Zanger M, Nebert DW, Gelboin HV, Harwick JP, Meyer UA. Characterization of the common genetic defect in humans deficient in debrisoquine metabolism. Nature 1988;331:442–46.
93. Kimura S, Umeno M, Skoda RC, Gelboin HV, Meyer UA, Gonzalez FJ. The human debrisoquin 4-hydroxylase (CYP2D) locus: sequence and

identification of the polymorphic CYP2D6 gene, a related gene and a pseudogene. Am J Hum Genet 1989;45:889–904.

94. Ayesh R, Idle JR, Ritshie JC, Crothers MJ, Hetzel MR. Metabolic oxidation phenotypes as markers for susceptibility to lung cancer. Nature (London) 1984;312:169–70.

95. Roots I, Drakoulis N, Plotch M, Heinmeyer G, Loddenkemper R, Minks T, Nitz T, Otte F, Koch M. Debrisoquin hydroxylation phenotype, acetylation phenotype, and ABO blood group as genetic host factors of lung cancer risk. Klin Wochenschr 1988;66:87–97.

96. Boobis AR, Davies DA. Debrisoquine oxidation phenotype and susceptibility to lung cancer. Br J Clin Pharmacol 1990;30:653–56.

97. Speirs CJ, Murray S, Davies DS, Biola Madadeje AF, Boobis AR. Debrisoquine oxidation phenotype and susceptibility to lung cancer. Br J Clin Pharmacol 1990;29:101–9.

98. Duché, J-C, Joanne C, Barré J, Decremoux H, Dalphin J-C, Depierre A, Brochard P, Tillement J-P, Bechtel P. Lack of a relationship between the polymorphism of debrisoquine oxidation and lung cancer. Br J Clin Pharmacol 1991;31(5):533–36.

99. Leeman T, Dayer P, Meyer UA. Single-dose quinidine treatment inhibits metoprolol oxidation in extensive metabolizers. Eur J Clin Pharmacol 1986;29:739–41.

100. Skoda RC, Gonzalez FJ, Demierre A, Meyer UA. Two mutant alleles of the human cytochrome dbl-gene (P450C2D1) associated with genetically deficient metabolism of debrisoquine and other drugs. Proc Natl Acad Sci USA 1988;85:5240–43.

101. Evans WE, Relling MV. XbaI 16- plus 9-kilobase DNA restriction fragment identify a mutant allele for debrisoquine hydroxylase: report of a family study. Mol Pharmacol 1990;37:639–42.

102. Gaedigk A, Blum M, Gaedigk R, Eichelbaum M, Meyer UA. Deletion of the entire cytochrome P-450 Cyp2D6 gene as a cause of impaired drug metabolism in poor metabolizers of the debrisoquine/sparteine polymorphism. Am J Hum Genet 1991;48:943–50.

103. Hanioka N, Kimura S, Meyer UA, Gonzalez FJ. The human *CYP2D* locus associated with a common genetic in drug oxidation: a G1934 to a base change in intron 3 of mutant *CYP2D6* allele results in an aberrant splice recognition site. Am J Hum Genet 1990;47:994–1001.

104. Broly F, Gaedigk A, Heim M, Eichelbaum M, Morike K, Meyer UA. Debrisoquine/sparteine hydroxylation genotype and phenotype: analysis of common mutation and alleles of CYP2D6 in a European population. DNA Cell Biol 1991;10:545–58.

105. Heim M, Meyer UA. Genotyping of poor metaboliser of debrisoquine by allele-specific PCR amplification. Lancet 1990;336:529–32.

106. Niznick HB, Tyndale RF, Sallee FR, Gonzalez FJ, Hardwick JP, Inaba T, Kalow W. The dopamine transporter and cytochrome P-450IID1 (debrisoquine 4-hydroxylase) in brain: resolution and identification of two distinct [$^3$H]GBR-12935 binding proteins. Arch Biochem Biophys 1990;276;424–32.

107. Guengerich FP. Characterization of human microsomal cytochrome P-450 enzymes. Am Rev Pharmacol Toxicol 1989;29:241–64.

108. Ged C, Rouillon JM, Pichard L, Combalbert J, Bressot N, Bories P, Michel H, Beaune P, Maurel P. The increase in urinary excretion of 6β-hydroxycortisol as a marker of human hepatic cytochrome P450IIIA induction. Br J Clin Pharmacol 1989;28:373–87.

109. Todorovic R, Devanesan PD, Cavalieri EL, Rogan EG, Park SS, Gelboin HV. A monoclonal antibody to rat liver cytochrome P450 IIC11 strongly and regiospecifically inhibits constitutive benzo(*a*)pyrene metabolism and DNA binding. Mol Carcinog 1991;4:308–14.

110. Nhamburo PT, Gonzalez FJ, McBride OW, Gelboiw HU, Kimura S. Identification of a new P450 expressed in human lung: complete cDNA sequence, cDNA directed expression, and chromosome mapping. Biochem. 1989;28:8060–66.

111. Nhamburo PT, Gonzalez FJ, McBride OW, Kozak CA, Gelboiw HU, Gonzalez FJ. The human CYP2F gene subfamily: identification of a new cytochrome P450, cDNA-directed expression, and chromosome mapping. Biochem 1990;29:5491–99.

# Part Four

## TOBACCO AND RESPIRATORY DISEASES

**ALBERT HIRSCH**

In the industrialized countries (1.2 billion inhabitants), tobacco smoking is responsible each year for 1.8 million deaths, of which 0.8 million were prior to age 65. Extrarespiratory cancers (laryngeal, orobuccal cavity, bladder), certain cardiovascular diseases (coronary heart disease, peripheral vascular disease, stroke), lung carcinoma, and chronic respiratory diseases (chronic bronchitis and emphysema) are causally related to tobacco. Chapter 21 is devoted to the epidemiologic methodology that has led to knowledge about this causal relationship between tobacco use and disease. Despite the possibility of misclassification of smoking status, it appears that self-report is a valid measure for assessing the adverse health effects of cigarette smoking and the health benefits of cessation. Epidemiologic methodology can provide the information necessary to develop preventive strategies, including information on the psychosocial factors that influence the smoking habit. The concept of the "healthy" smoker, as a phenomenon of natural selection by a person who takes up the smoking habit because his or her lungs are relatively resistant to the adverse health effects of tobacco, has to be studied rigorously to identify the characteristics of the susceptible smoker.

Chapters 22 through 24 concern the effect of environmental tobacco smoke (ETS). Passive smoking is related to adult respiratory function impairment, respiratory symptoms, and lung cancers, but biases in the categorization of passive smoking can be produced by active smoking among ETS-exposed subjects, socioeconomic status, susceptibility in some subgroups, estimations of exposure, and measures of diseases. In childhood, some data concerning the effects of ETS are very consistent, such as the effects on the fetus of smoking during pregnancy, and acute respiratory illness observed in young infants exposed to parents' tobacco smoking. But the effects of ETS on lung maturity, the consequences in adulthood of alteration of flow rates at birth, and chronic respiratory symptoms such as coughing and asthma are still controversial. A weak association has been found between bronchial hyperresponsiveness and active smoking in adults and for young children when passive smoking is clearly assessed, and may, in any case, depend on age, sex, and atopy.

Mechanisms in respiratory carcinogenesis and the epidemiology of smoking-related lung cancers are discussed in Chapters 25 and 26. The consequences of changes in cigarettes (e.g., lights, with reduced carcinogenic tars), the use of natural and synthetic agents to reduce cancer risk, and the refinement of the methods for biochemical markers to identify smokers who are at an especially high risk for cancer are reviewed. Among the data concerning the epidemiology of smoking, perhaps the most interesting is related to the importance of duration of smoking: Excess risk is principally dependent on the number of years spent smoking. Although risks decrease after quitting smoking, the annual excess risk for lung cancer remains roughly constant for many years thereafter.

Chapters 27 through 30 are devoted to the difficult problem of cessation of tobacco use. This has been studied from the pharmacological and behavioral perspectives, and the two approaches appear complementary. The role of health professionals, particularly general practitioners, pneumologists, and nurses are presented in a practical way, in terms of evaluated results from numerous published trials.

This part closes in Chapter 31 with an overview of tobacco control policy. To be efficient, an integrated policy should associate a complete ban of tobacco advertising, systematic increases in retail price through tax increases to dissuade youth from tobacco use, and protection of nonsmokers in closed public places. Evaluation of the impact of such a policy before and after its implementation could be made in terms of monitored tobacco products consumption and health consequences. Some examples of countries with significant results in terms of reduction of respiratory diseases are evoked.

# 21

# Respiratory Diseases and Tobacco
# Epidemiologic Methodology

MARGARET R. BECKLAKE

McGill University
Montreal, Quebec, Canada

## I. Introduction

### A. Definitions and Focus

Epidemiology has been defined as "the study of the distribution and determinants of health-related states and events in populations and the application of this study to control health problems" [1]. The target populations about whom inferences are to be made may be plant, animal, or human. Epidemiologic methods have been used to address a wide range of questions about natural phenomena in each of these fields of scientific endeavor. For these reasons epidemiology has been characterized as a discipline rather than a science, which is defined as an organized body of information about natural phenomena in a particular domain: for example, oncology, biochemistry, and respiratory disease [2]. As a result the epidemiology of particular conditions, such as cancer or respiratory disease (also referred to as content epidemiology), tends to be incorporated into textbooks about these conditions. By contrast, in textbooks of epidemiology, content epidemiology tends to be cited principally to illustrate applications of epidemiologic methods [3].

The focus of this volume is on the prevention of respiratory disease consequent on environmental exposures encountered in the air men and women breathe in their workplaces, in their communities, or in their personal environment. This part, the last in the volume, deals with tobacco smoke, and this chapter deals with the methodology of the discipline of epidemiology pertinent to the prevention of tobacco-related respiratory diseases. The information generated using this methodology (i.e., the content epidemiology of the respiratory diseases) is described in the subsequent chapters of this part.

### B. Uses of Epidemiology in the Study, Management, and Prevention of the Adverse Health Effects of Environmental Exposures

Epidemiologic studies are used (1) to identify and describe the adverse health effects of environmental exposures; (2) to establish dose–response relationships where possible, and if not, exposure–response relationships (preferably quantitative rather than qualitative); (3) based on an analysis of the resulting information, to develop control strategies for control of the adverse health effects; and once these are in place; (4) to evaluate their efficacy and/or effectiveness. *Efficacy* refers to the extent to which an intervention produces a beneficial result under ideal circumstances, effectiveness to the extent to which it meets its objectives in a defined population when deployed in the field [1]. This general approach can be used for all types of health outcome, respiratory or nonrespiratory, nonmalignant or malignant.

Important elements in the study methodology include the incorporation of the principles of toxicology, with emphasis on dose–response (or its surrogate exposure–response) relationships as key to establishing causality [4] as well as providing the scientific basis for setting environmental control levels [5]. Note that the concept and definition of dose in toxicology is the amount of agent delivered to the target organ and retained in contact with it long enough to produce a toxic effect.

Comparable epidemiologic methodology can be used in the study of the ill-health effects of exposure (1) to workplace pollution [6,7]; (2) to urban community pollution [8,9]; and (3) exposure to tobacco smoke [10–20]. Exposure levels tend to be higher and easier to measure quantitatively, and populations easier to characterize when the exposures of interest are pollution in the workplace, in contrast to when the exposures of interest are to community air pollution or tobacco smoke. Other methodologic differences in studies of the adverse health effects of tobacco smoke are dictated by (1) the nature of the exposure (being for the most part personally generated); (2) the fact that cumulative past exposure has of necessity to be self-reported, and based on recall of what is often a changing habit; (3) the addictive nature of the habit, and (4) the likelihood of underreporting exposure in the face of public pressure to quit. In addition, the emphasis in control of the smoking epidemic of the twentieth century is on elimination of the habit, whereas in occupational epidemiology the emphasis is on controlling the workplace pollution to levels such as to protect human health. Common features between occupational and tobacco epidemiology include (1) most of the exposure-related respiratory outcomes (lung cancer, bronchitis, chronic obstructive pulmonary disease); (2) the measurement tools to assess ill health (respiratory questionnaires, lung functions, death certificate information); and (3) recognition of the importance of making every effort to characterize exposure as completely as possible, including all potential factors influencing its intensity, variability, and duration.

## II.  Adverse Health Effects of Exposure to Tobacco Smoke: Epidemiologic Studies in Historical Perspective

Among the earliest studies to implicate smoking as a cause of illness and disease were clinical reports, and among the first diseases to be linked to smoking was lung cancer. In the 1930s, for instance, surgeons operating for lung cancer noted that their patients were invariably smokers [10]. In the 1940s, an analysis of insurance data linked smoking with premature mortality [11]. In addition, in the 1940s, data were gathered for two studies published in 1950, one carried out in the United States [12] and one in the United Kingdom [13], both of which had as their objectives an investigation of the cause(s) of lung cancer. The evolution of the British study [13,14] described by Sir Richard Doll in an interview in 1990 [15] also provides a fascinating insight into the origins of modern chronic disease epidemiology through the eyes of one of its most distinguished practitioners. In the U.K. study, a case-control design was used in a hypothesis-generating study: Suspected cases of lung and other cancers were interviewed in hospital to gather information about suspected determinants, including smoking and other exposures, and the cases then classified according to the final diagnosis, usually established by pathology. The striking finding, Doll recalls, was that cases in whom the diagnosis of lung cancer was not confirmed were invariably nonsmokers, those in which the diagnosis was confirmed were invariably smokers. This contrast with a control group, in whom interview bias was least likely to occur, was, in his view, the most convincing evidence of a causal association yielded by the study.

These findings led Doll and Hill to design and carry out the first planned epidemiologic study to test the hypothesis that smoking was a cause of lung cancer, a cohort mortality study of British doctors [14]. Within 29 months of follow-up, a statistically significant excess of lung cancer was demonstrated in smokers, and by 50 months, associations of smoking with bronchitis and coronary thrombosis were also demonstrable; for both conditions, this was the first time that such associations had been demonstrated [15]. Another important finding was, in Doll's view, the demonstration that quantitative risk estimates could be derived from a case-control approach; in the data, virtually the same risk estimates were obtained from the case-control as from the cohort data.

Over the next few years, support for these findings was greatly strengthened by other published data and led to a statement by the British MRC supporting the conclusion that tobacco smoking was a cause of lung cancer [15]. By the early 1960s, sufficient evidence had accumulated for the Royal College of Physicians in a report on smoking and health [16] to conclude that "cigarette smoking is an important cause of lung cancer." Their report, published in 1962, cited 216 references. Two years later, in 1964, a report of the U.S. Surgeon General [17] reached essentially the same conclusions, and cited 1011 references. It is also of interest that prior to the 1960s, a smoking history was rarely part of the medical record; as Doll comments, smoking was "normal" [15]. However, by the mid-1960s, smoking history was considered an obligatory part of the medical history. In other words, the medical profession has accepted the evidence of causality.

The 1964 Surgeon General's report was one in a series of comprehensive and landmark reports issued by the U.S. Surgeon General's office over the subsequent decades, each report focusing on a different smoking-related issue [17–28]. Conditions reviewed included other cancers [20], cardiovascular disease [21], and chronic lung diseases [22,23]; one report focused on the ill-health consequences of involuntary smoking and the risks for unborn, young, and adolescent children [24]. A more recent report documents the health benefits of smoking cessation [28] and deals with, among other things, the effects of smoking cessation on respiratory cancer and on nonmalignant respiratory disease. Although most of these reports focus on content (i.e., the health consequences of smoking), several, including one on the health benefits of smoking cessation [28], devote one or more chapters to the epidemiologic methodology, which was used to generate the information reviewed in the volume.

### III. Information Required for the Development of Preventive Strategies

#### A. Components of the Information Base

The twentieth-century epidemic of tobacco-related diseases is attributed to the use of tobacco as cigarettes, as much as to the greater use of tobacco [29]. Reasons include the lower pH of cigarette smoke compared to pipe and cigar smoke and the need to inhale more deeply to maximize nicotine absorption (the addictive agent); this inevitably increases the absorption of other toxic and carcinogenic agents in cigarette smoke [26,30].

Strategies for disease prevention are, or should be, developed from an information base: The more complete the information base and the more effectively it can be translated into action, the more likely that the preventive strategies will be successful. The information base on which preventive strategies for lung cancer and chronic nonmalignant respiratory disease should be developed comes mainly from epidemiologic studies and includes the following (see also Table 1):

1. Unequivocal evidence for the causal association of both diseases of interest with smoking

**Table 1** Information Base Required for the Development of Strategies for the Prevention of Tobacco-Related Respiratory Disease

| Issue or question | Information base[a] | Refs. |
|---|---|---|
| Unequivocal evidence of causality for the diseases of interest[b] | Comparison of outcomes in exposed and nonexposed; also comparing subjects by levels of exposure and by cumulative exposure; coherence with clinical and experimental data | [12–14, 17, 18, 22, 23, 29] |
| Uniquivocal evidence of the health benefits of eliminating exposure for the diseases of interest[b] | Comparison of outcomes by exposure category (never, ex, current), and of outcome in ex-smokers stratified by time since last exposure, time since quitting, and by status at quitting | [25,27,28,31] |
| Exposure response relationships (qualitative and quantitative), including the effect of duration since quitting | Comparison of outcomes in those exposed by category (never, ex, current) by level of current exposure (cigarettes/day) and by cumulative exposure (cigarettes/years, pack/years) | [22,25,28,31–33] |
| Characteristics of smokers | Comparison of personal characteristics of those who do (or do not) take up and/or maintain and/or quit the habit, including the reasons for their decision (psychological, social, pharmacological, etc.) | [28–38] |
| Identification and characterization of high- and/or low-risk smokers | Comparison of personal and exposure characteristics of those who do and do not exhibit ill-health effects of exposure | [36,38] |

[a]Should include epidemiologic studies addressing the issues, comparisons, or questions listed.
[b]Lung cancer and chronic nonmalignant lung disease.

2.  Unequivocal evidence of health benefits of smoking cessation for both the diseases of interest
3.  Evidence not only of qualitative but also of quantitative exposure–response relationships for both diseases
4.  Characteristics of smokers, in particular why they take up the habit, why they maintain it, and why they quit
5.  Identification of the high-risk smoker
6.  Evaluation of existing preventive programs with a view to improving their effectiveness

### B.  Health Benefits of Smoking Cessation, and Exposure–Response Relationships

As already indicated, epidemiologic studies have been responsible for contributing the major part of the information base pertinent to the issue of causality, starting with the landmark 1950 and 1954 studies of Doll and Hill [13,14]. A comprehensive review of the epidemiologic methodology used to generate this large information base is beyond the scope of the present chapter, and the reader is referred to the timely reviews in the reports of the U.S. Surgeon General [17–18].

Epidemiologic studies, for the most part carried out in the 1980s, have also contributed in a major way to the evidence, now considered unequivocal, of the health benefits of smoking cessation [28,31]. Since the chemical constituents of cigarette smoke, including carbon monoxide, hydrogen cyanode, and nicotine, can be detected in persons who smoke, either as inhaled or as metabolic products, these have been used to establish smoking status, in particular in studies of smoking cessation [28].

Estimates of exposure in most of these studies have been qualitative, based on smoking categories (never, ex, and current), and/or daily smoking level, and/or cumulative exposure (cigarette- or pack-years) and/or materials smoked (cigarettes, pipes, cigars) [20,22,32–34]. While qualitative exposure measurements are usually adequate to establish causality, they may theoretically result in sufficient misclassification to minimize the chances of detecting statistical interactions such as effect modification, information that may be pertinent to the identification of the high-risk smoker.

### C.  Smoking Career and Determinants of Smoking

The term *smoking career* has been introduced to convey the idea that "smoking is a complex, evolving process, the stages of which may be differentially influenced by the interplay of social or environmental, psychologic and biologic factors" [35]. Nicotine addiction [36], conditioning of smoking [35], marketing, economic factors, and social differentiation are all considered to influence the initiation of the habit. Factors thought to sustain the habit are stress, negative affect, weight, family and peer encouragement, and failure to hear or comprehend the strength of the evidence linking ill health to smoking.

Although the addictive properties of nicotine were dismissed in the first Surgeon General's report on smoking [17,35], the 1988 report recognized that "cigarettes and other forms of tobacco are addicting" [26]. This served to reinforce research into the basic and clinical psychopharmacology of nicotine and its effects on the automatic nervous system, on human cognitive function and performance, and on the use of clinical pharmacology methods to understand tobacco dependency and why people smoke [27]. The research approaches, methodology, and measurement instruments in research into smoking cessation are described elsewhere [35–37]. The information base furnished by this research has been used extensively in the development of preventive strategies.

In contrast to the strong information base on the addictive nature of cigarette smoking and why smokers maintain the habit, less effort has been directed at determining why people do or do not take up the habit. What research there is on why people take up smoking is concentrated in the psychosocial domain [35,36]. Virtually no research attention has been directed at the possibility that characteristics on the organs most immediately involved, (i.e., the lungs), might influence a person's choice. Indeed, implicit in the comparison of the character-istics of smokers and nonsmokers to establish risk, a common research approach, is the assumption that the decision to take up the habit is random in relation to health characteristics such as lung function used to measure disease outcome [22]. That this is unlikely to be the case, at least for nonmalignant respiratory disease, is suggested by a report on the "healthy" smoker which cited the evidence that those who elect to take up the habit have on average better levels of lung function than those who do not [38,39]. This implies a health selection process. Evidence for a health selection can be found in several studies published over the last two decades, although in most instances the phenomenon escaped comment by the authors [38]. The decision to take up smoking may also relate to the immediate responsiveness of a person's airways to exposure to cigarette smoke and the capacity to sense this responsiveness. There is also some evidence that the same selection factors may influence a person's decision to undertake employment in a dusty occupation [40]. A stronger information base on the health as opposed to psychosocial determinants of taking up the smoking habit might also contribute to improving preventive strategies.

### D. Identification and Characteristics of High-Risk Smoker

Not all people exposed to apparently similar levels of cigarette smoke develop disease, as tobacco industry spokesmen, among others, have pointed out. However, not a great deal of research attention has been directed at what puts some people at risk and protects others [41]. For instance, between-individual differences in deposition, retention, and clearance of dust particles appear to explain differences in the extent of fibrosis evoked by installation of comparable fiber loads in animal models of asbestosis [42]. The same might also be so for particles in cigarette smoke. Such differences, which could be related to airway geometry [43], would result in incorrect exposure assessment and affect the exposure side of exposure–response relationships. Alternatively, there could be differences in individual susceptibility that would affect the response side of the exposure–response relationship. Susceptibility can be examined as an effect modifier of exposure–response relationships. *Effect modification* has been defined as "a natural phenomenon which exists independently of a particular study"; it can be measured as a change in magnitude of an effect measure, according to the value of a third variable [44]. Effect modification can be detected by the use of interaction terms in multiple linear regression analyses, and can be examined quantitatively by examining risk in subgroups of the study population stratified according to the level of the potential effect modifier of interest. There has been considerable research interest but relatively little research activity into the between-individual differences in susceptibility to tobacco smoke [41]. Strengthening of this information base would also be pertinent to the planning of preventive strategies.

## IV. Preventive Strategies: Epidemiologic Methodology

The decades of the 1960s and 1970s saw the development of a strong data base documenting the adverse health effects of cigarette smoking [16–18]. The data base was further strengthened in the 1980s [19–29], a decade that also saw a spectacular increase in public awareness of the ill-health consequences of tobacco exposure, particularly in North America. In addition, the regular publication of the Surgeon General's reports documenting various aspects of the twentieth-century smoking epidemic, and more important, the obligatory labeling of cigarette packages with health warnings kept the matter in the public eye. With characteristic North American activism, many different preventive strategies were implemented [28,45]. At present, by far the most frequently employed preventive strategy is aimed at smoking cessation, with smoking prevention as the next most frequently employed strategy: some programs include both. This section reviews briefly the epidemiologic methodology used to develop the data base documenting the health benefits of smoking cessation, and the epidemiologic methodology in use to evaluate the success of smoking intervention programs.

### A. Study Designs

All the usual study designs, experimental as well as nonexperimental (observational), can be, and most have been, used to assess the health consequences of smoking cessation. In addition, the effectiveness of intervention trials to achieve smoking cessation has been evaluated using experimental study designs. A key feature of the experimental design is that the researcher control all aspects of the study, including assigning the participants to the exposure (or intervention) category, preferably by a random procedure. By contrast, in nonexperimental designs this assignment is the result of the subject's choice, explicit or not, or is due to some other factor or process. A current example of a randomized controlled intervention trial is the Lung Health Study, a multicenter trial to determine whether smoking intervention and bronchodilator therapy can favorably affect the natural history of chronic obstructive pulmonary disease (COPD) [46]. Almost 6000 people have been recruited in 10 participating centers. After careful baseline documentation, subjects were randomized into usual care, or intervention groups, with two arms in the intervention group, smoking intervention/active drug and smoking intervention/placebo [47].

Table 2 summarizes features of study designs in relation to their usefulness in the present context. An excellent discussion on their strengths and weaknesses can be found in the 1990 Surgeon General's report [28]. The various study designs are arranged in order of increasing strength in furnishing evidence for causality; all are potentially subject to selection, information, and confounding bias [28];

1. *Ecologic studies* are based on comparison of groups stratified for exposure by response characteristics (e.g., a comparison of countries for years since introduction of cigarette smoking and mortality due to lung cancer) [15]. Limitations are in the estimates of exposure and often inadequate control of confounding so that exposure–response relationships may be seriously biassed. Furthermore, there is no direct link at the level of the individual between exposure and outcome.

2. *Cross-sectional studies*, in which exposure and response are measured at the same point in time, are the workhorse of environmental and occupational epidemiology [3] and have provided much of the evidence for causality linking smoking with chronic nonmalignant respiratory disease. Inferences about causality and/or the benefits of cessation are based on comparisons of outcomes by smoking categories (e.g., never vs. ever and/or current and/or ex, never, or current vs. ex). Cross-sectional studies of the effects of smoking, or of quitting, on lung function measurements are subject to selection bias due to the "healthy" smoker effect [38]. Thus in a given study, if those who took up the habit had better prior lung function than those who did not, the study results will underestimate the potential ill-health effects of smoking or the potential benefits of cessation. Cross-sectional studies may also be subject to information bias. For instance, in addition to inaccuracy of recall of a possibly changing habit, recall bias of self-reported past exposure could occur, depending on the presence of symptoms and the subject's belief

**Table 2** Study Designs Used to Establish the Data Base on the Benefits of Smoking Cessation, as Well as to Assess the Efficacy and/or Effectiveness of Smoking Intervention Programs

| Design | Features | Potential sources of bias | Comment |
|--------|----------|---------------------------|---------|
| Ecologic | Analysis units are groups; exposure and responses may be based on existing data | Exposure misclassification; confounding (information not available); no link between exposure and response at the level of the individual | Inexpensive; feasible; inference based on between-group differences in response and the extent to which it parallels between-group differences in exposure |
| Cross-sectional | Exposure and outcome measurement at the same point in time | Time relationships may be obscured; selection bias may occur into exposure on basis of favorable characteristics (e.g., large lung volumes) or out of exposure (e.g., for reasons of ill health) | The workhorse of epidemiology: inference based on comparison of never with ever, current with ex-smokers; suitable for the study of chronic disease such as COPD for which onset time may be difficult to determine with precision |
| Case-control | Cases that exhibit the condition under study and controls that do not are compared; odds ratios approximate relative risk | Differential misclassification due to recall failure or bias, also to interviewer bias, exposure history not collected blind, or overmatching | Relatively quick and easy to perform; exposure response estimates not necessarily biased: case-control comparisons focus on exposure, or if matched for exposure, on host factors |
| Cohort | Study group defined by time, place, or person: subjects usually stratified by exposure (never, ex, current by level) and followed for outcome (e.g., lung cancer) | Differential loss to follow-up in relation to smoking status; misclassification due to changing smoking status over time with attenuation of exposure–response relationships | Repeated exposure measurements can be made during follow-up to minimize misclassification; suitable for the study of disease, for which onset time can usually be determined with reasonable precision |

| Intervention trial | Tests the causal hypothesis; preferable if assignment to intervention or not is randomized; neither subject nor observer can be blinded to intervention status in preventive trials of smoking cessation | In a trial of smoking cessation, power will depend on success rate in the intervention arm; misreporting of smoking status may increase under pressure to quit in a trial setting | Intervention can be at a personal, community, or national level, or from mass media; most studies examine only one source of intervention; the different sources of intervention can be examined in meta-analysis of several trials |
| --- | --- | --- | --- |
| Hybrid study designs | Usual example is the case control within a cohort | Information bias for exposure minimized by the use of the cohort framework | Exposure measurements for cases and controls can be explored in much greater detail than is possible for all cohort members |

*Source:* Based on information presented in Chapter 2 of ref. 28 and in refs. 25, 27, and 29.

as to their origin. The result could be exaggeration or underestimation of an association.

   3.   *Case-control studies* are based on subject selection according to outcome: cases for the presence of the condition of interest, and controls for its absence. Exposure and other information is then collected and inferences about causality are based on exposure comparisons in relation to case vs. control status. If cases and controls are also matched for exposure, the contrast can focus on host factors as determinants of disease. Case control data can contribute information on the effects of smoking cessation but may be subject to recall bias by cases compared to controls, with distortion of the effects of cessation. Selection of appropriate controls is crucial.

   4.   *Cohort studies* start with definition of a study population, usually characterized by time and/or place and/or person, for whom information exists to enable stratification of subjects by exposure category [e.g., never, ever; or ex, current (by level)]. The cohort is then followed to record incidence of disease(s), such as cancer, in which disease onset can be defined relatively precisely. By contrast, chronic nonmalignant respiratory diseases, for which it is hard to pinpoint the time of onset, are usually investigated by prevalence studies. The main sources of bias are differential loss to follow up in relation to exposure status, and misclassification due to changing smoking status over time, particularly in those who quit. Exposure can be reevaluated during follow-up to minimize misclassification.

   5.   *Intervention trials* may or may not conform to the experimental design, depending on whether or not assignment to the intervention is by a random process. Trials may be used to test the causal hypothesis (that smoking cessation confers health benefits) as well as to evaluate intervention programs.

   6.   *Hybrid study designs,* most common of which is the case control within the cohort, is a powerful design that exploits the structure of the cohort to identify case and controls and then examines their exposure contrasts in much greater detail than resources usually permit for all members of the cohort. If cases and controls are matched for exposure, the contrast can focus on host factors (see above under case-control studies).

### B.   Smoking Variable and Dynamic Nature of the Smoking Cessation Process

In epidemiologic terms, the independent variable, also called the exposure variable or explanatory variable [1], was smoking status in the studies that created the information base required for the development of strategies for the prevention of tobacco-related respiratory disease (see Table 1). Misclassification may occur, given that smoking status is based on self-reported information and is likely to be subject to recall failure or bias (inevitable where exposure covers a long period of the subject's life). Self-reporting as a method of measurement tends to be regarded with scepticism by epidemiologists and clinicians alike. Nevertheless, it is worth remembering that a self-completed questionnaire to determine the independent variable (i.e., smoking category or status) has furnished exposure information for most of the studies comprising this now very extensive data base documenting the adverse health effects of cigarette smoking. Also of interest is the fact that the 1990 Surgeon General's report concludes that other than in the context of intervention trials, self-report is a valid measure of smoking status for observational studies [28]. There are other examples of the strength of self-reported exposure data; for example, in occupational epidemiology, self-reported exposure to workplace pollutants has also provided some of the strongest evidence of a causal relationship between COPD and exposures to dusts and/or fumes at work [48].

The 1990 Surgeon General's report describes smoking cessation as a dynamic process that begins with the decision to stop smoking and ends with abstinence from cigarettes maintained over a long period of time [28]. Most people who eventually quit go through several cycles of quit and restart before they achieve abstinence [28,36]. Thus during the period of time they are subjects in an intervention trial, their smoking status is likely to change several times. Ex-smokers should therefore not be treated as a single group in the analysis of results [28]. Failure to take this into account may even have resulted in underestimation of the health benefits of cessation [28].

### C. Source of the Cessation Message

Smoking cessation messages may be promoted by governments, states, health authorities, nongovernmental associations, and religious groups. They may be community, clinic, or workplace based. They may also be promoted by physicians and other health professionals [28,36]. Whereas in a single study it is often not possible to assess the source of the cessation message as a determinant of a program's efficacy and/or effectiveness, this may be possible by combining the results of several studies. For instance, a meta-analysis [1] of the determinants of success of 39 controlled trials indicated that reinforcement, multiple interactions, and the involvement of the physician with other health professionals all improve the success of the intervention [49]. Other factors currently under investigation in France as determinants of program success include the physician-advisor's personal smoking status [50].

### D. Target Populations

The term *target population* is used to refer to the population from whom the study population was selected [1]. This also is usually the population about whom information is sought and/or to whom the results are to be applied, a more appropriate definition when considering preventive strategies. The wider and more detailed the information base in terms of the consequences (and/or benefits) of smoking cessation, the more precisely strategies aimed at cessation can be targeted. In general, the older the person, the more established the smoking habit is likely to be, and the greater the difficulty of achieving cessation.

Strategies aimed at smoking prevention imply a target population prior to taking up the habit, or at the time of considering taking up the habit. This usually means younger persons, today usually teenagers or even preteenagers. Strategies for smoking prevention require as detailed information as possible on the characteristics of those who take up the habit compared to those who do not and their reasons for doing so [35,36].

Psychosocial factors influencing people to take up the habit include (1) the addictive properties of nicotine; (2) parental and peer smoking habits [35]: parental smoking is thought to be one of the main determinants of a young person taking up the habit [51]; (3) psychological factors, including race, gender, education, and income: smoking tends to be taken up by the less successful, the less educated, and those with fewer resources [36]; and (4) the influence of personality (e.g., extroverts are more likely than introverts to become smokers) [51]. This information base is clearly pertinent to planning preventive strategies.

In contrast to the considerable volume of information into psychological determinants of smoking and the early respiratory ill-health effects of smoking on lung function [52], little information is available on health-related character-istics that might influence young persons to take up or avoid the habit. A report on the "healthy" smoker already referred to cited evidence to suggest that young persons who take up the habit have on average higher levels of lung function than those who do not [38]. A medline search on the titles *healthy smoker* or *susceptible smoker* yielded only three articles, including those cited here [38,41]. Nor, surprisingly, is this area targeted for future research in current reviews and/or reports [28,31,51], despite the fact that cigarette smoking is known to affect other personal characteristics, such as bronchial reactivity [53,54]. This information base clearly needs strengthening if it is to be useful in planning preventive strategies.

### E. Analytical Issues

In an excellent, clear, and succinct discussion of analytical issues in observational studies of the health consequences of smoking cessation, the 1990 Surgeon General's report points out that the complex associations between disease risk, age, and duration of active smoking, on the one hand (variables which are often collinear and/or interrelated), and abstinence(s), on the other hand, complicate the assessment of the health consequences of smoking cessation [28]. This will also be the case for intervention trials of smoking cessation, even though the irregular process of cessation may be better documented in the context of an intervention trial. In the 1990 Surgeon General's report, emphasis is also put on the fact that analytical approaches should be biologically appropriate, and preferably developed to address a study question appropriately framed to incorporate a pertinent biological hypothesis. Indeed, regardless of the type of data analyzed, the method of analysis should properly represent what is known about the underlying biologic process, both in terms of better understanding the disease process and of better planning of preventive strategies.

## V. Synthesis, Information Gaps, and Future Research

In this chapter on respiratory diseases and tobacco, the focus has been on epidemiologic methodology rather than on content, defined as the information generated by epidemiologic research. Epidemiologic methodology has furnished most of the information necessary for the development of strategies for the prevention of respiratory diseases due to tobacco. All standard epidemiologic study designs have been used to generate this information base, the choice being tailored to the particular research question and/or the population(s) available for, or accessible to study. The exposure variable, smoking status, is inevitably qualitative, based on self-report and recall for past smoking experience. Despite this potential source of misclassification, especially in the ex-smoking category, the adverse health effects of cigarette smoking and the health benefits of cessation have been unequivocally documented, and causality proven beyond doubt. Other than in intervention trials to promote cessation, self-report appears to be a valid measure of smoking status.

The information base necessary to develop preventive strategies includes unequivocal evidence of the adverse health effects of cigarette smoking and of the benefits of smoking cessation; documentation of exposure–response relationships using quantitative in addition to qualitative estimates of exposure, the characteristics of people who do (and do not) take up and/or maintain and/or quit the habit and the reasons for their smoking behavior, and identification of the high-risk smoker. Epidemiologic methodology has contributed to all aspects of this information base, including information on the psychosocial factors influencing the smoking habit. Least well researched appears to be the role of the characteristics of the lungs themselves as determinants of future smoking status.

The concept of the healthy smoker as a phenomenon of natural selection by a person who takes up the smoking habit because his or her lungs are relatively resistant to the adverse health effects of tobacco smoke is supported by published data. Personal characteristics that appear to be associated with this choice include better than average lung function and possibly less tendency to acute airway responses to inhaled pollutants of any sort. Future research should include studies designed to examine this concept more rigorously. Studies should be undertaken to determine whether the health characteristics that relate to the choice of a "smoking career" are also related to and/or determine the choice of an occupation which involves exposure to dust and fumes at work, and the obverse of this research, to identify the characteristics of the susceptible smoker.

Appreciation of the fact that only a limited number of those who smoke exhibit adverse effects in the form of respiratory or other disease remains a challenge to medical science and may be a reason why antismoking propaganda continues to be received with scepticism by certain members of the public. The publication of the present volume may serve to direct research attention to these pertinent but as yet largely unanswered questions.

## Acknowledgments

The writer, who is a Career Investigator of the MRC of Canada, thanks J. Hanley, P. Ernst, and R. Menzies of the Department of Epidemiology and Biostatistics, McGill University for critical comment of the text.

## References

1.  Last JM, ed. A dictionary of epidemiology. 2nd ed. New York: Oxford University Press, 1988.
2.  Miettinen O. Theoretical epidemiology: principles of occurrence research in medicine. New York: Wiley, 1985.
3.  Becklake MR. Evaluation of respiratory hazards in the working environment through environmental, epidemiologic and medical surveys. In: Proceedings of the 7th International Pneumoconiosis Conference, August 23–28, 1988. U.S. Department of Health and Human Services. Public Health Service. Centers for Disease Control. National Institute for Occupational Safety and Health. DHHS (NIOSH) Publication 90–108, Part 1:16–21, 1990.
4.  Hill AB. The environment and disease: association or causation? Proc R Soc Med 1965;58:7–12.
5.  McDonald JC. Epidemiology. In: Weill H, Turner-Warwick M, eds. Occupational lung diseases: research approaches and methods, New York: Marcel Dekker, 1981:373–404.
6.  Becklake MR. In: Witschi HP, Brain JD, eds. Toxicology of inhaled materials. Handbook of inhaled materials, Chapter 5: Epidemiologic studies in human populations. New York: Springer-Verlag, 1985:115–42.
7.  Monson RR. Occupational epidemiology. Boca Raton, FL: CRC Press, 1980.
8.  Speizer FE. Overview of epidemiologic studies on aerosols. In: Lee SD,

Shneider T, Grant LD, Venkerle PJ, Speizer FE, eds. Aerosols: research, risk assessment and control strategies. Chelsea MI, Lewis Publishers, 1986.
9. Holland WW. Chronic obstructive lung disease prevention. Br J Dis Chest 1988;82:32–44.
10. Oschsner A, De Bakey M. Carcinoma of the lung. Arch Surg 1941;42:209–258.
11. Pearl R. Tobacco smoking and longevity. Science 1938;87:216–17.
12. Wynder EL, Graham EA. Tobacco smoking as an etiologic factor in bronchogenic carcinoma. JAMA 1950;143:329–31.
13. Doll R, Hill AB. Smoking and carcinoma of the lung. Br Med J 1950;2:739–48.
14. Doll R, Hill AB. The mortality of doctors in relation to their smoking habits: a preliminary report. Br Med J 1954;1:1451–53.
15. Conversation with Sir Richard Doll. Br J Addict 1991;86:365–77.
16. Royal College of Physicians of London. Smoking and health. Summary of a report of the Royal College of Physicians of London on smoking in relation to cancer of the lung and other diseases. London: Pitman Medical Publishing Co., 1962.
17. U.S. Public Health Service. Smoking and health. Report of the Advisory Committee to the Surgeon General of the U.S. Public Health Service. PHS Publication 1103. U.S. Department of Health, Education and Welfare, PHS, CDC, 1964.
18. U.S. Department of Health, Education and Welfare. Smoking and health. A report of the Surgeon General. DHEW Publication (PHS) 79-50066. U.S. Department of Health Education, and Welfare, Public Health Service, Office of the Assistant Secretary of Health, Office on Smoking and Health, 1979.
19. U.S. Department of Health and Human Services. The health consequences of smoking for women. A report of the Surgeon General. DHEW Publications. U.S. Department of Health and Human Services, Public Health Service, Office of the Assistant Secretary for Health, Office on Smoking and Health, 1980.
20. U.S. Department of Health and Human Services. The health consequences of smoking: cancer. A report of the Surgeon General. DHHS Publication (PHS) 82-50179. U.S. Department of Health and Human Services, Public Health Service, Office on Smoking and Health, 1982.
21. U.S. Department of Health and Human Services. The health consequences of smoking: cardiovascular disease. A report of the Surgeon General. DHHS Publication 84-50204. U.S. Department of Health and Human Services, Public Health Services, Office on Smoking and Health, 1983.
22. U.S. Department of Health and Human Services. The health consequences

of smoking. Chronic obstructive lung disease. A report of the Surgeon General. DHHS Publication (PHS) 84-50205. U.S. Department of Health and Human Services, Public Health Service, Office on Smoking and Health, 1984.

23.   U.S. Department of Health and Human Services. The health consequences of smoking. Cancer and chronic disease in the workplace. A report of the Surgeon General. DHHS Publication (PHS) 84-50207. U.S. Department of Health and Human Services, Public Health Service, Office on Smoking and Health, 1985.

24.   U.S. Department of Health and Human Services. The health consequences of involuntary smoking. A report of the Surgeon General. DHHS Publication (CDC) 87-8398. U.S. Department of Health and Human Services, Public Health Service, Center for Disease Control, 1986.

25.   Schwartz JL. Review and evaluation of smoking cessation methods. United States and Canada 1978–1985. NIH Publication, 87-2940. U.S. Department of Health and Human Services, Public Health Service, National Institutes of Health, 1987.

26.   U.S. Department of Health and Human Services. The health consequences of smoking: nicotine addiction. A report of the Surgeon General. DHHS Publication (CDC) 88-8406. U.S. Department of Health and Human Services, Public Health Service, Center for Disease Control, Center for Health Promotion and Education, Office on Smoking and Health, 1988.

27.   U.S. Department of Health and Human Services. Reducing the health consequences of smoking: 25 years of progress. A report of the Surgeon General. DHHS Publication (CDC) 89-8411. U.S. Department of Health and Human Services, Public Health Service, Center for Disease Control, Center for Chronic Disease Prevention and Health Promotion, Office on Smoking and Health, 1989.

28.   U.S. Department of Health and Human Services. The health benefits of smoking cessation. A report of the Surgeon General. DHHS Publication (CDC) 90-8416. U.S. Department of Health and Human Services, Public Health Service, Center for Disease Control, Center for Chronic Disease Prevention and Health Promotion, Office on Smoking and Health, 1990.

29.   Sherman CB. Health effects of cigarette smoking. Clin Chest Med 1991;12:643–58.

30.   Burns DM. Cigarettes and cigarette smoking. Clin Chest Med 1991;12:631–42.

31.   Samet JM. Health benefits of smoking cessation. Clin Chest Med 1991;12:669–80.

32.   Peat JK, Woolcock AJ, Cullen K. Decline of lung function and development of chronic airflow limitation. A longitudinal study of nonsmokers and smokers in Busselton, Western Australia. Thorax 1990;45:32–37.

33. Jaakkola MS, Jaakkola JJK, Ernst P, Becklake MR. Ventilatory lung function in young cigarette smokers: a study of susceptibility. Eur Respir J 1991;4:643–60.
34. Jaakkola MS, Ernst P, Jaakkola JJK, Ng'ang'a LW, Becklake MR. Effect of cigarette smoking on the evolution of ventilatory lung function in young adults: an eight-year longitudinal study. Thorax 1991;40:907–13.
35. Haire-Joshu D, Morgan G, Fisher EB. Determinants of cigarette smoking. Clin Chest Med 1991;12:711–25.
36. Cohen C, Pickworth WB, Henningfile JE. Cigarette smoking and addiction. Clin Chest Med 1991;12:701–10.
37. Hovezec J, Benowitz NL. Basic and clinical psychopharmacology of nicotine. Clin Chest Med 1991;12:681–99.
38. Becklake MR, Lalloo U. The "healthy" smoker: a phenomenon of health selection? Respiration 1990;57:137–44.
39. Becklake MR. Epidemiologic evidence of varying susceptibility to inhaled substances. Pharmacogenetics 1991;1:98–101.
40. Bakke P, Eide GE, Gulsvik A. Occupational exposure to dust and gas in a general population. Eur Resp J 1988;1(Suppl):70S.
41. Farrow DC, Samet JM. Identification of the high risk smoker. Clin Chest Med 1991;12:659–68.
42. Bégin R, Massé S, Sébastien P, Bossé J, Rola-Pleszczynski M, Boctor M, Côté Y, Fabi D, Dalle D. Asbestos exposure and retention as determinants of airway disease and asbestos alveolitis. Am Rev Respir Dis 1986;134:176–81.
43. Becklake MR, Toyota B, Stewart M, Hanson R, Hanley J. Lung structure as a risk factor in adverse pulmonary responses to asbestos exposure: a case-referent study in Québec chrysotile asbestos miners and millers. Am Rev Respir Dis 1983;128:385–88.
44. Rothman KJ. Modern epidemiology. Boston: Little, Brown, 1986.
45. Fisher EB, Haire-Joshu D, Morgan GD, et al. State of the art: Smoking and smoking cessation. Am Rev Respir Dis 1990;142:702–20.
46. Anthonisen N. Lung health study. Am Rev Respir Dis 1989;140:871–72.
47. Connett JE, Kusek JW, Bailey WC, O'Hara P, Wu M. Design of the Lung Health Study: a randomized clinical trial of early intervention for chronic obstructive lung disease. Controlled Clinical Trials (in press) 1993.
48. Becklake MR. Occupational exposures: evidence for a causal association with chronic obstructive pulmonary disease. Am Rev Respir Dis 1989;140:S85–S91.
49. Rottke TE, Batista RN, De Friese GH, Brekke ML. Attributes of successful smoking cessation interventions in medical practice: a meta-analysis of 39 controlled trials. JAMA 1988;254:2883–89.
50. Slama K, Karsenty S, Hirsch A. Doctor recruitment and participation in

a primary care smoking cessation intervention. Presented at the 8th World Conference on Tobacco and Health, Buenos Aires, Argentina, March 30–April 3, 1992.

51.    Fielding JE. Smoking: health effects and control. N Engl J Med 1985;313:491–98.

52.    Wright JL. Small airway disease: structure and function. In: Hensley MJ, Saunders NJ, eds. Clinical epidemiology of chronic obstructive pulmonary disease. New York: Marcel Dekker, 1989:55–80.

53.    Pride NB. Smoking and bronchial hyperresponsiveness. In: Sluiter HJ, Van der Lende R, eds. Bronchitis IV. Assen, The Netherlands: Van Gorcum, 1989:71–79.

54.    O'Connor GT, Sparrow D, Weiss ST. The role of allergy and unspecific airway hyperresponsiveness in the pathogenesis of chronic obstructive lung disease. Am Rev Respir Dis 1989;140:225–52.

# 22

# Adult Respiratory Diseases and Environmental Tobacco Smoke

**ROBERT E. DALES**

University of Ottawa
Ottawa, Ontario, Canada

**GERRY B. HILL**

Laboratory Centre for Disease Control
Ottawa, Ontario, Canada

**WALTER O. SPITZER**

McGill University
Montreal, Quebec, Canada

## I. Introduction

Environmental tobacco smoke (ETS) is a combination of sidestream smoke, which comes from the burning end of a cigarette, smoke that diffuses through the cigarette paper, and exhaled mainstream smoke from the person actively smoking the cigarette [1–4]. ETS contributes substantially to indoor air pollution. It is the single most important source of respirable particulates and frequently the only present source of nicotine and some $N$-nitrosamines [2]. Like mainstream smoke, ETS probably contains over 4000 compounds in either particulate or vapor phases, many of which have known harmful properties. The effects of passive smoking cannot necessarily be extrapolated from dose–response information on active smoking because the compositions of mainstream and sidestream smoke are different [1–6]. Prior to inhalation, ETS compounds have more time than mainstream smoke to undergo aging, with resultant physical and chemical changes such as oxidation [1]. Compared to mainstream smoke, undiluted sidestream smoke contains higher concentrations of several toxic and carcinogenic compounds, including volatile nitrosamines, aromatic amines, and ammonia [1].

Inaccurate quantification of cumulative personal exposure is probably the greatest barrier to estimating the chronic health effects in passive smokers. For example, the majority of epidemiologic studies have used crude dichotomous indices of exposure [1–5]: the presence or absence of a spousal or household smoker.

The importance of ETS-related health effects in adults can be judged by the burden of illness due to respiratory disease in the population, the proportion of adults exposed to ETS, and the magnitude of risk conferred by ETS exposure.

The burden of respiratory illness is large and has been concisely summarized by Redline [7]. Based on the 1986 U.S. National Health Interview Survey, over 10 million Americans are estimated to have emphysema or chronic bronchitis. COPD accounted for more than 17 million office visits, 1 million hospitalizations, and 3.6% of all deaths. International variation in reported mortality exists with fourfold differences between Japan ($73/10^5$) and Romania ($433/10^5$). For the year 1991, Statistics Canada estimated that 32% of cancer deaths among men and 19% among women will be due to lung cancer [8].

ETS is ubiquitous and many people are exposed. A cross-Canada survey of 14,000 children revealed that approximately half lived in a household where there was smoking [9]. Among men from 18 U.S. cities who participated in the MRFIT study from 1973–1982, 20% of lifetime nonsmoking men were married to a smoker [10]. Residential exposure is more common among women. Forty percent of lifetime nonsmoking women from five U.S. cities and 54% from seven French cities were married to a smoker in the mid-1970s [11]. Workplace exposure is similarly prevalent. In the 1986 Canadian Labour Force Smoking Survey, 53% reported that smoking was permitted in their immediate work area. It was most common in transportation occupations (67%) and least likely in professions (34%) [12]. A German study of 1351 white-collar workers reported that 28% of lifetime nonsmokers were exposed to ETS at work or at home [13]. Recent legislation restricting smoking in public places and work sites has probably had a major impact upon work exposure, but its influence on residential exposure is unknown.

Does ETS exposure cause respiratory disease among adults? There exist several excellent reviews addressing this question [1–5]. Most experts believe there is a causal link between ETS and lung cancer [1–4] but are less certain about adult respiratory function, with opinions ranging from inconsistent and inconclusive [3,5] to a small effect of uncertain clinical significance [4]. The influence of ETS on adult respiratory symptoms and cancer of the respiratory system apart from lung have received relatively little attention. Even if the magnitude of effect or risk were small, the impact on population health is potentially important since both exposure to ETS and respiratory diseases are commonplace. Further, this health issue is of practical importance because a "cure" is available: avoidance.

In this chapter we concentrate on the effect of passive smoking on adult respiratory function impairment and lung cancer; attention is also given to respiratory symptoms. The studies of lung cancer have been analyzed exhaustively by traditional approaches [2], meta-analyses [1], and a "best-evidence synthesis" [4]. For this reason an overview of these reviews is presented in a historical context. In comparison, the studies of respiratory symptoms and function are fewer in number and have been less thoroughly criticized. They are difficult to summarize by meta-analysis because of differences between studies in potential biases of uncertain importance and differences in measurements of exposures and outcomes. For these reasons the relevant published data is described and then critically analyzed to allow the reader to reach his or her own conclusions.

Many studies concerning ETS and adult respiratory diseases other than cancer used population data initially collected for other purposes [10,11,14]. Several other epidemiologic data sets probably exist where collected information on ETS and respiratory health has not been reported because it was not of primary interest to the investigators. Therefore, this review of published data cannot be considered comprehensive. Further, it may not be "politically correct" [15,16] to report that cigarette smoke has no observable effect on respiratory health. This position could be construed as supporting an industry responsible for marketing the single most important preventable cause of death in our society [17]. This could contribute to the "file-drawer" [18] phenomenon, whereby more negative than positive studies are left unpublished inflating the proportion of published studies detecting an adverse health effect of ETS.

## II. Respiratory Symptoms and Function

### A. Epidemiologic Studies

*Summary of the Literature*

Symptoms

A small adverse effect of environmental tobacco smoke (ETS) on adult lower respiratory symptoms would be consistent with the overall experience based on eight reports of nine different study populations (11,14,19–24). Kauffman et al. compared results from the American Six Cities study to the French study, Population Atmosphérique et Affections Respiratoires Chroniques [11]. Eight studies were cross-sectional [11,14,19–23], and one was a prospective study by Schwartz and Zeger [24]. The majority of studies were restricted to adult lifetime nonsmokers, but two studies were of nonsmokers without differentiation between lifetime nonsmokers and former smokers [19,20]. Exposure was crudely assessed, often by whether or not the spouse currently smoked [11,19] or there was a smoker in the household [19,20]. Passive smoking at work and cumulative exposure were rarely considered [11,14]. Statistically significant associations between ETS and respiratory symptoms were detected in three study populations at $p < 0.05$ [14,20,24] and one at $p < 0.07$ [11]. Odds ratios were consistent across these studies, ranging from 1.1 to 1.4. Two other studies reported similar small effects which did not reach statistical significance [21,22]. Although the largest studies [14,20] detected statistically significant differences, relatively small sample sizes did not account for all of the studies failing to detect an association. Potentially confounding factors such as socioeconomic status and indoor and outdoor pollutants were infrequently considered [11,14,21,22].

One of the better studies was that of Euler et al. [14], based on 7037 nonsmokers at least 25 years of age selected from a California population of 37,000 Seventh-Day Adventist households. ETS exposure was measured by two items: "years working with a smoker" and "years living with a smoker." COPD was defined as being present if any one of the following were present: (1) cough and/or sputum on most days for at least 3 months per year for 2 years or more, (2) a personal history of wheezing and a physician's diagnosis of asthma, or (3) dyspnea when walking and a physician's diagnosis of emphysema. The odds ratios were 1.07 ($p < 0.01$) for each 10 years lived with a smoker and 1.11 ($p < 0.001$) for every 10 years worked with a smoker after adjusting for ambient exposure to total suspended particulates, occupational exposure to a variety of pollutants, personal active smoking in the past, age, sex, race, and occupation.

The one prospective study [24] reported a relative risk of 1.4 [95% confidence interval (CI) 1.1 to 1.9] for the association between ETs and "episodes of phlegm." This was based on a daily diary of respiratory symptoms kept for 3 years by approximately 100 student nurses with varied smoking habits and living in residence. Exposure was indicated simply by the presence of a smoking roommate.

## Respiratory Function

A detrimental effect of ETS on respiratory function is consistent with results of the studies summarized in Table 1. All studies measuring pulmonary function were cross-sectional in design with the exception of one case-control study from Greece [32]. The majority of studies were restricted to lifetime nonsmokers; four others did not differentiate between lifetime nonsmokers and ex-smokers [19,27–29]. Exposure was crudely assessed. Residential exposure was often defined by whether or not the spouse smoked [10,11,19,29,32]. Seven studies accounted for ETS both at home and work [11,13,25–27,29,31]; four studies made some attempt to estimate cumulative exposure [25,28,31,32], but only one used cumulative exposure in a continuous rather than a dichotomous fashion [25]. Whether or not inadequate attention to the respiratory function measurement technique could have influenced results could not be assessed. Statistically significant adverse effects of ETS at $p < 0.05$ were reported by seven studies [10,11,22,25–28], and a further three reported differences favoring a detrimental effect of ETS at $p > 0.05$ [21,31,32]. There were no reports of significant differences in the opposite direction. When measured, ambient respirable suspended particulates and carbon monoxide were higher in environments reported to contain tobacco smoke [27,29] and higher concentrations of expired carbon monoxide were detected in nonsmokers with smoking spouses [10]. Only the case-control study considered potentially susceptible populations, those with COPD. No studies comprehensively accounted for outdoor pollution levels or indoor environmental factors that could potentially influence respiratory function, such as the presence of pets, gas stove use, crowding, or the presence of home dampness and molds. The most comprehensive assessment of exposure was done by Masi et al. [25]. In 1980–1981, respiratory symptoms and function data were collected on students and bank employees in Montreal, Canada. Three years later, information concerning lifetime ETS exposure was collected by a mailed questionnaire. Analysis was restricted to 293 lifetime nonsmokers divided roughly between men and women whose average age was 24 years. The index of home ETS exposure used was the number of household smokers multiplied by the number of years they lived in the same household as the subject. The index of work exposure was duration of exposure multiplied by its concentration, which was subjectively assessed to be light (five cigarettes), moderate (15 cigarettes), or heavy (25 cigarettes). Using parameters derived from logistic regression analysis, it was determined that a man who had lived at home with two smoking parents for 20 years would have a 15% reduction in $FEF_{25-75}$ ($p < 0.01$). A woman exposed at work for 10 years would have a 13% decrease in single breath diffusing capacity ($p < 0.05$).

Another of the better studies was that of Kauffman et al. [11], who selected subjects from a large survey of over 7800 urban French from households where the head was not manually employed. The latter characteristic was used to exclude those exposed to occupational pollution. The assessment of residential exposure was limited to spousal smoking habits. For all nonsmokers combined, passive smoking did not appear to influence lung function. However, when the analysis was restricted to those at least 40 years old, a different picture emerged. Among nonsmokers, those living with smoking compared to nonsmoking spouses had slightly lower values of lung function that were not explained by age, town of residence, or social class [33]. Among men, these differences were 0.56 L/s for $FEF_{25-75}$ ($p = 0.01$) and 0.12 L for $FEV_1$ ($p > 0.10$). Among women, values were 0.17 L/s for $FEF_{25-75}$ ($p = 0.01$) and 0.09 L for $FEV_1$ ($p = 0.007$), respectively. A dose–response relation was found in women who did not work outside the home, a subgroup not exposed to occupational pollution, including tobacco smoke. Nonsmokers less than 40 years of age, who were excluded from the primary analysis, showed a trend opposite to the older age group analyzed; ETS exposure was associated with better lung function. This apparent inconsis-

**Table 1** Influence of Environmental Tobacco Smoke on Respiratory Symptoms and Function

| Population[a] | ETS exposure[b] | Results[c] (E vs. NE) | Comments[d] |
|---|---|---|---|
| Lebowitz, 1976 [23] Never-smokers $\geq$ 15 yr, random sample from Arizona | Household smoker E, $n = 267$ NE, $n = 991$ | Cough: $\downarrow$ 3% ($p > 0.05$) | Not adjusted for other home/work exposures |
| Schilling, 1977 [19] Nonsmoking spouses from survey of 3 U.S. towns | Smoking spouse E, $n = 114$ NE, $n = 138$ | Cough, phlegm, wheeze $\leftrightarrow$ FEV$_1$ residual $\downarrow$ 0.18 L in $\delta$ but $\uparrow$ 0.09 L in $\female$ | Symptom data not shown; FEV$_1$ $\downarrow$ in ETS—exposed $\delta$ confined to ex-smokers |
| Simecek, 1980 [20] Nonsmoking adults from census of Czech districts | Household smoker $n = 80,690$ | Chronic bronchitis $\uparrow$ ($p <$ 0.005) | $\delta$ affected primarily; stratified by work exposure |
| White, 1980 [27] Nonsmoking, nonresidentially exposed volunteers in Californian fitness study | $\geq$ 20-yr workplace exposure E, $n = 400$ NE, $n = 400$ | % predicted: FEV$_1$ $\downarrow$ 5% ($p > 0.05$) and FEF$_{25-75}$ $\downarrow$ 14% ($p < 0.005$) | E vs. NE differences in SES and other home/workplace exposures not shown |
| Comstock, 1981 [21] Census made from Maryland | Household smoker E, $n = 765$ NE, $n = 959$ | For lifetime nonsmokers: symptoms $\uparrow$ 5% ($p > 0.05$) FEV$_1$ impairment $\uparrow$ 1% | Adjusted for age, education, household crowding, cooking fuel, etc. |
| Kentner, 1984 [13] German never-smoking white-collar workers | Current home or work exposure E, $n = 383$ NE, $n = 208$ | Inconsistent results across FEF$_{25-75}$, FEF$_{75-85}$, MMEF | FEV$_1$ not mentioned |
| Lebowitz, 1984 [30] 117 families randomly sampled in Arizona | Smoking in home | Daily PEF not related to ETS | Number of adults and smoking status not mentioned; numeric results not shown |
| Salem, 1984 [31] Never-smoking Egyptians | Work or home exposure $\geq$ 4 h/day for $\geq$ 1 yr E, $n = 219$ NE, $n = 130$ | % predicted FEV$_1$ $\downarrow$ 1.5% ($p > 0.05$) | Source of subjects not described; not adjusted for SES, other home/work exposures |

| Study | Exposure | Results | Comments |
|---|---|---|---|
| Brunekreef, 1985 [28] Nonsmoking rural Dutch ♀ | A. ≥ 10 cigarettes/day currently smoked in household E, $n = 27$ NE, $n = 16$ B. ≥ 10 cigarettes/day smoked between 1965–82 E, $n = 19$ NE, $n = 16$ | A. $FEV_1$ ↓ 1%, PEF ↓ 10% ($p < 0.01$) B. $FEV_1$ ↓ 7%, PEF ↓ 10% ($p < 0.001$) | Small sample size; SES, other home/workplace exposures not considered |
| Hosein, 1986 [29] Nonsmoking U.S. ♀ homemakers, 25–44 years old | Packs/day smoked inside home E, $n = 72$ NE, $n = 42$ | $FEV_1$ ↑ 1% $p > 0.05$) | Adjusted for gas stoves, not SES; ↑ respirable particulates in homes with ETS ($p < 0.001$) |
| Euler, 1987 [14] Nonsmoking Californian Seventh-Day Adventists | Years lived or worked with smoker, $n = 7037$ | COPD: OR 1.1 per 10-yr exposure ($p < 0.01$) | Adjusted for ambient TSP, work exposures, prior active smoking, sex, race, education |
| Kalandidi, 1987 [32] ♀ Athenian never-smokers Cases: hospitalized with COPD ($n = 103$) Controls: hospital visitors ($n = 179$) | Spousal smoking current and cumulative | COPD: OR 1.7 (95% CI 0.8–3.4) for $> 3 \times 10^5$ cigarettes smoked by spouse | Smoking ♂ more likely to be hospitalized; therefore, visiting spouses may be more likely ETS exposed |
| Svendsen, 1987 [10] Married ♂ never smokers from 18 U.S. cities | Spouse smoked E, $n = 162$ NE, $n = 514$ | $FEV_1$ ↓ 3% or 99 mL (95% CI 5–192) | ↑ expired CO in ETS-exposed ♂ ($p = 0.001$); not adjusted for other home/work exposures |
| Masi, 1988 [25] Never-smoking Canadian students, bank employees | Cumulative exposure at work and home, $n = 293$ | ♂: $FEF_{25-75}$ ↓ 15% with 20-yr exposure to 2 vs. 0 smoking parents ($p < 0.01$) ♀: DLCO ↓ 13% with 10-yr work exposure $p < 0.05$) | Most comprehensive ETS exposure; not adjusted for SES |

**Table 1** Continued

| Population[a] | ETS exposure[b] | Results[c] (E vs. NE) | Comments[d] |
|---|---|---|---|
| Hole, 1989 [22] Never-smoking 45–64 years old from census sample of two Scottish urban areas | Household smoker or ex-smoker 45–64 year old E, $n$ = 1538 NE, $n$ = 917 | Dyspnea OR 1.1 (95% CI 0.8–1.5) Sputum OR 1.2 (95% CI 0.9–1.7) $FEV_1$ ↓ 3% ($p < 0.01$) | 21% of ♀ classified as NE lived with smoker who was not in survey |
| Kauffman, 1989 [11] Never-smoking ♀: 5 U.S., 7 French cities | Smoking spouse France: E, $n$ = 1476 NE, $n$ = 822 U.S.: E, $n$ = 451 NE, $n$ = 275 | France: wheeze OR 1.0 (95% CI 0.8–1.4) $FEV_1$ residual ↓ 0.04 L ($p > 0.05$) U.S.: wheeze OR 1.4 (95% CI 1.0–1.9) $FEV_1$ residual ↓ 0.4 L ($p > 0.05$) | French ♀ ≥ 40 yrs: $FEV_1$, 4% ↓ ($p < 0.007$) with dose–response for homemakers |
| Masjedi, 1990 [26] Never-smoking Iranians | Home/work exposure E = 132 NE = 143 | ♂: $FEV_1$ ↓ 10% with work ETS ($p < 0.05$) and ↓ 5% with home ETS ♀: $FEV_1$ ↓ 2% with home ETS | Subjects excluded if exposed to "hazardous substances" at work |
| Schwartz 1990 [24] California student nurses in residence | Smoking roommate, $n$ = 100 | Phlegm episode RR 1.4 (95% CI 1.1–1.9) | Adjusted for subjects' personal smoking habits |

[a]Describes populations studied for ETS-related health effects. They were often subgroups of larger populations studied for other reasons.
[b]Describes how ETS exposure was indicated or quantitated: E, exposed; NE, not exposed; E, $n$, number of subjects exposed to ETS; NE, $n$, number of subjects not exposed to ETS.
[c] ↓ (decreased), ↑ (increased), ↔ (similar) in the exposed group compared to the nonexposed group.
[d]Not a comprehensive list of strengths and weaknesses. See the text for further details.

tency was interpreted by the author to reflect the importance of cumulative exposure to ETS, presumably greater in the older age group.

### Critical Analysis

The reported respiratory health effects of environmental tobacco smoke must be interpreted in light of real or potential methodological weaknesses which could have contributed to an over- or underestimation of the true effect size.

#### Healthy Passive Smoker Effect

Particularly susceptible adults may take steps to avoid ETS exposure. Those who develop symptoms upon exposure may choose not to live with smokers, or alternatively, restrict household smoking to a relatively uninhabited part of the home (e.g., the basement). This behavior would reduce the estimated health effects from ETS in all of the above-described cross-sectional studies by matching healthier nonsusceptible people with ETS exposure, and vice versa. This phenomenon may explain the findings of Kauffman et al. [11]: Among younger women $FEF_{25-75}$ was better in the exposed than unexposed group ($p = 0.04$). Similar avoidance behaviors have been shown to minimized observed health effects from occupational pollution [34] (i.e., the healthy worker effect) and indoor allergens [35].

#### Active Smoking History of ETS-Exposed Subjects

The health effects of active personal cigarette smoking could easily confound the lesser but similar effects looked for in ETS-exposed subjects. A minority of study groups were nonsmokers without further differentiation into ex-smokers or lifetime nonsmokers. The former may be symptomatic and have impaired lung function due to prior active smoking, which in a cross-sectional study could be incorrectly attributed to ETS. Strong evidence for the existence of this bias can be found in data presented by Comstock et al. [21]: In the ETS-exposed group, 42% of nonsmokers had previously smoked, while in the unexposed group, only 25% of nonsmokers had previously smoked. Further evidence exists in the study of Shilling et al. [19]. An observed detrimental effect of ETS on nonsmoking men was reportedly due to the lower $FEV_1$ found only among those nonsmokers who were ex-smokers. This bias should not influence the majority of studies that reported reduced lung function among ETS-exposed lifetime nonsmokers. However, even restricting the assessment of health effects to reported lifetime nonsmokers has not escaped all criticism. Uberla [36] postulated that clandestine active smoking may explain the findings of Hirayama [37] that lung cancer among Japanese women was more frequent when the spouse smoked. The hypothesis is that Japanese women would tend to conceal or deny actively smoking because it was socially unacceptable. If household smoke were present, female spouses would find it easier to conceal their active smoking. Therefore, these women may have had a higher incidence of lung cancer due to clandestine active smoking rather than spousal smoking. The presence of this bias is unproven and would be less likely to occur in North America and Europe, where women are more liberated, and unlikely to occur in studies of ETS-exposed men.

## ETS and Socioeconomic Status

Other factors that affect respiratory symptoms and level of function may differ between ETS-exposed and nonexposed subjects. Active cigarette smoking is associated with lower socioeconomic status [17,38], which increases the risk of respiratory infections [39]. Smoking is also associated with dusty work conditions [40]. Consequently, reported ETS exposure may reflect pulmonary impairment due to respiratory infections and occupational hazards. When assessed, however, socioeconomic status did not appear to have influenced observed relations between ETS and respiratory disease. The results of Euler et al. [14] and Kauffman et al. [11] were not changed significantly by adjustment for educational level. White and Froeb [27] reported differences in lung function between exposure groups despite similar occupations and working and living locations. Thus a socioeconomic bias creating an observed effect seems unlikely although theoretically plausible.

## Susceptible Subgroups

Identification of susceptible adult subgroups has received little attention in epidemiologic studies apart from a report by Cummings et al. [41] that those with chronic respiratory illness found ETS to be more "bothersome" than those without respiratory disease. Perhaps those with preexistent severe pulmonary impairment and disability are more compromised by further small decrements in lung function. The nonspecific airways hyperresponsiveness of asthma may result in larger $FEV_1$ decrements due to the irritants in ETS, which include acrolein, formaldehyde, oxides of nitrogen, and respirable particulates [2].

Studies among children suggest that boys are more susceptible than girls [42], but gender differences have not been seen consistently in adults. Masjedi et al. [26] reported 6% $FEV_1$ decrements among exposed men ($p < 0.005$) and only 2% decrements among exposed women ($p < 0.05$). Masi et al. [25] detected associations between $FEF_{25-75}$ and passive smoking at home ($p < 0.01$) for males but not for females. Different exposure situations often confound assessment of gender susceptibility. Adult women are more likely to be exposed at home, and adult men, at work.

## Estimating Exposure

Due to the unavailability of accurate measures of ETS dose, exposure estimates in all epidemiologic studies were necessarily inaccurate. In order of sophistication, the following exposure definitions have been used: (1) a spouse who smoked, (2) the presence of at least one household smoker, (3) exposure occurring either at home or at work, and (4) current and cumulative residential and occupational exposure. True personal exposure is dependent on many other factors, which have not been accounted for in the epidemiologic studies. These include exposure to all forms of tobacco smoke combustion (cigarettes, cigars, pipes), proximity to the smoker, size of the enclosure and its air-exchange rate, and duration of exposure at home, work, social gatherings, and other public places, including transportation facilities. Assuming random misclassification, this inaccuracy would reduce the observed estimates of effect; ETS is probably causing a greater adverse health effect than has been reported.

## Measures of Disease

Questionnaires ascertaining both exposure and symptoms are susceptible to certain biases. If there exists a group of "yea-sayers" who tend to respond yes to questions (i.e., globally overreport) and a group of "nay-sayers" who tend to respond no (i.e., globally underreport), an artifactual relationship would be created between smoke exposure and symptoms [43]. This would not influence the majority of studies that have measured respiratory function. Alternatively, the presence of respiratory illness may increase the recall and reporting of prior exposure [44], an effect that could bias results of all cross-sectional studies. However, most studies have used very simple exposure estimates, such as current number of household smokers; it seems unlikely that illness would lead to overreporting on these simple questions.

## Authors' Interpretation

The differential effects in younger versus older ETS-exposed spouses reported by Kauffman et al. [11] could be interpreted to show the importance of cumulative exposure (greater in older women) or alternatively, to be an example of inconsistent findings and a null overall effect [5]. Furthermore, several studies have reported detectable health effects from environmental tobacco smoke among a few of many outcomes. Masi et al. [25] concluded that ETS reduced respiratory function; 40 associations were tested statistically, and four were found be significant at $p < 0.05$. Although the outcomes tested were not all independent of one another, the authors advised caution in the interpretation of their results. Without correcting for multiple comparisons or using a global summary statistic, associations due to chance become more likely. The large studies detecting an adverse effect of ETS reported approximate 3% changes in $FEV_1$. Negative results are rarely considered by the authors to be falsely negative due to low power.

In summary, the health-related effects of ETS exposure are probably greater than those measured in epidemiologic studies due to the self-selection of subjects and inaccurate assessment of ETS exposure. Biases that would artifactually create an observed effect of ETS that did not actually exist, such as active ex-smoking by passive smokers, workplace exposures, socioeconomic status, and questionnaire-associated problems, have been addressed in several of the studies.

## B.  Experimental Studies

### Summary of the Literature

#### Subjects with Asthma

Dahms et al. [45] exposed 20 patients with asthma and 10 control subjects without asthma to mechanically produced smoke for 60 min in an environmental chamber. Carboxyhemoglobin concentrations increased 0.43% in the control group and 0.38% among the asthmatic group. $FEV_1$ in the asthmatic group fell 9% by 15 min and 21% by 60 min, whereas there were no decrements in the control group ($p < 0.01$). Knight and Breslin [46] reported similar findings in six subjects with asthma and increased airways responsiveness to histamine. Exposure to mechanically produced cigarette smoke in an environmental chamber was associated with an 11% decrease in $FEV_1$. During a control period, inhaling smoke-free air for 1 h, the $FEV_1$ rose 4.6% from baseline. Stankus et al. [47] selected subjects who had physician-diagnosed asthma and also complained of respiratory symptoms on exposure to cigarette smoke. Bronchodilators were withheld for at least 8 h, and corticosteroids were withheld the morning of the challenge. During the 2-h period of cigarette exosure in an environmental chamber, atmospheric carbon monoxide ranged from 9 to 14 ppm. $FEV_1$ declines were $\geq$ 20% in seven subjects and 1 to 15% in the remaining 14 subjects. The authors concluded that only a subgroup of patients with asthma were "smoke sensitive."

Contrary to these previous four studies, Shephard et al. [48] reported that 2 h of exposure to cigarette smoke in an environmental chamber that produced a carbon monoxide level of 24 ppm did not significantly affect respiratory function in 14 asthmatic subjects. However, subjects with chronic bronchitis or pulmonary emphysema were not excluded; the usual medications were continued on experimental days, and two subjects had levels of bronchial reactivity outside the range commonly associated with clinical asthma; inhalation of 25 mg/mL of methacholine did not induce a 20% fall in $FEV_1$. Finally, Wiedemann et al. [49] exposed nine patients with asthma to 1 h of cigarette smoke in an environmental chamber. Carboxyhemoglobin levels increased from 1.71% to 2.57% during exposure and the $FEV_1$ fell from 3.48 L to 3.45 L during exposure ($p > 0.05$). The FVC fell from 4.65 L to 4.56 L ($p = 0.01$). Unexpectedly, there was a small improvement ($p = 0.05$) in airways reactivity. Medications were withheld prior to the test, and bronchial challenge tests were in the range commonly associated with asthma.

### Subjects Without Asthma

Among 88 lifetime smokers not described as having asthma, Salem et al. [31] reported that peak expiratory flow decreased ($p < 0.05$) following a 30-minute exposure to eight machine-smoked cigarettes in a $103^-$ $m^3$ chamber. Concentrations were not measured, but exposure was considered to be "rather heavy." Pimm et al. [50] also studied "healthy" lifetime nonsmokers without known allergic disease. Carboxyhemoblobin levels were 0.5% higher during exposure than during a control period breathing room air. Over the 2-h exposure period, there were no significant reductions in flows or lung volumes. A subsequent study by the same investigators employed similar conditions, but subjects exercised in the chamber to increase minute ventilation 2.5 times the resting value. FEV$_1$ was 3.3% ($p < 0.05$) lower on exposure compared to control days [51].

### Critical Analysis

Although both epidemiologic and experimental studies have investigated the influence of ETS on respiratory function, there are many differences between these two approaches. Experimental studies have tested only for acute reversible effects, usually in subjects with asthma. Epidemiologic studies have addressed the effects of chronic exposure in the general population, leaving questions concerning susceptible subgroups and reversibility of effect unanswered. The experimental studies were largely free of the methodologic problems hampering interpretation of the epidemiologic studies. These chamber studies accurately quantified both exposure and response. Measurement of baseline function obviated the potentially confounding influences of prior active or passive smoking and socioeconomic status. However, results obtained from small groups of volunteer subjects are difficult to generalize to defined population subgroups. Previous responses to ETS may determine volunteers' interest in, and self-selection for, these studies. Medication usage could have protected subjects with asthma from an FEV$_1$ response, and including subjects without asthma would also make acute FEV$_1$ responses less likely. Physical exercise will increase the individual's dose by increasing minute ventilation and may result in larger FEV$_1$ decrements. This possibility was rarely investigated.

Results from these experimental studies support an acute reversible effect of ETS on FEV$_1$ in some subjects with asthma. The lack of a detectable effect in a few studies may be due to methodologic weaknesses or the existence of differential susceptibilities between subjects.

## III.  Lung and Other Cancers

Over the past 10 years, epidemiological studies of the association between environmental tobacco smoke (ETS) and cancer in nonsmokers have accumulated, and with them a series of reviews, critical analyses, and acrimonious debates. Most studies have focused on lung cancer in nonsmokers, especially women, with residential exposure to ETS from smoking spouses. Fewer data have been garnered on the association of ETS with other types of cancer or on ETS exposure outside the home. The studies that fuel this debate are observational studies in humans, although there is evidence from experimental studies in rodents that inhalation of mainstream smoke produces tumors [52] and that the tar from sidestream smoke is carcinogenic when applied to the skin [53]. Before discussing the controversy surrounding the epidemiologic studies, it might be useful to place the problem within the broader context of active tobacco smoking and cancer.

As shown in Table 2, the cancer death rate in England and Wales increased sharply for males, but not for females, during the first half of the twentieth century. Much of the increase in males was due to an exponential rise in the mortality from cancer of the lung. In what was probably the first formal case-control study of cancer, published in 1933, Stocks and Karn [54] found no elevated risk of cancer from cigarette smoking. (Parenthetically, theirs was the first report of a preventive effect of frequent consumption of vegetables). However, as Clemmesen [55] noted: "In England and Wales and the United States the increase in bronchial carcinoma had during the 1940's reached a level which permitted more extensive studies, and no less than five major papers on the association between tobacco smoking and this disease appeared in 1950." By 1954, Dorn [56] had collected 14 case-control studies of smoking and lung cancer, and over the next 10 years the results of several large cohort studies [57] added weight to the evidence incriminating cigarette smoking. From the

**Table 2**  Cancer Mortality in England and Wales, 1911–1965[a]

|           | All cancer[b] | | Lung cancer | |
|-----------|------|--------|------|--------|
|           | Male | Female | Male | Female |
| 1911–1915 | 118.8 | 126.5 | 1.6  | 1.0 |
| 1921–1925 | 131.3 | 128.0 | 2.4  | 1.0 |
| 1931–1935 | 141.6 | 128.0 | 8.4  | 2.4 |
| 1941–1945 | 140.9 | 117.1 | 19.7 | 3.8 |
| 1951–1955 | 159.5 | 111.0 | 46.0 | 6.2 |

*Source:* McKenzie A, Case RAM, Pearson JT. General Register Office. Cancer statistics for England and Wales 1901–1955. Studies in Medical and Population Subjects No. 13. London: Her Majesty's Stationery Office, 1957.
[a]Age-standardized rates per 100,000 by gender [Segi's standard world population (Segi M, Kurihara M. Cancer mortality for selected sites in 24 countries. Sendai, Japan: Tohoku University School of Medicine, 1966: 3)].
[b]Excluding leukemia and Hodgkin's disease.

beginning, the validity of this epidemiological evidence was fiercely attacked; the resulting controversy was instrumental in sharpening the methodological and statistical rigor of epidemiological studies of chronic disease in the postwar period. Several potential sources of bias in such studies were identified: in the selection of control groups, in the misclassification of disease or exposure status, and in the presence of confounding factors. Methods of statistical analysis became more sophisticated, with emphasis on the estimation of relative risk, rather than simple comparisons of proportions. Methods of multivariate analysis to adjust for confounding factors were developed, and Cornfield [58] showed how to combine the results of sets of studies statistically to give a combined estimate of relative risk, a procedure that was later termed *meta-analysis* [59]. The need for samples large enough to provide power for hypothesis testing and precision of estimation was realized.

Eventually, the sheer weight of the epidemiologic evidence, and increasing familiarity with the methods used, convinced most professionals and public health authorities that active cigarette smoking caused carcinoma in the epithelia of the respiratory and urinary tracts [17]. Public health campaigns aimed at reducing smoking had some success, especially in males, although the impact of this on lung cancer death rates is only recently being felt, due to the 20-year latency between tobacco consumption and lung cancer mortality [8].

Ten years ago the cycle of controversy began again as toxicologists and epidemiologists became interested in the possible carcinogenic effects of ETS. By 1986, sufficient evidence had accumulated to warrent two federally sponsored reports in the United States. The review by the National Research Council (NRC) [1] identified 18 studies of lung cancer and ETS, primarily in nonsmoking women with smoking spouses. After excluding five studies, chiefly because of incomplete information, the NRC subjected the remaining studies, 10 case-control and three cohort studies, to a formal meta-analysis. The overall relative risk (95% confidence interval) was 1.24 (1.04, 1.50) for 10 case-control studies and 1.44 (1.20, 1.72) for the cohort studies. The relative risk was 1.34 (1.18, 1.53) when these two groups of studies were combined. In five of the studies, three case-control and two cohort, a dose–response relationship was seen (i.e., an increasing relative risk with increasing amounts smoked by the spouse). However, when the analysis was restricted to the four case-control studies and one cohort study from the United States, the overall relative risk was 1.14 (0.92, 1.40). The same 13 studies were reviewed by the U.S. Surgeon General (2) without a formal meta-analysis. Both reviews paid special attention to the possibility of bias in the studies: in particular, information bias due to unblinded interviewing and to misclassification of the smoking status of the subjects. If misclassification is nondifferential, affecting cases and controls alike, the true relative risk is underestimated. However, if the spouses of smokers are more likely to falsely claim nonsmoking status than the spouses of nonsmokers, the estimate of relative risk would be biased upwards [36]. Bias due to confounding factors such as diet and occupation are also possible but of unknown significance. After consideration of possible biases, and despite the generally small excess risk observed in most studies, both official reports concluded that a true increase in risk of lung cancer exists for nonsmokers exposed to residential ETS.

The evidence up to 1989 on the adverse health effects of ETS, including cancer, was also reviewed by Spitzer et al. [4]. Rather than a formal meta-analysis or traditional literature review, a *best evidence synthesis* [60] was employed. The working group considered only studies deemed methodologically sound as assessed by well-defined a priori criteria. There were 16 admissible studies relating to spousal smoking and lung cancer: 13 case-control [61–73] and three cohort studies [74–76]. Seven of the admissible case-control studies were positive [61–67] (i.e., detecting on association between passive smoking and lung cancer), of which six provided evidence of a dose–response relation [61–63,65–67]. Four case-control studies were negative with inadequate power [68–71], and two were negative [72,73] with adequate power. Among spouses of men who smoked at least 20 cigarettes daily, the large Japanese cohort study [74] detected an increased risk of lung cancer, relative risk 1.9 (1.3, 2.7), but the large American cohort study [75] did not, relative risk 1.1 (0.8, 1.6). The third cohort study [76], of Scottish women, was considered inconclusive because of a small sample size. The working group concluded that a causal relation between exposure to ETS and lung cancer was "plausible and even likely" based on the preponderance of positive studies, cross-cultural consistency, evidence of a dose–response relation, and biological plausibility.

Since these extensive reviews, several additional case-control studies have been reported. Lee [77] listed 18 studies in which it was possible to calculate relative risks for both passive and active smoking. For females, the median relative risk among these studies was 1.60 for passive smoking and 4.54 for active smoking. In seven of the studies, a similar comparison was possible for males, with a median relative risk of 2.10 for passive smoking and 12.02 for active smoking. Lee noted that the excess risk for passive smoking was over 10% of that for active smoking in both sexes, a proportion which exceeded that expected from the cotinine levels found in passive smokers.

A recent study of particular interest is that by Janerich et al. [78], a population-based case-control study of lung cancer in nonsmokers involving 191 matched case/control pairs. Although no increased risk was found for ETS exposure in adult life, heavy exposure (25 or more smoker-years) during childhood and adolescence doubled the risk of lung cancer, relative risk 2.07 (1.16, 3.68). This is the first study pointing out the importance of childhood exposure in this context.

The meta-analysis of studies in the 1986 NRC report [1] was roundly criticized by Letzel et al. [79] chiefly on the grounds of possible errors of misclassification. Similar criticisms have been expressed by Fleiss and Gross [80], who went on to perform a meta-analysis on nine American epidemiological studies, five of them included in the NRC analysis and four published later. The overall relative risk was 1.12 (0.95, 1.30), similar to that quoted in the NRC report for studies in the United States.

The evidence for an increased risk of cancer, other than lung cancer, among nonsmokers exposed to ETS is very sparse. The only solid evidence comes from the large cohort study in Japan by Hirayama [57]. Significant and dose-related relative risks for cancer of the nasal sinuses and brain were found in nonsmoking wives of smokers. The increased risk for sinonasal cancer is consistent with the increased risk of such tumors among active smokers reported by Elwood [81]. The significance of the increased risk of brain cancer for passive smoking in Hirayama's study remains to be determined; this type of cancer has not previously been associated with active smoking. Unlike the elevated risks from active smoking, no association between laryngeal cancer and passive smoking has been reported.

In general, there is fair evidence that residential exposure to ETS produces cancer in the epithelium of the respiratory tract of nonsmokers, as would be expected from the presence of carcinogens in ETS and the strong evidence of carcinogenicity of active smoking in humans. However, the excess risk of lung cancer, the only respiratory cancer of numerical importance, is likely to be very small, perhaps 30%. Such an increase could be important from a public health point of view because of the prevalence of the exposure, at least in the past. For example, if half of the women who do not smoke themselves are exposed to ETS at home, the 30% excess risk translates into 13% of lung cancers among such women being attributable to residential ETS. However, there is no such evidence that the incidence of lung cancer among nonsmokers is increasing, and the recent changes of smoking prevalence imply that exposure to ETS will be less of a problem in the future.

## IV. Conclusions

A causal relation between environmental tobacco smoke and respiratory disease has biological plausibility: ETS contains irritants, toxins, and carcinogens that can affect lung function and cause cancer. Among children, ETS causes respiratory disease, which if not reversible must affect adult lung function. The contents of ETS are similar to mainstream smoke, an important cause of respiratory disease in our society. This high "prior probability" that ETS causes disease, combined with the supporting empirical evidence, leaves little doubt that ETS causes impairment of lung function and cancer among adults. Two unanswered questions remain. What is the magnitude of the effect, and what is its clinical relevance?

The observed effect on respiratory symptoms was small at most, and reductions in FEV$_1$ were approximately 3% from either household or workplace exposure. The true magnitude is probably larger than that observed because of self-selection and inaccuracy of exposure measurements (discussed in Section II.A). Prospective studies and accurate exposure measures could address these problems. The study by Masi et al. [25] provides an example of how exposure can potentially be better assessed in epidemiologic studies, but objective validation of questionnaire-assessed exposure is needed.

The clinical relevance of minimally increased symptoms and small reductions in lung function is uncertain. Studies of potentially susceptible subgroups are needed. Subjects with preexisting severe airflow limitation may not tolerate further small decrements in lung function. Those with bronchial hyperresponsiveness may respond with larger decrements in lung function. Active smoking and grain dust exposure act additively or synergistically to cause airflow obstruction [82]. Active smoking similarly enhances the risks of lung cancer from radon and asbestos exposure. Synergism between ETS and these exposures have not yet been assessed. There is also a need to study other meaningful outcomes: use of respiratory medications, absence from work or school due to respiratory illness, physician visits, and hospital admissions for respiratory diseases. All of these simple indicators reflect quality of life and financial cost to the individual and to society.

Apart from assessing the clinical relevance of exposure to environmental tobacco smoke, more resources should be invested in strategies to minimize exposure to tobacco smoke. Western society's belief that nonsmokers have the right to inhale clean air has resulted in a reduction in passive smoking. ETS exposure will continue to be restricted because it "bothers" a majority of adults, 75% according to Cummings et al. [41]. Further research is not likely to change this perception. Reducing the number of active smokers through education, increased tobacco taxes, and therapy for addiction should reduce passive exposure. Legislation restricting smoking in workplaces and public areas, including transportation facilities, has been effective in reducing exposure outside the home. Within the home, passive smoking will be reduced if the number of active smokers can be reduced through current methods or alternatively, by a ban on cigarettes. Efforts are currently being made to provide families with an appreciation of the pollution levels they experience when tobacco is smoked inside the home. Examples of public education statements could be: "Do you worry about health problems from lead in paint and gasoline . . . and about mercury in food? Cigarettes smoked in your home expose your entire family to both lead and mercury" or "Cigarettes smoked in your home may expose you and your family to more formaldehyde than if your home were insulated with urea-formaldehyde foam insulation (UFFI)." Householders should also know that low-tar cigarettes are not "low-pollution" cigarettes. They have ventilated filters that reduce mainstream smoke but increase sidestream smoke [83]. Hopefully, this type of information will encourage household smokers to smoke outside the home, or preferably, quit. Exposure reduction would deal effectively with the effects on children's and adults' health as well as the noxious and disagreeable experiences of those exposed.

### Acknowledgments

The authors with to thank Pierre Ernst, associate professor of medicine and epidemiology and biostatistics, McGill University, Montreal, Canada, and Dr. Murray J. Kaiserman, Tobacco Products Section, Health and Welfare, Canada for their assistance in the preparation of this chapter.

### References

1. National Research Council, Committee on Passive Smoking. Environmental tobacco smoke: measuring exposures and assessing health effects. ISBN 0-309-03730-1. Washington, DC; National Academy Press, 1986.
2. U.S. Department of Health and Human Services. The health consequences of involuntary smoking. A report of the Surgeon General. U.S. Department of Health and Human Services, Public Health Service, Centers for Disease Control, Center for Health Promotion and Education, Office on Smoking and Health, 1986.
3. Fielding JE, Phenow KJ. Health effects of involuntary smoking. N Engl J Med 1988;319:1452–60.
4. Spitzer WO, Lawrence V, Dales R, Hill G, Archer MC, Clark P, Abenhaim L, Hardy J, Sampalis J, Pinfold SP, Morgan PP. Links between passive smoking and disease: a best-evidence synthesis. Clin Invest Med 1990;13:17–42.
5. Witorsch P. Effects of ETS exposure on pulmonary function and respiratory health in adults. In: Ecobichon DJ, Wu JM, eds. Environmental tobacco smoke. Proceedings of the International Symposium at McGill University, 1989. Lexington, MA: Lexington Books, 1990;169–85.
6. Adams JD, O'Mara-Adams KJ, Hoffmann D. Toxic and carcinogenic agents in undiluted mainstream smoke and sidestream smoke of different types of cigarettes. Carcinogen 1987;8:729–31.
7. Redline S. The epidemiology of COPD. In: Cherniack NS, ed. Chronic obstructive pulmonary disease. Philadelphia: WB Saunders, 1991:225–34.
8. Canadian cancer statistics 1991. Toronto, Ontario, Canada: National Cancer Institute of Canada, 1991.
9. Dales RE, Zwanenburg H, Burnett R, Franklin CA. Respiratory health

effects of home dampness and molds among canadian children. Am J Epidemiol 1991;134:196–203.

10. Svendsen KH, Kuller LH, Martin MJ, Ockene JK. Effects of passive smoking in the multiple risk factor intervention trial. Am J Epidemiol 1987;126:783–795.

11. Kauffmann F, Dockery DW, Speizer FE, Ferris BG Jr. Respiratory symptoms and lung function in relation to passive smoking; a comparative study of American and French women. Int J Epidemiol 1989;18:334–344.

12. Health and Welfare Canada, 1988. The smoking behavior of Canadians—1986, by WJ Millar. ISBN 0-662-16517-9. Ottawa, Ontario, Canada: Minister of Supply and Services, Canada.

13. Kentner M, Triebig G, Weltle D. The influence of passive smoking on pulmonary function: a study of 1,351 office workers. Prev Med 1984;13:656–69.

14. Euler GL, Abbey DE, Magie AR, Hodgkin JE. Chronic obstructive pulmonary disease symptom effects of long-term cumulative exposure to ambient levels of total suspended particulates and sulphur dioxide in California Seventh-Day Adventist residents. Arch Environ Health 1987;42:213–22.

15. Salutin R. Loose canons (political correctness). Saturday Night 1991;106:20,22.

16. Fennell T, Jenish D. The growing threat of political correctness: across Canada and the United States, repression is sweeping through the universities. Readers Digest 1991;139:55,56.

17. U.S. Department of Health and Human Services. Reducing the health consequences of smoking: 25 years of progress. A report of the Surgeon General. DHHS Publication (CDC) 89-8411. U.S. Department of Health and Human Services, Public Health Service, Centers for Disease Control, Center for Chronic Disease Prevention and Health Promotion, Office on Smoking and Health, prepublication version, January 11, 1989.

18. Rosenthal R. "File drawer problem" intolerance for null results. Psychol Bull 1979;86:638–41.

19. Schilling RSF, Letai AD, Hui SL, Beck JB, Schoenberg JB, Bouhuys A. Lung function, respiratory disease, and smoking in families. Am J Epidemiol 1977;106:247–83.

20. Simecek C. Reflection of passive exposure to smoking in the home on the prevalence of chronic bronchitis in non-smokers. Czech Med 1980;3:308–10.

21. Comstock GW, Meyer MB, Helsing KJ, Tockman MS. Respiratory effects of household exposures to tobacco smoke and gas cooking. Am Rev Respir Dis 1981;124:143–48.

22. Hole DJ, Gillis CR, Chopra C, Hawthorne VM. Passive smoking and cardiorespiratory health in a general population in the West of Scotland. Br Med J 1989;299:423–27.
23. Lebowitz MD, Burrows B. Respiratory symptoms related to smoking habits of family adults. Chest 1976;69:48–50.
24. Schwartz J, Zeger S. Passive smoking, air pollution, and acute respiratory symptoms in a diary study of student nurses. Am Rev Respir Dis 1990;141:62–67.
25. Masi MA, Hanley JA, Ernst P, Becklake MR. Environmental exposure to tobacco smoke and lung function in young adults. Am Rev Respir Dis 1988;138:296–99.
26. Masjedi M-R, Kazemi H, Johnson DC. Effects of passive smoking on the pulmonary function of adults. Thorax 1990;45:27–31.
27. White JR, Froeb HF. Small airways dysfunction in nonsmokers chronically exposed to tobacco smoke. N Engl Med 1980;302:720–23.
28. Brunekreef B, Fischer P, Remijn B, Van der Lende R, Schouten J, Quanjer P. Indoor air pollution and its effect on pulmonary function of adult non-smoking women. III. Passive smoking and pulmonary function. Int J Epidemiol 1985;14:227–30.
29. Hosein HR, Corey P. Domestic air pollution and respiratory function in a group of housewives. Can J Public Health 1986;77:44–50.
30. Lebowitz MD. Influence of passive smoking on pulmonary function: a survey. Prev Med 1984;13:645–55.
31. Salem ES, El Zahby M, Senna GA, Malek A. Pulmonary manifestations among passive smokers. Bull Int Union Tuberc 1984;59:50–53.
32. Kalandidi A, Trichopoulos D, Hatzakis A, Tzannes S, Saracci R. Passive smoking and chronic obstructive lung disease (letter to the editor). Lancet 1987;2:1325–26.
33. Kauffman F, Tessier J-F, Oriol P. Adult passive smoking in the home environment: a risk factor for chronic airflow limitation. Am J Epidemiol 1983;117:269–80.
34. Eisen EA, Wegman DH, Louis TA. Effects of selection in a prospective study of forced expiratory volume in Vermont granite workers. Am Rev Respir Dis 1983;128:587–91.
35. Brunekreef B, Hoek G, Groot G. Pets, allergy and respiratory symptoms in children. Int J Epidemiol 1992;21:338–42.
36. Uberla K. Lung cancer from passive smoking: hypothesis or convincing evidence? Int Arch Occup Environ Health 1987;59:421–37.
37. Hirayama T. Cancer mortality in non-smoking women with smoking husbands based on a large-scale cohort study in Japan. Prev Med 1984;13:680–90.

38. Stephens T. Canadians and smoking: an update. ISBN 0-662-18656-7. Prepared for the Tobacco Programs Unit, Health Promotion Directorate, Health Services and Promotion Branch, Health and Welfare Canada, 1991.

39. Graham NMH. The epidemiology of acute respiratory infections in children and adults: a global perspective. Epidemiol Rev 1990;12:149–78.

40. Sterling T, Weinkam J. The confounding of occupation and smoking and its consequences. Soc Sci Med 1990;30:457–67.

41. Cummings KM, Zaki A, Markello S. Variation in sensitivity to environmental tobacco smoke among adult non-smokers. Int J Epidemiol 1991;20:121–25.

42. Murray AB, Morrison BJ. Passive smoking by asthmatics: its greater effects on boys and girls and on older than on younger children. Pediatrics 1989;84:541–49.

43. Ilfeld FW Jr. Further validation of a psychiatric symptom index in a normal population. Psychol Rep 1976;39:1215–28.

44. Feinstein AR. Clinical epidemiology: the architecture of clinical research. Philadelphia: WB Saunders, 1985:299–300.

45. Dahms TE, Bolin JF, Slavin RG. Passive smoking: effects on bronchial asthma. Chest 1981;80:530–34.

46. Knight A, Breslin ABX. Passive cigarette smoking and patients with asthma. Med J Aust 1985;142:194–95.

47. Stankus RP, Menon PK, Rando RJ, Glindmeyer H, Salvaggio JE, Lehrer SB. Cigarette smoke-sensitive asthma: challenge studies. J Allergy Clin Immunol 1988;82:331–38.

48. Shepard RJ, Collins R, Silverman F. "Passive" exposure of asthma subjects to cigarette smoke. Environ Res 1979;20:392–402.

49. Wiedemann HP, Mahler DA, Loke J, Virgulto JA, Snyder P, Matthay RA. Acute effects of passive smoking on lung function and airway reactivity in asthmatic subjects. Chest 1986;89:180–85.

50. Pimm PE, Silverman F, Shephard RJ. Physiological effects of acute passive exposure to cigarette smoke. Arch Environ Health 1978;33:201–13.

51. Shephard RJ, Collins R, Silverman F. Responses of exercising subjects to acute "passive" cigarette smoke exposure. Environ Res 1979;19:279–91.

52. IARC Working Group on the Evaluation of the Carcinogenic Risk of Chemicals to Humans. Biologic data relevant to the evaluation of carcinogenic risk to humans. In: IARC Monograph. Vol. 38. Lyon, France: IARC, 1986:127–98.

53. Wynder EL, Hoffman D. Biologic tests for tumorigenic and ciliatoxic activity. In: Wynder EL, Hoffman D, eds. Tobacco and tobacco smoke:

studies in experimental carcinogenesis. New York: Academic Press, 1967:181–250.

54. Stocks P, Karn MN. A cooperative study of the habits, home life, dietary and family histories of 450 cancer patients and of an equal number of control patients. Ann Eugen 1933;5:237–80.

55. Clemmesen J. Statistical studies in the aetiology of malignant neoplasms. Acta Pathol Microbiol Scand 1965;(Suppl 174)I:1–543.

56. Dorn HF. The relationship of cancer of the lung and the use of tobacco. Am Stat 1954;8:7–13.

57. Hirayama T. Health effects of active and passive smoking. In: Aoki M, ed. Smoking and health 1987. New York: Elsevier Science Publishers, 1987:75–86.

58. Cornfield J. A statistical problem arising from retrospective studies. Proc 3rd Berkeley Symp 1956;4:135–48.

59. Glass GV. Primary, secondary and meta-analysis of research. Educ Res 1976;5:3–8.

60. Slavin RE. Best evidence synthesis: an alternative to meta-analytic and traditional reviews. Educ Res 1986;15:5–11.

61. Akiba S, Kato H, Blot WJ. Passive smoking and lung cancer among Japanese women. Cancer Res 1986;46:4804–7.

62. Dalager NA, Pickle NW, Mason TJ, et al. The relation of passive smoking to lung cancer. Cancer Res 1986;46:4808–11.

63. Garfinkel L, Auerbach O, Joubert L. Involuntary smoking and lung cancer: a case-control study. J Natl Cancer Inst 1985;75:463–69.

64. Humble CG, Samet JM, Pathak DR. Marriage to a smoker and lung cancer risk. Am J Public Health 1987;77:598–602.

65. Lam TH, Kung ITM, Wong CM, et al. Smoking, passive smoking and histological types in lung cancer in Hong Kong Chinese women. Br J Cancer 1987;56:673–78.

66. Sandler DP, Wilcox AJ, Everson RB. Cumulative effects of lifetime smoking on cancer risk. Lancet 1985;1:312–14.

67. Trichopoulos D, Kalandi A, Sparros L. Lung cancer and passive smoking: conclusion of a Greek study. Lancet 1983;2:677–78.

68. Kabat GC, Wynder EL. Lung cancer in nonsmokers. Cancer 1984;53:1214–21.

69. Koo LC, Ho JH-C, Saw D. Active and passive smoking among female lung cancer patients and controls in Hong Kong. J Exp Clin Cancer Res 1983;4:367–75.

70. Wu AH, Henderson BE, Pike MC, Yu MC. Smoking and other risk factors for lung cancer in women. J Natl Cancer Inst 1985;74:747–51.

71. Lee PN, Chamberlain J, Alderson MR. Relationship of passive smoking

to risk lung cancer and other smoking-associated diseases. Br J Cancer 1986;54:97–105.

72. Chan WC, Colborne MJ, Fung SC, Ho HC. Bronchial cancer in Hong Kong 1976–1977. Br J Cancer 1979;39:182–92.

73. Pershagen G, Hrubec Z, Svensson C. Passive smoking and lung cancer in Swedish women. Am J Epidemiol 1987;125:17–24.

74. Hirayama T. Passive smoking and cancer: an epidemiologic review. In: Kurinhara M, Aoki K, Miller RW, Muir C, eds. Changing cancer patterns and topics in cancer epidemiology. Gann Monogr Cancer Res 1987;33:127–35.

75. Garfinkel L. Time trends in lung cancer among nonsmokers and a note on passive smoking. J Natl Cancer Inst 1981;66:1061–66.

76. Gillis CR, Hole DJ, Hawthorne VM, Boyle P. The effect of environmental tobacco smoke in two urban communities in the west of Scotland. Eur J Respir Dis (Suppl) 1984;133:121–26.

77. Lee P. Lung cancer and passive smoking. Br J Cancer 1991;63:161–62.

78. Janerich DT, Thompson WD, Varela LR, Greenwald P, Chorost S, Tucci C, Zaman MB, Melamed MR, Kiely M, McKneally MF. Lung cancer and exposure to tobacco smoke in the household. N Engl J Med 1990;323:632–36.

79. Letzel H, Blumner E, Uberla K. Meta-analyses on passive smoking and lung cancer: effects of study selection and misclassification of exposure. Environ Technol Lett 1988;9:491–500.

80. Fleiss JL, Gross AJ. Meta-analysis in epidemiology, with special reference to studies of the association between exposure to environmental tobacco smoke and lung cancer: a critique. J Clin Epidemiol 1991;44:127–39.

81. Elwood JM. Wood exposure and smoking: association with cancer of the nasal cavity and parnasal sinuses in British Columbia. Can Med Assoc J 1981;124:1573–77.

82. DoPico GA, Reddan W, Tsiatis A, Peters ME, Rankin J. Epidemiologic study of clinical and physiologic parameters in grain handlers of northern United States. Am Rev Respir Dis 1984;130:759–65.

83. Kaiserman MJ, Rickert WS, Collishaw NE. Smoking in the home environment: a controlled room study. Presented at Indoor Air '90, the 5th International Conference on Air Quality and Climate, Toronto, Ontario, Canada, 1990.

# 23

## Childhood Respiratory Diseases and Environmental Tobacco Smoke

SCOTT T. WEISS and JOHN P. HANRAHAN

Brigham and Women's Hospital
and Harvard Medical School
Boston, Massachusetts

## I. Introduction

1986 was a benchmark year for research into the health effects of environmental tobacco smoke. In that year the National Research Council [1] and the U.S. Surgeon General [2] issued summary reports of the health effects of environmental tobacco smoke upon a wide range of medical conditions. The purpose of this chapter is to examine critically the health effects of environmental tobacco smoke and its relationship to childhood respiratory diseases.

Children may be particularly susceptible to the effects of environmental tobacco smoke because their immunologic and respiratory systems are still under development, and the dose of exposure relative to their size may be greater than for adults. In addition, proximity to exposure, and thus effective dose, may be greater in very young children. In this chapter we review newer, more quantitative, measures of exposure and research reports that enhance or change recommendations made in the 1986 reports.

## II. Measures of Exposure

The accurate assessment of exposure to environmental tobacco smoke and linkage to health outcomes in children is complex and is complicated by absence of knowledge at many steps along the pathway from exposure to disease. ETS is known to be composed of several thousand compounds in either gas [3] or particulate phase [4]. Specific associations between particular health outcomes and individual chemical constituents of ETS are largely unknown. Moreover, environmental concentrations of these constituents are likely to vary substantially based on a number of factors, including tobacco source of the smoke, time from production to inhalation, and environment in which the exposure takes place [5]. As is the case with the many exposure–response relationships, there are important host-related issues for both the effective dose received and host susceptibility to the individual constituents of environmental tobacco smoke. All these factors combine to cause imprecise definition of the specific inciting or causative chemical agents, even for the health outcomes clearly associated with ETS. In lieu of a precise link between individual ETS constituents and health outcomes, associations are usually drawn between surrogates or markers of ETS exposure. These surrogates are generally selected as exposure measures because they are present in high concentrations in ETS, and/or the technical capability to measure them exists [1].

In studies performed to date examining health outcomes associated with ETS, exposure assessment has generally taken one of three forms: (1) modeling exposure based on (a) questionnaires or (b) air sampling of the environment where the preponderance of exposure took place, (2) personal air monitoring of the exposure environment, or (3) measurement of a biological marker of exposure. Each of these methodologies entails certain difficulties and advantages, enumerated briefly below.

## A.  Questionnaires

Until recently, interview or questionnaire assessment of ETS exposure has been the standard assessment tool for epidemiologic studies. This methodology has numerous obvious limitations, including being subject to recall bias and providing only a crude quantitation of exposure. Nonetheless, this exposure assessment method offers some compelling advantages over more objective methods. First, many of the health outcomes in both children and adults that are postulated to be associated with ETS exposure are believed to result from long-term, low-level exposure. These exposures cannot be summarized and could even be misrepresented by environmental sampling or biomarkers, both of which assess recent exposure levels. Exposure assessment by questionnaire also does not employ a single or multiple surrogate markers of exposure. The use of a surrogate marker in environmental sampling or as a biomarker requires that the ETS constituent(s) which impact the health outcome under investigation must have levels that correlate with the marker being used to quantitate exposure. Furthermore, most factors related to the uptake and elimination of the surrogate marker may vary between exposed individuals, so that measurements of a surrogate do not accurately reflect the effective biologic dose. Finally, questionnaire data are essential in identifying confounding or modifying exposures or host factors that may influence the health outcome being evaluated.

In a recent paper, Coultas and colleagues (1989) evaluated the validity of ETS exposure history by determining the reliability of two responses obtained 4 months apart [6]. In these nonsmoking adults, their investigators found high concordance between responses as to whether or not maternal and parental smoking occurred during pregnancy and childhood. However, the reliability of quantitative estimates of the amount smoked by parents during childhood or spouses during adulthood was poor. Similarly, mean urine cotinine levels increased with report of more prolonged recent ETS exposure, although there was wide variability of levels within exposure categories.

### B. Environmental Sampling

Chamber and field studies have demonstrated that a variety of tracers can be used to measure ETS levels. Carbon monoxide (CO), respirable suspended particulates (RSPs), aromatic hydrocarbons, and tobacco specific nitrosomines are among the compounds that have been found to be elevated in indoor environments with ETS exposure. A recent study among children attending a day care center in North Carolina demonstrated that nicotine levels in the home environment were correlated with children's urinary cotinine levels when obtained in day care the day after air sampling in the home [7]. In general, fixed environmental monitoring for ETS has limited applicability in epidemiologic studies, as cumulative individual exposures are better assessed by questionnaire or biomarkers.

A limited number of studies have utilized personal air sampling monitors to evaluate ETS exposure. Several of these studies have employed measurements of respirable particulates (RSP) and found that ETS-exposed subjects have a consistently higher level of RSP than those of unexposed individuals [8–12]. Nonetheless, the nonspecific nature of this measure and high background levels in many in unexposed subjects make quantitation of individual exposure difficult by this method. More recently, passive personal exposure devises that collect and quantify nicotine have been developed and validated [11,12]. However, these have yet to be employed on any wide-scale basis in epidemiologic studies of health outcomes.

### C. Biomarkers

While environmental sampling and questionnaire reporting of ETS exposure continue to be used, the use of biologic markers of exposures has become an important tool in epidemiologic studies. Biomarkers offer the advantage of providing a quantitative estimate of exposure and summing exposure of an individual over many potentially different microenvironments. Many constituents of ETS have been evaluated for potential usefulness as biomarkers. The ideal biomarker would be both a sensitive and specific indicator of total ETS exposure, measurable in biological fluids at low expense, and itself a cause or highly correlated with the health outcome of interest. Unfortunately, no single biomarker has met all of these criteria. Thiocyanate is found in plasma, urine, and saliva of ETS exposed subjects, but lacks specificity and sensitivity [13]. Other compounds, including hydroxyproline, $n$-nitrosoproline (NPRO), aromatic amines, and DNA adducts of environmental carcinogens, have been detected in biological fluids of active smokers. However, these compounds have yet to be demonstrated to be of use in discerning ETS exposure. Carbon monoxide (CO) also has utility as a biomarker of active smoking measured either as the exhaled alveolar air concentration or as carboxyhemoglobin levels (COHb) in the blood [1,13]. Carbon monoxide is produced both endogenously and by exogenous sources unrelated to smoking (such as home heating devices), causing this marker to lack specificity for ETS exposure. While effective in detecting active smokers, carbon monoxide does not have suitable discriminant ability at low levels of environmental exposure to reliably separate ETS exposed from unexposed nonsmokers.

Measurement of nicotine and its metabolites in human biological fluids has been adopted most widely in epidemiologic studies over the last 10 years to quantify active and passive cigarette smoking exposure. Nicotine and cotinine have the advantage of being more specific indicators of cigarette smoking than other biomarkers. In addition, measurement techniques for cotinine using gas chromotography or immunoassay have become widely available which can detect levels as low as 0.5 ng/mL in biological fluids [14]. Advantageous, too, is the elimination kinetics of cotinine from biological fluids, persisting with a half-life of between 18 to 36 h for both urine and serum measures [1].

Several studies have confirmed the utility of cotinine as a biomarker in epidemiologic studies of ETS exposure in children. Jarvis and co-workers in a 1985 study of 569 nonsmoking British schoolchildren found a progressive increase in salivary cotinine levels in groups with zero, one, and two smoking parents [15]. Henderson and colleagues in the above-mentioned study of North Carolina children attending a day care center found that mean urinary cotinine levels (corrected for creatinine) were higher in 12 children exposed to smoking parents (geometric mean 86.5 ng/mg creatinine) than in 12 infants in nonsmoking households (geometric mean 13.7 ng/mg), with little overlap of individual measurements [7]. They found that a cutoff of 30 ng/mg creatinine was optimal to separate ETS exposed from unexposed children. A study by Cummings et al. of 663 nonsmokers attending a cancer screening clinic in Buffalo, New York [16], found a significant correlation between urinary cotinine levels and the number of reported contacts with smokers in the 4-day prior to specimen collection. Cotinine levels collected from November through April were also significantly higher than those collected during the remainder of the year. Nonetheless, these authors found wide variability in urinary cotinine levels within exposure strata. In a population-based survey of more than 2000 children and adults in Albuquerque, New Mexico, mean salivary cotinine levels were found to parallel increases in the number of smokers in the home [17]. In addition, the presence of a smoking mother in the home increased the odds of detecting salivary cotinine levels in children compared to the presence of a father who smoked. Finally, Greenberg and co-workers studied 433 neonates from central North Carolina [18], 60% of whom were found to have cotinine detectable in their urine during a home interview approximately 3 weeks after birth. Correlates of infant urine cotinine level included both the amount of maternal smoking and the amount of exposure to other household smokers.

While these and other studies establish cotinine as the biomarker that performs best in assessing ETS exposure in children, it is not without its potential limitations [19]. Cotinine demonstrates wide within-subject variability even when exposure is rigidly controlled in chamber studies. This is thought to be due to temporal differences in uptake and the rate of metabolism of nicotine by the cytochrome P450 system. Cotinine has also found to be present in certain foodstuffs, including tomatoes, powdered tea, green peppers, and eggplant, calling its specificity as a smoking exposure measure into question. Despite these difficulties, a growing number of studies suggest that it does correlate with nicotine levels and/or number of smokers in the home and is therefore the best biochemical marker yet available to assess ETS exposure.

Moreover, optimal assessment of ETS exposure at present requires a combined approach of careful questionnaire documentation of exposure, especially in epidemiologic studies of health outcomes associated with chronic exposures, in addition to an objective exposure measure, preferably a biomarker such as cotinine. The latter will serve to both sum recent exposure over all microenvironments and to smokers. This can allow characterization of exposure–response relationships with ETS and will permit better elucidation of potential confounders of ETS exposure such as covert active smoking.

## III. Cotinine and Respiratory Outcomes

Two recent studies have utilized cotinine as a biomarker of ETS exposure when looking at respiratory outcomes. Lieberman and co-workers studied 87 women who had third-trimester amniocenteses performed because of preterm delivery [20]. Of these 87 women, 22 had some level of clotinine in their amniotic fluid (range 2 to 459 ng/mL; mean ± SE, 136 ± 26.2 ng/mL). The authors examine the relationship of amniotic fluid cotinine to indices of lung maturity. Fetal lung maturity was determined by measurement of the amniotic fluid lecithin sphingomyelin (L/S) ratio and the level of saturated phosphatidylcholine (SPC), the major component of pulmonary surfactant in amniotic fluid. Both L/S ratio and SPC concentration have been noted to be powerful predictors of lung maturity and the risk of RDS in infants. Mean lung maturity, as measured by L/S ratio and SPC level, was greater in the smoke-exposed fetuses, despite the fact that mean gestational age at which the amniotic fluid sample was obtained was obtained was actually slightly lower in that group than in the group without cotinine. Linear regression analyses demonstrated that amniotic fluid cotinine was a significant predictor of SPC independent of gestational age. The regression model predicted that a fetus with an amniotic fluid cotinine level of 100 ng/mL would on average have an SPC level that was 4 µg/dL higher than that of an unexposed fetus of a comparable gestational age. This translated into roughly a 1-week increase in lung maturity in fetuses exposed to maternal cigarette smoke. The regression model for SPC versus gestational age for cotinine positive and negative fetuses is shown in Figure 1. The results for L/S ratio were similar. These results were also statistically significant. The predicting model for change in L/S with gestational age in exposed and unexposed fetuses is shown in Figure 2. The authors speculate that the observed increase in lung maturity associated with maternal cigarette smoking is a form of dismaturity, the long-term implication of which is currently unknown. Studies looking as L/S ratio and its relationship to respiratory outcomes in infants exposed to ETS in utero would be of interest.

Recent data also suggest that prenatal maternal cigarette smoking can have an influence on measures of lung function at birth. A recently completed study examined the effect of prenatal maternal cigarette smoking on pulmonary function in 80 healthy infants tested shortly after birth (mean $4.2 \pm 1.9$ weeks) [21]. In this study, maternal smoking during pregnancy was measured by a questionnaire and by urine cotinine concentrations (corrected for creatinine) obtained at each prenatal visit. The infant's pulmonary function was assessed by partial expiratory flow volume curves and by helium dilution measurement functional residual capacity (FRC). There was an extremely high correlation between mean prenatal cigarettes per day and mean prenatal urine cotinine expressed as nanograms per milligram of creatinine (Fig. 3). Measures of forced expiratory flow were statistically significantly lower in infants born to smoking mothers. $V_{max}$ FRC, a measure of forced expiratory flow, and $V_{max}$ FRC/FRC were significantly lower in infants born to smoking mothers (Fig. 4). These results persisted after controlling for infant size, age, gender, and passive exposure to environmental smoke between birth and the time of pulmonary function testing. No differences in flow were evident in infants exposed and unexposed to ETS in the home after stratifying by prenatal exposure status. The implication is that maternal smoking during pregnancy is associated with significant reductions in forced expiratory flow rates in young infants at birth. The results suggest that maternal smoking during pregnancy may impair in utero airway development and/or alter lung

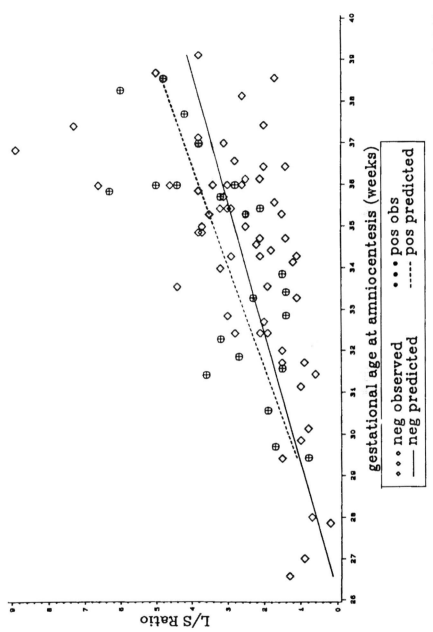

**Figure 1** Lecithin-sphingomyelin ratio (L/S) as a measure of lung maturity according to gestational age at amniotic fluid sampling, as predicted by linear regression. Dotted lines = cotinine present; solid lines = cotinine absent.

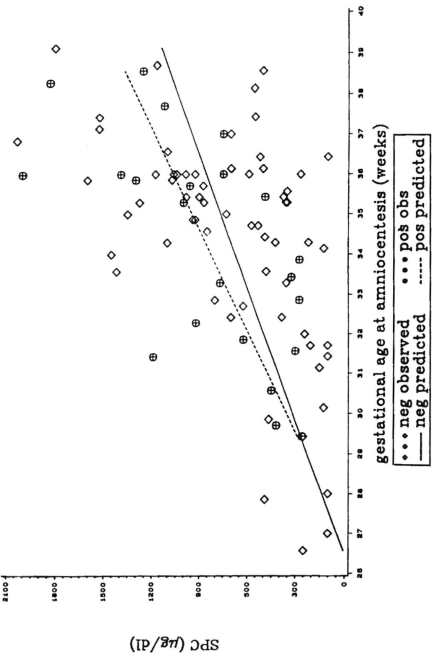

**Figure 2**  Saturated phosphatidylcholine as a measure of lung maturity according to gestational age of amniotic fluid sampling, as predicted by linear regression. Dotted line = cotinine present; solid line = cotinine absent.

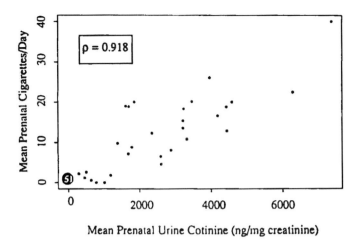

**Figure 3** Mean reported cigarettes per day vs. mean urine cotinine valves (corrected for urine creatinine) during pregnancy for 80 women. (From reference 21.)

elastic recall properties. The study does not exclude the possibility that additional adverse effects of postnatal smoking exposure could be present as well, especially with more prolonged exposure.

Taken together these data would suggest that maternal cigarette smoking during pregnancy has measurable effects on lung maturity and flow rates at birth. What remains unknown is the relationship of these studies to subsequent studies of older children where postnatal exposure is also a factor. The results of these studies should be considered in reviewing the studies on acute respiratory illness, chronic respiratory symptoms, and chronic respiratory disease that follow.

## IV. Acute Respiratory Illness

Two important methodologic problems need to be considered when evaluating studies of the effect of ETS on acute respiratory illnesses in children. For children under the age of 10 years, parents usually report both exposure and respiratory illness outcomes for their children, and some investigators feel that the presence of symptoms or infections in parents may lead to recall bias or result in exaggerated reporting of children's respiratory symptoms by symptomatic parents. Since parental symptoms are more likely to occur in cigarette smokers, adjusting for this potential bias may result in overadjustment. An additional factor that needs to be considered is that acute respiratory illnesses, specifically bronchitis and pneumonia, are substantially more frequent during the first few years of life than later in childhood and are also more common in male children.

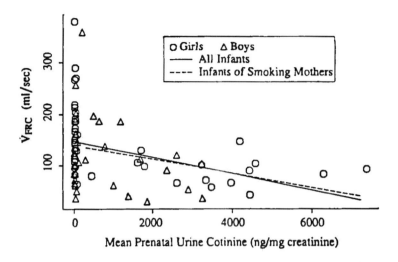

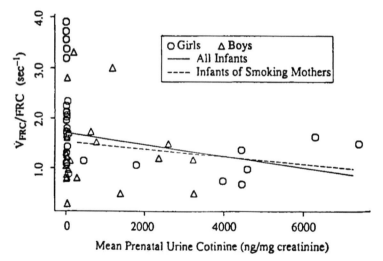

**Figure 4**  Flow at FRC (top) and flow of FRC corrected for FRC volume (bottom) vs. mean prenatal maternal urine cotinine concentration (corrected for creatinine) for 80 infants tested at ≤50 post-conception weeks. Solid line = regression relationship for all infants, dashed line = infants of smoking mothers alone.

Thus in examining studies of acute respiratory illness, both potential recall bias and secular trends with age and gender need to be considered.

The classic study in this area is the paper of Harlap and Davies [22]. These investigators performed a longitudinal study of 10,672 live births in Israel between the years 1965 and 1968. They observed that infants whose mother reported that they smoked at a prenatal visit had a 27.5% higher hospital admission rate for pneumonia and bronchitis than that of children with nonsmoking mothers. In light of the data presented in Section III, this study cannot differentiate between the residual effects of in utero vs. postnatal exposure, and no biomarkers of exposure were investigated.

Ogston and co-workers investigated 1565 infants enrolled in the Tayside Morbidity and Mortality Study in England [23]. Prospective information was collected on parental smoking habits and upper and lower respiratory infections, later confirmed by chart review. Increased respiratory illnesses during the first year of life were predicted by the presence of parental smoking, and this influence persisted after adjustment for the age of the parents, the method of heating and cooking in the home, and the social class of the family. Drawbacks of this study include the absence of adjustment for prenatal smoking, the fact that the number of cigarettes smoked per day was not recorded, and the fact that parents were simply divided into smokers and nonsmokers. However, an exposure–response relationship was present, where the respiratory infection rate increased from nonsmoking families to those with only a father smoking, to those families with a mother or both parents smoking.

Stern and colleagues (1987) studied 4099 aged 7 to 12 years old [24]. This retrospective study found that children whose mothers smoked during the first 2 years of life were more likely to be hospitalized at least once before the age of 2 years for a respiratory illness than were children of nonsmoking mothers. Again, this study cannot differentiate the effects of in utero vs. postnatal exposure and is retrospective in nature.

Perhaps the best performed study from the methodologic point of view is the work of Chen and co-workers [25–27]. These investigators studied the influence of ETS exposure on hospitalization for bronchitis and pneumonia during the first 18 months of life in 2227 Chinese children. What is interesting about this report is that of the 1746 smoking families, there were no mothers who smoked. These investigators found a dose–response relationship of father's smoking to hospitalization for respiratory illness during the first 18 months. There was a dose–response relationship to the number of cigarettes smoked, which persisted after adjustment for sex, birth weight, nursery care, father's education, coal used for cooking, and parental report of respiratory symptoms. Most susceptible were infants who were less than 6 months of age, had low birth weight, or were bottle fed. This report also suggests that passive smoking and artificial feeding work synergistically to produce a detrimental effect much greater than that produced by separate action of either one. This finding takes on added significance when coupled with the information that smoking mothers tend to be less likely to breast feed, and if they do breast feed, to have less breast milk than that of nonsmoking mothers. Use of father's smoking as the index of exposure does not completely address the prenatal vs. postnatal exposure issue.

Finally, a large study of 4800 English and Scottish children aged 5 to 11 years old participating in the national study of health and growth demonstrated that the effects of ETS are not limited to infants [28]. This investigation demonstrated that even in 5- to 11-year-old children, an exposure–response relationship was evident between number of cigarettes smoked by mother and father and bronchitis attacks in the last 2 months, even after controlling for numbers of members in the household, parental education, and age and gender of the child.

None of the post-1986 studies examining ETS effect on acute respiratory illness utilize biomarkers of exposure. In addition, none of the new studies, with the possible exception of Chen, adequately differentiate between prenatal and postnatal exposure. Thus they confirm the findings summarized in the Surgeon General's report, but provide no additional information beyond what is already known.

In summary, it appears that there is an increased risk of hospitalization for severe bronchitis and pneumonia associated with parental smoking, which ranges from 20 to 40% during the first year or two of life. Although younger children appear to represent the most susceptible group for these acute respiratory illnesses, data do exist to suggest that older children may also be at risk. Although recall bias is a potential explanation for these results, a substantial number of studies have controlled for parental symptoms and illness reporting in examining these relationships, and the results still hold. In addition, the exposure–response nature of the relationship, its biologic plausibility, and its persistence after control for confounding variables would suggest that the relationship is causal. What remains unknown is precise quantification of dose, the relationship between in utero prenatal and postnatal exposure, and the interrelationship with this association of low birth weight, allergy, and breast feeding.

## V. Chronic Respiratory Symptoms

Methodologic concerns in evaluating studies relating ETS exposure to respiratory symptoms in children include the aforementioned bias of overreporting of children's symptoms by symptomatic parents. The potential exists for other variables, such as social class, crowding, home cooking fuel to bias the association of ETS with chronic symptoms, and finally, underreporting of active smoking on the part of children, particularly those over the age of 10. All three of these effects can potentially lead to an overestimate of the effect of ETS on respiratory symptoms on children of smoking parents. Prior studies [29,30] have demonstrated that adjustment for parental symptoms or illnesses decreased the strength of the association between ETS exposure and respiratory symptoms in the child but did not eliminate it.

## A. Cough/Phlegm

Since the original reports of Colley et al. [31,32], a number of studies have demonstrated an exposure–response relationship between the number of smokers in the home and the prevalence of cough. Age is an important factor to consider in evaluating these investigations because respiratory symptom prevalence changes dramatically over age in children, with younger children showing high prevalence rates, which declines as the child ages. This is, in part, accounted for by lung maturation but is also influenced by the marked increase in lung size associated with the growing child. In addition, time activity patterns in the home, specifically, proximity to the mother, decrease with increasing age, suggesting that the influence of ETS exposure will probably be greatest in young children. Finally, children of parents who smoke are more likely to become smokers themselves than are children of nonsmokers.

Stern and colleagues examined the effect of maternal cigarette smoking on chronic respiratory symptoms in 4000 Canadian school children [24]. Both cough and phlegm were reported more frequently in children whose mothers smoke than among children whose mothers did not. This report cannot differentiate between prenatal and postnatal exposure. Marks conducted a study of inner-city preschool 5-year-olds [33]. Children in smoking households were more likely to experience cough with physical activity. The National Study of Health and Growth in England also found a relationship between chronic cough and the number of cigarettes smoked per day at home by parents [28]. This effect persisted in these older children after adjustment for all potential confounding variables. No independent measure of exposure was utilized in any of these investigations. These studies of cough demonstrate that an exposure–response relationship persists after adjustment for potential confounding variables in both young (<2 years), preschool (<5 years) and in older (5 to 11 years) children. Longitudinal data are also present, but there is no independent biomarker of exposure, no potential control for the child's own smoking, and no identification of any unique, susceptible subgroup.

## B. Wheeze

There are no studies that look at wheezing in infants. Marks did demonstrate a dose–response relationship of exercise-induced wheeze to maternal cigarette smoke in preschool 5-year-olds [33]. The National Study of Health and Growth demonstrated a dose–response relationship of persistent wheezing between number of cigarettes smoked at home by parents that persisted after adjustment for a variety of confounding variables [28]. The deficiencies of these studies have been summarized above.

McConnochie and Roghmann examined the effects of passive smoking of ETS exposure on wheezing on children aged 6 to 10 [34]. In this longitudinal investigation maternal cigarette smoking was an important determinant of wheezing only among children who had a prior family history of allergy. These investigators also controlled for gender, breast feeding, and other potential confounding variables. However, no attempt was made to determine whether any of these children were active smokers. Chen and coinvestigators compared 121 7-year-old children with a prior history of low birth weight to an unselected reference group of schoolchildren of the same age [25]. The investigators controlled for a variety of potential confounding variables such as socioeconomic status, neonatal oxygen scores, allergy, and family history of asthma. A significant association between maternal smoking and wheeze in these children was found. Again, no attempt was made to control for potential active smoking in this age group.

Neuspiel et al. studied the effect of ETS on wheezing symptoms in a cohort of 9670 British children between the ages of birth and 10 years [35]. This longitudinal study demonstrated that children of smoking mothers had an increased cumulative incidence of wheezy bronchitis that demonstrated an exposure–response relationship. The increase in wheezy bronchitis was 14% if the mother smoked more than 4 cigarettes per day, but increased to 49% if the mother smoked more than 14 cigarettes per day. This analysis controlled for a variety of potential confounding variables, including parental smoking, social status of the family, gender, history of family allergy, crowding, breast feeding, type of cooking and heating in the home, and bedroom dampness. However, the child's own smoking, maternal prenatal smoking, and maternal symptoms were not controlled for.

### C. Summary

The Surgeon General's report concluded that a 30 to 80% excess prevalence of chronic cough or phlegm compared in children of smoking parents compared to children with nonsmoking parents [2]. Studies of the effect of ETS on wheezing varied from no increase in risk to a sixfold increase in risk, depending on the study and the age as a child [2]. New studies reported since the 1986 Surgeon General's report confirm these findings and demonstrate increased cough over all ages from birth to age 14. The bulk of these studies were done in children under 10 years of age, suggesting that active cigarette smoking by these children is not likely to be a major factor confounding the results. In addition, although biomarkers of exposure have not been used in any study, a dose–response relationship has been observed. These new studies do not afford any significant methodological advances over pre-1986 work. Specifically, they do not control for parental respiratory symptoms or illnesses or utilize biomarkers of ETS exposure. Prior studies, however, that have controlled for parental symptoms yield similar results.

With regard to wheeze symptoms, it appears that the variable results reported up to the 1986 Surgeon General's Report may be related to specific susceptibility in children who have increased airways responsiveness or a family history of allergy. Thus with regard to wheezing symptoms in particular, family history of allergy or asthma may be an important confounding variable in interpreting these data. This issue needs further investigation. Again, it is clear that the issue of family history, or adjustment for parental symptoms, may represent some genetically susceptible phenotype or may be important methodologically to control for potential reporting bias. A correlation between family history and household exposure to ETS and subsequent adjustment for family history will tend to lead to an understatement of the statistical significance of ETS. Again, it is clear that in reviewing these studies that there are significant methodologic advances to be made. Particularly important is independent ascertainment of personal smoking status in older children to eliminate exposure misclassification and obtain unbiased estimates of the effect of ETS exposure on chronic respiratory symptoms.

## VI. Chronic Respiratory Disease: Asthma

Studies on the effect of passive smoking on asthma in children can be divided into three groups: those studies that examine the effect of passive smoking on asthma severity as a potential exacerbating factor, those subjects that look at passive smoking as an etiologic factor causing the occurrence of asthma in children, and finally, those studies that look at bronchial responsiveness per se and whether ETS is causal or an exacerbating factor.

### A. Passive Smoking as an Exacerbating Factor for Asthma in Children

Existing studies leave little question that passive smoking is an important exacerbating factor for symptom occurrence and lower levels of lung function among children with asthma. Murray and Morrison [36] initially studied 94 nonsmoking asthmatic children between the ages of 7 and 17 who were referred to their allergy clinic. Symptom score was significantly greater and pulmonary function was significantly lower among the smoke-exposed children. The ETS effect is seen from maternal cigarette smoke exposure but not for a paternal source. In a cross-sectional study of 240 consecutively referred asthmatic subjects between the ages of 7 and 17 years, these authors [37] observed that there were seasonal differences in the passive smoking effect, which appeared to predominate in the cold, wet season when the children were primarily indoors. These authors' largest investigation studied a population of 415 nonsmoking asthmatic children between the ages of 1 and 17 [38]. The children were referred to the two pediatric allergists at the Children's Hospital in Vancouver. The children were stratified according to their maternal cigarette smoking status based on maternal self-report. Asthma was defined as a doctor's diagnosis of this condition. The asthmatic children of smoking mothers were comparable to the asthmatic children of nonsmoking mothers in terms of their mean age, sex ratio, duration of asthma, family history of asthma, wood stove use, and overall skin test positivity. Asthmatic children of smoking mothers were more likely to have higher asthma symptom scores and lower levels of $FEV_1$ and $FEF_{25-75}$ than nonmaternal smoking-exposed asthmatic children. The effects were greater in children over the age of 7 and in boys. Limitations of this study include potential selection bias in that the patients were not drawn from a community sample, and that exposure assessment was simply by questionnaire, without independent validation of maternal or child exposure by cotinine or another biomarker.

These studies clearly support the concept that exacerbations of asthma and lower levels of pulmonary function in asthmatic children are significantly worse than in asthmatic children with nonsmoking mothers. This conclusion must be tempered by the possibility of selection bias, and the need for objective validation of exposure and careful control of potential confounders such as social class.

Corroborative evidence for an effect of passive smoking on asthma exacerbations comes from the work of Evans and co-workers [39]. These investigators investigated 276 children with a doctor's diagnosis of asthma from 259 low-income families in New York City. Passive smoking was assessed by parental questionnaire. Outcome variables in this study included emergency room visits, hospitalizations, and level of pulmonary function ($FEV_1$ and $FEF_{25-75}$). The investigators utilized multiple linear regression techniques to control for other potential confounding variables that might influence outcome, including smoking by the children themselves, the presence of other irritants or allergens in the child's home, and the type of home heating. Age and gender were not controlled for in the analyses. Passive smoke exposure (expressed as the presence of any smoker in the home) was positively (and significantly) associated with emergency room visits but not with hospitalizations or abnormalities of pulmonary function. The frequency of days with asthma symptoms per month was also related directly with emergency room visits, independent of the effect of passive smoking. The authors estimate a 63% mean annual increase in ER visits attributable to the presence of one or more smokers in the household compared to nonsmoking households.

### B.  Relationship of Passive Smoking to the Occurrence of Childhood Asthma

The relationship of maternal cigarette smoking to the occurrence of asthma has been examined in two longitudinal studies, which have yielded conflicting results. Fergusson and colleagues [40] studied a birth cohort of children born in the urban region of Christchurch, New Zealand. The initial cohort consisted of 1265 children that was reduced to 1115 children at follow-up at age 6 years. Parental smoking was assessed by a questionnaire administered to the child's mother. Asthma was assessed with a variety of different questions and physician's reports. Although maternal cigarette smoking was associated with more frequent lower respiratory illness and greater medical consultation, there was no association between maternal cigarette smoking and the occurrence of asthma in this study.

In contrast to this negative report, Weitzman and co-workers analyzed data on 4331 children aged 0 to 5 years collected during the National Health Interview Survey [41]. In a multivariate analysis controlling for race, income, and education, these authors found that children whose mothers smoked more than or equal to half a pack of cigarettes a day were more likely to have asthma [odds ratio (OR) = 2.1], to be taking asthma medication (OR = 4.6), and more likely to have asthma develop during the first year of life (OR = 2.6). Although maternal cigarette smoking was associated with increased numbers of hospitalizations for asthma by virtue of its association with increased risk of asthma, among asthmatic children, children of smoking mothers were not more likely to be hospitalized. Because of the cross-sectional nature of this investigation it is unclear whether maternal smoking is simply an exacerbating factor or one of the causal factors for the development of asthma in children. Again, the importance of maternal smoking during pregnancy versus postnatal ETS exposure in explaining these findings is also unclear.

In a longitudinal study, Martinez and co-workers, using data from the Tucson Epidemiologic Study, did find an association between parental smoking and subsequent development of asthma before the age of 12 years [42]. In this study, maternal cigarette smoking was assessed by a self-reported questionnaire, and asthma in children was defined by doctor's diagnosis reported on maternal questionnaires. Subjects were followed up over a 14-year period and 89 incident cases of asthma were diagnosed. The risk of developing asthma was roughly 60% greater among children with mothers who smoked 10 or more cigarettes per day after adjusting for gender and parental symptoms (relative risk = 1.59, 95% CI, 1.03, 22.44). The authors found that the effect was restricted to families where mothers had fewer than 12 years of education. This report also found significantly larger FVC values in the female children of smoking mothers.

Taken together, these reports yield conflicting results. Lack of biomarkers of exposure, misclassification of personal smoking, different-aged children, and lack of control for prenatal in utero effects may confound the results of these studies. In addition, prior investigations have suggested that maternal smoking may be a risk factor only in those strongly genetically predisposed (i.e., those children with strong parental asthma histories). Better identification of the asthma phenotype in terms of allergy and airways responsiveness may provide more precise understanding as to the role of passive smoke exposure on the development of asthma.

### C. Effects of Passive Smoking on Bronchial Responsiveness

At least two studies have documented that passive smoking influences nonspecific bronchial responsiveness among asthmatic children. In both of their previous reports, Murray and Morrison have demonstrated that bronchoreactivity to histamine was significantly greater in children of smoking mothers [37]. In their most recent report this effect seems to predominate in boys [38].

O'Connor and co-workers [43] studied 292 children from a population-based sample of subjects aged 6 to 21 years of age. Bronchial responsiveness was tested with eucapnic hyperpnea to subfreezing air. Asthma was by self-report of a doctor's diagnosis, and passive smoke exposure was assessed by maternal report on questionnaire. These investigators found that bronchial responsiveness was increased among asthmatic children of smoking mothers. This effect was independent of level of $FEV_1$ and age. Social class was not assessed in this analysis, nor were there any gender differences in the effect. Biomarkers of exposure were also not assessed.

These reports suggest that the influence of passive smoke exposure is primarily children with already established asthma. The report of Martinez et al. suggests an effect of parental smoking and bronchial responsiveness that is independent of asthma status [44]. In this study, investigators in Italy studied 172 9-year-old children from three Italian towns. Asthma was defined as a doctor's diagnosis of that condition and parental self-report was used to assess passive smoke exposure. Bronchial responsiveness was assessed with carbachol. Bronchial responsiveness was increased significantly among male children of smoking parents (OR = 4.3, $p = 0.009$). In female children of smoking parents, however, there was no significant increase in bronchial responsiveness (OR = 1.5, $p = 0.4$). Although the relationship between bronchial responsiveness in children and parental cigarette smoking was stronger in asthmatic children, the results were still significant after controlling for asthma and atopy.

Skin test reactivity among male children of smoking parents was also increased ($p = 0.001$). This report suggests that male children are differentially affected by parental cigarette smoke, particularly maternal cigarette smoke, in terms of both bronchial responsiveness and skin test reactivity, but that this effect was not limited to children with already diagnosed asthma.

## VII. Conclusions

Exposure assessment is complex. Existing epidemiologic studies have utilized questionnaires exclusively in studies of respiratory health effects in children over 1 year of age. A small number of studies are just beginning to appear that utilize urinary cotinine as a biomarker to validate questionnaire information on exposure. To date, few epidemiologic studies have relied exclusively on air sampling as an index of exposure. Although studies in infancy have documented a relationship between amniotic fluid cotinine and L/S ratio and maternal urinary cotinine and pulmonary function, no study with biomarkers is available for older children. In addition, it remains exceedingly difficult to separate the effects of postnatal from prenatal maternal cigarette smoke exposure in examing the influence on respiratory symptoms.

It is clear that acute respiratory illnesses and chronic respiratory symptoms, specifically cough, phlegm, and wheeze in children, are related to ETS. The magnitude of prenatal vs. postnatal effect, however, is currently unknown. In addition, in children older than the age of 10, studies using biomarkers to identify personal smoking by children have not yet been performed. Studies on asthmatic children and wheezing children suggest that children with an atopic diathisis may be at particular risk for an adverse effect of maternal smoking during childhood. The issue of whether ETS is a true risk factor for the development of asthma, or whether it is simply an exacerbating factor, is currently unsettled. Finally, it is unclear whether ETS causes increased bronchial responsiveness in all children or simply exacerbates or worsens bronchial responsiveness among asthmatic children. It is likely that investigations ongoing into the twenty-first century will increasingly utilize biomarkers of exposure, with further refinement of our understanding of these scientific issues.

## References

1. National Research Council. Environmental tobacco smoke: measuring exposures and assessing health effects. Washington, DC: National Academy Press, 1986.
2. U.S. Surgeon General. The health consequences of involuntary smoking. U.S. Department of Health and Human Services, Public Health Service, 1986.
3. Eatough DJ, Benner CL, Bayona JM, Richards G, Lamb JD, Lee ML, Lewis EA, Hansen L. Chemical composition of environmental tobacco

smoke. 1. Gas-phase acids and bases. Environ Sci Technol 1989;23:679–87.

4.  Benner CL, Bayona JM, Caka FM, et al. Chemical composition of environmental tobacco smoke. 2. Particulate-phase compounds. Environ Sci Technol 1989;23:688–99.

5.  Proctor CJ, Smith G. Considerations of the chemical complexity of ETS with regard to inhalation studies. Exp Pathol 1989;37:164–69.

6.  Coultas DB, Peake GT, Samet JM. Questionnaire assessment of lifetime and recent exposure to environmental tobacco smoke. Am J Epidemiol 1989;130:338–47.

7.  Henderson FW, Holly FR, Morris R, et al. Home air nicotine levels and urinary cotinine excretion in preschool children. Am Rev Respir Dis 1989;140:197–201.

8.  Spengler JP, Treitman RD, Tosteson TD, Mage DJ, Soczek ML. Personal exposures to respirable particulates and implications for air pollution epidemiology. Environ Sci Technol 1985;19:700–707.

9.  Schenker MD, Smith T, Muñoz A, Woskie S, Speizer FE. Diesel exposure and mortality among railway workers: results of a pilot study. Br J Ind Med 1984; 41:320–22.

10. Sexton R, Spengler JD, Treitman RD. Personal exposure to respirable particulates: a case-study in Waterbury, Vermont. Atmos Environ 1984;18:1385–1398.

11. Muramatsu M, Umemura S, Okada T, Tomita H. Estimation of personal exposure to tobacco smoke with a newly developed nicotine personal monitor. Environ Res 1984;35:218–27.

12. Hammond SK, Leaderer BP. A diffusion monitor to measure exposure to passive smoking. Environ Sci Technol 1987;31:494–97.

13. Jarvis MJ, Tunstall-Pedoe H, Feyerabend C, Vesey C, Saloojee Y. Comparison of tests used to distinguish smokers from nonsmokers. Am J Public Health 1987;77:1435–38.

14. Watts RR, Langone JJ, Knight GJ, Lewtas J. Cotinine analytical workshop report: consideration of analytical methods for determining cotinine in human body fluids as a measure of passive exposure to tobacco smoke. Environ Health Perspect 1990;84:173–82.

15. Jarvis MJ, Russell MAH, Feyerabend C, Eiser JR, Morgan M, Gammage P, Gray EM. Passive exposure to tobacco smoke: saliva cotinine concentrations in a representative population sample of non-smoking schoolchildren. Br Med J 1985;291:927–29.

16. Cummings KM, Markello SJ, Mahoney M, Bhargave AK, McElroy PD, Marshall JR. Measurement of current exposure to environmental tobacco smoke. Arch Environ Health 1990;45(2):74–79.

17. Coultas DB, Howard CA, Peake GT, Skipper BJ, Samet JM. Salivary

cotinine levels and involuntary tobacco smoke exposure in children and adults in New Mexico. Am Rev Respir Dis 1987;136:305–9.

18. Greenberg RA, Bauman KE, Glover LH, et al. Ecology of passive smoking by young infants. J Pediatr 1989;114:774–80.

19. Idle JR. Titrating exposure to tobacco smoke using cotinine: a minefield of misunderstandings. J Clin Epidemiol 1990;43:313–17.

20. Lieberman E, Torday J, Barbieri R, Cohen A, Van Vunakis H, Weiss ST. The association of in utero cigarette smoke exposure to fetal lung maturation. Obstet Gynecol 1992;79:564–70.

21. Hanrahan JP, Tager IB, Segal MR, Castile RG, Van Vunakis H, Weiss ST, Speizer FE. The effect of maternal smoking during pregnancy on early infant lung function. Am Rev Respir Dis 1992;145:1129–35.

22. Harlap S, Davies AM. Infant admissions to hospital and maternal smoking. Lancet 1974;1(7857):529–32.

23. Ogston SA, Florey C, Du V, Walker CHM. Association of infant alimentary and respiratory illness with parental smoking and other environmental factors. J Epidemiol Community Health 1987;41:21–25.

24. Stern B, Raizenne M, Burnett R, Kearney J. Respiratory effects of early childhood exposure to passive smoke. Indoor Air '87. Proceedings of the 4th International Conference on Indoor Air Quality and Climates. New York: Springer-Verlag, 1987.

25. Chen Y. Synergistic effect of passive smoking and artificial feeding on hospitalization for respiratory illness in early childhood. Chest 1989;5:1004–7.

26. Chen Y, Li W-X, Yu S. Influence of passive smoking on admissions for respiratory illness in early childhood. Br Med J 1986;293:303–6.

27. Chen Y, Li W-X, Yu S, Qian W. Chang-Ning epidemiological study of children's health. I. Passive smoking and children's respiratory diseases. Int J Epidemiol 1988;17(2):348–55.

28. Somerville SM, Rona RJ, Chinn S. Passive smoking and respiratory conditions in primary school children. J Epidemiol Community Health 1988;42(2):105–10.

29. Lebowitz MD, Knudson RJ, Burrows B. The Tucson epidemiology study of chronic obstructive lung disease. I. Methodology and prevalence of disease. Am J Epidemiol 1975;102:137–52.

30. Ferris BG, Ware JH, Berkey CS, Dockery DW, Spiro A, Speizer FE. Effects of passive smoking on health of children. Environ Health Perspect 1985;62:289–95.

31. Colley JRT. Respiratory symptoms in children and parental smoking and phlegm production. Br Med J 1974;2(5912):201–4.

32. Colley JRT. Respiratory disease in childhood. Br Med Bull 1971;27(1):9–14.

33.  Marks BE. Respiratory illness and home environment. Br Med J 1988;296(6638):1740.
34.  McConnochie KM, Roghmann KJ. Breast feeding and maternal smoking as predictors of wheezing in children age 6 to 10 years. Pediatr Pulmonol 1986;2:260–68.
35.  Neuspiel DR, Rush D, Butler NR, Golding J, Bijur PE, Kurzon M. Parental smoking and post-infancy wheezing in children: a prospective cohort study. Am J Public Health 1989;79(2):168–71.
36.  Murray AB, Morrison BJ. The effect of cigarette smoke from the mother on bronchial responsiveness and severity of symptoms. J Allergy Clin Immunol 1986;77:575–81.
37.  Murray AB, Morrison BJ. Passive smoking and the seasonal difference of severity of asthma in children. Chest 1988;94:701–8.
38.  Murray AB, Morrison BJ. Passive smoking by asthmatics: its greater effect on boys than on girls and on older than on younger children. Pediatrics 1989;84:451–49.
39.  Evans D, Levison MJ, Feldman CH, Clark NM, Wasilewski Y, Levin B, Mollins RB. The impact of passive smoking on emergency room visits of urban children with asthma. Am Rev Respir Dis 1987;735:567–72.
40.  Fergusson DM, Hons BA, Horwood LJ. Parental smoking and respiratory illness during early childhood: a six-year longitudinal study. Pediatr Pulmonol 1985;1:99–106.
41.  Weitzman M, Gortmaker S, Walker DK, Sobol A. Maternal smoking and childhood asthma. Pediatrics 1990;85:505–11.
42.  Martinez FD, Cline M, Burrows B. Increased incidence of asthma in children of smokers. Pediatrics 1992;80:21–26.
43.  O'Connor GT, Weiss ST, Tager IB, Speizer FE. The effect of passive smoking on pulmonary function and nonspecific bronchial responsiveness in a population based sample of children and young adults. Am Rev Respir Dis 1987;135:800–804.
44.  Martinez FD, Antognoni G, Macri F, et al. Parental smoking enhances bronchial responsiveness in nine-year-old children. Am Rev Respir Dis 1988;138:518–23.

# 24

## Tobacco Smoke and Bronchial Responsiveness

**FRANCINE KAUFFMANN and ISABELLA ANNESI**

INSERM U169
Villejuif, France

**DONALD A. ENARSON**

University of Alberta
Alberta, Canada

## I. Introduction

To assess asthma objectively, Dautrebande et al. [1] proposed bronchial provocation tests which were considered to reflect an endogenous characteristic and only recently have been seen as expressing an acquired trait [2]. Hence environmental factors related to asthma have primarily been considered to be risk factors triggering (activating) or worsening bronchial hyperresponsiveness. Initially, tobacco smoking was not proposed as playing a role in bronchial hyperresponsiveness [3], as the few case series reports led to contradictory results [4,5]. During the past decade, the renewal of interest in the *Dutch hypothesis* [6,7], according to which bronchial hyperresponsiveness may predispose some subjects to chronic airflow limitation, a major cause of which is tobacco smoking, has given birth to numerous epidemiological investigations on bronchial responsiveness. Thus bronchial hyperresponsiveness has become one candidate in the delineation of the smoker susceptible to develop chronic airflow limitation [7,8], and preventive strategies directed to hyperresponsive smokers might then be envisaged.

In the present chapter we assess evidence regarding the association between active and passive tobacco smoke exposure and bronchial hyperresponsiveness in adults and children using, for the most part, results from epidemiological studies and taking into account both the factors (such as age, atopy, or airway caliber) that may interact with this association and selection bias (the "healthy smoker effect") [9,10], which may obscure it.

## II.    Tobacco Smoke Exposure and Bronchial Hyperresponsiveness in Adults

Epidemiological studies conducted in both population-based and work force–based samples allow us to examine whether existing evidence is compatible with an association of smoking to bronchial hyperresponsiveness. The first epidemiological study on this topic, by Van der Lende in 1972 in the general population of Vlaardingen in the Netherlands, did not show any association of smoking with bronchial responsiveness [11]. Ten years later, Kabiraj et al. [12] showed a positive association between smoking habits and bronchial hyperresponsiveness in a nested case (PIMZ, protease inhibitor MZ) control (PIM) study conducted on 65 persons in Malmö (Sweden). Since then, a series of surveys have observed associations between smoking habits and bronchial hyperresponsiveness (Table 1). Significant associations were observed in the entire group studied [14–16] or only in subgroups [17], for both current and past smoking or only some category of smoking habits, for any index of bronchial hyperresponsiveness [20] or only for a quantitative index [22]. However, the lack of standardization for the stimulus chosen, the dose given, or the expression of the results limits comparison among studies.

In occupational cohorts (Table 2), Pham et al. [24] conducted the first study and noted a lack of association in a comparison of reactors and nonreactors in four groups of smokers (non, ex, moderate, and heavy). However, there was some trend ($p = 0.10$), and an analysis contrasting current smokers vs. nonsmokers and ex-smokers vs. nonsmokers showed significant differences. This study illustrates the dependence of the results according to the method of classifying smoking habits. To standardize the results of the various surveys, the odds ratios (OR) for having increased responsiveness were computed using the same crude definition of smoking, namely current and ex-smokers vs. nonsmokers, respectively. Table 3 gives the results for the studies from which data are available. As some reports have used four- or five-class variables for smoking and others mainly underlined results in subgroups, the picture given may be slightly different from the main conclusions of the authors described in Tables 1 and 2. For community-based studies, odds ratios ranged from 1.1 to 2.9. It is important to notice that no study had an odds ratio lower than 1.0 for current smoking. The lowest OR [22] was observed for the study with the highest prevalence of response to bronchoprovocation, which varied from 6.1 to 30.9%

among studies. Similar results were observed for current smoking for work force–based studies which showed odds ratios (except one) between 1.4 and 2.9. The odds ratio greater than 7 (with a large confidence interval) observed by Taylor et al. [25] corresponds to a rather mixed population. Prevalences varied between 5.0 and 37.5%.

As differences in prevalence of responders might be critical, summary statistics were computed retaining in each study a definition of hyperresponsiveness giving a prevalence close to 20%. These summary statistics (Table 3) show significant relationships for current smoking in both population- and work force–based studies and a significant association for ex-smoking in work force–based studies. The OR values for current smoking were rather similar in both types of surveys (1.50 and 2.06, with overlapping confidence intervals). However, these ORs should not be considered a real measure of an effect of tobacco smoke exposure on bronchial hyperresponsiveness, but only as an indicative value (in particular for current smoking, in population-based studies, for which there was a significant heterogeneity between surveys).

Results obtained from studies using continuous indices, such as the $PD_{20}$ value or the dose–response slope [17], further support the observations based on dichotomous variables. As expected, various results have been observed when various cutoffs of hyperresponsiveness were used. The association of bronchial hyperresponsiveness was stronger in some studies [21,36] and weaker in others [15,33] when the cutoff was changed to define a greater degree of hyperresponsiveness. Associations of smoking with continuous indices of responsiveness were always observed when an association was present for a dichotomous definition of hyperresponsiveness in the same study. Furthermore, some studies showed an association with a continuous parameter, whereas the association with a dichotomous one was less clear [36,37], an observation not surprising, as using a cutoff for a variable with a (log)normal distribution [15,37] represents a loss of information [38].

Overall, the consistency of the results from epidemiological studies supports the hypothesis of an association between smoking and bronchial hyperresponsiveness. However, the exact nature of this association, causal or not, has yet to be determined. Arguments in favor of a causal association include increasing responsiveness with the amount smoked and decreasing responsiveness after cessation of exposure.

The highest prevalence of bronchial hyperresponsiveness was observed for the heaviest smokers in several studies [16,21,29,39], in particular in the population of French policemen, in which the association was restricted to smokers of at least 30 g/day [29]. Significant relations were observed, with the amount smoked expressed by the current amount [16,21,29,39], pack-years [16,40], or the duration of smoking [16]. The significant increase with age of bronchial hyperresponsiveness in current smokers in the population-based study

**Table 1** Population-Based Studies on the Relationship of Smoking Habits to Bronchial Hyperresponsiveness

| Author | Population | Smoking | Bronchial hyper-responsiveness[a] | Results[b] | Comments |
|---|---|---|---|---|---|
| Van der Lende et al., 1973, Netherlands [11] | Men and women, Vlaardingen, 25% sample, 18–61 yr | 95 nonsmokers, 165 smokers | Histamine, $PC_{20} \leq$ or 32 mg/mL | No association | |
| Kabiraj et al., 1982, Sweden [12] | Malmö, nested design PIM [31] and PIMZ [34], 48 yr | 19 nonsmokers, 23 ex-smokers, 23 smokers | Methacholine, $PC_{15}$ | Association with current smoking | No role of PIMZ |
| Welty et al., 1984, United States [13] | East Boston, 171 subjects, median age 38 yr | 43 nonsmokers, 128 ex- and current smokers | Hyperpnea with cold air, $PD_9$ | $p = 0.10$ for ever vs. never smokers | |
| Burney et al., 1987, United Kingdom [14] | Southampton, 511 subjects, 18–64 yr | 259 nonsmokers, 116 ex-smokers, 136 smokers | Histamine, $PD_{20} \leq$ 8 $\mu$mol, log $PD_{20}$ | Association with current smoking (24% vs. 12% for ex- and 10% for nonsmoking), role of smoking after 40 years of age | Age dependence of the relationship |
| Woolcock et al., 1987, Australia [15] | Rural, 917 subjects, 18–88 yr | 483 nonsmokers, 240 ex-smokers, 194 smokers | Histamine, $PD_{20} \leq$ 3.9 $\mu$mol | Association with current smoking (13.7% vs. 11.7% for ex- and 10.1% for nonsmoking) ($p < 0.001$) | |

| Reference | Population | Subjects | Measure | Results | Comments |
|---|---|---|---|---|---|
| Cerveri et al., 1989, Italy [16] | Lombardy town, 415 subjects, 15–64 hr | 295 nonsmokers, 50 ex-smokers, 70 smokers, all "normal" | Methacholine, $PD_{15}$ ≤ 4800 µg, ln $PD_{15}$ | Difference between smokers and nonsmokers, dose effect of smoking (amount more than duration), past smoking since 1 yr similar to nonsmokers | Asymptomatic and all subjects $FEV_1$ > 85% predicted; adjustment for age and $FEV_1$ |
| O'Connor et al., 1989, United States [17] | Veterans Study, 778 men, 41–86 yr | 299 nonsmokers, 375 ex-smokers, 104 smokers | Methacholine, slope | Association only among atopics, which remained after adjustment for $FEV_1$ | Middle-aged and elderly |
| Trigg et al., 1990, United Kingdom [18] | Kingston, random general practices, 314 subjects, 18–75 yr | 142 nonsmokers, 76 ex-smokers, 96 smokers | Methacholine, $PD_{20}$ ≤ 11 µmol | Association with smoking OR = 1.2 (CI: 0.6–2.5) for ex- vs. nonsmokers and OR = 2.2 (CI: 1.2–4.1) ($p < 0.01$) for current vs. nonsmokers | 35% response rate |
| Lebowitz and Quackenboss, 1990, United States [19] | Pima County, 216 subjects, 18–65 yr | Environmental exposure to smoking, questionnaire, and measures of particulates ($PM_{10}$) | Peak flow variability, reactivity = out of the reference range of asymptomatic nonsmokers | Relation of diurnal variability with environmental tobacco smoke when high $PM_{10}$ is measured in home environment | |

*(continued)*

**Table 1** Continued

| Author | Population | Smoking | Bronchial hyper-responsiveness[a] | Results[b] | Comments |
|---|---|---|---|---|---|
| Sparrow et al., 1991, United States [20] | Veterans study, 914 men, 41–86 yr | 342 nonsmokers, 448 ex-smokers, 124 smokers | Methacholine, $PD_{20}$ ≤ 8.6 μmol, slope | Relation with age among ex-smokers (using either dichotomous variable or slope) | This relation remained after adjustment for FEV1 |
| Bakke et al., 1991, Norway [21] | Bergen, 490 subjects, 18–73 yr | 186 nonsmokers, 109 ex-smokers, 195 smokers | Methacholine, ≤32 mg/mL and ≤8 mg/mL | Association with ≤8 mg/mL and not for ≤32 mg/mL of methacholine | Does not remain after adjustment for FEV1 (personal communication) |
| Rijcken et al., 1991, Nederlands [22] | Vlaardwedde and Vlaardingen, 1967–1987 1177 men (2780 obs.) and 1039 women (2232 obs.) | 1039 nonsmokers, 459 ex-smokers, 718 smokers | Histamine, $PC_{20}$ ≤ 16 mg/mL, continuous ($\log_2 PC_{20}$) | Association with continuous, not with dichotomous variable | Association decreases ($p = 0.10$) after adjustment for FEV1; no interaction with atopy or symptoms |

| Dow et al., 1992, United Kingdom [23] | Southampton, initially random sample from three general practices, 65–98 yr; sample enriched in subjects with "bronchial irritability symptoms" | 131 nonsmokers, 133 ex-smokers, 60 smokers | Methacholine, $PD_{20}$ ≤ 6.4 $\mu$mol | No association; OR = 0.4 (CI: 0.2–1.0) for ex- vs. nonsmoking and OR = 1.5 (CI: 0.5–4.1) for current vs. nonsmoking | High proportion without test for cardiorespiratory disease |
| | | | Salbutamol, 200 $\mu$g, increased $FEV_1$ ≥ 15% | OR = 0.3 (CI: 0.1–1.3) for ex- vs. nonsmoking and OR = 0.4 (CI: 0.1–2.2) for current vs. nonsmoking | All associations were studied after adjustment for symptoms of "bronchial irritability" |

[a]$PC_y$, provocative concentration of bronchoconstrictor provoking a y% fall in $FEV_1$; $PD_{20}$, provocative dose of bronchoconstrictor provoking a 20% fall in $FEV_1$; slope, % of change in $FEV_1$ per mg/mL of bronchoconstrictor.
[b]OR, odds ratio; CI, 95% confidence interval.

**Table 2** Work Force-Based Studies on the Relationship of Smoking Habits to Bronchial Hyperresponsiveness

| Author | Population | Smoking | Bronchial hyper-responsiveness[a] | Results | Comments |
|---|---|---|---|---|---|
| Pham et al., 1984, France [24] | 1040 iron miners, 35–55 yr | 173 nonsmokers, 91 ex-smokers, 441 < 20 cigarettes/day, 335 > cigarettes/day | Acetylcholine, $PD_{10} \leq 1200 \ \mu g$ | Association ($p = 0.10$ with a four-class variable for smoking | |
| Taylor et al., 1985, United Kingdom [25] | 227 workers, mixed group | 39 nonsmokers, 71 ex-smokers, 117 smokers | Histamine, $PC_{10} \leq 16 mg/ml$ | Current and ex-smokers more responsive (29.6% and 24.3%) than nonsmokers (5.3%) ($p = 0.01$ and $0.06$, respectively) | Association between smokers and nonsmokers remains among men with $FEV_1 > 80\%$ predicted |
| | | | $400 \ \mu g$ salbuta-mol, % increase $FEV_1$ | Current smokers more responsive (4.7% increase) than nonsmokers (3.0% increase) ($p = 0.02$) | |
| Enarson et al., 1985, Canada [26] | 504 grainhandlers, mean age 37 yr | 143 nonsmokers, 141 ex-smokers, 220 smokers | Methacholine, $PC_{20} \leq 8 \ mg/mL$ | Current and ex-smokers more responsive (16.8% and 14.3% than nonsmokers (10.1%), but not significantly | Adjustment for age, employment, and allergy |

| Study | Population | | Measure | Result | Comments |
|---|---|---|---|---|---|
| Vollmer et al., 1985, United States [27] | 351 country employees, 444 screening cohort | | Isoproterenol, % increase $FEV_1$ | Distribution more skewed toward high values for current and ex-smokers than for nonsmokers (significant for ex-smokers) | Adjustment for atopy, leucocyte count [28], and $FEV_1$ (see below) |
| Annesi et al., 1987, 1988, France [28,29] | 320 policemen, 27–58 yr | 111 nonsmokers, 82 ex-smokers, 127 smokers | Methacholine, $PD_{10} \leq 6$ mg, $PD_{20} \leq 6$ mg | Association with a four-class variable for smoking ($\chi^2$ of trend, $p = 0.04$); heavy smokers more responsive than other men ($p = 0.01$) | |
| Ernst et al., 1989, Canada [30] | 246 insulators, 20–50 yr | Pack-years | Methacholine, $PC_{15}$ | Pack-years unrelated to $PC_{15}$ (with adjustment for $FEV_1$) | |
| Kennedy et al., 1990, Canada [31] | Five surveys in foundry, cedar saw mill, office workers, 654 nonasthmatics, mean age 42 yr | 208 nonsmokers, 195 ex-smokers, 251 smokers | Methacholine, $PC_{20} \leq 16$ mg/mL, $PC_{20} \leq 8$ mg/mL slope | Current and ex-smokers more hyperresponsive than nonsmokers | Association only among non atopics which disappears after adjustment for $FEV_1$ level; among hyperresponsive, smokers less responsive than nonsmokers |
| Iversen and Pedersen, 1990, Denmark [32] | 181 farmers (124 pig, 57 dairy), mean age 43 yr | Pack-years | Histamine, $PC_{20} \leq 32$ mg/mL | Significant association with pack years | Remains after adjustment for $FEV_1$ |

*(continued)*

**Table 2** Continued

| Author | Population | Smoking | Bronchial hyper-responsiveness[a] | Results | Comments |
|---|---|---|---|---|---|
| Kongerud and Soyseth, 1991, Norway [33] | 337 aluminum potroom workers | 83 nonsmokers, 30 ex-smokers, 224 smokers | Methacholine, $PC_{20} \leq 32$ mg/mL | Current and ex-smokers more responsive than nonsmokers (significant for ex-smokers | Remains after adjustment for $FEV_1$ |
| Neukirch et al., 1992, France [34] | 117 detergent industry, mean age 39 yr | 45 nonsmokers, 25 ex-smokers, 47 smokers | Peakflow variability, amplitude % mean | No significant association (% of responders: heavy smokers 12.2%, moderate 10.6%, ex-smokers 10.6%, nonsmokers 9.9%) | |

[a]$PC_x$, provocative concentration of bronchoconstrictor provoking a $y\%$ fall in $FEV_1$; PD, provocative dose of bronchoconstrictor provoking a $y\%$ fall in $FEV_1$; amplitude % mean, [(highest peak flow – lowest peak flow)/mean peak flow] × 100.

**Table 3** Bronchial Hyperresponsiveness and Smoking Habits: Odds Ratios in Epidemiological Studies Conducted in Adults

| Study | Definition of bronchial hyperresponsiveness[a] | Prevalence [% (n)][b] | Current vs. never-smokers (odds ratio)[c,d] | | Ex- vs. never-smokers (odds ratio)[c,d] | |
|---|---|---|---|---|---|---|
| **Community-based studies** | | | | | | |
| Netherlands 1988 [35] | $PC_{20} \leq 16$ mg/mL (H) | 23.7 (2156) | 1.18 | (0.94–1.47) | 0.71 | (0.51–1.01) |
| 1991 [22] | $PC_{20} \leq 16$ mg/mL (H) | 30.9[e] (5012)[f] | 1.11 | (0.97–1.26) | 0.96 | (0.81–1.12) |
| United States [20] | $PD_{20} \leq 8$ µmol (MC) | 12.7 (914) | 1.88* | (1.07–3.29) | 1.18 | (0.76–1.83) |
| United Kingdom [14] | $PD_{20} \leq 8$ µmol (H) | 14.3 (511) | 2.64*** | (1.53–4.58) | 1.18 | (0.59–2.34) |
| Australia [15] | $PD_{20} \leq 3.9$ µmol (H) | 11.3[e] (917) | 1.43 | (0.87–2.36) | 1.17 | (0.72–1.91) |
| | $PD_{10} \leq 3.9$ µmol | 21.4 | 2.11*** | (1.44–3.09) | 1.40 | (0.95–2.05) |
| Italy [16] | $PD_{15} \leq 4.8$ mg (MC) | 30.1 (415) | 1.93* | (1.13–3.31) | 1.41 | (0.74–2.66) |
| Norway [21] | $PC_{20} \leq 8$ mg/mL (MC) | 6.1[e] (490) | 2.87* | (1.14–7.18) | 2.06 | (0.69–6.17) |
| | $PC_{20} \leq 32$ mg/mL (MC) | 19.6 | 1.30 | (0.77–2.20) | 1.71[g] | (0.96–3.06) |
| Summary statistic | | 20.7 (5403) | 1.50*** | (1.28–1.75)[h] | 1.11 | (0.92–1.34) |
| **Work force–based studies** | | | | | | |
| Iron miners [24] | $PD_{10} \leq 1.2$ mg (AC) | 18.9 (1040) | 1.69* | (1.05–2.72) | 2.04* | (1.10–3.76) |
| Policemen [28,29] | $PD_{20} \leq 6$ mg (MC) | 15.0 (320) | 1.45 | (0.70–2.99) | 1.19 | (0.52–2.73) |
| | $PD_{10} \leq 6$ mg | 37.5[e] | 1.38 | (0.82–2.33) | 1.05 | (0.58–1.92) |
| Mixed [25] | $PC_{20} \leq 16$ mg/mL (H) | 23.8 (227) | 7.56** | (2.06–27.69) | 5.77** | (1.44–23.24) |
| Grainhandlers [26] | $PC_{20} \leq 8$ mg/mL (MC) | 14.3 (504) | 1.73[g] | (0.91–3.26) | 1.41 | (0.69–2.88) |

*(continued)*

**Table 3** Continued

| Study | Definition of bronchial hyper-responsiveness[a] | Prevalence [% (n)][b] | Current vs. never-smokers (odds ratio)[c,d] | | Ex- vs. never-smokers (odds ratio)[c,d] | |
|---|---|---|---|---|---|---|
| Mixed [31] | $PC_{20} \leq 16$ mg/mL (MC) | 24.3 (654) | 2.34*** | (1.48–3.70) | 2.00** | (1.23–3.26) |
| Potroom workers [33] | $PC_{20} \leq 8$ mg/mL (MC)[e] | 5.0 (337) | 2.29 | (0.52–10.08) | 4.50 | (0.82–24.86) |
| | $PC_{20} \leq 32$ mg/mL | 12.2 | 2.94[g] | (1.04–8.28) | 7.18** | (2.24–23.05) |
| Summary statistic | | 18.5 (3082) | 2.06*** | (1.59–2.66) | 2.00*** | (1.50–2.68) |

[a]AC, acetylcholine; MC, methacholine, H, histamine.

[b]n, number of observations.

[c]95% confidence interval.

[d*], $p \leq 0.05$, **, $p \leq 0.01$; ***, $p \leq 0.001$.

[e]Not considered in the summary statistic. In case of various definitions of hyperresponsiveness, the category considered in the summary statistic was that with a prevalence the closest to 20%.

[f]5012 observations were obtained from 2216 different subjects. These odds ratios are adjusted for age, log(eos), gender, symptoms, city, and the nonindependence of several measures in the same subjects. All other odds ratios in this table are unadjusted.

[g]$p \leq 0.10$ (Fisher exact test when appropriate).

[h]Breslow and Day test for heterogeneity of the odds ratios between studies $p = 0.02$.

conducted by Burney et al. [14] in subjects aged 18 to 64 years is a strong argument in favor of a cumulative effect of tobacco smoke. In that study there was also an increase with age of bronchial hyperresponsiveness of borderline significance in ex-smokers, but no relation of age with responsiveness in nonsmokers. Similar conclusions were drawn by Sparrow et al. [20] from a study conducted in a much older group (41 to 86 years) in which they observed a significant relation of bronchial hyperresponsiveness with age in former smokers, which remained after adjustment for total pack-years, years since quitting, and $FEV_1$ level. They suggested that the lack of association in current smokers was due to the small number of subjects concerned or the selected nature of current smoking at this age. Cohort effects or differences between countries may also explain discordances between studies. In contrast to Sparrow et al., Dow et al. [23], also in an aged population, did not observe an association (and even a reverse trend) of bronchial hyperresponsiveness with ex-smoking. Differences in the population studied may explain these findings, as in the Veterans study [20] subjects with asthma 20 years earlier were excluded, and in the Dow et al. study, the sample was enriched with subjects with symptoms of "bronchial irritability." At variance with the hypothesis of long duration or high cumulative dose required are the conclusions from Cerveri et al. from an Italian population survey [16]. They observed a stronger relation of bronchial hyperresponsiveness with the daily amount of smoking than with its duration, which would favor the hypothesis of an acute noxious effect of tobacco smoke.

The hypothesis of an acute effect of smoking on responsiveness done by Cerveri et al. [16] was partially supported by some trend (not significant) of return to normal of bronchial responsiveness 1 year after cessation of smoking. However, this hypothesis has not yet been tested in an epidemiological study that includes longitudinal data on bronchial hyperresponsiveness after cessation of smoking. The few clinical reports focused on short-term cessation have led to unclear conclusions [41]. Most epidemiological studies have reported data on ex-smoking, independently of the amount smoked, duration of smoking, or since cessation. With the exception of the Dutch study (Table 3), all studies exhibit ORs greater than 1 for ex-smoking compared to nonsmoking in population-based studies. In work force–based studies, all odds ratios were greater than 1, often significantly and the summary statistic gave an odds ratio of 2, similar to that observed for current smoking. Overall, observations from population-based studies only exhibit a marginal effect for ex-smoking. This suggests that people have not smoked enough before cessation (according to a cumulative hypothesis) and/or that stopping smoking had a beneficial effect. Furthermore, the healthy smoker effect may have been efficient enough to remove the susceptible smokers from smoking groups. In work force–based studies, it is striking that ex-smoking and current smoking were observed to have similar associations with bronchial hyperresponsiveness. It is possible that the healthy *worker* effect has removed the susceptible subjects (in particular, the susceptible smokers) out of the work force, masking the beneficial effect of stopping smoking in these working populations. In a study by Kongerud et al. [33], an association was even observed for ex-smoking and not for current smoking, a finding interpreted by the authors as being due to selection bias.

## III.   Environmental Tobacco Smoke and Bronchial Hyperresponsiveness in Children

In children, there have been only a limited number of studies of bronchial responsiveness because of the reluctance of investigators to use pharmacological stimuli. As epidemiological data are scanty, clinical reports are included in results on children described in Table 4. In a clinical study conducted on 41 asthmatics aged 7 to 17 years, Murray and Morrison [44] showed a significantly increased level of responsiveness to histamine in children according to maternal smoking. The differences between the children of smoking and nonsmoking mothers were greater in older than in younger children. They later extended [48] these findings in a larger group of 104 asthmatics, among whom they observed a significant relation of the duration of maternal smoking with $PC_{20}$, suggesting as for adults a cumulative effect of smoking. In a population-based sample of 292 subjects aged 6 to 21 years, O'Connor et al. [45] confirmed this finding, observing a significant association of maternal smoking with cold air challenge response in asthmatics. There was no relation in nonasthmatics. Using carbachol in a population-based sample of 166 schoolchildren aged 9 years, Martinez et al. [47] showed that hyperresponsiveness, as defined by $PD_{20} \leq 1200$ μg of carbachol, was increased in children whose mothers smoked in comparison with those whose mothers did not smoke. The overall odds ratio for having increased bronchial hyperresponsiveness was 2.4. The association was restricted to boys [OR = 3.9 (CI 1.1 to 13.6) in boys and OR = 1.0 (CI 0.3 to 3.1) in girls], confirming the sex difference already observed among asthmatics by Murray and Morrison [48]. Differences according to the sex of the child may relate to the sex-specific dysanaptic growth (inequal growth of parenchyma and airways) [6,51]. A similar association of bronchial hyperresponsiveness with paternal smoking was observed for boys in the study by Martinez et al. Similarly, Forastiere et al. [36 and personal communication] in a population-based sample of 1770 children aged 7 to 11 years, found that the OR for being a strong responder ($PD_{20} \leq 4$ mg/mL) to methacholine if exposed to maternal or paternal smoking was significantly greater than 1. In contrast to the findings of Martinez et al., girls were at much greater risk if exposed to maternal smoking [OR = 2.7 (CI: 1.3 to 5.5)] than boys [OR = 1.0 (CI: 0.5 to 1.9)] (F. Forastiere, personal communication).

**Table 4** Relationship of Environmental Tobacco Smoke Exposure to Bronchial Hyperresponsiveness Among Children

| Author | Population | Smoking | Bronchial hyper-responsiveness[a] | Results[b] | Comments |
|---|---|---|---|---|---|
| Ekwo et al., 1983, United States [42] | Iowa City, 183 school children, 6–12 yr | Parental smoking (50%) | Isoproterenol | Significant ($p <$ 0.001) increases in $FEF_{75}$, $FEV_1$, and $FEF_{25-75}$ after iso-proterenol in children from smoking families compared to others | No longer significant when expressed as a % of the pre-bronchodilator value |
| Weiss et al., 1985, United States [43] | East Boston, 173 teenagers, 12–16 yr | Mother (67%) | Hyperpnea with cold air ($\Delta FEV_1$/pred $FEV_1$) $\geq$ 9% (23%) | No association (OR = 0.81) | |
| Murray and Morrison, 1986, Canada [44] | Allergy clinic, 41 children with wheezing or asthma, 7–17 yr | Mother (24%), father (37%), both (49%) | Histamine, log $PC_{20}$ $FEV_1$ | Maternal smoking related to log $PC_{20}$ ($p < 0.01$) | |
| O'Connor et al., 1987, United States [45] | East Boston, 286 subjects, 6–21 yr | Mother (61%) | Hyperpnea with cold air ($\Delta FEV_1$/pred $FEV_1$) % | Significant ($p =$ 0.02) regression coefficient for maternal smoking as a predictor of $\Delta FEV_1$ in asthmatics | Wide range of age |
| Corbo et al., 1987, Italy [46] | Central Italy, 255 students, 11–14 yr | Mother (32%) | Methacholine, $PC_{20}$ $FEV_1$ $\leq$ 64 mg/mL (16%) | No association (OR = 0.77) | |

*(continued)*

477

**Table 4** Continued

| Author | Population | Smoking | Bronchial hyper-responsiveness[a] | Results[b] | Comments |
|---|---|---|---|---|---|
| Martinez et al., 1988, Italy [47] | Central Italy, 166 schoolchildren, 9 yr | Mother (10%), father (39%), both (26%) | Carbachol, $PD_{20}$ $FEV_1 \leq 1200\ \mu g$ (45%) | Association only with maternal smoking (OR = 2.39; $p$ < 0.05) | Males at much greater risk than females |
| Murray and Morrison, 1989, Canada [48] | Allergy clinic, 104 children with wheezing or asthma, 7–17 yr | Mother (25%) | Histamine, log $PC_{20}$ | Association of log $PC_{20}$ in boys ($p$ < 0.01) but not in girls; relation of duration of exposure with $PC_{20}$ | |
| Strachan et al., 1990, United Kingdom [49] | Edinburgh, 770 children, 7 yr | Salivary cotinine (41% with $\geq$ 1.3 ng/mL) | Exercise, $\Delta FEV_2 \geq$ 20% (5%) | No association with salivary cotinine, $\geq$ 13 ng/mL (OR = 0.92) | |
| Lebowitz and Quackenboss, 1990, United States [19] | Pima County, Arizona, 108 children of employees, 5–15 yr | 1–20 cigarettes/day exposure (25%) >20 cigarettes exposure (17%) | Daily peak flow variability | Association with familial smoking, >20 cigarettes/day (OR = 3.6; $p$ < 0.05) | |
| Young et al., 1991, Australia [50] | Prenatal clinic, 63 normal infants, 4–5 weeks | Parental smoking (52%) | $PC_{40}$ $V_{max}FRC$ g/L | Lower median $PC_{40}$ $V_{max}FRC$ in exposed vs. nonexposed without family history of asthma (0.52 g/L vs. 2.75 g/L; $p$ < 0.05) | Early age |

478

| Forastiere et al., 1991, Italy [36, and personal communication] | Central Italy, 1777 children, 7–11 yr | Mother (11%), father (30%), both (26%) | Methacholine, $PC_{20}$ $FEV_1 \leq 64$ mg/mL (49%) and $\leq 4$ mg/mL (15%), dose–response slope, and area under the curve | Correlation of the slope with parental smoking ($p < 0.01$); relation of $PC_{20}$ $FEV_1 \leq 4$ mg/mL with mother (OR = 1.6 (CI 1.1–2.2), father OR = 1.5 (CI 1.0–2.5) and both parents OR = 1.1 (CI 0.7–1.6) smoking | Females at significantly greater risk than males |

[a]$PC_y$, provocative concentration of bronchoconstrictor provoking a y% fall in $FEV_1$;
[b]$PD_{20}$, provocative dose of bronchoconstrictor provoking a 20% fall in $FEV_1$; $\Delta FEV_1$, initial $FEV_1$ – postchallenge $FEV_1$; slope, % of change in $FEV_1$ per mg/mL of bronchoconstrictor. OR, odds ratio; CI, 95% confidence interval.

Smoking during pregnancy might be one explanation for an effect of maternal smoking, but very few authors have reported observations, since studies need to be performed soon after birth or concern mothers who smoke only during pregnancy, a rare occurrence, to properly assess the in utero effect of smoking. The role of maternal smoking during pregnancy is supported by the study by Young et al. [50], who found an increase in the level of responsiveness to histamine in a sample of 63 normal infants soon after birth. In the population-based sample of children studied by Martinez et al., it should be noticed that hyperresponsiveness was present in seven out of the 10 children whose mothers acknowledged having smoked regularly during pregnancy compared with 29% of children whose mothers did not smoke. Further studies on this topic [52] could both help the understanding of the mechanisms involved in bronchial hyper-responsiveness and have practical consequences in terms of prevention.

No relationship was observed between bronchial hyperresponsiveness and reported environmental exposure to tobacco smoke in older children studied by Martinez et al. [47] and Forastiere et al. [36]. Among teenagers, Corbo et al. [46] did not find any association (even a reverse trend) between $PC_{20} \leq 64$ mg/mL to methacholine and maternal smoking in 261 students aged 11 to 14 years. In the same way, the odds ratio was even below 1 in 173 teenagers challenged with cold air studied by Weiss et al. [43]. Several reports have emphasized that cold air or exercise challenge do not assess the same bronchial hyperresponsiveness as do direct stimuli of the smooth muscle (histamine, acetylcholine, carbachol, and methacholine) and that cold air may be particularly insensitive in nonasthmatics [53]. In adults, too, the study conducted by Welty et al. [13] with cold air challenge was rather inconclusive. Similarly, the type of test used may explain the lack of association observed by Strachan et al. [49] with exercise challenge in a study conducted in 770 children aged 7 to 11 in which (recent) environmental exposure to tobacco smoke was assessed precisely by cotinine levels.

Overall, data are sufficiently consistent to support the hypothesis that environmental tobacco smoke, in particular maternal smoking, contributes to heightened childhood bronchial hyperresponsiveness. Differences in the reported associations between passive smoking and bronchial hyperresponsiveness relate to difficulties in quantifying passive smoking and, more than in adults, in the lack of standardization of bronchial hyperresponsiveness among children and adolescents. Environmental exposure to tobacco smoke depends on the number of cigarettes smoked in the family, ventilation, and meteorological conditions, as well as on the time spent at home. Objective assessment of this exposure by cotinine measurements [49] or environmental measures [19] only allows assessment of current exposure. Whether boys (or girls) or asthmatics are more susceptible needs to be confirmed. The role of other indoor or outdoor exposures intervening in the relation of smoking to hyperresponsiveness should be studied.

The role of dampness has already been suggested to act synergically with maternal smoking for asthma and exercise-induced cough, a potential indirect estimate of bronchial hyperresponsiveness [54].

## IV. Assessment of Bronchial Lability Without Bronchoconstriction Challenge

A number of measures other than bronchoconstriction response may be assumed to indicate bronchial lability. These include response to bronchodilator, variation in peak expiratory flow rate, or short-term variation in $FEV_1$ (e.g., measurement before and after a work shift). Although it is possible to identify responders, it is not at all certain that they measure the same thing as methacholine or histamine bronchoprovocation response. This is particularly true for the last two measurements. Several studies using bronchodilator tests reported associations with smoking in both adults [25,27] (Table 3) and children [42] (Table 4). The study reported in 1983 by Ekwo et al. [42] using a bronchodilator was the first epidemiological study conducted on the relationship of parental smoking to bronchial hyperresponsiveness. Among 183 children aged 6 to 12 years drawn from a general population of primary schoolchildren, postdilator $FEV_1$ values were significantly higher than predilator $FEV_1$ values in children from smoking families but not in those from nonsmoking families. The increase in $FEV_1$ after use of a bronchodilator in the smoking families did not remain significant, however, when the results were expressed as a percentage of the prebronchodilator value. This illustrates the question of whether absolute or proportional response is the most appropriate way of analyzing provocation test responses.

Whereas the association of occupational or air pollution with peak flow variability has been the topic of a large number of reports [55], data on smoking habits are scanty and preliminary. So far, they did not show an association between smoking and peak flow variability [34,56,57] (Table 2). However, reported environmental tobacco smoke was associated with peak flow variability in children 5 to 15 years [19]. Among adults, peak flow variability was related to tobacco smoke when subjects were also exposed to high-particulate-matter concentrations ($PM_{10} \geq 50$ $\mu g/m^3$) [19] or to formaldehyde in the home [58].

Short-term changes in $FEV_1$ have been used for research into physiological assessment of occupational lung disease and did show some association with occupational exposures. A number of studies [59–62] evaluating the relationship of tobacco smoking with short-term changes in $FEV_1$ have failed to demonstrate such a relationship. Two studies of swine confinement workers [63,64] showed adverse effects of tobacco smoking on change in $FEV_1$ values over the course of a working day, one of which was statistically significant and the other of which was not. One other study, standardized for the time of day, and including unexposed workers, showed a significant negative relationship of smoking on change in $FEV_1$ [65].

Overall, results observed for peak flow variability or $FEV_1$ changes over a work shift are less clear-cut than for provocation tests. Further studies are needed in particular for peak flow variability, which may become a tool used much more widely in epidemiology [55].

## V.  Healthy Smoker Effect

Two questions should be addressed to assess the relation between smoking and bronchial hyperresponsiveness: Does smoking cause (or exacerbate) bronchial hyperresponsiveness, and does bronchial hyperresponsiveness influence smoking habits? The second question refers to one aspect of the *healthy smoker effect.* This term, by analogy to the *healthy worker effect,* corresponds to the fact that susceptible subjects may refrain from smoking, and this bias may mask the deleterious effect of smoking (9). As for the healthy worker effect, longitudinal studies are the method of choice to assess and circumvent such bias. After a 5-year follow-up study on 183 nonasthmatics aged 13 to 23 years at the first survey, Tashkin et al. [66] observed that young males (but not females) who remained nonsmokers had significantly lower $FEV_1$ values than those who subsequently initiate the habit of smoking regularly. They suggested that this discordance between male and female factors in relation to starting smoking may be due to social forces but also to a greater airway reactivity to nonspecific stimuli, which could then influence subjects not to take up smoking habits. This hypothesis is not supported by the preliminary results from 261 nonsmoking children and adolescents followed for an average of 3.5 years after a cold air challenge [67]. Starting smoking did not relate to either $FEV_1$ level or cold air challenge. Male passive smokers, nonsmokers with a smoking spouse, represent a rather interesting insight into the choice of nonsmoking related to asthma in a general population in France (17.2% of these passive smokers compared to 7.8% among true nonsmokers reported a history of asthma $p = 0.07$) [68]. As stated by Becklake and Lalloo [9], the number of people susceptible to the effect of smoking is probably higher among any group of nonsmokers than among a group of smokers drawn from the same population. Allergic symptoms and bronchial hyperresponsiveness may induce selection bias more than do chronic symptoms or low $FEV_1$ values, because these acute characteristics are more easily perceived. Consequently, it is extremely difficult to show a positive association of active smoking with allergy or asthma [10,69], even more than with hyperresponsiveness. This does not imply that smoking may not be a risk factor for allergy or asthma. In the more "experimental" situation of environmental tobacco smoke exposure, it has already been shown in several reports that there is an association of exposure with childhood asthma [70,71]. However, environmental exposure to tobacco smoke in children may also be less common in asthmatics or diagnosed allergic subjects [19]. Volunteers may participate in a study because of their symptoms, whereas choosing asymptomatic subjects may select subjects not susceptible to tobacco smoke. Therefore, opposite selection biases may potentially explain the discordant results on the association of smoking to hyperresponsiveness in clinical reports [4–6]. As for occupational exposures [72], follow-up designs are needed to assess the role of factors highly concerned by selection bias. These designs, however, are methodologically very difficult because of the changes resulting from exposure and/or change in exposure and the difficulty in studying those who cease employment.

Because of the healthy smoker effect, some authors have examined the relation between the degree of responsiveness and the amount smoked, restricting the analysis either among the smokers [39] or among the responders [31]. Whereas the association with "ever-smoked" or current smoking was not obvious in the study conducted by Rijcken et al. [39], they showed a relation between the amount smoked and hyperresponsiveness. Similarly, Kennedy et al. [31] observed that smokers cluster around a moderate level of the responsiveness distribution. They suggest that at the high level of responsiveness experienced by asthmatics, the level may determine smoking habit rather than the other way around. Furthermore, studies of employed populations should consider whether the study group is already biased to exclude more responsive subgroups, a situation likely to occur in exposed occupations, such as in miners [73].

## VI. Physiological Interpretations

Numerous mechanisms have been proposed to explain the association between tobacco smoke and bronchial hyperresponsiveness and are summarized in Figure 1. The interrelationships between bronchial hyperresponsiveness, airway caliber,

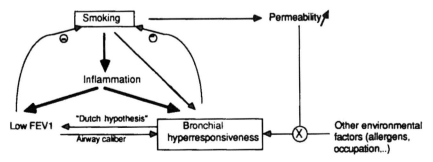

**FIGURE 1**   Potential pathways between tobacco smoke and bronchial hyperresponsiveness.

and airway inflammation are not well understood, but the role of inflammation, direct and/or indirect, is generally considered to be a key phenomenon. Furthermore, other factors may modify the relationship of smoking to bronchial hyperresponsiveness, such as age (see above), atopy, genetic factors, or other environmental factors.

Data on the potential role of genetic factors modifying the relation of smoking to responsiveness are scanty. Kabiraj et al. [12] failed to find any role of PIMZ. In a clinical report [74], smoking among siblings of atopic asthmatics was related to bronchial hyperresponsiveness as strongly as was atopy, which may reflect a particular susceptibility of these subjects to smoking. More studies are urgently needed on these aspects.

There are various specific mechanisms by which exposure to tobacco smoke might increase the risk of developing bronchial hyperresponsiveness in childhood, such as a toxic effect of carbon monoxide or nicotine during fetal life, which may induce perturbations in lung growth and maturation [75]. Bronchial hyperresponsiveness, triggered by exposure to allergen, virus, or irritant may become persistent following exposure to tobacco smoke. Infections are favored by active and passive smoking. Excluding some short-term exacerbations of bronchial hyperresponsiveness, infections seem to play little role in explaining natural variations in hyperresponsiveness [6,76].

The lack of a clear association between smoking and bronchial hyperresponsiveness assessed by indirect stimuli of the airway smooth muscle (cold air, exercise) in adults [13] and in children [43,49] may relate to the different relation of airway caliber with cold air or exercise challenge response [53]. As $FEV_1$ level may be associated with bronchial hyperresponsiveness due to a diminished airway caliber and, conversely, bronchial hyperresponsiveness may be a risk factor for $FEV_1$ decline (Dutch hypothesis), there is no definite way of analyzing epidemiological data to clarify the respective relations of smoking, $FEV_1$ level, and bronchial hyperresponsiveness. Several studies have addressed the question by looking at the association of smoking to bronchial hyperresponsiveness after adjusting for $FEV_1$ level. They have led to conflicting results: The relations were no longer significant in several studies [22,31; Bakke, personal communication] but did not change in others [14,20], including the study on French policemen (Table 5). However, such an adjustment may represent an overadjustment according to the Dutch hypothesis. Assessment of the role of bronchial hyperresponsiveness in $FEV_1$ decline is a difficult issue [6], in particular because there might be some heterogeneity between individuals [8]. Pride has suggested that there may be an acquired type of bronchial hyperresponsiveness in smokers in late middle age of a different significance for the development of chronic airflow limitation than that associated with "endogenous" bronchial hyperresponsiveness as proposed by the original Dutch hypothesis [77]. Furture studies should assess the role of airway caliber in children as it has been done in adults.

**Table 5** Relationship of Bronchial Hyperresponsiveness to Smoking Habits Before and After Adjustment for $FEV_1$ Level[a] and Leucocyte Count in 313 Policemen (Logistic Models)

| Risk factor | Coefficient (β) | Odds ratio[b] |
|---|---|---|
| Model 1 | | |
| Ex-smokers vs. nonsmokers | 0.10 ± 0.43 | 1.19 |
| Smokers <10 g/day vs. nonsmokers | 0.24 ± 0.57 | 1.27 |
| Smokers 10–19 g/day vs. nonsmokers | −0.78 ± 0.78 | 0.46 |
| Smokers 20–29 g/day vs. nonsmokers | −0.15 ± 0.60 | 0.86 |
| Smokers ≥ 30 g/day vs. nonsmokers | 1.59 ± 0.50 | 4.90** |
| Model 2 | | |
| $FEV_1$ level | −0.82 ± 0.18 | 2.27[c],*** |
| Ex-smokers vs. nonsmokers | −0.04 ± 0.46 | 0.96 |
| Smokers <10 g/day vs. nonsmokers | 0.17 ± 0.61 | 1.19 |
| Smokers 10–19 g/day vs. nonsmokers | −0.57 ± 0.80 | 0.57 |
| Smokers 20–29 g/day vs. nonsmokers | −0.33 ± 0.62 | 0.72 |
| Smokers ≥ 30 g/day vs. nonsmokers | 1.26 ± 0.54 | 3.53* |
| Model 3 | | |
| $FEV_1$ level | −0.78 ± 0.18 | 2.18[c],*** |
| $Log_{10}$ leucocytes/mm$^3$ | 3.31 ± 1.64 | 1.15[d],* |
| Ex-smokers vs. nonsmokers | −0.12 ± 0.47 | 0.89 |
| Smokers <10 g/day vs. nonsmokers | 0.06 ± 0.62 | 1.06 |
| Smokers 10–19 g/day vs. nonsmokers | −0.95 ± 0.83 | 0.39 |
| Smokers 20–29 g/day vs. nonsmokers | −0.50 ± 0.63 | 0.61 |
| Smokers ≥30 g/day vs. nonsmokers | 0.88 ± 0.56 | 2.41 (p = 0.12) |

[a] $FEV_1$ level, adjusted residual on age and height.
[b] *, $p \le 0.05$; **, $p \le 0.01$; ***, $p \le 0.001$.
[c] Per 1 SD decrease.
[d] Per 10% leucocyte increase [i.e., $\log_{10} 1.1$, OR = exp (3.31 $\log_{10}1.1$)].

There is no question that smoking induces inflammation and a significant correlation between the amount smoked and peripheral leucocyte count has been established [78,79]. Evidence of an association of cellular inflammation with bronchial hyperresponsiveness comes from animal models, morphological studies, and analyses of bronchoalveolar lavages of asthmatics (recently reviewed in ref. 80). However, the causal nature of this association has not been demonstrated [81] nor has it been determined which are the specific cells and mediators involved in the various forms and stages of bronchial hyperresponsiveness [82]. Epidemiological evidence of the role of inflammation on bronchial hyperresponsiveness is limited. In the study conducted in middle-aged policemen, associations between bronchial hyperresponsiveness and both leucocyte count and haptoglobin (an acute-phase protein) level were observed [29,83]. In the veterans study [17], bronchial hyperresponsiveness related significantly to markers of allergic inflammation (IgE level and eosinophils) but not to total leucocyte count. However, distinctions between allergy and inflammation are less clear cut than considered previously [2]. The relation of smoking with bronchial hyperresponsiveness observed in the veterans study remained after adjustment for IgE and eosinophils. In the French policemen study, it was shown that the association between heavy smoking and bronchial hyperresponsiveness remained after adjustment for both positive skin prick tests and leucocyte count [29]. These observations favor the hypothesis that inflammation (allergic or not) is not the sole explanation of the relation between smoking and hyperresponsiveness. Anti-inflammatory drugs have not so far been shown to cause a clear decrease of bronchial hyperresponsiveness among smokers [76,84]. Whether airway inflammation may play a direct or an indirect role in inducing bronchial hyperresponsiveness is extremely difficult to assess, as bronchial hyperresponsiveness and $FEV_1$ are particularly strongly related in smokers [2,76,80], and a raised leucocyte count in relation with a lower $FEV_1$ has been observed in several epidemiological studies [85,86]. After adjustment for both leucocyte count and $FEV_1$ level, the association between heavy smoking and bronchial hyperresponsiveness in the French policemen study, was no longer significant (although the odds-ratio remained greater than 2) (table 5). Some indications from a morphological study by Mullen et al. [40] suggest that cigarette smoking, airway caliber and airway inflammation exert an independent effect on bronchial hyperresponsiveness. More studies, which would benefit for a multidisciplinary approach, are needed on this question.

Burney et al. have suggested that atopy, a factor highly related to bronchial responsiveness, may play a major role on responsiveness in the young ages and that current smoking plays an important role in middle-aged and elderly subjects [14,76]. In their study conducted on veterans, O'Connor et al. [17] observed that bronchial hyperresponsiveness was related to current smoking only in atopics. However, several studies have reported that the associations of responsiveness with smoking remained after adjustment for allergic markers, such as positive skin prick test [14,29,31] or eosinophils [22]. As atopics are more likely not to take up smoking, as well as to quit smoking [10,69], the interrelations of atopy, smoking, and bronchial hyperresponsiveness are likely to be complex [87]. Smoking, which has already been shown to interact in the development of occupational allergy [10,88], may play a role in bronchial hyperresponsiveness through increasing a predisposition to allergy [6,10]. Smoking exerts a permissive effect on acid anhydride–specific IgE antibody production [88] and might interfere in bronchial hyperresponsiveness as persistent acid anhydride hyperresponsiveness correlates with both histamine bronchial hyperresponsiveness and specific IgE level. The direct effect of smoking on the immune system, such as the suppression of regulator T-cell function [6,89] and increased permeability due to smoking have been proposed to explain the relation of smoking to bronchial hyperresponsiveness [6,10]. Epithelial damage may increase the accessibility of stimuli to receptor sites and play a role in the interactions of respiratory epithelial cells and bronchial smooth muscle, but the role of smoking in these interactions is not known [6]. Bronchial hyperresponsiveness may appear through a cascade involving inflammation, increased permeability, and sensitization to allergens. Increased permeability may also be one mechanism involved in the relation of smoking to bronchial hyperresponsiveness, independent of allergen sensitization. Several studies have shown an increased epithelial permeability in relation to smoking of small and large molecules [6,90–92]. However, in the study conducted by Kennedy et al. in 10 smokers and eight nonsmokers, the observed increased permeability in smokers did not relate to increased responsiveness to histamine. The small sample size or differing physical locus for permeability and responsiveness [92] may explain these findings, which are likely to be complex.

Assessment of tobacco smoke hypersensitivity by changes in lung function after tobacco smoke challenge have led to discordant results. Whereas Wiedemann et al. [93] did not show any change in $FEV_1$ value after 1-h challenge among nine asymptomatic adults, Dahms et al. [94] reported an average 21.4% change in $FEV_1$ value among 10 asthmatics and no change among 10 controls. In children, Oldigs et al. did not show any decrease in $FEV_1$ value after challenge in 11 asthmatics [95]. Menon et al. [96] showed a good reliability of a positive response to cigarette smoke challenge 2 years apart. No late-phase reaction occurred according to 24-h peak flow recording after tobacco smoke challenge. Decrease in $FEV_1$ value appeared after 30 min for Dahms and 60 min for Menon, which is longer than with histamine or methacholine challenges. Menon et al. [96] did not show a correlation between methacholine sensitivity and airway responsiveness to environmental tobacco smoke. Tobacco smoke hypersensitivity fails to explain the association between smoking and markers of allergy [4]. Similarly, tobacco smoke hypersensitivity (an acute phenomenon) is not likely to be the explanation for the role of smoking in persistent bronchial hyperresponsiveness.

## VII. Conclusions

Overall, existing evidence clearly supports the hypothesis of an association of bronchial hyperresponsiveness with active smoking in adults and with passive smoking in young children. The association is consistent among studies, although rather weak. A certain amount of exposure is needed for expressing the effect, which may depend on age, sex, and atopy. The magnitude of the association observed may well be notably decreased by the healthy smoker effect, a phenomenon difficult to assess and even more difficult to quantitate. It is very possible that the healthy smoker effect will increase in relation to efficient preventive strategies. Therefore, in the presently changing world of tobacco consumption it is likely that associations between tobacco smoke and bronchial responsiveness may change according to time and differently in various countries. Whether the association is truly causal is difficult to know because of the interrelations of bronchial hyperresponsiveness with baseline levels of lung function.

Future studies, especially with longitudinal design, are clearly needed to better assess the role of active and passive exposure to tobacco smoke on bronchial responsiveness and to delineate subgroups of individuals more susceptible to the development of smoking-related bronchial hyperresponsiveness. Biological or environmental assessment of current tobacco smoke exposure may be useful but cannot take the place of questionnaires allowing retrospective assessment of exposure. Smoking during pregnancy, various types of tobacco or inhalation habits, and potential interactions with other indoor or outdoor environmental exposures should be explored further. In developing countries where indoor exposure is high and tobacco consumption is increasing, studies might help in establishing specific preventive strategies. Various types of challenge on the same subjects as well as peak flow variability measures should be undertaken. Risk factors (such as genetic factors according to animal data) [97] may be different for various types of hyperresponsiveness, and tobacco smoke may relate preferentially to one type of hyperresponsiveness. Taking sensitivity and reactivity into account [98] may add to an understanding of differences in smoking-induced hyperresponsiveness and asthma-related hyper-responsiveness [2,80]. The delineation of smokers more likely to develop hyperresponsiveness may come by a better assessment of the role of personal characteristics, such as atopy, sex, age, and growth stage, as well as genetic factors. In addition to asthmatics or atopics, cystic fibrosis patients and even heterozygous subjects for this disease may be at risk [99,100].

Screening smokers for bronchial hyperresponsiveness is premature, as no specific treatment for smoking-related hyperresponsiveness has so far been shown to be effective, and it is still disputed whether hyperresponsive subjects are at greater risk to develop chronic airflow limitation [2,6,101]. However, bronchial hyperresponsiveness may be one of the markers that allow us to identify susceptible smokers. As these subjects probably constitute a heterogeneous group, other markers are needed. The next step will be evaluation of the usefulness of specific preventive strategies directed to potential susceptible smokers.

### References

1. Dautrebande L, Philippot E. Crise d'asthme expérimental par aérosols de carbaminoylcholine chez l'homme traité par dispersat de phényl amino-propane. Presse Med 1941;49:942–46.
2. Pride NB. Bronchial hyperreactivity in smokers. Eur Respir J 1988;1:485–87.
3. Boushey HA, Holtzman MJ, Sheller JR, Nadel JA. Bronchial hyper-reactivity. Am Rev Respir Dis 1980;121:389–413.
4. Gerrard JW, Cockroft DW, Mink JT, Cotton DJ, Poonawala R, Dosman JA. Increased nonspecific bronchial reactivity in cigarette smokers with normal lung function. Am Rev Respir Dis 1980;122:577–81.
5. Brown NE, McFaden ER Jr, Ingram RH Jr. Airway responses to inhaled histamine in asymptomatic smokers and nonsmokers. J Appl Physiol 1977;42:508–13.
6. Weiss ST, O'Connor GT, Sparrow D. The role of allergy and airway responsiveness in the natural history of chronic airflow obstruction (CAO). In: Weiss S, Sparrow D, eds. Airway responsiveness and atopy in the development of chronic lung disease. New York: Raven Press, 1989:181–240.
7. Pride N. Smoking, allergy and airways obstruction: revival of the "Dutch hypothesis." Clin Allergy 1986;16:3–6.
8. Burrows B. Airways obstructive diseases: pathogenetic mechanisms and natural histories of the disorders. Med Clin North Am 1990;74:547–59.
9. Becklake MR, Lalloo U. The "healthy smoker": a phenomenon of health selection? Respiration 1990;57:137–44.
10. Kauffmann F, Annesi I, Oryszczyn MP. The relationship between smoking and allergy. In: Sluiter HJ, Van der Lende R, Gerritsen J, Postma DS, eds. Bronchitis IV. Assen, The Netherlands: Van Gorcum, 1989:57–70.
11. Van der Lende R, Visser BF, Wever-Hess J, DeVries K, Orie NGM. Distribution of histamine threshold values in a random population. Rev Inst Hyg Mines 1973;28:186–90.
12. Kabiraj MU, Simonsson BG, Groth S, Björklund A, Bülow K, Lindell SE. Bronchial reactivity, smoking, and $\alpha_1$-antitrypsin. A population-based study of middle-aged men. Am Rev Respir Dis 1982;126:864–96.
13. Welty C, Weiss ST, Tager IB, Muñoz A, Becker C, Speizer FE, Ingram RH. The relationship of airways responsiveness to cold air, cigarette smoking, and atopy to respiratory symptoms and pulmonary function in adults. Am Rev Respir Dis 1984;130:198–203.
14. Burney PGJ, Britton JR, Chinn S, Tattersfield AE, Papacosta AO, Kelson MC, Anderson F, Corfield DR. Descriptive epidemiology of bronchial

reactivity in an adult population: results from a community study. Thorax 1987;42:38–44.

15. Woolcock AJ, Peat JK, Salome CM, Yan K, Anderson SD, Schoeffel RE, McCowage G, Killalea T. Prevalence of bronchial hyperresponsiveness and asthma in a rural adult population. Thorax 1987;42:361–86.

16. Cerveri I, Bruschi C, Zoia MC, Maccarini L, Grassi M, Lebowitz MD, Rampulla C, Grassi C. Smoking habit and bronchial reactivity in normal subjects. A population-based study. Am Rev Respir Dis 1989;140:191–96.

17. O'Connor GT, Sparrow D, Segal MR, Weiss ST. Smoking, atopy and methacholine airway responsiveness among middle-aged and elderly men. Am Rev Respir Dis 1989;140:1520–26.

18. Trigg CJ, Bennett JB, Tooley M, Sibbald B, D'Souza MF, Davies RJ. A general practice based survey of bronchial hyperresponsiveness and its relation to symptoms, sex, age, atopy, and smoking. Thorax 1990;45:866–72.

19. Lebowitz MD, Quackenboss JJ. The effects of environmental tobacco smoke on pulmonary function. Int Arch Occup Environ Health 1990(Suppl):147–52.

20. Sparrow D, O'Connor G, Rosner B, Segal MR, Weiss ST. The influence of age and level of pulmonary function on nonspecific airway responsiveness. The normative aging study. Am Rev Respir Dis 1991;143:978–82.

21. Bakke PS, Baste V, Gulsvik A. Bronchial responsiveness in a Norwegian community. Am Rev Respir Dis 1991;143:317–22.

22. Rijcken B, Schouten JP, Mensiga TT, Weiss ST, deVries K, Van der Lende R. Factors associated with bronchial responsiveness to histamine in a population sample of adults. In: Rijcken B, ed. Bronchial responsiveness and COPD risk; an epidemiological study. Thesis Groningen, 1991:37–52.

23. Dow L, Coggon D, Holgate ST. Respiratory symptoms as predictors of airways lability in an elderly population. Respir Med 1992;86:27–32.

24. Pham QT, Mur JM, Chau N, Gabiano M, Henquel JC, Teculescu D. Prognostic value of acetylcholine challenge test: a prospective study. Br J Ind Med 1984;41:267–71.

25. Taylor RG, Joyce H, Gross E, Holland F, Pride NB. Bronchial reactivity to inhaled histamine and annual rate of decline in $FEV_1$ in male smokers and ex-smokers. Thorax 1985;40:9–16.

26. Enarson DA, Chan-Yeung M, Tabona M, Kus J, Vedal S, Lam S. Predictors of bronchial hyperexcitability in grain handlers. Chest 1985;87:452–55.

27. Vollmer WM, Johnson LR, Buist AS. Relationship of response to a bronchodilator and decline in forced expiratory volume in one second in population studies. Am Rev Respir Dis 1985;132:1186–93.

28. Annesi I, Neukirch F, Orvoen-Frija E, Oryszczyn MP, Korobaeff M, Doré

M, Kauffmann F. The relevance of hyperresponsiveness but not of atopy to FEV$_1$ decline. Preliminary results in a working population. Bull Eur Physiopathol Respir 1987;23:397–400.

29. Annesi I, Kauffmann F, Oryszczyn MP, Neukirch F, Orvoen-Frija E, Lellouch J. Leukocyte count and bronchial hyperresponsiveness. J Allergy Clin Immunol 1988;82:1006–11.

30. Ernst P, Dales RE, Nunes F, Becklake MR. Relation of airway responsiveness to duration of work in a dusty environment. Thorax 1989;44:116–20.

31. Kennedy SM, Burrows B, Vedal S, Enarson DA, Chan-Yeung M. Methacholine responsiveness among working populations. Relationship to smoking and airway caliber. Am Rev Respir Dis 1990;142:1377–83.

32. Iversen M, Pedersen B. Relation between respiratory symptoms, type of farming, and lung function disorders in farmers. Thorax 1990;45:919–23.

33. Kongerud J, Soyseth V. Methacholine responsiveness, respiratory symptoms and pulmonary function in aluminium potroom workers. Eur Respir J 1991;4:159–66.

34. Neukirch F, Liard R, Segala C, Korobaeff M, Henry C, Cooreman J. Peak expiratory flow variability and bronchial responsiveness to methacholine: an epidemiological study in 117 workers. Am Rev Respir Dis 1992;146:71–75.

35. Rijcken B, Schouten JP, Weiss ST, Speizer FE, Van der Lende R. The relationship between airway responsiveness to histamine and pulmonary function level in a random population sample. Am Rev Respir Dis 1988;137:826–32.

36. Forastiere F, Pistelli R, Michelozzi P, Corbo GM, Agabiti N, Bertollini R, Ciappi G, Perucci CA. Indices of nonspecific bronchial responsiveness in a pediatric population. Chest 1991;100:927–34.

37. Rijcken B, Schouten JP, Weiss ST, Meinesz AF, De Vries K, Van der Lende R. The distribution of bronchial responsiveness to histamine in symptomatic and in asymptomatic subjects. A population-based analysis of various indices of responsiveness. Am Rev Respir Dis 1989;140:615–23.

38. Kauffmann F. Means or cut-offs? Bull Eur Physiopathol Respir 1983;19:73p–75p.

39. Rijcken B, Schouten JP, Weiss ST, Speizer FE, Van der Lende R. The relationship of nonspecific bronchial responsiveness to respiratory symptoms in a random population sample. Am Rev Respir Dis 1987;136:62–68.

40. Mullen JBM, Wiggs BR, Wright JL, Hogg JC, Paré PD. Nonspecific airway reactivity in cigarette smokers. Relationship to airway pathology and baseline lung function. Am Rev Respir Dis 1986;133:120–25.

41. Buczko GB, Vanderdoelen JL, Boucher R, Zamel N. Effects of cigarette

smoking and short-term smoking cessation on airway responsiveness to inhaled methacholine. Am Rev Respir Dis 1984;129:12–14.

42. Ekwo EE, Weinberger MM, Lachenbruch PA, Huntley WH. Relationship of parental smoking and gas cooking to respiratory disease in children. Chest 1983;84:662–68.

43. Weiss ST, Tager IB, Muñoz A, Speizer FEZ. The relationship of respiratory infections in early childhood to the occurrence of increased levels of bronchial responsiveness and atopy. Am Rev Respir Dis 1985;131:573–78.

44. Murray AB, Morrison BJ. The effect of cigarette smoke from the mother on bronchial hyperresponsiveness and severity of symptoms in children with asthma. J Allergy Clin Immunol 1986;77:575–81.

45. O'Connor GT, Weiss ST, Tager IB, Speizer FE. The effect of passive smoking on pulmonary function and nonspecific bronchial responsiveness in a population-based sample of children and young adults. Am Rev Respir Dis 1987;135:800–804.

46. Corbo GM, Foresi A, Valente S, Bustacchini S. Maternal smoking and bronchial responsiveness in children. Am Rev Respir Dis 1987; 127(Suppl):245.

47. Martinez FD, Antognoni G, Macri F, Bonci E, Midulla F, De Castro G, Ronchetti R. Parental smoking enhances bronchial responsiveness in nine-year old children. Am Rev Respir Dis 1988;138:518–23.

48. Murray AB, Morrison BJ. Passive smoking by asthmatics: its greater effect on boys than on girls and an older than on younger children. Pediatrics 1989;84:451–59.

49. Strachan DP, Jarvis MJ, Feyerbend C. The relationship of salivary cotinine to respiratory symptoms, spirometry and exercise-induced bronchospasm in seven-year old children. Am Rev Respir Dis 1990;142:147–51.

50. Young S, Le Souëf PN, Geelhoed GC, Stick SM, Turner KJ, Landau LI. The influence of a family history of asthma and parental smoking on airway responsiveness in early infancy. N Engl J Med 1991;324:1168–73.

51. Kauffmann F. Sex-specific dysanapsis and the effect of passive smoking among asthmatics. Pediatrics 1990;86:646–47.

52. Tager IB. Passive smoking, bronchial responsiveness and atopy. Am Rev Respir Dis 1988;138:507–9.

53. Hargreave FE, Gibson PG, Ramsdale EH. Airway hyperresponsiveness, airway inflammation, and asthma. Immunol Allergy Clin North Am 1990;10:439–48.

54. Andrae S, Axelson O, Björksten B, Fredriksson M, Kjellman NIM. Symptoms of bronchial hyperreactivity and asthma in relation to environmental factors. Arch Dis Child 1988;63:473–78.

55. Lebowitz MD. The use of peak expiratory flow rate measurements in respiratory disease. Pediatr Pulmonol 1991;11:166–74.
56. Higgins BG, Britton JR, Chinn S, Burney PGJ, Tattersfield AE. A comparison of the $PD_{20}$ and the dose response slope as measures of bronchial reactivity in epidemiological surveys. Am Rev Respir Dis 1989;139(Suppl):A31.
57. Quackenboss JJ, Lebowitz MD, Hayes C, Young CL. Respiratory responses to indoor/outdoor air pollutants: combustion pollutants, formaldehyde and particulate matter. In: Harper JP, ed. Combustion processes and the quality of the indoor environment. Pittsburgh PA: AWMA, 1989:280–93.
58. Krzyzanowski M, Quackenboss JJ, Lebowitz MD. Chronic respiratory effects of indoor formaldehyde exposure. Environ Res 1990;52:117–25.
59. McKerrow C, McDermott M, Gislon JC, Shilling RSF. Respiratory function during the day in cotton workers: a study in byssinosis. Br J Ind Med 1958;15:75–83.
60. Ghio AJ, Castellan RM, Kinsley KB, Hankinson JL. Changes in forced expiratory volume in one second and peak expiratory flow rate across a work shift among unexposed blue collar workers. Am Rev Respir Dis 1991;143:1231–34.
61. Corey P, Hutcheon M, Broder I, Mintz S. Grain elevator workers show work-related pulmonary function changes and dose–effect relationships with dust exposure. Br J Ind Med 1982;39:330–37.
62. Tweeddale PM, Alexander F, McHardy GJR. Short term variability in $FEV_1$ and bronchodilator responsiveness in patients with obstructive ventilatory defects. Thorax 1987;42:487–90.
63. Donham KJ, Zavala DC, Merchant J. Acute effects of the work environment on pulmonary functions of swine confinement workers. Am J Ind Med 1984;5:367–75.
64. Donham K, Haglind P, Peteson Y, Rylander R, Belin L. Environmental and health studies of farm workers in Swedish swine confinement buildings. Br J Ind Med 1989;46:31–37.
65. Enarson DA, Yeung M. Determinants of changes in $FEV_1$ over a workshift. Br J Ind Med 1985;42:202–4.
66. Tashkin DP, Clark VA, Coulson AH, Bourque LB, Simmons M, Reems C, Detels R, Rokaw S. Comparison of lung function in young nonsmokers and smokers before and after initiation of the smoking habit. A prospective study. Am Rev Respir Dis 1983;128:12–16.
67. O'Connor G, Tager I, Weiss ST, Speizer FE. Prospective evaluation of smoking initiation by children and young adults. Am Rev Respir Dis 1987;135(Suppl):A339.

68. Kauffmann F, Tessier JF, Oriol P. Adult passive smoking in the home environment: a risk factor for chronic airflow limitation. Am J Epidemiol 1983;117:269–80.
69. Oryszczyn MP, Annesi I, Neukirch F, Doré MF, Kauffmann F. Relationships of total IgE level, skin prick test response and smoking habits. Ann Allergy 1991;67:355–58.
70. Weitzman M, Gortmaker S, Klein Walker D, Sobol A. Maternal smoking and childhood asthma. Pediatrics 1990;85:505–11.
71. Landau LI. Smoking and childhood asthma. Med J Australia 1991;154:715–16.
72. Kauffmann F, Drouet D, Lellouch J, Brille D. Occupational exposure and 12-year spirometric changes among Paris area workers. Br J Ind Med 1982;39:221–32.
73. Mannino D, Daniloff E, Peck A, Petsonk E. Do miners select jobs based on airway responsiveness? Am Rev Respir Dis 1991;143(Suppl)A264.
74. Grainger DN, Stenton SC, Avery AJ, Duddridge M, Walters EH, Hendrick DJ. The relationship between atopy and non-specific bronchial responsiveness. Clin Exp Allergy 1990;20:181–87.
75. Wang NS, Cheng MF, Schrauf-Nagel DE, Yao YT. The accumulative scanning EM changes in baby mouse lungs following prenatal and postnatal exposure to nicotine. J Pathol 1984;144:89–100.
76. Burney PGJ, Anderson HR, Burrows B, Chan-Yeung M, Pride NB, Speizer FE. Epidemiology. In: Holgate ST, ed. The role of inflammatory processes in airway hyperresponsiveness. Oxford: Blackwell Scientific, 1989:222–50.
77. Pride NB. Smoking and bronchial hyperresponsiveness. In: Sluiter HJ, Van der Lende R, Gerritsen J, Postma DS, eds. Bronchitis IV. Assen, The Netherlands: Van Gorcum, 1989:71–82.
78. Corre F, Lellouch J, Schwartz D. Smoking and leucocyte count. Results of an epidemiological survey. Lancet 1971;2:632–34.
79. Taylor RG. Smoking and the leucocyte count. Eur J Respir Dis 1987;71:35–38.
80. Holgate ST, ed. The role of inflammatory processes in airway hyperreponsiveness. Oxford: Blackwell Scientific, 1989.
81. Drazen JM. Physiology. In: Holgate ST, ed. The role of inflammatory processes in airway hyperresponsiveness. Oxford: Blackwell Scientific, 1989:108–50.
82. Kay AB. Cellular mechanisms In: Holgate ST, ed. The role of inflammatory processes in airway hyperresponsiveness. Oxford: Blackwell Scientific, 1989:151–78.
83. Kauffmann F, Frette C, Annesi I, Oryszczyn MP, Doré MF, Neukirch F.

Relationships of haptoblobin level to FEV₁, wheezing, bronchial hyper-responsiveness and allergy. Clin Exp Allergy 1991;21:669–74.

84. Lim TK, Turner NC, Watson A, Joyce H, Fuller RW, Pride NB. Effects of nonsteroidal anti-inflammatory drugs on the bronchial hyperreponsiveness of middle-aged male smokers. Eur Respir J 1990;3:872–79.

85. Chan Yeung M, Abboud R, dy Buncio A, Vedal S. Peripheral leukocyte count and longitudinal decline in lung function. Thorax 1988;43:462–66.

86. Frette C, Annesi I, Doré MF, Korobaeff M, Kauffmann F, Neukirch F. Circulating leucocytes and FEV1. Eur Respir J 1983;2(suppl 369s).

87. Burrows B, Martinez FD. Bronchial responsiveness, atopy, smoking and chronic obstructive pulmonary disease. Am Rev Respir Dis 1989;140:1515–17.

88. Newman Taylor AJ, Venables KM, Durham SR, Graneek BJ, Topping MD. Acid anhydrides and asthma. Int Arch Allergy Appl Immunol 1987;82:435–39.

89. Tollerud DJ, Clark JW, Morris-Brown LM, Neuland CY, Mann DL, Pankin-Trost LK, Blattner WA, Hoover RN. Association of cigarette smoking with decreased numbers of circulating natural killer cells. Am Rev Respir Dis 1989;139:194–98.

90. Mason GR, Uszler JM, Effros RM, Reid E. Rapidly reversible alterations of pulmonary epithelial permeability induced by smoking. Chest 1983;83:6–1.

91. Hogg JC. The effect of smoking on airway permeability. Chest 1983;83:1–2.

92. Kennedy SM, Elwood RK, Wiggs BJR, Paré JC. Increased airway mucosal permeability of smokers. Relationship to airway reactivity. Am Rev Respir Dis 1984;129:143–48.

93. Wiedemann HP, Mahler DA, Loke J, Virgulto JA, Snyder P, Matthay RA. Acute effects of passive smoking on lung function and airway reactivity in asthmatic subjects. Chest 1986;89:180–88.

94. Dahms TE, Bolin JF, Slavin RG. Passive smoking. Effects on bronchial asthma. Chest 1981;80:530–34.

95. Oldigs M, Jörres R, Magnussen H. Acute effect of passive smoking on lung function and airway responsiveness in asthmatic children. Pediatr Pulmonol 1991;10:123–31.

96. Menon PK, Stankus RP, Rando RJ, Salvaggio JE, Lehrer SB. Asthmatic responses to passive cigarette smoke: persistence of reactivity and effect of medications. J Allergy Clin Immunol 1991;88:861–69.

97. Pauwels RA. Genetic factors controlling airway responsiveness. Clin Rev Allergy 1989;7:235–43.

98. Sterk PJ, Bel EH, Bronchial hyperresponsiveness: the need for a distinction

between hypersensitivity and excessive airway narrowing. Eur Respir J 1989;2:262–74.

99. Davis PB. Airway responsiveness and atopy in cystic fibrosis. In: Weiss S, Sparrow D, eds. Airway responsiveness and atopy in the development of chronic lung disease. New York: Raven Press, 1989:293–313.

100. Rubin BK. Exposure of children with cystic fibrosis to environmental tobacco smoke. N Engl Med 1990;323:782–88.

101. Rijcken B. Bronchial responsiveness and COPD risk; an epidemiological study. Thesis Groningen, 1991.

# 25

## Tobacco Smoke as a Respiratory Carcinogen

DIETRICH HOFFMANN
and ILSE HOFFMANN

American Health Foundation
Valhalla, New York

### I. Introduction

Epidemiologic studies have clearly established that smoking of cigarettes, cigars, and pipes is causally associated with cancer of the lung and cancer of the upper respiratory tract [1,2] (see Chapter 26). Laboratory studies have substantiated epidemiologic observations with bioassays and by identifying specific carcinogens, cocarcinogens, and tumor promoters in tobacco smoke. Such investigations have also helped to elucidate mechanisms involved in cancer causation by tobacco smoke and its constituents. Since many millions of people continue to smoke cigarettes despite health warnings and health promotion efforts, laboratory studies should monitor new tobacco products and provide an impetus and guidance for reducing toxic and carcinogenic agents in tobacco smoke. In addition, there is the challenge and the opportunity for exploring the chemoprevention of cancer of the respiratory tract.

### II. Physicochemical Nature of Tobacco Smoke

The burning of tobacco generates mainstream smoke (MS) during puff drawing and sidestream smoke (SS) during smoldering between puffs. The physicochemical nature of these smoke aerosols, and the concentrations of carcinogens in them, are functions of several factors: the type of tobacco burned, the temperatures during puff drawing (860 to 900°C) and during smoldering (500 to 650°C), the intensity of puff drawing, the characteristics of the reducing atmospheres in the burning cone, and the overall physical design of the tobacco product (e.g., length; circumference; nature and porosity of wrapper, pipe bowl, or cigarette paper; type of filter tip).

The chemical and physical makeup of the tobacco in cigarettes has a profound influence on the composition, toxicity, and tumorigenic activity of the smoke. Cigarettes in the United States, Japan, and most European countries are composed of blends of bright, burley, and oriental tobaccos, while most cigarettes in the United Kingdom and Finland contain exclusively bright (flue-cured) tobaccos. These bright and blended cigarettes deliver a weakly acidic mainstream smoke (pH 5.5 to 6.2) in which nicotine occurs in its protonated form in the particulate matter. In France, some parts of Germany, Switzerland, Italy, North Africa, and South America, a high percentage of the cigarettes contain mainly burley (air-cured) tobaccos. Smoke of burley and black cigarettes is initially neutral but later puffs produce weakly alkaline smoke (pH 6.8 to 7.5), and at that point a portion of the nicotine is present in the vapor phase. The smoke of cigars is neutral to alkaline (pH 6.5 to 8.0); thus it also contains primarily unprotonated nicotine. Sidestream smoke of cigarettes and cigars has a pH range of 6.8 to 8.5 [3]. Unprotonated nicotine is more rapidly absorbed in the buccal mucosa than is protonated nicotine [4]; this is probably one of the reasons why the primary cigar smoker tends not to inhale the smoke.

MS and SS components are generated along different pathways. Some compounds are partially transferred unchanged from the tobacco into the smoke (e.g., nicotine, some wax constituents), others are products of pyrolysis and pyrosynthesis from nonspecific precursors (e.g., carbon monoxide, benzo[a]pyrene), and still others are partially transferred and partially pyrosynthesized (e.g., nitrosamines, volatile aldehydes). However, most smoke constituents are produced by partial degradation or by oxidation of specific precursors (e.g., furans, indoles, flavor components from specific tobacco terpenoids); some may also stem entirely from specific tobacco constituents (e.g., hydrogen cyanide, nitrogen oxides, ammonia) [5–7].

Tobacco smoke is an aerosol composed of volatile compounds present in the gas phase and of semivolatiles and nonvolatiles in the particulate phase. The 400 to 500 mg of mainstream smoke emerging from the mouthpiece of a cigarette contains about $10^9$ particles per milliliter, ranging in diameter from 0.1 to 1.0 μm (mean diameter 0.25 μm) [8]. About 95% of the MS of a nonfilter cigarette is comprised of 400 to 500 individual gaseous compounds, of which nitrogen, oxygen, and carbon dioxide constitute the major ones. The remainder of the smoke weight is given by more than 3500 individual components in the particulate phase [9].

For chemical analysis, cigarette smoke is separated arbitrarily into a vapor phase and a particulate phase. Individual compounds, of which more than 50% appear in the vapor phase of freshly generated MS, are considered volatile smoke components, all others belong to the particulate phase (Fig. 1). Tables 1 and 2 list the major types of compounds identified and their estimated concentration in the smoke of one cigarette [1,5,7,11–14]. The quantitative data presented here are derived from cigarettes that were machine smoked under standardized laboratory conditions [15]. These data do not fully reflect the yields obtained when humans smoke cigarettes. This applies especially to the smoking of low-yield cigarettes, during which the smoker tends to compensate for the low nicotine delivery by drawing puffs more intensely and by inhaling the smoke more deeply [16–18].

Tobacco contains at least 30 metals, with potassium, calcium, and magnesium as the major metals [19]. These metals are not listed in Table 2 because less than 1% of them transfer from the tobacco into the smoke [20]. Tables 1 and 2 also lack a description of the chemical nature and a listing of the concentrations in smoke of agricultural chemicals and pesticides which occur as a result of their use in tobacco cultivation and/or postharvest treatments [11,21]. Information about the specific chemicals and their applied amounts varies greatly from country to country and is therefore excluded from the tables. One has to

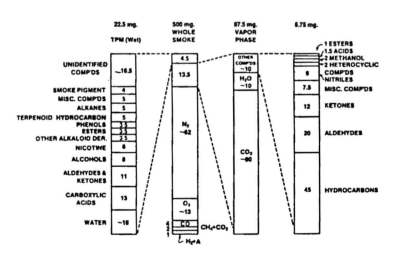

**Figure 1**  Total cigarette composition (% w/w). (From ref. 10.)

**Table 1**  Major Constituents of the Vapor Phase of the Mainstream Smoke of Nonfilter Cigarettes

| Compound[a] | Concentration/cigarette (% of total effluent) |
|---|---|
| Nitrogen | 280–320 mg (56–64%) |
| Oxygen | 50–70 mg (11–14%) |
| Carbon dioxide | 45–65 mg (9–13%) |
| Carbon monoxide | 14–23 mg (2.8–4.6%) |
| Water | 7–12 mg (1.4–2.4%) |
| Argon | 5 mg (1.0%) |
| Hydrogen | 0.5–1.0 mg |
| Ammonia | 10–130 μg |
| Nitrogen oxides (NO$_x$) | 100–600 μg |
| Hydrogen cyanide | 400–500 μg |
| Hydrogen sulfide | 20–90 μg |
| Methane | 1.0–2.0 mg |
| Other volatile alkanes (20) | 1.0–1.6 mg[b] |
| Volatile alkenes (16) | 0.4–0.5 mg |
| Isoprene | 0.2–0.4 mg |
| Butadiene | 25–40 μg |
| Acetylene | 20–35 μg |
| Benzene | 12–50 μg |
| Toluene | 20–60 μg |
| Styrene | 10 μg |
| Other volatile aromatic hydrocarbons (29) | 15–30 μg |
| Formic acid | 200–600 μg |
| Acetic acid | 300–1700 μg |
| Propionic acid | 100–300 μg |
| Methyl formate | 20–30 μg |
| Other volatile acids (6) | 5–10 μg |
| Formaldehyde | 20–100 μg |
| Acetaldehyde | 400–1400 μg |
| Acrolein | 60–140 μg |
| Other volatile aldehydes (6) | 80–140 μg |
| Acetone | 100–650 μg |
| Other volatile ketones (3) | 50–100 μg |
| Methanol | 80–180 μg |
| Other volatile alcohols (7) | 10–30 μg |
| Acetonitrile | 100–150 μg |
| Other volatile nitriles (10) | 50–80 μg[b] |
| Furan | 20–40 μg |
| Other volatile furans (4) | 45–125 μg[b] |
| Pyridine | 20–200 μg |
| Picolines (3) | 15–80 μg |
| 3-Vinylpyridine | 10–30 μg |
| Other volatile pyridines (25) | 20–50 μg[b] |
| Pyrrole | 0.1–10 μg |
| Pyrrolidine | 10–18 μg |
| N-Methylpyrrolidine | 2.0–3.0 μg |
| Volatile pyrazines (18) | 3.0–8.0 μg |
| Methylamine | 4–10μg |
| Other aliphatic amines (32) | 3–10 μg |

[a]Numbers in parentheses represent the individual compounds identified in a given group.
[b]Estimate.

**Table 2** Major Constituents of the Particulate Matter of the Mainstream Smoke of Nonfilter Cigarettes

| Compound[a] | μg/cigarette[b] |
|---|---|
| Nicotine | 1000–3000 |
| Nornicotine | 50–150 |
| Anatabine | 5–15 |
| Anabasine | 5–12 |
| Other tobacco alkaloids (17) | n.a. |
| Bipyridyls (4) | 10–30 |
| n-Hentriacontane ($n$-$C_{31}H_{64}$)[c] | 100 |
| Total nonvolatile hydrocarbons (45)[c] | 300–400[c] |
| Naphthalene | 2–4 |
| Naphthalenes (23) | 3–6[c] |
| Phenanthrenes (7) | 0.2–0.4[c] |
| Anthracenes (5) | 0.05–0.1[c] |
| Fluorenes (7) | 0.6–1.0[c] |
| Pyrenes (6) | 0.3–0.5[c] |
| Fluoranthenes (5) | 0.3–0.45[c] |
| Carcinogenic polynuclear aromatic hydrocarbons (11)[d] | 0.1–0.25 |
| Phenol | 80–160 |
| Other phenols (45)[c] | 60–180[c] |
| Catechol | 200–400 |
| Other catechols (4) | 100–200[c] |
| Other dihydroxybenzenes (10) | 200–400[c] |
| Scopoletin | 15–30 |
| Other polyphenols (8)[c] | n.a. |
| Cyclotenes (10)[c] | 40–70[c] |
| Quinones (7) | 0.5 |
| Solanesol | 600–1000 |
| Neophytadienes (4) | 200–350 |
| Limonene | 30–60 |
| Other terpenes (200–250)[c] | n.a. |
| Palmitic acid | 100–150 |
| Stearic acid | 50–75 |
| Oleic acid | 40–110 |
| Linoleic acid | 150–250 |
| Linolenic acid | 150–250 |
| Lactic acid | 60–80 |
| Indole | 10–15 |
| Skatole | 12–16 |
| Other indoles (13) | n.a. |
| Quinolines (7) | 2–4 |
| Other aza-arenes (55) | n.a. |
| Benzofurans (4) | 200–300 |
| Other O-heterocyclic compounds (42) | n.a. |
| Stigmasterol | 40–70 |
| Sitosterol | 30–40 |
| Campesterol | 20–30 |
| Cholesterol | 10–20 |
| Aniline | 0.36 |
| Toluidines | 0.23 |
| Other aromatic amines (12) | 0.25 |
| Tobacco-specific N-nitrosamines (6)[d] | 0.34–2.7 |
| Glycerol | 120 |

[a]Numbers in parentheses represent individual compounds identified.
[b]n.a., Not available.
[c]Estimate.
[d]For details, see Table 3.

bear in mind, though, that some portions of the residues of such chemicals remain on the tobacco and transfer into the smoke. Flavor additives have also been omitted from these tabulations. Such aromatic compounds are employed especially in the manufacture of low-yield cigarettes [22]. Except for menthol, which does not seem to decompose during smoking ($\leq$ 10 mg/U.S. cigarette [23]), the flavor additives appear in the smoke either unchanged or partially altered by combustion [22]. The nature of flavor additives is a trade secret; thus little is published about them or their transfer rates into the smoke and their fate during combustion. However, it is well known that the use of coumarin as a flavor additive to tobacco has been discontinued in many countries because it is carcinogenic in rats.

## III. Bioassays

Since the early 1960s remarkable progress has been achieved in respiratory carcinogenesis. We have become well aware of the existence of carcinogens with organ specificity for the respiratory tract of laboratory animals, and bioassays of aerosols and volatilized chemicals have also provided considerable evidence for their potential to induce tumors in the respiratory tract of mice, rats, and hamsters [24].

Three decades ago, the Leuchtenbergers reported the first extensive inhalation experiments in which mice were exposed daily to air-diluted cigarette smoke in specially designed chambers [25]. This smoke exposure led to early histological, cytological, and cytochemical changes in the major bronchi of the mice. The smoke exposure also caused various degrees of bronchitis associated with atypical proliferation of the bronchial epithelium. The investigators reported that after long-term exposure to cigarette smoke aerosols, all mice showed extracellular deposition of brown pigment in the lung. After about 12 to 15 months, smoke-exposed mice began to develop lung adenoma and lung adenocarcinoma in significantly higher numbers than did the control mice. In inhalation studies with the gas phase of cigarette smoke, lung adenomas have also been observed, though to a significantly lesser extent than with the whole smoke [26]. The findings of the Leuchtenbergers [25,26] were confirmed by Otto, who passively exposed inbred albino mice to cigarette smoke on a daily basis. After at least 12 months of smoke exposure, 23 of 60 mice developed lung adenomas, whereas only 3 of 60 control mice were found with such tumors. One mouse in the exposed group developed a squamous cell carcinoma of the lung after 16 months [27]. Several criticisms have been voiced with regard to the induction of lung adenoma and lung adenocarcinoma in mice by passive exposure to cigarette smoke. Concerns include the fact that such exposures caused tumors in the peripheral lung, not in the bronchi, and that some of the tested strains of mice had a relatively high rate of spontaneous lung adenomas. Today we are aware that the incidence of lung adenocarcinoma (and not only carcinoma in the bronchi) is significantly increased in cigarette smokers and that such tumors are even seen in nonsmokers who have been exposed to environmental tobacco smoke, to carcinogenic chemicals, or to radiation [2]. In the past it was also not understood how the topical application of tobacco "tar" to the skin of these strains of mice could lead to the development of lung adenoma and adenocarcinoma. Today, we are aware that tobacco smoke contains agents such as the tobacco-specific *N*-nitrosamines which induce lung adenoma and adenocarcinoma upon topical application to the skin of mice [28].

A major breakthrough in inhalation assays came through the development of new smoke-inhalation devices that facilitate inhalation of diluted tobacco smoke aerosols [29–31]. When 80 rats were exposed seven times daily for intermittent periods (8.4 × 30 seconds) to 10% cigarette smoke aerosol for up to 2.5 years, most animals developed hyperplastic and metaplastic changes in the nasal turbinals, larynges, and tracheas. Seven of the 80 smoke-exposed F344 female rats developed tumors in the respiratory tract, including one adenocarcinoma and one squamous cell carcinoma in the lung, compared to one alveologenic carcinoma only in the 93 control rats [32].

Dontenwill and associates developed the Hamburg II smoke inhalation device, in which small animals can be exposed to air-diluted smoke (Fig. 2). Eighteen groups, each consisting of 80 female and 80 male random-bred Syrian golden hamsters, comprised this cigarette smoke inhalation lifetime assay. Animals in group 1 were exposed once a day for about 10 min to air-diluted smoke (7:1), those in group 2 had twice-daily exposures to diluted smoke, hamsters in group 3 had three exposures to diluted smoke, those in group 4 were exposed twice daily to the gas phase of diluted smoke, and group 5 consisted of sham-treated controls. In group 1, 38 animals developed papilloma and one animal had a carcinoma of the larynx (total 24%), hamsters in group 2 developed 69 papillomas and 17 carcinomas of the larynx (total 54%), corresponding tumor yields in group 3 were 77 papillomas and 11 carcinomas of the larynx (total 55%), and laryngeal tumors were not observed in group 4 (gas phase only) or in group 5 (controls). Three hamsters in group 2 developed papilloma of the pharynx; tumors of the lung were not seen in any of the hamsters in this study [33].

In another assay, male Syrian golden hamsters from two inbred lines were exposed five times a week for up to 100 weeks to air-diluted smoke. In one inbred strain, 7 of 102 hamsters developed papilloma in the larynx, 9 had microinvasive cancer; in the second inbred strain, 11 of 102 animals had papilloma and 2 microinvasive cancers occurred in the larynx; none of the control hamsters developed laryngeal tumors [34]. In a dose–response lifetime study with hamsters of a strain that is susceptible to the induction of laryngeal tumors,

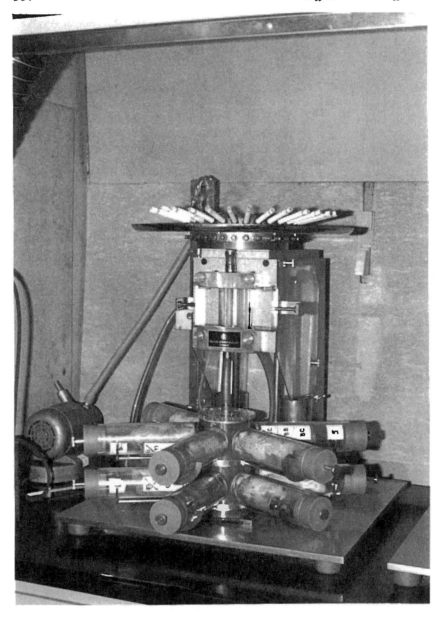

**Figure 2**   Hamburg II smoke inhalation device for 10 hamsters. (From ref. 44.)

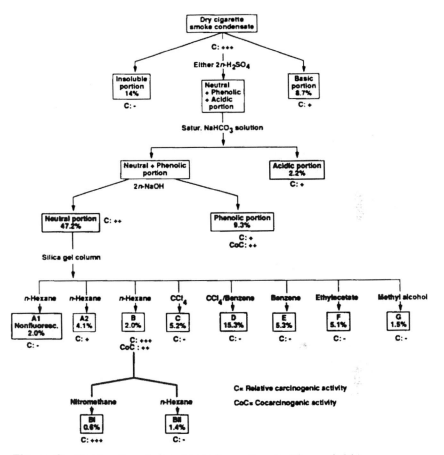

**Figure 3** Fractionation of cigarette smoke condensate. (From ref. 36.)

70% of the animals responded to twice-daily exposures to 22% cigarette smoke with papilloma and 47% with carcinoma of the larynx. The corresponding incidences in the hamsters exposed to 11% cigarette smoke twice daily were 27% and 7%, and in the control group 6% and 0%, respectively. In the high-dose group, 3 of 62 hamsters developed also tracheal papillomas [35].

## IV. Respiratory Carcinogens in Tobacco Smoke

Inhalation studies with Syrian golden hamsters have demonstrated that only whole smoke induces benign and malignant tumors of the respiratory tract in a

**Table 3** Tumorigenic Agents in Tobacco and Tobacco Smoke

| Compound | In processed tobacco[a] (per gram) | In mainstream smoke[a] (per cigarette) | IARC evaluation of evidence of carcinogenicity[b] | |
|---|---|---|---|---|
| | | | In laboratory animals | In humans |
| PAHs[c] | | | | |
| Benz[a]anthracene | | 20–70 ng | Sufficient | |
| Benzo[b]fluoranthene | | 4–22 ng | Sufficient | |
| Benzo[j]fluoranthene | | 6–21 ng | Sufficient | |
| Benzo[k]fluoranthene | | 6–12 ng | Sufficient | |
| Benzo[a]pyrene | 0.1–90 ng | 20–40 ng | Sufficient | Probable |
| Chrysene | | 40–60 ng | Sufficient | |
| Dibenz[a,h]anthracene | | 4 ng | Sufficient | |
| Dibenzo[a,i]pyrene | | 1.7–3.2 ng | Sufficient | |
| Dibenzo[a,l]pyrene | | present | Sufficient | |
| Indeno[1,2,3-cd]pyrene | | 4–20 ng | Sufficient | |
| 5-Methylchrysene | | 0.6 ng | Sufficient | |
| Aza-arenes | | | | |
| Quinoline | | 1–2 μg | | |
| Dibenz[a,h]acridine | | 0.1 ng | Sufficient | |
| Dibenz[a,j]acridine | | 3–10 ng | Sufficient | |
| 7H-Dibenzo[c,g]-carbazole | | 0.7 ng | Sufficient | Sufficient |
| N-Nitrosamines | | | | |
| N-Nitrosodimethylamine | ND–215 ng | 0.1–180 ng | Sufficient | |
| N-Nitrosoethylmethylamine | | 3–13 ng | Sufficient | |
| N-Nitrosodiethylamine | | ND–25 ng | Sufficient | |
| N-Nitrosonornicotine | 0.3–89 μg | 0.12–3.7 μg | Sufficient | |
| 4-(Methylnitrosamino)-1-(3-pyridyl)-1-butanone | 0.2–7 μg | 0.08–0.77 μg | Sufficient | |
| N'-Nitrosoanabasine | 0.01–1.9 μg | 0.14–4.6 μg | Limited | |
| N-Nitrosomorpholine | ND–690 ng | | Sufficient | |

| | | | | |
|---|---|---|---|---|
| Aromatic amines | | | | |
| 2-Toluidine | | 30–200 ng | Sufficient | Inadequate |
| 2-Naphthylamine | | 1–22 ng | Sufficient | Sufficient |
| 4-Aminobiphenyl | | 2–5 ng | Sufficient | Sufficient |
| Aldehydes | | | | |
| Formaldehyde | 1.6–7.4 µg | 70–100 µg[d] | Sufficient | Limited |
| Acetaldehyde | 1.4–7.4 µg | 18–1400 µg[d] | Sufficient | Inadequate |
| Crotonaldehyde | 0.2–2.4 µg | 10–20 µg | | |
| Miscellaneous organic compounds | | | | |
| Benzene | | 12–48 µg | Sufficient | Sufficient |
| Acrylonitrile | | 3.2–15 µg | Sufficient | Limited |
| 1,1-Dimethylhydrazine | 60–147 µg | | Sufficient | |
| 2-Nitropropane | | 0.73–1.21 µg | Sufficient | |
| Ethylcarbamate | 310–375 ng | 20–38 ng | Sufficient | |
| Vinyl chloride | | 1–16 ng | Sufficient | Sufficient |
| Inorganic compounds | | | | |
| Hydrazine | 14–51 ng | 24–43 ng | Sufficient | Inadequate |
| Arsenic | 500–900 ng | 40–120 ng | Inadequate | Sufficient |
| Nickel | 2000–6000 ng | 0–600 ng | Sufficient | Limited |
| Chromium | 1000–2000 ng | 4–70 ng | Sufficient | Sufficient |
| Cadmium | 1300–1600 ng | 41–62 ng | Sufficient | Limited |
| Lead | 8–10 µg | 35–85 ng | Sufficient | Inadequate |
| Polonium-210 | 0.2–1.2 pCi | 0.03–1.0 pCi | Sufficient | Sufficient |

[a]ND, not detected.

[b]No designation indicates that an evaluation by IARC has not been carried out.

[c]PAHs, polynuclear aromatic hydrocarbons.

[d]The 4th report of the Independent Scientific Committee on Smoking and Health (1988) published values for the 14 leading British cigarettes in 1986 (51.4% of the market) of 20 to 105 µg/cigarette (mean 59 µg) for formaldehyde and 550 to 1150 µg/cigarette (mean 910 µg) for acetaldehyde.

**Table 4**  Likely Causative Agents for Tobacco Smoke-Related Cancers

| Organ(s) | Carcinogen or tumor initiator[a] | Enhancing agents |
|---|---|---|
| Respiratory tract, including larynx | NNK<br>PAHs<br>Polonium-210 (minor factor)<br>Acetaldehyde, formaldehyde | Catechol (cocarcinogen)<br>Weakly acidic tumor promoters<br>Acrolein |
| Esophagus | NNN<br>Volatile nitrosamines (?) | Ethanol<br>Catechols |
| Pancreas | NNK, NNAL | Nutrition |
| Bladder | 4-Aminobiphenyl<br>2-Naphthylamine<br>2-Toluidine | Infectious-agents (?) |
| Oral cavity | NNN, NNK<br>PAHs | Ethanol<br>HSV-1 and HSV-2<br>Nutrition |

[a]PAHs, polynuclear aromatic hydrocarbons; NNN, $N'$-nitrosonornicotine; NNK, 4-(methylnitrosamino)-1-(3-pyridyl)-1-butanone; NNAL, 4-(methylnitrosamino)-1-(3-pyridyl)-1-butanol.

dose-dependent fashion; however, inhalation of smoke that is free of particulate matter (tar) does not lead to tumors. This indicates that the dose of carcinogens in the gas phase by itself is not sufficient to induce tumors and that the majority of the carcinogens reside in the particulate matter of tobacco smoke. This consideration has led to in-depth fractionation studies and bioassays in mice, rats, and rabbits with tobacco smoke condensate [11,36,37]. The neutral subfractions B and B1, which contain a concentrate of the polynuclear aromatic hydrocarbons (PAHs), harbor the major tumor initiators (Fig. 3). The PAH subfraction is also the only portion of the tar that upon repeated intratracheal instillation elicits tumors in the respiratory tract of rats [38]. However, assays of the PAH concentrate explain only a small fraction of the total carcinogenicity of the tar. Results from bioassays of the PAH subfraction in combination with the weakly acidic, noncarcinogenic fraction explain 75 to 90% of the total carcinogenicity of the tar [36,37]. The weakly acidic fraction contains the major tumor promoters, the volatile phenols, and the major cocarcinogens, the catechols. In addition to tumor initiators, tumor promoters, and cocarcinogens, tobacco smoke contains carcinogens with organ specificity. These act independent of the mode of exposure or site of application by inducing benign and malignant tumors in specific organs. Table 3 presents a list of the known tumorigenic agents in tobacco smoke, their concentrations in the smoke of one cigarette, and the evaluation of evidence of their carcinogenicity by the International Agency for Research on Cancer [39,40]. Table 4 is a list of the likely causative agents for tobacco smoke-related cancers on the basis of organ specificity of carcinogens and their various biological activities and concentrations in cigarette smoke.

The agents in tobacco smoke most likely to cause induction of cancer of the respiratory tract are PAHs, the tobacco-specific *N*-nitrosamine 4-(methylnitrosamino)-1-(3-pyridyl)-1-butanone (NNK), volatile aldehydes, acetylaldehyde, formaldehyde, and to a minor extent, polonium-210 (which stems from agricultural and environmental sources).

### A. Polynuclear Aromatic Hydrocarbons

It has been established that PAHs induce tumors in the respiratory tract of hamsters upon intratracheal instillation [41]. PAHs also induce lung tumors upon implanation in the lung with beeswax as a carrier. This protocol has also been employed successfully with tobacco smoke condensates [42,43]. The PAH concentrate of cigarette smoke condensate is the only fraction that upon repeated intratracheal instillation induces squamous cell tumors in the lungs of rats [38]. Pretreatment of hamsters with a tumor-initiating PAH by intratracheal instillation followed by tobacco smoke exposure leads to a high incidence of respiratory tract tumors, consistent with the initiation (PAH) promotion model [44]. The levels of exposure to PAHs experienced by smokers are not inconsistent with their potential role as causative agents for respiratory tract cancer.

### B. Tobacco-Specific *N*-Nitrosamines

During the processing of tobacco and during smoking, the *Nicotania* alkaloids are partically N-nitrosated to tobacco-specific *N*-nitrosamines (TSNAs). So far, seven TSNAs have been identified in tobacco products (Fig. 4) [7]. Of these *N'*-nitrosonornicotine (NNN), 4-(methylnitrosamino)-1-(3-pyridyl)-1-butanone (NNK), and its reduction product 4-(methylnitrosamino)-1-(3-pyridyl)-1-butanol (NNAL) derive directly from the major tobacco alkaloid, nicotine. Their formation depends primarily on the nitrate/nitrite content of the tobacco. The smoke of one cigarette yields 0.025 to 1.0 μg of NNN and 0.02 to 0.5 μg of NNK per cigarette [7]. Of the seven known TSNAs, NNN, NNK, and NNAL are powerful carcinogens that induce benign and malignant tumors of the lung, nasal cavity, esophagus, pancreas, and/or liver of mice, rats, and hamsters (Table 5). NNK, a specific lung carcinogen in laboratory animals, causes benign and malignant tumors in the bronchi and peripheral lungs. A single dose of 0.7 mg of NNK/rat (9 μmol/kg) is sufficient to induce a significant number of lung tumors [46]. The cumulative dose of this carcinogen that reaches the respiratory tract of a heavy smoker (40 cigarettes daily) during 40 years amounts to 10 μmol of NNK/kg body weight [47]. Although a comparison of human and animal data is based on some assumptions and disregards the fact that additional exposure may come from endogenously formed NNN and NNK (inhaled nicotine may be nitrosated) [48], this computation supports

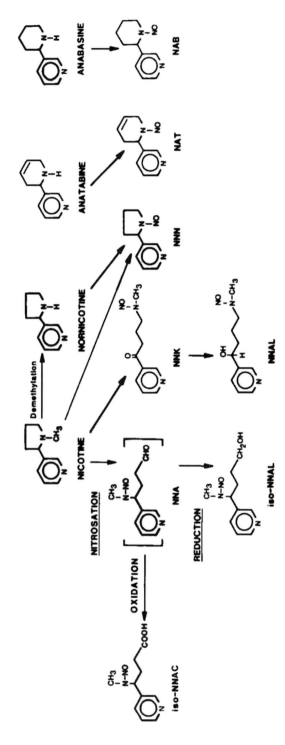

**Figure 4** Formation of tobacco-specific *N*-nitrosamines.

**Table 5** Carcinogenicity of Tobacco-Specific *N*-nitrosamines (TSNAs)

| TSNA[a] | Animal (strain) | Route of application | Principal target organ | Dose (mmol/animal) |
|---|---|---|---|---|
| NNN | | | | |
| | Mouse | Topical (TI)[b] | None | 0.028 |
| | Mouse (A/J) | Intraperitoneal | Lung | 0.1 |
| | Rat (F344) | Subcutaneous | Nasal cavity, esophagus | 0.2–3.4 |
| | | Oral | Esophagus, nasal cavity | 1.0–3.6 |
| | Rat (Sprague–Dawley) | Oral | Nasal cavity | 8.8 |
| | Syrian golden hamster | Subcutaneous | Trachea, nasal cavity | 0.9–2.1 |
| NNAL | | | | |
| | Mouse (A/J) | Intraperitoneal | Lung | 0.12 |
| | Rat (F344) | Oral (drinking water) | Lung, pancreas | 0.32 |
| NAB | | | | |
| | Rat (F344) | Oral | Esophagus | 3–12 |
| | Syrian golden hamster | Subcutaneous | None | 2 |
| NAT | | | | |
| | Rat (F344) | Subcutaneous | None | 2.8 |
| iso-NNAC | | | | |
| | Mouse (A/J) | Intraperitoneal | None | 0.2 |
| NNK | | | | |
| | Mouse(Sencar) | Topical (TI) | Skin | 0.028 |
| | | Topical | Lung | 0.6–1.2 |
| | Mouse (A/J) | Intraperitoneal | Lung | 0.01–0.12 |
| | Rat (F344) | Subcutaneous | Lung, nasal cavity, liver | 0.2–2.8 |
| | | Oral (drinking water) | Lung, liver, pancreas | 0.075–0.31 |
| | | Oral (gavage) | Liver, lung | 1.3 |
| | | Intravesical | Lung, liver | 1.5 |

*Source*: Ref. 45.
[a]NNN, *N*'-nitrosonornicotine; NNAL, 4-(methylnitrosamino)-1-(3-pyridyl)-1-butanol; NAB, *N*'-nitrosoanabasine; NAT, *N*'-nitrosoanatabine; iso-NNAC, 4-(methylnitrosamino)-4-(3-pyridyl)butyric acid. NNK, 4-(methylnitrosamino)-1-(3-pyridyl)-1-butanone.
[b]TI, tumor-initiating assay with TPA as promoter.

the concept that NNK, and possibly other TSNAs, play a major role in respiratory carcinogenesis in tobacco smokers. Biochemical studies (discussed later) strengthen this view.

### C.  Volatile Aldehydes

Studies of the chronic inhalation of formaldehyde (14 ppm) and acetaldehyde (1000 to 3000 ppm) have demonstrated that these compounds cause tumors of the nasal cavity in rats [49]. Since rats are obligatory nose breathers, one may deduce that the aldehydes are contact carcinogens. As such they would be expected to affect the lungs in humans. In 40 years of smoking at a rate of 40 cigarettes per day, exposure to formaldehyde (100 μg/cigarette) and acetaldehyde (1000 μg/cigarette) would amount to about 58 g and 580 g, respectively. These doses are at least 100- to 1000-fold higher than those of PAHs and $N$-nitrosamines, the other major respiratory carcinogens in tobacco smoke. Together with hydrogen cyanide, the volatile aldehydes are also the major ciliatoxic agents in tobacco smoke that inhibit lung clearance [11].

### D.  Polonium-210 ($^{210}$Po)

Tobacco smoke contains 0.03 to 1.0 pCi polonium-210 ($^{210}$Po) per cigarette. The sources of $^{210}$Po, which transfers from the tobacco into the smoke, are certain fertilizers with high $^{210}$Po content [50] and/or airborne $^{210}$Po, which is trapped by the glandular hair (trichomes) found on the surface of tobacco leaves [51]. The $\alpha$-particle-emitting element $^{210}$Po induces lung tumors upon inhalation in rats and upon intratracheal instillation in Syrian golden hamsters. The levels of $^{210}$Po measured in the lungs of smokers are generally three times higher than those in nonsmokers [52]. The U.S. National Council on Radiation Protection and Measurement ascribed about 1% of the risk of lung cancer after 50 years of cigarette smoking to polonium-210 inhaled from the smoke [53].

## V.  Environmental Tobacco Smoke

Epidemiologic studies have incriminated exposure to environmental tobacco smoke (ETS) as a risk factor for lung cancer in nonsmokers [54–58]. In fact, it has been estimated that nonsmokers living with cigarette-smoking spouses have an about 30% higher risk for lung cancer than do nonsmokers who live with nonsmoking spouses [54]. However, this estimate has been challenged. In 1985, the IARC considered the available epidemiologic data as inconclusive [1]. Nevertheless, a biological basis for an association between ETS exposure and lung cancer clearly exists. Agents resulting from the incomplete combustion of tobacco, which are known carcinogens, are inhaled as indoor air pollutants and are retained in the respiratory tract of the nonsmoker. The IARC concluded its review by stating that "because of its physicochemical nature and in view of known concepts of chemical carcinogenesis, passive smoking gives rise to some risk of cancer" [1]. This evaluation emphasizes that epidemiologic methods may not be sufficiently sensitive for establishing a risk factor for cancer from environmental smoke exposure.

The smoke generated between puff drawing is sidestream smoke (SS) [54]. When it is obtained under standardized laboratory conditions, fresh undiluted SS contains far higher concentrations of toxic and tumorigenic agents than does mainstream smoke (MS). The release of carcinogenic volatile N-nitrosamines and aromatic amines into SS is remarkably high [1,54,55,59,60]. Table 6 presents

**Table 6** Some Toxic and Tumorigenic Agents in Undiluted Cigarette Sidestream Smoke

| Compound | Type of toxicity[a] | Amount of sidestream smoke per cigarette | Sidestream/mainstream smoke ratio |
|---|---|---|---|
| Vapor phase | | | |
| Carbon monoxide | T | 26.8–61 mg | 2.5–14.9 |
| Carbonyl sulfide | T | 2–3 $\mu$g | 0.03–0.13 |
| Benzene | C | 240–490 $\mu$g | 8–10 |
| Formaldehyde | C | 1500 $\mu$g | 50 |
| 3-Vinylpyridine | T | 330–450 $\mu$g | 24–34 |
| Hydrogen cyanide | T | 14–110 $\mu$g | 0.06–0.4 |
| Hydrazine | C | 90 ng | 3 |
| Nitrogen oxides ($NO_x$) | T | 500–2000 $\mu$g | 3.7–12.8 |
| N-Nitrosodimethylamine | C | 200–1040 ng | 20–130 |
| N-Nitrosopyrrolidine | C | 30–390 ng | 6–120 |
| Particulate phase | | | |
| Tar | C | 14–30 mg | 1.1–15.7 |
| Nicotine | T | 2.1–4.6 mg | 1.3–21 |
| Phenol | TP | 70–250 $\mu$g | 1.3–3.0 |
| Catechol | CoC | 58–290 $\mu$g | 0.67–12.8 |
| o-Toluidine | C | 3 $\mu$g | 18.7 |
| 2-Naphthylamine | C | 70 ng | 39 |
| 4-Aminobiphenyl | C | 140 ng | 31 |
| Benz[a]anthracene | C | 40–200 ng | 2–4 |
| Benzo[a]pyrene | C | 40–70 ng | 2.5–20 |
| Quinoline | C | 15–20 $\mu$g | 8–11 |
| NNN | C | 0.15–1.7 $\mu$g | 0.5–5.0 |
| NNK | C | 0.2–1.4 $\mu$g | 1.0–22 |
| N-Nitrosodiethanolamine | C | 43 ng | 1.2 |
| Cadmium | C | 0.72 $\mu$g | 7.2 |
| Nickel | C | 0.2–2.5 $\mu$g | 13–30 |
| Polonium-210 | C | 0.5–1.6 pCi | 1.06–3.7 |

[a]C, carcinogenic; CoC, cocarcinogenic; T, toxic; TP, tumor promoter.

data for agents in SS that are known carcinogens, tumor promoters, or cocarcinogens. In the Ames assay, SS appears to be slightly more genotoxic than does MS [62]. On a gram-to-gram basis, the particulate matter of SS is more carcinogenic on mouse skin than is the particulate matter of MS [11].

SS is the major source of ETS. Other sources are those gas-phase components that diffuse through the cigarette paper, the aerosol that escapes from the burning cone into the air, and that portion of MS that is not retained but is exhaled by the smoker. Table 7 presents published data on toxic and carcinogenic agents in smoke-polluted indoor environments [1,54,55,63,64]. The concentration of toxic agents in ETS appears quite low by comparison to their levels in undiluted smoke, but one needs to take into account the fact that the active inhalation of tobacco smoke is limited to the time it takes to smoke a cigarette, whereas inhalation of ETS may occur over several hours each day.

**Table 7**  Some Toxic and Tumorigenic Agents in Indoor Environments Polluted by Tobacco Smoke

| Pollutant | Location | Concentration/$m^3$ |
|-----------|----------|---------------------|
| Nitric oxide | Workrooms | 50–440 $\mu$g |
| | Restaurants | 17–240 $\mu$g |
| | Bar | 80–520 $\mu$g |
| | Cafeteria | 2.5–48 $\mu$g |
| Nitrogen dioxide | Workrooms | 68–410 $\mu$g |
| | Restaurants | 40–190 $\mu$g |
| | Bar | 2–116 $\mu$g |
| | Cafeteria | 67–200 $\mu$g |
| Hydrogen cyanide | Living room | 8–122 $\mu$g |
| Benzene | Public places | 20–317 $\mu$g |
| Formaldehyde | Living room | 23–50 $\mu$g |
| Acrolein | Public places | 30–120 $\mu$g |
| Acetone | Public places | 360–5800 $\mu$g |
| Phenols (volatile) | Coffee houses | 7.4–11.5 ng |
| *N*-Nitrosodimethylamine | Restaurants, public places | 0–240 ng |
| *N*-Nitrosodiethylamine | Restaurants, public places | 0–200 ng |
| Nicotine | Public places | 1–6 $\mu$g |
| | Restaurants | 3–10 $\mu$g |
| | Workrooms | 1–13.8 $\mu$g |
| Benzo[*a*]pyrene | Restaurants, public places | 3.3–144 ng |
| *N*'-Nitrosonornicotine | Bar, restaurant, car | 4–32 ng |
| 4-(Methylnitrosamino)-1-(3-pyridyl)-1-butanone | Bar, restaurant, car | 1–120 ng |

*Source*: Data from refs. 1, 54, 61, 63, and 64.

This is reflected in comparative measurements of the uptake of nicotine by active and passive smokers. In blood serum and in the urine of passive smokers, the concentration of cotinine, a major nicotine metabolite, amounts to about 0.5% of that of heavy cigarette smokers, reaching up to 2% in more heavily exposed persons [65–68]. Indicators other than nicotine and its metabolites which are also used to reflect the uptake of ETS are carboxyhemoglobin, thiocyanate, and 4-aminobiphenyl or TSNA adducts. These are not significantly elevated in the physiologic fluids of ETS-exposed persons, primarily because the levels of their corresponding indoor air pollutants are relatively low or can be derived from sources other than tobacco combustion [54,55,69]. It is highly desirable to develop other specific markers of uptake of tobacco constituents by passive smokers, especially biochemical markers for the uptake of carcinogenic agents from ETS.

## VI. Mechanism of Tobacco Carcinogenesis

An important task of the laboratory scientist is to elucidate the mechanisms involved in the causation of cancer by tobacco smoke and its constituents. This concept should also lead to a rationale for the prevention of cancer in tobacco smokers and beyond this to the reduction of cancer in the population at large. The major cancer-causing agents in tobacco smoke are procarcinogens, agents that require metabolic activation for exerting their genotoxic activity. Thus a major objective of carcinogenesis is to understand the enzymatic activation and detoxification of procarcinogens, binding of the activated species with cellular components, activation of proto-oncogenes by these adducts, and the inhibition of tumor suppressor genes. Since the active forms of the carcinogens react not only with DNA but also with protein, the latter adducts have been explored as markers for the exposure of the smoker to specific tobacco carcinogens.

### A. Polynuclear Aromatic Hydrocarbons

The mechanisms by which PAHs are metabolically activated (by P450 isozymes), interact with DNA, activate proto-oncogenes, and initiate the carcinogenic process have been reviewed in detail [70–72]. Studies have shown that diol epoxides with one carbon terminus of the epoxide ring in the bay region, such as (+)7α,8β-dihydroxy-9β,10β-epoxy-7,8,9,10-tetrahydrobenzo[a]pyrene [(+)-anti-BPDE] (Fig. 5), are major ultimate carcinogens of several carcinogenic PAHs that have been identified in MS and SS (Table 3). Similar mechanisms of activation are seen with carcinogenic methylated PAHs in tobacco smoke, such as 5-methylchrysene, with the additional structural requirement that the highly tumorigenic bay region diol epoxides have a methyl group and an epoxide ring in the same bay region [73]. These aspects are of importance in regard to tobacco

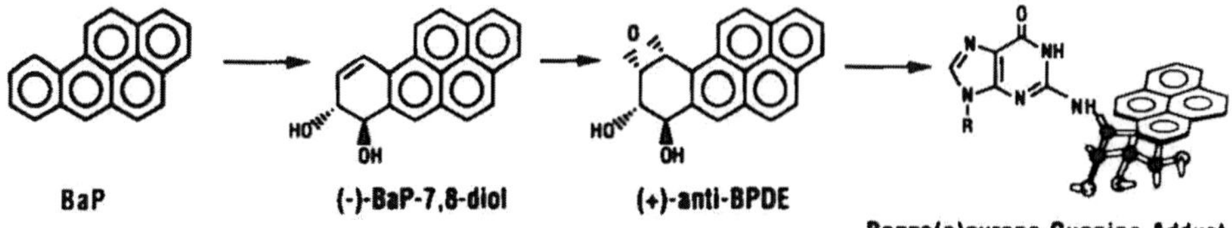

**Figure 5**   Benzo[a]pyrene: metabolic activation and binding to guanine. (From ref. 70.)

carcinogenesis because they provide a rationale for the high tumorigenicity on mouse and rabbit skin and in the lung of rats of the PAH-enriched subfraction of tobacco smoke condensate [36,38,74,75].

As discussed earlier, the carcinogenic activity of the PAH concentrate of tobacco smoke condensate is greatly accelerated when it is applied together with the inactive weakly acidic fraction. This observation is of major significance for the role of PAHs in tobacco carcinogenesis. Extensive fractionation studies have clearly shown that the weakly acidic fraction has both promoting and cocarcinogenic activities that accelerate the carcinogenic effects of PAHs [76]. The cocarcinogenic activity of tobacco smoke condensate, when measured on mouse skin, can largely be attributed to catechols [77,78], whereas the chemical nature of the tumor promoters remains largely unknown, although phenols contribute to this activity [76]. Studies of the effects of smoke condensate subfractions on normal human bronchial epithelial cells have led to the conclusion that the polaric neutral fraction is also likely to contain compounds with promoting activities [79].

The metabolically activated species of the carcinogenic PAHs are capable of covalently binding to cellular macromolecules (DNA, RNA, and proteins). In laboratory animals the carcinogenic potency of several types of genotoxic carcinogens, including PAHs, is generally correlated with their potential to form adducts with DNA [70,80].

Studies using the $^{32}$P-labeling method have shown that the DNA from lung tissue of smokers and nonsmokers contains multiple adducts, with levels and patterns varying greatly between individuals [81,82]. However, DNA adducts that were measured with the $^{32}$P-labeling method in tissues of the lung and larynx have generally demonstrated an association with cigarette smoking [81,82].

## B.   Tobacco-Specific N-Nitrosamines

The metabolism of TSNAs, especially that of $N'$-nitrosonornicotine (NNN) and 4-(methylnitrosamino)-1-(3-pyridyl)-1-butanone (NNK), has been investigated in vivo in laboratory animals as well as in vitro in subcellular fractions, cultured cells, and cultured tissues from animals and humans [45,83]. These studies have revealed various metabolic transformations, among which α-hydroxylation appears to be a key reaction since ultimately, it leads to the formation of adducts of TSNA metabolites with DNA and proteins. The metabolic pathways for NNN and NNK are summarized in Figure 6. In vivo assays with NNK in rats have shown that 7-methylguanine, $O^6$-methylguanine, and $O^4$-methylthymidine are formed in lung, liver, and nasal mucosa but not in other organs, such as esophagus, spleen, and kidney [83–85]. It is remarkable that DNA methylation has been detected consistently only in tissues that are known to be targets for tumor induction by NNK. This finding strengthens the concept of organ specificity of NNK for the lungs of rats, mice, and hamsters. Studies on $O^6$-methylguanine levels in lung DNA during chronic dosing with NNK have shown that this alkylated base accumulates and persists in part due to inhibition of the repair enzyme, $O^6$-methylguanine-DNA methyltransferase by high doses of NNK [85,86]. $O^6$-Methylguanine formation is particularly efficient in Clara cells.

These studies with the lung carcinogen NNK give rise to the mechanistic link between nicotine exposure and the formation of promutagenic adducts. In mice, NNK forms not only $O^6$-methylguanine in the lung and thereby causes miscoding due to DNA adduct formation and leads to lung adenoma, but importantly, these lung adenomas contain activated K-*ras* proto-oncogene [87]. Activated K-*ras* oncogene has also been found in specimens of lung adenocarcinomas from 41 of 141 cigarette smokers, and tobacco carcinogens appear to activate K-*ras* by point mutation on codon 12, [88]; thus K-*ras* oncogene activation is probably an important event in the pathogenesis of adenocarcinoma in the human lung. In a recent study the presence of K-*ras* point mutations at high frequency has been defined as occurring in a subgroup of lung cancer patients with very poor prognosis [89]. Figure 7 depicts the linkage of nicotine with lung tumor induction by means of the formation of NNK and its DNA adducts, which cause activation of the K-*ras* proto-oncogene. α-Hydroxylation of NNK leads not only to the formation of methyl diazohydroxide (compound 6, Fig. 6) but also to 4-(3-pyridyl)-4-oxobutyl diazohydroxide (compound 7). This intermediate is also formed by α-hydroxylation of NNN (Fig. 6). In vivo it can react with DNA and protein, as does the methylating intermediate methyl diazohydroxide. The formation of the keto alcohol (compound 9) upon hydrolysis of DNA and hemoglobin from animals treated with NNK or NNN is consistent with 4-(3-pyridyl)-4-oxybutylation by compound 7 [90–92].

The adduct formation of the metabolites of NNK and NNN with protein led to studies on dosimetry of exposure to the carcinogenic TSNAs in tobacco chewers and smokers by measuring hemoglobin adducts. Although there is a strong overlapping of the levels of hemoglobin-TSNA adducts in smokers and nonsmokers (including passive smokers), 7 of 40 smokers showed adduct levels

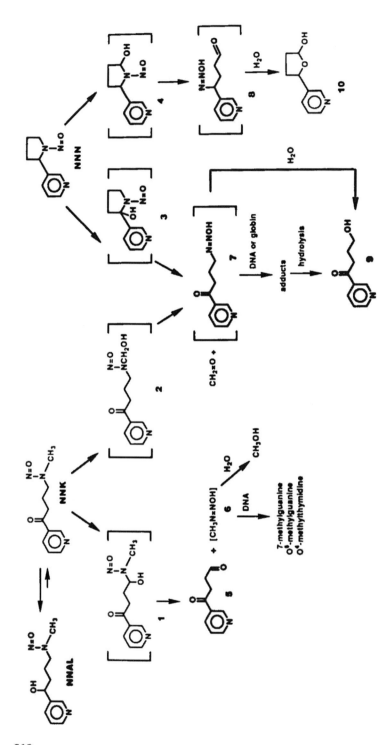

**Figure 6** Metabolic activation of NNK and NNN to hypothetical intermediates (shown in brackets) which bind to DNA and protein. (From ref. 45.)

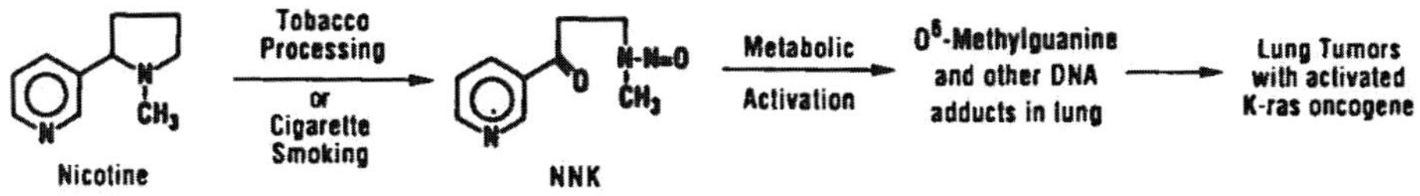

**Figure 7** Scheme linking nicotine to formation of DNA adducts including $O^6$-methylguanine. The latter leads to DNA miscoding and activation of K-*ras* oncogene and lung tumors.

to be clearly elevated above those in nonsmokers [93]. This suggests that some persons activate NNK and/or NNN more efficiently than others. One could conceivably develop methods that permit the identification of smokers with greater metabolic potential and/or with greater capacity for the endogenous nitrosation of alkaloids after inhalation or ingestion of *Nicotiana* alkaloids.

## VII. Reduction of Exposure to Tobacco Carcinogens

The commitment to create a smoke-free society deserves the full support of the medical and scientific community. Unfortunately, recent statistics on tobacco use do not appear to support this goal for the near future. According to the World Health Organization, the percentile increase in cigarette consumption from 1971–1975 to 1979–1981 in all parts of the world, except in Europe, has exceeded the increases in population. In Africa with a 23.4% population increase, there was a 41.5% increase in cigarette consumption, in Latin America the population grew by 24.5% and cigarette consumption by 31.4%, and in Asia these figures were 21.8% and 28.5%, respectively [94]. The trend of an increased cigarette consumption appears to continue throughout the world with the exception of Europe and North America. These statistics reinforce the need for health education about the harmful effects of cigarette smoking and for the widest availability of smoking cessation programs. These aspects are discussed more fully in Chapters 9 to 12 of this book. However, these figures also show that a strong case can be made for the need to reduce exposure to tobacco carcinogens. Principal approaches to this goal are (1) modification of tobacco products, and (2) inhibition of the metabolic activation of tobacco carcinogens and of endogenous formation of TSNAs by certain nutrients and chemopreventive agents.

### A. The Changing Cigarette

In a 1991 article we reviewed "Lung Cancer and the Changing Cigarette" [95]. Thus this topic is discussed only briefly here. Epidemiological studies have clearly shown a dose–response relationship between daily cigarette consumption and the risk of cancer of the lung, upper digestive tract, pancreas, and the urinary bladder (see Chapter 26). These findings on smokers are supported by dose–response observations in bioassays with whole cigarette smoke and with its particulate matter. Thus the reduction of smoke yields by cigarette modification was seen as the first practical approach to a reduction of the carcinogenicity of cigarette smoke. It was achieved primarily by changes in the design of cigarettes, most notably by the use of cellulose acetate filter tips, and by altering the composition of the cigarette tobacco and tobacco blends. Other changes in the makeup of manufactured cigarettes include utilization of porous cigarette paper and incorporation of reconstituted tobacco sheets, expanded tobacco lamina, and expanded tobacco midribs. In the past decade, reductions in smoke yields have also been achieved by reducing the diameter of cigarettes and especially, by using perforated filter tips. The latter dilute cigarette smoke up to 50% with air while maintaining the consumer acceptability of the cigarettes. The result is a drastic reduction in the sales-weighted tar and nicotine yields of commercial cigarettes in many developed countries, especially in Canada, the United States, the United Kingdom, Sweden, France, Germany, and Austria [95]. For example, the sales-weighted average tar and nicotine yields of American cigarettes have been reduced from 38 mg and 2.7 mg in 1955 to 13 mg and 1.0 mg, in 1991, respectively. In other countries, the tar yields of popular cigarettes are still higher than 22 mg [96,97].

Changes in the makeup of commercial cigarettes have also led to selective removal of certain toxic agents from the smokestream. The semivolatile phenols, for example, are removed from the mainstream smoke to a far greater extent than is tar by cellulose acetate filter tips with plasticizers. Carbon monoxide and other volatile toxic smoke components are selectively reduced by perforated filter tips, and the levels of carcinogenic PAHs in smoke can be selectively lowered by using tobacco that is rich in nitrate [95]. However, the reduction of PAHs in the smoke of high-nitrate tobaccos (1 to 2%) leads to an undesirable increase in the smoke levels of carcinogenic, volatile nitrosamines, and tobacco-specific $N$-nitrosamines [7]; thus the reduction of PAHs in tobacco smoke must be achieved by other means. While there is clearly some success in reducing harmful agents in the smoke of the low-yield cigarette, there are also concomitant undesirable effects. For example, to make the low-yield cigarette acceptable to the consumer, the tobacco blends formulated for these cigarettes are enhanced with flavor by selecting certain aromatic tobacco types and/or by adding aromatic concentrates from other tobaccos or other plants, or by adding synthetic flavoring compounds. This practice can inadvertently lead to the introduction of carcinogenic agents, as was the case with coumarin [98]. Since the formulations of flavoring agents are by and large trade secrets, governmental regulations are needed with respect to monitoring of products and setting permissible levels.

Also, it is important that scientists outside industrial laboratories who are concerned with the toxicology of tobacco products are made aware of this issue.

Finally, one has to be aware that the cigarette smoke yields reported for tar, nicotine, and other smoke components are obtained by machine smoking of cigarettes under standardized conditions; thus consideration needs to be given to the fact that most smokers of low-yield cigarettes compensate for the low nicotine delivery by smoking more intensely [16–18,99]. Nevertheless, these smokers do not generally compensate fully for low smoke yields, as is reflected by the fact that prolonged use of low-yield cigarettes reduces the risk of cancer to some extent [95] (see Chapter 26). However, the reduction in risk is only minor compared to the benefits of giving up cigarette smoking altogether.

### B. Chemopreventive Approaches

The use of natural and synthetic agents is a relatively recent attempt to reduce cancer risk. This approach to cancer prevention is based primarily on epidemiologic observations of protective effects exerted by certain vegetables and fruits. Such observations have been strengthened by findings from bioassays in laboratory animals and by biochemical studies. Nontoxic agents that hold promise as inhibitors of carcinogenesis, as well as micronutrients with such properties, are now being evaluated.

In the United States and in other developed nations, chemoprevention appears generally more acceptable than does the absolute elimination of carcinogens. This applies especially in cases where the reduction of exposure to carcinogens would require a change in diet, a reduction in alcohol consumption, or elimination of tobacco chewing or tobacco smoking. Micronutrients that are effective chemopreventive agents and appear to decrease the risk of cancer at various sites are vitamin A, $\beta$-carotene, and synthetic retinoids. Vitamins C and E, which are antioxidants, may at least partially prevent the generation of nitrosamines and mutagens during food formation and during the manufacture of consumer products; these antioxidants may also inhibit the endogenous formation of genotoxic agents upon consumption of their precursors. In the case of cigarette smokers, vitamin C clearly inhibits the endogenous formation of $N$-nitrosamines, as is reflected in a reduced urinary excretion of $N$-nitrosoproline [101]. Folic acid and folates, vitamin $B_{12}$, and other B vitamins may prevent the induction of cancerous lesions. Selenium may possibly have an anticancer effect [101–104].

In 1987, the U.S. National Cancer Institute had already sponsored 24 intervention trials with selected chemopreventive agents that were or are being tested as inhibitors of a variety of types of cancers in humans, including cancer of the lung, oral cavity, and esophagus [105]. So far we are not aware of chemopreventive trials specifically designed for smokers. That there is hesitation in exploring chemopreventive measures for smokers is understandable, since cessation of smoking is a proven effective alternative that leads to remarkable reduction of cancer risk in the lung and upper respiratory tract.

Nevertheless, model studies in laboratory animals have proven the feasibility of inhibiting the carcinogenic effects of NNK and NNN. As discussed earlier, upon metabolic activation these carcinogenic nitrosamines form adducts with DNA and hemoglobin. Phenylethylisothiocyanate (PEITC), which occurs in cruciferous vegetables, was found to inhibit the metabolic activation, DNA binding, and tumorigenicity of NNK in mice and rats [106–108]. The inhibition of metabolic activation of NNK and of its induction of lung tumors in mice is increasingly more efficient when the chain length of the hydropholic moiety is extended from benzylisothiocyanate ($C_6H_5$–$CH_2$–NCS) to phenylbutylisothiocyanate ($C_6H_5$–$CH_2$–$CH_2$–$CH_2$–$CH_2$–NCS) [109]. At this time, the inhibition of the carcinogenicity of TSNA by the isothiocyanates is being studied in rats. Biochemical studies and bioassays also hold promise for several other chemical inhibitors of the carcinogenicity of NNN and NNK, including indole-3-carbinol [110], ellagic acid, a polyphenol abundant in edible fruits, butylated hydroxyanisole (BHA), a food antioxidant [111], and D-limonene and citrus fruit oils [112].

It has been discussed that consumption of green tea may play some role in the lower cancer incidence rates of Japanese and Japanese-American cigarette smokers compared to those of American cigarette smokers [113,114]. This has led to a study in chemoprevention in which strain A mice were given green tea extract (2%) or the major polyphenol of tea, (-)epigallocatechin-3-gallate (EGCG, 0.056%), in drinking water prior to treatment of the mice with subcutaneous injection of NNK. The mice given the tea extract, or the polyphenol plus NNK, developed significantly fewer lung adenomas than did the mice receiving NNK only. While green tea and EGCG had little effect on the $O^6$-methylguanine formation in the lung by NNK, both suppressed the increase of 8-hydroxydeoxyguanosine levels in mouse lung DNA that is usually seen with NNK [115].

These model studies with chemopreventive agents appear most promising for the inhibition of the carcinogenic effects of tobacco and tobacco smoke, especially for the inhibition of lung, oral, and esophageal cancer. Their thorough investigation should be actively pursued.

## VIII. Perspectives

Bioassays with cigarette smoke and its particulate matter as well as biochemical studies have strongly supported the conclusions from epidemiological observations that tobacco smoking, especially cigarette smoking, is causally associated with cancer of the lung and upper aerodigestive tract. As long as society condones tobacco smoking, laboratory studies are needed to provide a more complete understanding of the mechanisms and factors involved in tobacco carcinogenesis. The polynuclear aromatic hydrocarbons and the tobacco-specific *N*-nitrosamines are recognized major contributors to the increased risk of tobacco smokers for cancer of the respiratory tract; therefore, emphasis should be placed on the biochemistry and molecular biology of these carcinogens, which are involved in the development of cancer in smokers. These studies are not only of academic interest but will lead to the development and application of preventive methods. Such methods will help those who will not give up their smoking habit despite public health information and despite the availability of smoking cessation programs. Beyond these studies we attach great importance to refinement of the methods for biochemical markers which will help to identify those smokers who are at especially high risk for cancer of the lung, aerodigestive tract, and other sites.

Although the medical and scientific communities strongly support public health measures that are expected to lead to a smoke-free society, it must be realized that statistics on tobacco use at this time do not indicate that this goal will be reached in the near future. Thus, we must support the development of the low-yield cigarette and encourage public health authorities to set upper permissible limits for the delivery of tar of commercial cigarettes. This has already been done for the European community where 15 and 12 mg of tar have been set as upper limits of tar delivery for 1993 and 1998, respectively. Greater emphasis should also be placed on the reduction of known toxic and carcinogenic agents in cigarette smoke.

Another more recent approach to the reduction of cancer risk among smokers has been initiated by the application of chemopreventive measures. This is an area of great promise not only for the reduction of tobacco-related cancer. There exists a strong social case for development of the low-yield cigarette and chemoprevention as long as society condones tobacco smoking.

## Acknowledgment

We are grateful to Ernst L. Wynder for his support and encouragement of our studies in tobacco carcinogenesis and for the extensive contributions of our colleagues at the American Health Foundation: Klaus D. Brunnemann, Fung-Lung Chung, Stephen S. Hecht, and Abraham Rivenson. We thank Jennifer D. Johnting for editorial assistance. Our studies are supported by Grants CA-29580, CA-32391, and CA-44161, from the U.S. National Cancer Institute.

## References

1. International Agency for Research on Cancer. Tobacco smoking. IARC Monographs on the Evaluation of the Carcinogenic Risk of Chemicals to Humans. 1986;38:421.

2. U.S. Surgeon General. Reducing the health consequences of smoking. 25 years of progress. DHHS Publication (CDC) 89–8411. 1989:703.
3. Brunnemann KD, Hoffmann D. The pH of tobacco smoke. Food Cosmet Toxicol 1974;12:115–24.
4. Armitage AK, Turner DM. Absorption of nicotine in cigarette and cigar smoke through the oral mucosa. Nature 1970;226:1231–32.
5. Green CR. Some relationship between tobacco leaf and smoke composition. Proceedings of the American Chemical Society Symposium. Recent advances in the chemical composition of tobacco and tobacco smoke. New Orleans, LA, 1977:426–70.
6. Johnson WR. The pyrogenesis and physicochemical nature of tobacco smoke. Recent Adv Tobacco Sci 1977;3:1–27.
7. Brunnemann KD, Hoffmann D. Analytical studies on *N*-nitrosamines in tobacco and tobacco smoke. Recent Adv Tobacco Sci 1991;17:71–112
8. Ingebrethsen BJ. Aerosol studies of cigarette smoke. Recent Adv Tobacco Sci 1986;12:54–142.
9. Roberts DL. Natural tobacco flavor. Recent Adv Tobacco Sci 1988;14:49–81.
10. Dube MF, Green CR. Methods of collection of smoke for analytical purposes. Recent Adv Tobacco Sci 1982;8:42–102.
11. Wynder EL, Hoffmann D. Tobacco and tobacco smoke. Studies in experimental carcinogenesis. New York: Academic Press, 1967.
12. Enzell CR, Wahlberg I, Aasen AJ. Isoprenoids and alkaloids of tobacco. Chem Organ Nat Prod 1977;34:1–79.
13. Schmeltz I, Hoffmann D. Nitrogen containing compounds in tobacco and tobacco smoke. Chem Rev 1977;77:295–311.
14. Wahlberg I, Enzell CR. Tobacco isoprenoids. Nat Prod Rep 1987:237–76.
15. DeBardeleben MZ, Wickham JE, Kuhn WF. Determination of tar and nicotine in cigarette smoke from an historical perspective. Recent Adv Tobacco Sci 1991;17:115–48.
16. Herning RI, Jones RT, Bachman J, Mines AH. Puff volume increases when low-nicotine cigarettes are smoked. Br J Med 1981;183:187–89.
17. Haley NJ, Sepkovic DW, Hoffmann D, Wynder EL. Cigarette smoking as a risk factor for cardiovascular disease. VI. Compensation with nicotine availability as a single variable. Clin Pharmacol Ther 1985;38:164–70.
18. Augustine A, Harris RE, Wynder EL. Compensation as a risk factor for lung cancer in smokers who switch from nonfilter to filter cigarettes. Am J Public Health 1989;79:188–91.
19. Norman V. An overview of the vapor phase, semivolatile and nonvolatile components in cigarette smoke. Recent Adv Tobacco Sci 1977;3:28–58.
20. Jenkins RW Jr, Goldberg C, Williams TG. Neutron activation analysis in

tobacco and tobacco smoke studies: 2R1 cigarette composition, smoke transference and butt filtration. Beitr Tabakforsch 1985;13:59–65.

21. Sheets TJ. Pesticide residues on tobacco: perceptions and realities. Recent Adv Tobacco Sci 1991;17:33–68.

22. Leffingwell JC, Young HJ, Bernasek E. Tobacco flavoring for smoking products. Winston Salem, NC: R.J. Reynolds Tobacco Company, 1972.

23. Perfetti TA, Gordin HH. Just noticeable difference studies of mentholated cigarette products. Tobacco Sci 1985;29:57–66.

24. Nettesheim P, Griesemer RA. Experimental models for studies of respiratory tract carcinogenesis. In: Harris CC ed. Pathogenesis and therapy of lung cancer. New York: Marcel Dekker, 1978:75–188.

25. Leuchtenberger C, Leuchtenberger R, Doolin PF. A correlated histological, cytological and cytochemical study of tracheobronchial trees and lungs of mice exposed to cigarette smoke. I, II, and III. Cancer 1958;11:490–506; 1960;13:721–32; 1960;13:956–58.

26. Leuchtenberger C, Leuchtenberger R. Einfluss chronischer Inhalationen von frischem Zigarettenrauch und dessen Gasphase auf die Entwicklung von Lungentumoren bei Snell's Maeusen. Z Praeventivmed 1970;17:457–62.

27. Otto H. Experimentelle Untersuchungen an Maeusen mit passiver Zigarettenrauchbeatmung. Frankf Z Pathol 1963;73:10–23.

28. LaVoie EJ, Prokopczyk G, Rigotty J, Czech A, Rivenson A, Adams JD. Tumorigenic activity of the tobacco-specific nitrosamines 4-(methylnitrosamino)-1-(3-pyridyl)-1-butanone (NNK), 4-(methylnitrosamino)-1-(3-pyridyl)-1-butanol (iso-NNAL) and $N'$-nitrosonornicotine (NNN) on topical application to Sencar mice. Cancer Lett 1987;37:277–83.

29. Dontenwill W. Experimental investigations on the effect of cigarette smoke inhalation on small laboratory animals. In: Hanna MG Jr, Nettesheim R, Gilbert P Jr, eds. Inhalation Carcinogenesis. AEC Symp Ser 1970;18:389–412.

30. Hoffmann D, Wynder EL. Chamber development and aerosol dispersion. In: Hanna MG Jr, Nettesheim P, Gilbert P Jr, eds. Inhalation carcinogenesis. AEC Symp Ser 1970;18:173–89.

31. Maddox WL, Dalbey WE, Guerin MR, Stockley JR, Creasia DA, Kendrick J. A tobacco smoke inhalation exposure device for rodents. Arch Environ Health 1978;33:64–71.

32. Dalbey, WE, Nettesheim P, Griesemer R, Caton JE, Guerin MR. Chronic inhalation of cigarette smoke by F344 rats. J Natl Cancer Inst 1980;64:383–90.

33. Dontenwill W, Chevalier H-J, Harke H-P, Lafrenz U, Reckzeh G, Schneider B. Investigations on the effect of chronic cigarette smoke inhalation in Syrian golden hamsters. J Natl Cancer Inst 1973;51:1781–1832.

34ʹ  Bernfeld P, Homburger F, Russfield AB. Strain differences in the response of inbred Syrian hamsters to cigarette smoke inhalation. J Natl Cancer Inst 1974;53:1141–57.

35.  Bernfeld P, Homburger F, Soto E, Pai KJ. Cigarette smoke inhalation studies in inbred Syrian golden hamsters. J Natl Cancer Inst 1979;63:675–89.

36.  Hoffmann D, Wynder EL. A study of tobacco carcinogenesis. XI. Tumor initiators, tumor accelerators, and tumor promoting activity of condensate fractions. Cancer 1971;27:848–64.

37.  Dontenwill W, Chevalier H-J, Harke H-P, Klimisch H-J, Brune H, Fleischmann B, Keller W. Experimentelle Untersuchungen ueber die tumorerzeugende Wirkung von Zigarettenrauch-Kondensaten an der Maeusehaut. VI. Untersuchungen zur Fraktionierung von Zigarettenrauch-Kondensat. Z Krebsforsch 1976;85:155–67.

38.  Davis BR, Whitehead JK, Gill ME, Lee PN, Butterworth AD, Roe FJC. Response of rat lung to tobacco smoke condensate or fractions derived of it administered repeatedly by intratracheal instillation. Br J Cancer 1975;31:453–61.

39.  International Agency for Research on Cancer. Overall evaluations of carcinogenicity: an updating of IARC Monographs 1 to 42. IARC Monographs on the Evaluation of the Carcinogenic Risk of Chemicals to Humans. Lyon, France: IARC, Suppl. 7. 1987:440.

40.  International Agency for Research on Cancer. Radon. IARC Monographs on the Evaluation of the Carcinogenic Risks of Chemicals to Humans. Vol. 43. Lyon, France: IARC, 1988:173–259.

41.  Saffiotti U, Stinson SF, Keenan KP, McDowell EM. Tumor enhancement factors and mechanisms in the hamster respiratory tract carcinogenesis model. In: Mass MJ, Kaufman DG, Siegfried JM, et al., eds. Carcinogenesis, a Comprehensive Survey. Vol. 8. New York: Raven Press, 1985:63–92.

42.  Stanton MF, Miller E, Wrench C, Blackwell R. Experimental induction of epidermoid carcinoma in the lungs of rats by cigarette smoke condensate. J Natl Cancer Inst 1972;49:867–77.

43.  Deutsch-Wenzel RP, Brune H, Grimmer T, Dettbarn G, Misfeld J. Experimental studies in rat lungs on the carcinogenicity and dose–response relationships of eight frequently occurring environmental polycyclic aromatic hydrocarbons. J Natl Cancer Inst 1983;71:539–44.

44.  Hoffmann D, Rivenson A, Hecht SS, Hilfrich J, Kobayashi N, Wynder EL. Model studies in tobacco carcinogenesis with the Syrian golden hamster. Progr Exp Tumor Res (Karger, Basel) 1979;24:370–90.

45.  Hecht SS, Hoffmann D. The relevance of tobacco-specific nitrosamines to human cancer. Cancer Surv 1989;8:273–94.

46.  Belinsky SA, Foley YF, White CM, Anderson MW, Maronpot RR. Dose

response relationship between $O^6$-methylguanine formation in Clara cells and induction of pulmonary neoplasia in the rat with 4-(methylnitrosamino)-1-(3-pyridyl)-1-butanone. Cancer Res 1990;50:3772–80.

47. Hoffmann D, Rivenson A, Chung F-L, Hecht SS. Nicotine-derived *N*-nitrosamines (TSNA) and their relevance in tobacco carcinogenesis. Crit Rev Toxicol 1991;21:305–11.

48. Tsuda M, Kurashima Y. Tobacco smoking, chewing and snuff dipping. Factors contributing to the endogenous formation of *N*-nitroso compounds. Crit Rev Toxicol 1991;21:243–53.

49. International Agency for Research on Cancer. Formaldehyde(gas). IARC Monographs on the Evaluation of the Carcinogenic Risk of Chemicals to Humans. Suppl. 4. Lyon, France: IARC, 1982:131–32.

50. Tso TC, Harley N, Alexander LT. Source of lead-210 and polonium-210 in tobacco. Science 1966;153:880–82.

51. Martell EA. Radioactivity of tobacco trichomes and insoluble cigarette smoke particles. Nature 1974;249:215–17.

52. U.S. Surgeon General. The health consequences of smoking: cancer. DHHS Publication (OHS) 82-50179. 1982:322.

53. Ionizing radiation exposure of the population of the United States. Report 93. Bethesda, MD: National Council on Radiation Protection and Measurement. 1987.

54. National Research Council. Environmental tobacco smoke. Measuring exposure and assessing health effects. Washington, DC: National Academy Press, 1986:337.

55. U.S. Surgeon General. The health consequences of involuntary smoking. DHHS Publication (CDC) 87-8398. 1987.

56. Effects of passive smoking on health. Canberra, Australia: National Health and Medical Research Council Australia, 1986.

57. Health and Welfare Canada. Involuntary exposure to tobacco smoke. Publication 87-EHD-138. Ottawa, Ontario, Canada: National Health Welfare, 1987.

58. Saracci R, Riboli E. Passive smoking and lung cancer: current evidence and ongoing studies at the International Agency for Research on Cancer. Mutat Res 1989;222:117–27.

59. Hoffmann D, Wynder EL. Chemical constituents and bioactivity of tobacco smoke. IARC Scientific Publication 74. Lyon, France: IARC, 1986:145–65.

60. Guerin MR. Formation and physicochemical nature of sidestream smoke. IARC Scientific Publication 81. Lyon, France: IARC, 1987:11–23.

61. Klus H, Kuhn H. Verteilung verschiedener Tabakrauchbestandteile auf Haupt- und Nebenstromrauch. (Eine Uebersicht). Beitr Tabakforsch 1982;11:229–65.

62. Lewtas J, Williams K, Loefroth G, Hammond K, Laederer B. Environmental tobacco smoke. Mutagenic emission rates and their relationship to other emission factors. Proceedings of the 4th International Conference on Indoor Air Quality and Climate, Vol. 2, Berlin, 1987:8–12.
63. Klus H, Begutter H, Ball M, Introp I. Environmental tobacco smoke in real life situations. Proceedings of the 4th International Conference on Indoor Air Quality and Climate, Vol. 2, Berlin, 1987:137–41.
64. Brunnemann KD, Cox JE, Hoffmann D. Analysis of tobacco-specific N-nitrosamines in indoor air. Carcinogenesis 1992;13:2415–18.
65. Greenberg RA, Haley NJ, Etzel RA, Loda FA. Measuring the exposure of infants to tobacco smoke: nicotine and cotinine in saliva and urine. N Engl J Med 1984;310:1075–78.
66. Russell MAH. Estimation of smoke dosage and mortality of nonsmokers from environmental tobacco smoke. Toxicol Lett 1987;35:9–18.
67. Sepkovic DW, Axelrad CM, Colosimo SG, Haley NJ. Measuring tobacco smoke exposure: clinical applications and passive smoking. Proceedings of the 80th Annual Meeting of the Air Pollution Control Association, New York, 1987, 87-80.2.
68. Jarvis MJ. Application of biochemical intake markers to passive smoking measurements and risk estimation. Mutat Res 1989;222:101–10.
69. Bartsch H, Caporaso N, Cods M, Kadlubar G, Malaveille C, Skipper P, Talaska G, Tannenbaum SR, Vineis P. Carcinogen hemoglobin adducts, urinary mutagenicity, and metabolic phenotype in active and passive cigarette smokers. J Natl Cancer Inst 1990;82:1826–31.
70. Hall M, Grover PL. Polycyclic aromatic hydrocarbons: metabolism, activation and tumor initiation. In: Cooper CS, Grover PL, eds. Chemical carcinogenesis and mutagenesis. Vol. 1. Berlin: Springer-Verlag, 1990:327–72.
71. Cooper CS. The role of oncogene activation in chemical carcinogenesis. In: Cooper CS, Grover PL, eds. Chemical carcinogenesis and mutagenesis. Vol. 2. Berlin: Springer-Verlag, 1990:319–52.
72. Perera FP, Santella R, Brandt-Rauf P, Kahn S, Jiang W, Mayer J. Molecular epidemiology of lung cancer. In: Brugge J, Curran T, Harlow E, McCormick F, eds. Origins of human cancer: a comprehensive review. Cold Spring Harbor, NY: Cold Spring Harbor Laboratory Press, 1991:219–36.
73. Hecht SS, Melikian AA, Amin S. Methyl bay region epoxides: key intermediates in the metabolic activation of carcinogenic methylated polynuclear aromatic hydrocarbons. In: Politzer P, Martin JR, eds. Bioactive molecules. Vol. 5. 1988:291–311.
74. Wynder EL, Wright GA. A study of tobacco carcinogenesis. I. The primary fractions. Cancer 1957;10:255–71.

75. Grimmer G, Brune H, Dettbarn G, Naujack K-W, Mohr U, Wenzel-Hartung R. Contribution of polycyclic aromatic compounds to the carcinogenicity of sidestream smoke of cigarettes evaluated by implantation into the lung of rats. Cancer Lett 1988;43:173–77.
76. Hoffmann D, Schmeltz I, Hecht SS, Wynder EL. Polynuclear aromatic hydrocarbons in tobacco carcinogenesis. In: Gelboin G, T'so PO, eds. Polynuclear hydrocarbons and cancer. Vol. 1. New York: Academic Press, 1978:86–117.
77. Van Duuren BL, Goldschmidt BM. Cocarcinogenic and tumor promoting agents in tobacco carcinogenesis. J Natl Cancer Inst 1976;58:1237–42.
78. Hecht SS, Carmella S, Mori H, Hoffmann D. Role of catechol as a major cocarcinogen in the weakly acidic fraction of smoke condensate. J Natl Cancer Inst 1981;66:163–69.
79. Willey JC, Grafstrom RC, Moser CE Jr, Oyanne C, Sandqvist K, Harris CC. Biochemical and morphological effects of cigarette smoke condensate and its fractions on normal human bronchial epithelial cells in vitro. Cancer Res 1987;47:2045–49.
80. Pelkonen O, Vahakangas KN, Nebert DW. Binding of polycyclic aromatic hydrocarbons to DNA. Comparison with mutagenesis and tumorigenesis. J Toxicol Environ Health 1980; 6:1009–20.
81. Phillips DH, Hewer A, Martin CN, Garner RC, King MM, Correlation of DNA adduct levels in human lung with cigarette smoking. Nature 1988;336:790–92.
82. Randerath E, Miller RH, Mittal D, Avitts TA, Dunsford HA, Randerath K. Covalent DNA damage in tissues of cigarette smokers as determined by $^{32}$P-postlabeling assay. J Natl Cancer Inst 1989;81:341–47.
83. Hecht SS, Hoffmann D. 4-(Methylnitrosamino)-1-(3-pyridyl)-1-butanone, a nicotine-derived tobacco-specific nitrosamine, and cancer of the lung and pancreas in humans. In: Brugge J, Curran T, Harlow E, McCormick, F, eds. Origins of human cancer: a comprehensive review. Cold Spring Harbor, NY: Cold Spring Harbor Laboratory Press, 1991:745–55.
84. Castonguay A, Foiles PG, Trushin N, Hecht SS. A study of DNA methylation by tobacco-specific N-nitrosamines. Environ Health Perspect 1985;62:197–202.
85. Belinsky SA, White CM, Devereux TR, Swenberg JA, Anderson MW. Cell selective alkylation of DNA in rat lung following low dose exposure to the tobacco specific carcinogen 4-(N-methyl-N-nitrosamino)-1-(3-pyridyl)-1-butanone. Cancer Res 1987;47:1143–48.
86. Belinsky SA, White CM, Boucheron GA, Richardson FC, Swenberg JA, Anderson MW. Accumulation and persistence of DNA adducts in respiratory tissue of rats following multiple applications of the tobacco specific

carcinogen 4-(*N*-methyl-*N*-nitrosamino)-1-(3-pyridyl)-1-butanone. Cancer Res 1986;46:1280–84.

87. Belinsky SA, Devereux TR, Stoner GD, Anderson MW. Activation of the K-*ras* proto-oncogene in lung tumors from mice treated with 4-(*N*-methyl-*N*-nitrosamino)-1-(3-pyridyl)-1-butanone (NNK) and nitrosodimethylamine (NDMA). Cancer Res 1988;49:5303–11.

88. Rodenhuis S, Sletos RJC. Clinical significance of *ras* oncogene activation in human lung cancer. Cancer Res 1992;52:2665s–2669s.

89. Slebos RJC, Kibbelaar RE, Daleiso O, Kooistra A, Stam J, Meijer CJLM, Wagenaar SSC, Vanderschueren RGJR, Van Zandwijk N, Mooi WJ, Bos JL, Rodenhuis S. K-*ras* oncogene activation as a prognostic marker in adenocarcinoma of the lung. N Engl J Med 1990;323:561–65.

90. Carmella SG, Hecht SS. Formation of hemoglobin adducts upon treatment of F344 rats with the tobacco-specific nitrosamines 4-(methlynitrosamino)-1-(3-pyridyl)-1-butanone and *N'*-nitrosonornicotine. Cancer Res 1987;47: 2626–30.

91. Hecht SS, Spratt TE, Trushin N. Evidence for 4-(3-pyridyl)-4-oxobutylation of DNA in F344 rats treated with the tobacco-specific nitrosamines 4-(methylnitrosamino)-1-(3-pyridyl)-1-butanone and *N'*-nitrosonornicotine. Carcinogenesis 1988;9:161–65.

92. Peterson LA, Hecht SS. $O^6$-Methylguanine is a critical determinant of 4-(methylnitrosamino)-1-(3-pyridyl)-1-butanone tumorigenesis in A/J mouse lung. Cancer Res 1991;51:5557–64.

93. Carmella SG, Kagan SS, Kagan M, Foils PG, Palladino G, Quart AM, Quart E, Hecht SS. Mass spectrometric analysis of tobacco-specific nitrosamine hemoglobin adducts in snuff dippers, smokers, and nonsmokers. Cancer Res 1990;50:5438–45.

94. Change in apparent cigarette consumption and adult population size, by regions. WHO Health Statistics. Geneva: WHO, 1986:16–19.

95. Hoffmann D, Hoffmann I, Wynder EL. Lung cancer and the changing cigarette. In: O'Neil IK, Chen J, Bartsch H, eds. Relevance to human cancer of *N*-nitroso compounds, tobacco smoke and mycotoxins. IARC Scientific Publication 105. Lyon, France: IARC, 1991:449–59.

96. Djordjevic, MV, Sigountos CW, Hoffmann D, Brunnemann KD, Kagan MR, Bush LP, Safaev RD, Belitsky GA, Zaridze D. Assessment of major carcinogens and alkaloids in the tobacco and mainstream smoke of USSR cigarettes. Int J Cancer 1991;47:348–51.

97. Mitacek EJ, Brunnemann KD, Polednak AP, Hoffmann D, Suttajit M. Composition of popular tobacco products in Thailand, and relevance to disease prevention. Prev Med 1991;20:764–73.

98. International Agency for Research on Cancer. Coumarin. IARC Mono-

graphs on the Evaluation of the Carcinogenic risk of Chemicals to Humans. Vol. 10. Lyon, France: IARC, 1976:113–19.

99. Haley NJ, Sepkovic DW, Hoffmann D, Wynder EL. Cigarette smoking as a risk factor for cardiovascular disease. VI. Compensation with nicotine availability as a single variable. Clin Pharmacol Ther 1985;38:164–70.

100. Hoffmann D, Brunnemann KD. A study of tobacco carcinogenesis. XXVI. Endogenous formation of *N*-nitrosoproline in cigarette smokers. Cancer Res 1983;43:5570–74.

101. Peto R, Doll T, Buckley JD. Can dietary β-carotene materially reduce human cancer rates? Nature 1981;290:201–8.

102. Hennekens CH, Stampfer MJ, Willet W. Micronutrients and cancer chemoprevention. Cancer Detect Prev 1984;7:147–58.

103. Buring JE, Hennekens CH. Current issues in cancer chemoprevention. IARC Scientific Publication 103. Lyon, France: IARC, 1990:185–93.

104. El-Bayoumy K. The role of selenium in cancer prevention. In: DeVita V, Hellman S, Rosenberg SA, eds. Cancer principles and practice of oncology. 4th ed. Philadelphia: JB Lippincott, 1991:1–15.

105. Greenwald P, Cullen JW, McKenna JW. Cancer prevention and control: from research through applications. J Natl Cancer Inst 1987;79:389–400.

106. Morse MA, Wang CX, Stoner CD. Inhibition of 4-(methylnitrosamino)-1-(3-pyridyl)-1-butanone-induced DNA adduct formation and tumorigenicity in the lung of F344 rats by dietary phenethylisothiocyanate. Cancer Res 1989;49:549–53.

107. Morse MA, Amin S, Hecht SS, et al. Effects of aromatic isothiocyanates on tumorigenicity, $O^6$-methylguanine formation, and metabolism of the tobacco-specific nitrosamine 4-(methylnitrosamino)-1-(3-pyridyl)-1-butanone in A/J mouse lung. Cancer Res 1989;49:225–30.

108. Morse MA, Reinhardt JC, Amin SG, Hecht SS, Stoner GD, Chung F-L. Effects of dietary aromatic isothiocyanates fed subsequent to administration of 4-(methylnitrosamino)-1-(3-pyridyl)-1-butanone on lung tumorigenicity in mice. Cancer Lett 1990;49:225–30.

109. Morse MA, Eklind KI, Amin SG, Hecht SS, Chung F-L. Effects of alkyl chain length on the inhibition of NNK-induced lung neoplasia in A/J mice by aryl isothiocyanates. Carcinogenesis 1989;10:1757–59.

110. Morse MAW, Wang C-X, Amin SG, Hecht SS, Chung FL. Effects of dietary sinigrin or indole-3-carbinol on $O^6$-methylguanine-DNA-transmethylase activity and 4-(methylnitrosamino)-1-(3-pyridyl)-1-butanone-induced DNA methylation and tumorigenicity in F344 rats. Carcinogenesis 1988;9:1891–95.

111. Wattenberg LW, Coccia JB. Inhibition of 4-(methylnitrosamino)-1(pyr-

idyl)-1-butanone carcinogenesis in mice by D-limonene and citrus fruit oils. Carcinogenesis 1991;12:115–17.

112. Pepin P, Possignol G, Castonguay A. Inhibition of NNK-induced lung tumorigenesis in A/J mice by ellagic acid and butylated hydroxyanisole. Cancer J 1990;3:266–73.

113. Wynder EL, Fujita Y, Harris RE, Hiraguma T, Hiyarnor T. Comparative epidemiology of cancer between the United States and Japan: a second look. In: Sasaki R, Aoki K, eds. Epidemiology and prevention of cancer. Nagoya, Japan: University of Nagoya Press, 1990:103–27.

114. International Agency for Research on Cancer and International Association of Cancer Registries. Cancer incidence in five continents. Vol. 5. Lyon, France: IARC, 1987:868.

115. Cheng F-L, Xu Y, Ho C-T, Han C. Inhibition of tobacco-specific nitrosamine-induced lung tumorigenesis in A/J mice by green tea and its major polyphenol as antioxidants. Cancer Res 1992;52:3875–79.

# 26

## Tobacco and Lung Cancer Epidemiology

**SIMONE BENHAMOU**
and **CATHERINE HILL**

INSERM U351
and Institut Gustave Roussy
Villejuif, France

**SERGE KOSCIELNY**

Institut Gustave Roussy
Villejuif, France

## I. Introduction

The association between lung cancer and tobacco smoking has been suspected at least since the 1930s. A pioneer study published in 1940, which has not often been cited showed an increased risk of lung cancer among smokers compared to nonsmokers (reference quoted in ref. 1). This study was followed by two landmark case-control studies published in 1950 [2,3]. Numerous cohort and case-control studies have since confirmed the increased risk for lung cancer among smokers compared to nonsmokers. The epidemiological evidence on smoking-related cancers was reviewed extensively in a report of the Surgeon General in 1964 [4] and updated in successive reports [5–7]. In all studies, lung cancer risks were found to be increased with increased daily consumption, longer duration of smoking, inhalation, and early age at first cigarette, and decreased when individuals had stopped smoking for a long time. Other characteristics of cigarette smoking, such as the use of a filter, the type of tobacco (dark or light), and the level of tar, were studied less extensively. The epidemiological evidence on the associations between the risk of lung cancer and the type of tobacco product and inhalation, the daily consumption of cigarettes and the duration of smoking, the use of a filter, dark or light tobacco use, and tar levels is reviewed in the first part of this chapter. Variations in risk according to the histological type are also described.

Lung cancer was a relatively rare disease at the beginning of this century and is the leading cause of death and illness from cancer today in many industrialized countries. The variations in lung cancer death rates over time in France, the United Kingdom, and the United States, as well as the variations in per capita consumption of cigarettes in these countries, are presented in the second part of the chapter.

## II. Tobacco Smoking and Risk of Lung Cancer

### A. Type of Tobacco Product and Inhalation

Several studies have shown that lung cancer mortality is higher among cigarette, pipe, and cigar smokers than among nonsmokers and highest among cigarette smokers [5–7]. The results of a recent large case-control study [8] on lung cancer are presented in Table 1 for each tobacco product. Increased risks of lung cancer were observed among lifetime male cigar smokers and lifetime pipe smokers compared to nonsmokers [relative risk (RR) = 2.9 and 2.5, respectively]; these risks were lower than for lifetime cigarette smokers (RR = 9.0). Smokers who had smoked both cigars and cigarettes or both a pipe and cigarettes were at intermediate levels of risk (RR = 6.9 and 8.1, respectively).

In most studies performed on the association between lung cancer and the

**Table 1**  Risk of Lung Cancer According to Type of Tobacco Product

| Type of tobacco product | Males | | | Females | | |
|---|---|---|---|---|---|---|
| | Cases | Controls | RR$^a$ | Cases | Controls | RR$^a$ |
| Never smoked | 3% | 19% | 1.0 | 38% | 68% | 1.0 |
| Cigarettes only | 87% | 69% | 9.0** | 62% | 32% | 3.9* |
| Cigarettes and cigars | 3% | 3% | 6.9** | 0.1% | 0.1% | 3.3 |
| Cigarettes and pipes | 5% | 4% | 8.1** | 0.1% | 0% | — |
| Cigars only | 1% | 1% | 2.9** | 0% | 0% | — |
| Cigars and pipes | 0.3% | 1% | 4.6** | 0% | 0% | — |
| Pipes only | 1% | 2% | 2.5** | 0% | 0% | — |
| Cigarettes, cigars, and pipes | 1% | 1% | 7.5** | 0% | 0% | — |
| Total number | 6919 | 13,458 | | 884 | 1747 | |

**, $p < 0.05$; **, $p < 0.001$.
*Source:* Ref. 8.

degree of inhalation, a higher risk was observed in smokers who inhaled the smoke than in smokers who did not inhale [5–7]. The difference in risk, observed according to the type of tobacco product used, can be explained by inhalation patterns: the vast majority of exclusive cigarette smokers inhale the smoke, whereas most exclusive cigar or pipe smokers do not. The proportion of inhalers is higher among smokers of both cigars and cigarettes than among exclusive cigar smokers and lower than among exclusive cigarette smokers [9]. These differences in inhalation could be explained by the greater alkalinity of pipe or cigar smoke, which increases respiratory tract irritation and is therefore conducive to a reduced depth of inhalation.

## B. Daily Consumption of Cigarettes and Duration of Smoking

All epidemiological studies have shown consistent dose–response relationships between lung cancer risk and both the daily consumption of cigarettes and the duration of smoking in men and women (results summarized in refs. 5 to 7). In many studies, the risk for smokers who consume more than two packs per day in about 15 times higher than for nonsmokers.

The annual incidence of lung cancer in smokers can be separated into the annual incidence in nonsmokers, which depends on age, and an annual excess incidence related to smoking, which depends on the number of years of cigarette smoking. From a cohort study on British male doctors, Doll and Peto [10] estimated the annual excess incidence of lung cancer related to tobacco according to the duration and intensity of smoking (Table 2). The annual increase in lung cancer risk related to smoking is 20 times higher after 30 years of cigarette smoking than after 15 years, and 100 times higher after 45 years than after 15 years. Once smoking has stopped, the annual excess risk of lung cancer appears to remain roughly constant for many years thereafter [11]. This means that a moderate smoker who stops smoking after 30 years of cigarette smoking will be

**Table 2**  Annual Excess Incidence[a] of Lung Cancer in Smokers Compared to Nonsmokers According to Duration of Smoking

| Duration of smoking (yr) | Annual excess incidence/100,000 | |
|---|---|---|
| | *Moderate smokers* | *Heavy smokers* |
| 15 | 5 | 10 |
| 30 | 100 | 200 |
| 45 | 500 | 1000 |

[a]Estimated by Doll and Peto [10] from a model fitted to incidence data for male U.K. doctors.
*Source:* Adapted from ref. 7.

exposed 15 years later to an annual excess risk of lung cancer of 100 per 100,000 compared to a nonsmoker; if he had not stopped smoking, he would have been exposed to an excess risk of 500 per 100,000 [7].

It is quite common practice to combine the daily consumption and the duration of smoking to define lifetime smoking exposure in pack-years. For instance, smoking one pack of cigarettes per day for 30 years or smoking 2 packs per day for 15 years are summarized by a smoking history of 30 pack-years. The use of pack-years as a summary of smoking history must be avoided in the estimation of lung cancer risk because the risk is roughly proportional to the daily consumption multiplied by the duration raised to a power of 4 or 5: the risk of lung cancer is multiplied by 2 when the daily consumption increases twofold, and multiplied by about 20 ($2^4$ or $2^5$) when the duration is doubled.

### C.  Use of a Filter, Type of Tobacco (Light or Dark), and Tar Levels

Filtered cigarettes were introduced in the early 1960s in Western countries; therefore, the effect of a filter could not be studied in epidemiological studies before the late 1970s [7]. Recent studies have shown a fairly consistent tendency for the risk of lung cancer to be lower among smokers of filtered cigarettes than among smokers of nonfiltered cigarettes [7]. The results of the study of Lubin et al. [8] are presented in Table 3. A 2.5-fold excess risk was found in both males and females for lifetime smokers of nonfiltered cigarette compared to lifetime smokers of filtered cigarettes. However, the risk of lung cancer was not significantly lower in smokers who switched from nonfiltered to filtered cigarettes than in lifetime smokers of nonfiltered cigarettes [8].

Few studies have compared the risk of lung cancer incurred by smokers of dark tobacco compared to the risk incurred by smokers of light tobacco. The paucity of studies can be explained by the geographical distribution of dark and light tobacco use all over the world: Most studies on lung cancer and cigarette

**Table 3**  Risk of Lung Cancer According to Filter or Nonfilter Use

|                                               | RR$^a$ (95%CI)   |                |
| --------------------------------------------- | ---------------- | -------------- |
|                                               | *Males*          | *Females*      |
| Lifetime filter cigarette smokers             | 1.0              | 1.0            |
| Mixed filter and nonfilter cigarette smokers  | 1.6 (1.3–1.8)    | 1.8 (1.3–2.6)  |
| Lifetime nonfilter cigarette smokers          | 1.8 (1.5–2.1)    | 2.5 (1.2–5.2)  |

$^a$Adjusted for duration of smoking and years since subjects stopped smoking.
*Source:* Ref. 8.

smoking have been conducted in countries such as the United States or England, where light tobacco use is predominant, whereas dark tobacco is common in southern Europe and Latin America. Four studies have considered the different effects of dark and light tobacco [12–15], and their results are summarized in Table 4. All studies showed a higher risk for lifetime dark tobacco smokers and for smokers of mixed light and dark tobacco than for lifetime light tobacco smokers. However, no significant decrease was observed in smokers who switched from dark to light tobacco compared to lifetime dark tobacco smokers [16].

The average tar content of cigarettes has decreased regularly with time in industrialized countries [17]. Data on tar contents were practically nonexistent before the 1950s, and between the 1950s and the 1970s few and irregular measurements were performed. The results of some recent studies in which tar exposure and lung cancer risks were analyzed [8,14,18,19] are presented in Table 5. The risks associated were generally found to be higher with cigarettes containing a high tar content than with low-tar cigarettes. However, because tar levels are reduced by the use of a filter and are generally lower in light tobacco cigarettes than in dark tobacco cigarettes, some results have to be interpreted with caution because the use of filtered cigarettes and/or the type of tobacco were not taken into account in analyses.

**Table 4**  Risk of Lung Cancer (95% CI) According to Type of Tobacco Among Male Cigarette Smokers

| | Type of tobacco | | |
|---|---|---|---|
| *References* | *Light*[a] | *Mixed*[b] | *Dark*[b] |
| Benhamou et al. [12][c] | 1.0 | 1.6 (0.7–3.4) | 1.9 (1.0–4.0) |
| Berrino [13][d] | 1.0 | 1.1–1.2* | 1.6* |
| Joly et al. [14][e] | 1.0 | 1.2 (0.4–3.6) | 1.3 (0.6–3.0) |
| de Stefani et al. [16][f] | 1.0 | 1.6 (1.1–2.4) | 1.6 (1.2–2.2) |

[a]$\geq$ 80% lifetime light tobacco in de Stefani et al [16] and 100% lifetime light tobacco in all other studies.
[b]*, $p < 0.05$.
[c]Squamous cell, small-cell, and large-cell carcinomas. Adjusted for duration of smoking, daily consumption, social class, use of filter, current smoking, use of hand-rolled cigarettes, and inhalation. Matched on age, sex, date of diagnosis, hospital, and interviewer.
[d]All histological types. Adjusted for age, residence, daily consumption, use of filter, and years since subjects stopped smoking.
[e]All histological types. Ajusted for daily consumption.
[f]Squamous cell type. Adjusted for age, county, socioeconomic status, hospital, respondent (patient or surrogate), daily consumption, duration of smoking, years since subjects stopped smoking, use of filter, and use of hand-rolled cigarettes.

**Table 5** Lung Cancer Risk[a] According to Tar Exposure

| Reference | Tar exposure | | Males | Females | Males and females |
|---|---|---|---|---|---|
| Lubin et al. [8] | *Proportion of smoking history[b]* | | | | |
| | *Years of smoking* | *Tar level (mg/cig)* | | | |
| | 100% low-tar brands | <16.4 | 1.0 | 1.0 | |
| | 99–75% low-tar brands | <16.4 | 1.2 | — | |
| | All other cases | All others | 1.5 | 5.9 | |
| | 99–75% high-tar brands | ≥ 19.2 | 1.8 | 4.0 | |
| | 100% high-tar brands | ≥ 19.2 | 1.7 | 7.7 | |
| Joly et al. [14] | *Cumulative lifetime tar exposure[c] (mg)* | | | | |
| | *Males* | *Females* | | | |
| | < 15.56 | < 11.00 | 1.0 | 1.0 | |
| | 15.56–24.08 | ≥ 11.00 | 1.1 | 1.6 | |
| | > 24.08 | | 1.2 | | |
| Kaufman et al. [18] | *Average tar content (mg/cigarette)[d]* | | | | |
| | < 22.0 | | | | 1.0 |
| | 22.0–28.0 | | | | 1.9 |
| | > 28.0 | | | | 3.1 |
| Hammond et al. [19] | *Average tar content (mg/cigarette)* | | | | |
| July 1, 1960– | <17.6 | | 1.0 | 1.0 | |
| June 30, 1966 | 17.6–25.7 | | 1.2 | 1.5 | |
| | 25.8–35.8 | | 1.2 | 1.8 | |
| July 1, 1966– | <17.6 | | 1.0 | 1.0 | |
| June 1972 | 17.6–25.7 | | 1.2 | 1.2 | |
| | 25.8–35.7 | | 1.3 | 1.6 | |

[a]Mortality ratio in Hammond et al. [19] and relative risk in all other studies.
[b]Adjusted for duration of smoking, number smoked per day, and years since subjects stopped smoking.
[c]Adjusted for duration of smoking.
[d]Cigarette brand identified for at least 75% of years of smoking. Adjusted for sex, age, ethnic group, geographic region, years of education, year of interview, number of cigarettes per day, and age when subjects started smoking.

### D. Variation in Risk According to Histological Type

The risk of lung cancer is increased by smoking for the following histological types: squamous cell, small-cell, and adenocarcinomas. The risk is higher for squamous and small-cell carcinomas than for adenocarcinomas.

## III. Time Trends

### A. Lung Cancer Mortality and Incidence

Lung cancer was a relatively rare disease at the beginning of this century. In France, lung cancers accounted for only 5% of cancer deaths (7% in males and 3% in females) in 1950 [21,22]. The variations in lung cancer death rates between 1960 and 1989 in France, in the United States, and in the United Kingdom are shown in Figure 1 for males [23]. In France, lung cancer death rates increased regularly over time. The situation is different in the United Kingdom, where a substantial decrease in lung cancer mortality has been observed between 1960 and 1989; this decrease is the result of the reduction in tar levels in cigarettes, which is partially related to the use of a filter. In the United States, lung cancer

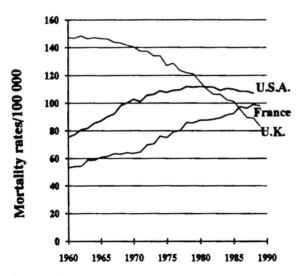

**Figure 1** Trends in lung cancer death rates/100,000 (standardized on the European population). Males aged 35 to 64. (Calculated from computed files provided by WHO [23].)

death rates increased until the 1975s and remained stable thereafter. The variations in lung cancer death rates for females are shown in Figure 2. No marked increase in lung cancer mortality has yet been detected in France. This situation is different from that observed in the United States. Lung cancer mortality rates among American females increased regularly over time. In France, women were traditionally nonsmokers. It is only in the cohorts born after 1960 that a similar proportion of smokers is observed among men and women. In older cohorts, the proportion of smokers was much smaller among women than among men, and these female smokers smoked less, inhaled less, and had been smokers for a shorter time than their male counterparts; they also smoked lighter cigarettes or filtered cigarettes more often [24].

Today, lung cancer is the leading cause of death and illness from cancer in the Western world and is the first cause of death from cancer among American women. Lung cancers accounted for 15% of cancer deaths (22% in males and 5% in females) in France in 1985. The number of new cases in 1980 worldwide was estimated at about 700,000 (10% of all new cancers diagnosed), and this figure is increasing at a rate of about 0.5% per year [20]. The dramatic lung cancer mortality observed today in many industrialized countries is the result of high tobacco consumption in these countries 30 years ago.

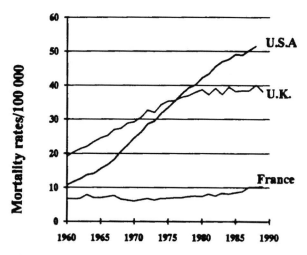

**Figure 2**  Trends in lung cancer death rates/100,000 (standardized on the European population). Females aged 35 to 64. (Calculated from computed files provided by WHO [23].)

## B. Tobacco Use

The evolution of the daily consumption of cigarettes per adult aged 15 or more in France, in the United States, and in the United Kingdom [25] is shown in Figure 3. There has been a substantial increase in per capita consumption of cigarettes since World War I. The daily consumption was similar in the United States and the United Kingdom until the 1940s. In France, cigarette smoking is a more recent phenomenon: During the 1930s and 1940s cigarette consumption in the United Kingdom was four times that in France. After 1975, a marked decrease in daily consumption was observed in the United Kingdom and the United States while it remained stable in France. However today, per capita consumption of cigarettes is higher in the United States than in France.

Trends in tobacco use in Europe have recently been reported by Hill [25]. Sales of manufactured cigarettes per adult (age 15 or over) and per day for EEC countries and the United States are given in Table 6. In 1950, daily cigarette consumption was greater in the United States than in any of the EEC countries. Ireland and the United Kingdom were the only European countries where at least 6 cigarettes per day were smoked. In all other countries, the daily consumption was fewer than 4 cigarettes per day. In 1989, the variation was much smaller, between 3.5 in Netherlands and 10.1 in Greece. In the countries where consumption was high in 1950, the maximum consumption was reached around

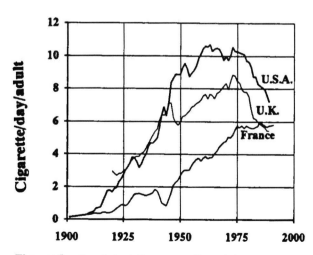

**Figure 3** Trends in daily consumption of cigarettes per adult (≥ 15 years). (Adapted from ref. 25.)

**Table 6**  Sales of Manufactured Cigarettes per Adult and per Day

| Country | 1950 | 1989 | Maximum (year) |
|---------|------|------|----------------|
| Belgium | 3.4 | 5.0 | 7.5 (1973) |
| Denmark | 3.5 | 5.2 | 6.4 (1976) |
| France | 2.5 | 5.7 | 6.0 (1985) |
| FRG | 1.7 | 6.4 | 7.3 (1975) |
| Greece | 4.4 | 10.1 | 10.2 (1987) |
| Ireland | 6.9 | 7.3 | 9.7 (1974) |
| Italy | 2.2 | 5.8 | 6.8 (1985) |
| Netherlands | 3.1 | 3.5 | 8.4 (1977) |
| Portugal | 1.7 | 5.2 | 5.5 (1987) |
| Spain | 1.8 | 6.7 | 7.4 (1987) |
| United Kingdom | 6.0 | 5.5 | 8.8 (1973) |
| United States | 8.9 | 8.0 | 10.7 (1963) |

*Source:* Ref. 25.

1975, followed by stabilization or a reduction in consumption. In other countries where consumption was low in 1950, it is still increasing [25].

## IV.  Conclusion

The increase in lung cancer death rates in many industrialized countries is the result of the increase in tobacco consumption in these countries. However, changes in smoking habits and cigarette content, such as use of a filter and a reduction in tar levels, have led to decreasing rates in young men in the United Kingdom, for instance. In Central and Eastern Europe, cigarette smoking is a relatively recent phenomenon in very young people and in female populations. The consequences of tobacco smoking on lung cancer mortality are just beginning to be detectable in the female population in France. However, because of the massive increase in the prevalence of smoking among young people and among women, it is relatively easy to predict the future evolution of the lung cancer epidemic in these populations.

### Acknowledgments

The authors thank Ms. L. Saint Ange for revising the manuscript.

### References

1.  Correa P. The new era of cancer epidemiology. Cancer Epidemiol Biomarkers Prev 1991;1:5–11.
2.  Wynder EL, Graham EA. Tobacco smoking as a possible etiologic factor

in bronchogenic carcinoma. A study of six hundred and eighty-four proved cases. JAMA 1950;143:329–34.

3. Doll R, Hill AB. Smoking and carcinoma of the lung. Preliminary report. Br Med J 1950;2:739–48.

4. Smoking and health. A report of the Surgeon General. DHEW Publication (PHS) 1103. Washington, DC: U.S. Department of Health and Human Services, 1964.

5. Smoking and health. A report of the Surgeon General. DHEW Publication (PHS) 79-50066. Washington, DC: U.S. Public Health Service, Office of Smoking and Health, 1979.

6. The health consequences of smoking. Cancer. A report of the Surgeon General. DHHS Publication (PHS) 82-50179. Washington, DC: U.S. Department of Health and Human Services, Public Health Service, Office of Smoking and Health, 1982.

7. IARC monographs on the evaluation of the carcinogenic risk of chemicals to humans. Vol. 38. Tobacco smoking. Lyon, France: IARC, 1986.

8. Lubin JH, Blot WJ, Berrino F, Flamant R, Gillis CR, Kunze M, Schmähl D, Visco G. Patterns of lung cancer risk according to type of cigarette smoked. Int J Cancer 1984;33:569–76.

9. Lubin JH, Richter BS, Blot WJ. Lung cancer risk with cigar and pipe use. Int J Cancer 1984;73:377–81.

10. Doll R, Peto R. Cigarette smoking and bronchial carcinoma: dose and time relationships among regular smokers. J Epidemiol Community Health 1978;32:303–13.

11. Doll R, Peto R. Mortality in relation to smoking: 20 years' observations on male British doctors. Br Med J 1976;2:1525–36.

12. Benhamou S, Benhamou E, Tirmarche M, Flamant R. Lung cancer and use of cigarettes: a French case-control study. J Natl Cancer Inst 1985;74:1169–75.

13. Berrino F. Lung cancer and tobacco smoking: analysis of a case-control study in North Italy. Unpublished.

14. Joly OG, Lubin JH, Caraballoso M. Dark tobacco and lung cancer in Cuba. J Natl Cancer Inst 1983;70:1033–39.

15. de Stefani E, Correa P, Carzoglio J, Deneo-Pellegrini H, Zavala D, Fierro L, Levin R, Fontham E. Black tobacco as a risk factor for squamous cell carcinoma of the lung. Unpublished.

16. Benhamou E, Benhamou S, Auquier A, Flamant R. Changes in patterns of cigarette smoking and lung cancer risk: results of a case-control study. Br J Cancer 1989;60:601–4.

17. Wald N, Doll R, Copeland G. Trends in tar, nicotine and carbon monoxide yields of UK cigarettes manufactured since 1934. Br Med J 1981;282:763–65.

18. Kaufman DW, Palmer JR, Rosenberg L, et al. Tar content of cigarettes in relation to lung cancer. Am J Epidemiol 1989;129:703–11.
19. Hammond EC, Garfinkel L, Seidman H, et al. "Tar" and nicotine content of cigarette smoke in relation to death rates. Environ Res 1976;12:263–74.
20. International Agency for Research on Cancer. Cancer: causes, occurrence and control. IARC Scientific Publication 100. Lyon, France: IARC, 1990.
21. Hill C, Benhamou E, Doyon F. Trends in cancer mortality, France 1950–1985. Br J Cancer 1991;63:567–90.
22. Hill C, Benhamou E, Doyon F, Flamant R. Evolution de la mortalité par cancer en France entre 1950 et 1985. Paris: INSERM, 1989.
23. World health statistics annual. Genèva: WHO, 1968 to 1989.
24. Hirsch A, Hill C, Frossart M, Tassin JP, Péchabrier M. Lutter contre le tabagisme. Paris: La Documentation Française, 1987.
25. Hill C. Trends in tobacco use in Europe. J Natl Cancer Inst Monogr 1992;12:21–24.

# 27

## Pharmacologic Characteristics of Tobacco Dependence

CAROLINE COHEN

Groupe Pharmacology SNC
Synthelabo Recherche, L.E.R.S.
Bagneux, France

WALLACE B. PICKWORTH
and JACK E. HENNINGFIELD

Addiction Research Center
National Institute on Drug Abuse
Baltimore, Maryland

## I. Introduction

The adverse effects of tobacco smoking include not only an increased risk for developing any of a wide range of diseases (e.g., chronic obstructive lung disease, cancers, heart disease, complications of pregnancy) but also the development of a dependence. The classification of tobacco as an addictive substance by regulatory agencies such as the U.S. Public Health Service and the World Health Organization is relatively recent, however. Until 1964, addiction was characterized by a physical withdrawal syndrome that follows cessation of chronic drug use. At this time, the tobacco withdrawal syndrome had not been identified and tobacco was not included among the addictive substances. With the widespread use of drugs that produced compulsive self-administration without producing a withdrawal syndrome, the concept of addiction was revised. According to the current definition, drug dependence is a state characterized by a compulsive use of a psychoactive drug in order to experience its psychic effects. Tolerance and physiological withdrawal may or may not be present [1–3].

Increased knowledge of the psychopharmacology of tobacco dependence allows for characterization of features of smoking behavior. Evidence that cigarette smoking is an addictive behavior is provided by epidemiologic studies and by clinical studies that assessed in humans and animals the rewarding effects of tobacco and the withdrawal syndrome following tobacco smoking cessation.

Three issues are discussed in the present chapter: why tobacco is considered an addictive substance, the psychopharmacology of tobacco dependence, and the pharmacologic treatments developed or under investigation to treat tobacco addiction.

## II. Tobacco Smoking: An Addictive Behavior

The main characteristic of drug dependence is a consistent pattern of drug administration. Numerous surveys have shown that elements of the pattern of cigarette smoking across individuals are highly consistent. The same observation has been made in laboratory settings in which it is possible to monitor volunteers' cigarette consumption [4,5]. Regular drug-taking behavior maintains a constant biological impregnation by the drug and by doing so, prevents either the onset of a withdrawal syndrome or acute intoxication. When biological concentrations of the drug are experimentally manipulated, subjects tend to change their drug-taking behavior to compensate for the effects of the manipulation. The most commonly employed experimental manipulation is to vary tobacco smoke composition and measure subsequent smoking. The composition of tobacco smoke can be varied by using ventilated filters that dilute the tobacco smoke, shortened cigarettes, or different types of tobacco. Extensive clinical studies have clearly demonstrated that smokers adapt their smoking behavior in response to an experimental manipulation of smoke concentration or composition [6–10]. Smokers increased or decreased the number, frequency, and volume of puffs per cigarette. They modified the volume of smoke inhaled. Eventually, they modified the number of cigarettes they usually smoked per day. Cigarette manufacturers developed a new kind of cigarette that under certain smoking conditions produced a smoke with low nicotine and tar contents. These cigarettes are still often considered by smokers to be safer. Unfortunately, because smokers adapt their smoking according to smoke concentration, such an attempt is inefficient to reduce intake of tobacco products. Although a change to cigarettes very low in tar and nicotine may reduce the hazards of smoking, subjects rated these cigarettes as unsatisfying [11–13].

Rather than varying the tobacco smoke composition, it is possible in volunteers to restrict the number of cigarettes smoked or the frequency [4,14,15]. Using this strategy, it was demonstrated that smokers changed their behavior to compensate for the effects of tobacco deprivation. For example, increases in the interval between smoking bouts were associated with increased puffs per bout.

Similarly, deprivation of tobacco decreased the latency to smoke when the opportunity arose.

These studies do not provide any information concerning which constituents of tobacco smoke are relevant in producing a compensatory behavior. This can be done only with studies in which constituents are manipulated independently. Whereas there is extensive literature on nicotine dose manipulation, only a few studies have manipulated other tobacco smoke components. "Tar," the dry particulate matter of tobacco smoke (nicotine not included), has been investigated. Sutton and collaborators [16] found that the tar yield of cigarettes (determined by cigarette smoking machine testing) determined the volume of smoke inhaled by smokers. When nicotine yield was controlled, smokers of lower-tar cigarettes puffed more smoke from their cigarettes than did smokers of higher-tar cigarettes. They also had higher plasma nicotine concentrations. By contrast, Woodman and colleagues [17] showed that with cigarettes of the same nicotine level, the total inhaled smoke volume was lower with the lower-tar cigarettes. It is difficult to draw a conclusion from these contradictory results as to the role of tar in tobacco smoking behavior. However, it is likely that the tar fraction contributed to the taste and smell of smoke and that these sensory stimuli may act as reinforcers for tobacco smoking [18].

Because nicotine is a powerful pharmacological agent contained in all tobacco products, its addictive properties have been studied extensively. Early reports demonstrated that smokers were able to perceive differences in the nicotine yield of cigarettes [19–21]. In other studies [22,23], smokers adjusted their smoking behavior based on the nicotine yield of the cigarettes. Using nicotine-enriched cigarettes, Fagerström showed that the more nicotine dependent the smoker, the more likely he or she was to compensate for changes in nicotine yield [24].

Supplemental nicotine can also be administered via an oral, subcutaneous, or intravenous route. Several nicotine delivery systems are now available: polacrilex gum, aerosol, and transdermal patch. Using these delivery systems, it was demonstrated that supplemental nicotine administration decreased cigarette smoking [25–29]. Smokers increased and then decreased the number of intravenous nicotine injections when saline was substituted for nicotine [30]. This is a typical adaptive behavior seen with other abused drugs.

Compensatory smoking behavior was also seen when a nicotinic antagonist was administered to block the effects of nicotine. The administration of the central nicotinic antagonist mecamylamine attenuated nicotine discrimination [31] and increased the number of cigarettes smoked and the number of puffs taken [32]. Subjects showed greater increases in plasma nicotine following cigarette smoking when pretreated with mecamylamine than when pretreated with placebo [33]. The peripheral nicotinic antagonist pentolinium did not affect smoking behavior in these conditions [32].

Animal studies can also provide useful data concerning the addictive effects of a drug. Intravenous nicotine self-administration has been induced in rats, dogs, squirrel monkeys, and baboons [34]. In all these species, however, the conditions under which nicotine self-administration was established were more limited than those of other drugs. For instance, nicotine self-administration was more consistent when nicotine was not continuously available, or was paired with conditioned stimuli, or during food deprivation.

Using another paradigm, the place preference procedure, it was possible to demonstrate that nicotine established a drug-seeking behavior in rats. During the training phase, the rat was placed in one environment when nicotine was given and in another environment when a placebo was given. After some exposure to both nicotine and placebo, the rat was given free access to either environment to determine which it preferred. Fudala and colleagues showed that rats preferred the environment paired with nicotine injections, and the central nicotinic antagonist mecamylamine blocked the nicotine-induced place preference [35,36].

The theory that smokers change their behavior to avoid either a low plasma nicotine level associated with the occurrence of tobacco withdrawal syndrome or a high plasma nicotine level producing intoxication is termed the *nicotine titration hypothesis*. The behavioral adaptations are often termed "downward" or "upward" compensation [37]. It is likely that the upper and lower limits of nicotine intake vary across individuals. Such individual characteristics should be taken into account in studying smoking behavior. They are also important parameters when prescribing nicotine replacement therapy to ease smoking cessation. Situational factors such as stress can also affect nicotine intake regulation [38,39].

## III.  Psychopharmacology of Tobacco Dependence

The importance of both psychosocial and physiological factors in drug addiction have long been appreciated [40]. However, a series of expert committees of the World Health Organization, in the 1950s, seemed to assume that the primary or at least most powerful biobehavioral mechanism by which drug addiction occurred was the establishment of physical dependence. When physical dependence had been established, drug deprivation would be accompanied by an aversive withdrawal syndrome, which in turn would motivate the drug-seeking behavior [2]. Although physical dependence continues to be recognized as an important aspect of drug dependence syndromes, it is now understood to be neither a necessary nor a sufficient factor in the establishment or maintenance of compulsive drug-seeking behavior [3]. This conclusion followed from a variety of observations, including the following: drugs may cause exceeding powerful states of drug seeking when insufficient doses are taken to engender physical dependence; treatment of withdrawal symptoms is rarely sufficient as the sole strategy to prevent drug-seeking behavior from continuing or from reemerging; relapse to drug dependence frequently occurs months or years after cessation; and not all drugs that produce physical dependence are sought by people who show other signs and symptoms of withdrawal [41].

It is now understood that drug self-administration is a behavior controlled strongly by the rewarding or reinforcing effects of the drug. These effects appear related to its euphoriant effects in humans. The strength of the reinforcing effects is related to such factors as drug deprivation, dose, past history of use, psychiatric state, genetic factors, tolerance, and physical dependence. The reinforcing effects of drugs may be assessed in the absence of a state of drug dependence as described elsewhere by assessing the possibility that humans or animals will self-administer the drug under standardized test conditions [3,42,43].

### A.  Tolerance and Withdrawal Syndrome

#### Tobacco Withdrawal Syndrome

A long list of tobacco withdrawal symptoms can be generated from reports of smokers who attempt to quit smoking. Complaints most often include "craving" for tobacco, irritability, restlessness, anxiety, difficulty in concentrating, increased appetite and food intake, and weight gain. Only about one-fourth of smokers report having experienced no withdrawal symptoms [3]. Clinical studies that have examined the tobacco withdrawal syndrome [44–48] have found similar symptoms: desire to smoke that peaked within the first 24 h of deprivation, falling heart rate, and performance deficits that were only partially recovered by the tenth day of tobacco deprivation. Changes in the resting electroencephalogram (EEG) (i.e., increased theta power, decreased alpha frequency) were evident as early as 12 h after tobacco deprivation and persist for up to 7 days. These EEG changes were consistent with changes in arousal levels.

It is possible that a withdrawal syndrome can be precipitated when a drug antagonist is given. Precipitated tobacco withdrawal responses have not yet been demonstrated, although Stolerman and colleagues [32] and Pickworth and co-workers [49] have shown that mecamylamine enhanced EEG signs and hand-steadiness responses that typically accompany early signs of tobacco withdrawal.

#### Tolerance to the Effects of Nicotine

Animal studies have demonstrated that tolerance develops to several effects of nicotine, including the initial depressant effect of nicotine on locomotor activity, and some physiological responses [3,50–52]. In human subjects, tolerance also develops to the aversive properties of tobacco. The first exposure to tobacco is generally a bad experience, and it is necessary to repeat tobacco smoking episodes before the individual experiences the rewarding properties of tobacco. The same observation was made in a recent study using nicotine polacrilex gum: never-smokers reported the most dysphoria from nicotine, ex-smokers were intermediate, and current smokers reported the least dysphoria from nicotine. Consistent with these results, never-smokers self-administered less nicotine than did ex-smokers or current smokers [53]. After repeated intravenous injections of nicotine, it was found that rapid tolerance develops to the subjective and cardiac effects of nicotine [54]. Acute nicotine tolerance was also shown after a single subcutaneous injection of nicotine [55].

## B. Rewarding Properties of Nicotine

The reinforcing effects of nicotine have been directly assessed in several species of animals tested in laboratory studies as well as in humans using intravenous drug self-administration strategy [34]. These studies showed that nicotine could serve to maintain behavior leading to its own self-administration, and that the reinforcing effects of nicotine were dependent on nicotine's actions at receptors in the brain. The testing strategy relied upon by the World Health Organization for assessing abuse potential or the propensity of a drug to serve as a reinforcer in humans is to assess its subjective effects according to standardized procedures [56]. Specifically, these effects of nicotine were assessed in volunteers by using a drug-liking scale and the morphine-benzedrine-group (MBG) scale of the Addiction Research Center Inventory (ARCI). The MBG scale or euphoriant scale is of particular interest for abuse liability testing. It was developed by Haertzen and his colleagues [57] from subjects' responses after the administration of prototypic drugs of abuse (e.g., opiates, amphetamines, barbiturates). Most addictive drugs elevate the MBG scale scores [58]. Tobacco smoke and nicotine given intravenously were shown to be euphoriants, as evidenced by increases in scores on the drug-liking scale and the MBG scale [25,59]. Volunteers with histories of drug abuse were used as subjects because they could accurately identify drugs with a potential for abuse and could compare the effects of nicotine to those of other abused drugs.

The maintenance of tobacco smoking may also be promoted by other actions of nicotine. Smokers report that smoking helps them to cope with feelings of anxiety, tension, and anger, to feel energized, alert, and attentive, and to keep body weight under control [60]. However, since the tobacco withdrawal syndrome is characterized by increased anxiety, tension, drowsiness, and body weight, it is possible that the effects reported by smokers are due to an alleviation of a withdrawal syndrome [3,61].

## IV.  Pharmacologic Treatments

### A.  Replacement Therapy

The principle of replacement therapy is to substitute a medication for the abused drug. The ideal medication is not toxic, does not induce dependence, and alleviates signs and symptoms of withdrawal by acting on the same neurobiological system as the abused drug. To the extent that nicotine is the addictive substance in tobacco, alternative forms of nicotine delivery should be able to block signs and symptoms of withdrawal and craving. They should also have a lower carcinogenic potential than tobacco products. Several forms of nicotine replacement have been used: intravenous administration of nicotine, nicotine polacrilex gum, nicotine transdermal patch, nasal nicotine solution, and nicotine aerosols [3,62,63]. Nicotine polacrilex gum reversed most of the tobacco withdrawal signs and symptoms, including heart rate decreases, EEG changes, cognitive impairments, and subjective discomfort [47,48,64,65]. However, the efficacy of nicotine polacrilex gum varies widely across studies and is sometimes weak. Furthermore, craving for tobacco is not reliably diminished by nicotine polacrilex gum. It has been argued that the speed at which a drug is delivered to the central nervous system affects the reinforcing efficacy of the drug [66]. For example, the inhaled form of cocaine ("crack") is considered more reinforcing and dependence producing than are other forms of cocaine delivery. Similarly, nicotine taken by the slow release of polacrilex gum would appear to be less reinforcing than cigarette smoking. Stimuli associated with tobacco smoking can be important determinants in maintaining tobacco dependence. In alcoholic patients, the desire to use alcohol is increased by presentation of alcohol-associated stimuli [67], and in opioid-dependent persons, an opioid withdrawal syndrome can be elicited by environmental stimuli associated with drug administration [68]. The same conditioned phenomena can be expected with nicotine, the effects of which are associated with a number of stimuli: tobacco smoke taste, harshness, smell, or cigarette sight [69]. It should be emphasized that the lack of effects of nicotine polacrilex gum reported by some patients can also be due to inappropriate instructions for its use. Beneficial effects from nicotine polacrilex gum depend on obtaining adequate dose levels. Any factor that diminishes nicotine absorption, such as salivary pH or chewing rate, could limit the efficacy of nicotine polacrilex [70,71].

The nicotine transdermal patch is another replacement therapy. Early results suggest that it could be a useful aid to smoking cessation [64,72]. Although its efficacy has not yet been proven, lobeline sulfate, an alkaloid with nicotine-like ganglionic effects, is used in several over-the-counter aids for quitting smoking [3].

The main issue that has been raised with nicotine replacement therapies is whether these forms of nicotine delivery will lead to dependence. However, it can be assumed that any dependence on nicotine delivery systems is actually a continued dependence on nicotine that originated with smoking [3,73,74].

### B.  Symptomatic Treatment Therapies

Several medications have been used to reduce withdrawal symptoms [3,64,75–77]: (1) alprazolam reduced anxiety, irritability, restlessness, and tension; (2) clonidine also reduced these withdrawal symptoms and reduced the craving for tobacco; (3) doxepin reduced craving for cigarettes and increased success rate at 1 and 9 weeks following cessation; and (4) buspirone reduced craving, anxiety, and fatigue.

### C.  Nicotine Blockade Therapy and Deterrent Therapy

Blockade therapy is using a drug (an antagonist) that blocks the addictive effects of the abused drug. The prototypical application is the use of naltrexone, a long-acting opiate antagonist, to treat opiate dependence. The central nicotinic antagonist mecamylamine has been proposed as an aid to smoking cessation [78]. Preliminary results indicated that mecamylamine blocked the subjective and physiological effects of tobacco, including craving. Mecamylamine increased the number of cigarettes smoked when subjects were not motivated to stop smoking; it reduced cigarette consumption after a few days in motivated patients. The main limitation of the blockade therapy is the low rate of patients' compliance. Based on the same principle of deterrent therapy as that used in treatment of alcoholism (disulfiram treatment), silver acetate has been administered to induce aversive effects when smoking. The efficacy of this strategy has not been validated.

## V.  Conclusions

The treatment of tobacco dependence appears more promising since the psychopharmacology of tobacco smoking behavior is better known. The notion that nicotine is the addictive substance in tobacco is generally accepted. Animal and human studies have shown that (1) nicotine could maintain self-administration and induce seeking behavior in animals, (2) nicotine intake was regulated to avoid either an intoxication or a withdrawal syndrome, (3) nicotine could induce euphoria, and (4) nicotine administration could block several tobacco withdrawal signs and symptoms. To the extent that nicotine is the addictive substance in tobacco products, nicotine substitution therapies have been developed. Their efficacy is not fully satisfactory, but further research is expected to lead to improvements on current substitution therapies.

Several factors are known to affect the success rate of nicotine substitution therapy: for instance, patients' compliance with the recommendations for use of nicotine delivery systems, or patients' need for nicotine. Tobacco smoking behavior is also determined by nonpharmacological factors (cigarette sight, smell, taste of smoke). Therefore, it may be expected that most replacement therapy would involve a nicotine delivery system that also involves sensory stimuli. As the reinforcing components of tobacco products are not those inducing the most health damage, it is theoretically possible to manufacture a safe substitute (although nicotine itself is not devoid of undesirable effects). Such a device would reduce the health problem of tobacco smoking but would not free the smoker of his or her compulsive behavior.

Symptomatic treatment of nicotine withdrawal would be enhanced if a better understanding of the psychopharmacology of tobacco smoking is known. Several pharmacological classes of drugs (sedative, tranquilizer, antidepressant, stimulant) have been tested for their efficacy to relieve the tobacco withdrawal syndrome. Some drugs reduce some signs and symptoms of withdrawal, although they should be used with caution due to their undesirable effects. Research in this area has recently been oriented toward drugs that reduced craving because available nicotine delivery systems reduced signs and symptoms of withdrawal but were unable to reduce craving for tobacco.

Finally, increased knowledge of the psychopharmacology of tobacco dependence should lead to the characterization of pharmacological determinants of vulnerability to abuse tobacco. Once this is accomplished, preventive strategies for tobacco dependence may be developed. Whereas studies are undertaken to investigate this aspect, the preventive applications are still to be defined.

## References

1. American Psychiatric Association. Diagnostic and statistical manual of mental disorders. 3rd ed. DSM-III-R. Washington, DC: American Psychiatric Association, 1987.
2. WHO Expert Committee on Addiction-Producing Drugs. 13th Report. Technical Report Series 273. Geneva: WHO, 1964.
3. The health consequences of smoking: nicotine addiction. A report of the Surgeon General. DHHS Publication (CDC) 88-8406. Washington, DC: U.S. Department of Health and Human Services, 1988.
4. Griffiths RR, Henningfield JE, Bigelow GE. Human cigarette smoking: manipulation of number of puffs per bout, interbout interval, and nicotine dose. J Pharmacol Exp Ther 1982;220:256–65.
5. Gust SW, Pickens RW, Pechacek TF. Relation of puff volume to other topographical measures of smoking. Addict Behav 1983;8:115–19.
6. Sutton SR, Feyerabend C, Cole PV, Russell MAH. Adjustment of smokers

to dilution of tobacco smoke by ventilated cigarette holders. Clin Pharmacol Ther 1978;24:395–405.

7. Henningfield JE, Griffiths RR. Effects of ventilated cigarette holders on cigarette smoking by humans. Psychopharmacology 1980;68:115–19.

8. Russell MAH, Sutton SR, Feyerabend C, Saloojee Y. Smokers' response to shortened cigarettes: dose reduction without dilution of tobacco smoke. Clin Pharmacol Ther 1980;27:210–18.

9. Chait LD, Griffiths RR. Smoking behavior and tobacco smoke intake: response of smokers to shortened cigarettes. Clin Pharmacol Ther 1982;32:90–97.

10. Zacny JP, Stitzer ML, Yingling JE. Cigarette filter vent blocking: effects on smoking topography and carbon monoxide exposure. Pharmacol Biochem Behav 1986;25:1245–52.

11. Turner JAM, Sillett RW, Ball KP. Some effects of changing to low-tar and low-nicotine cigarettes. Lancet 1974;September 28:737–39.

12. Rickert WS, Robinson JC. Estimating the hazards of less hazardous cigarettes. II. Study of cigarette yields of nicotine, carbon monoxide, and hydrogen cyanide in relation to levels of cotinine, carboxyhemoglobin, and thiocyanate in smokers. J Toxicol Environ Health 1981;7:391–403.

13. Bättig K, Buzzi R, Nil R. Smoke yield of cigarettes and puffing behavior in men and women. Psychopharmacology 1982;76:139–48.

14. Henningfield JE, Griffiths RR. A preparation for the experimental analysis of human cigarette smoking behavior. Behav Res Methods Instrum 1979;11:538–44.

15. Zacny JP, Stitzer ML. Effects of smoke deprivation interval on puff topography. Clin Pharmacol Ther 1985;38:109–15.

16. Sutton SR, Russell MAH, Iyer R, Feyerabend C, Saloojee Y. Relationship between cigarette yields, puffing patterns, and smoke intake: evidence for tar compensation? Br Med J 1982;285:600–603.

17. Woodman G, Newman SP, Pavia D, Clarke SW. The separate effects of tar and nicotine on the cigarette smoking manoeuvre. Eur J Respir Dis 1987;70:316–21.

18. Rose JE, Tashkin DP, Ertle A, Zinser MC, Lafer R. Sensory blockade of smoking satisfaction. Pharmacol Biochem Behav 1985;23:289–93.

19. Finnegan JK, Larson PS, Haag HB. The role of nicotine in the cigarette habit. Science 1945;102:94–96.

20. Goldfarb TL, Jarvik ME, Glick SD. Cigarette nicotine content as a determinant of human smoking behavior. Psychopharmacologia (Berlin) 1970;17:89–93.

21. Goldfarb T, Gritz ER, Jarvik ME, Stolerman IP. Reactions to cigarettes as a function of nicotine and "tar." Clin Pharmacol Ther 1976;19:767–72.

22. Herning RI, Jones RT, Bachman J, Mines AH. Puff volume increases when low-nicotine cigarettes are smoked. Br Med J 1981;283:187–89.

23. Gust SW, Pickens RW. Does cigarette nicotine yield affect puff volume? Clin Pharmacol Ther 1982;32:418–22.

24. Fagerström KO. Effects of a nicotine-enriched cigarette on nicotine titration, daily cigarette consumption, and levels of carbon monoxide, cotinine, and nicotine. Psychopharmacology 1982;77:164–67.

25. Henningfield JE, Miyasato K, Jasinski DR. Cigarette smokers self-administer intravenous nicotine. Pharmacol Biochem Behav 1983;19:887–90.

26. Rose JE, Herskovic JE, Trilling Y, Jarvik ME. Transdermal nicotine reduces cigarette craving and nicotine preference. Clin Pharmacol Ther 1985;38:450–56.

27. Nemeth-Coslett R, Henningfield JE. Effects of nicotine chewing gum on human cigarette smoking and subjective and physiologic effects. Psychopharmacology 1986;89:261–64.

28. Nemeth-Coslett R, Henningfield JE, O'Keeffe MK. Griffiths RR. Nicotine gum: dose-related effects on cigarette smoking and subjective ratings. Psychopharmacology 1987;92:424–30.

29. Lucchesi BR, Schuster CR, Emley GS. The role of nicotine as a determinant of cigarette smoking frequency in man with observations of certain cardiovascular effects associated with the tobacco alkaloid. Clin Pharmacol Ther 1967;8:789–96.

30. Henningfield JE, Goldberg SR. Control of behavior by intravenous nicotine injections in human subjects. Pharmacol Biochem Behav 1983;19:1021–26.

31. Henningfield JE, Miyasato K, Johnson RE, Jasinski DR. Rapid physiologic effects of nicotine in humans and selective blockade of behavioral effects of mecamylamine. In: Harris LS, ed. Problems of drug dependence. NIDA Research Monograph 43. DHHS Publication (ADM) 83-1264. Washington, DC: U.S. Department of Health and Human Services, 1983.

32. Stolerman IP, Goldfarb T, Fink R, Jarvik ME. Influencing cigarette smoking with nicotine antagonists. Psychopharmacologia 1973;28:247–59.

33. Pomerleau CS, Pomerleau OF, Majchrzak MJ. Mecamylamine pretreatment increases subsequent nicotine self-administration as indicated by changes in plasma nicotine level. Psychopharmacology 1987;91:391–93.

34. Henningfield JE, Goldberg SR. Nicotine as a reinforcer in human subjects and laboratory animals. Pharmacol Biochem Behav 1983;19:989–92.

35. Fudala PJ, Teoh KW, Iwamoto ET. Pharmacologic characterization of nicotine-induced conditioned place preference. Pharmacol Biochem Behav 1985;22:237–41.

36. Fudala PJ, Iwamoto ET. Further studies on nicotine-induced conditioned place preference in the rat. Pharmacol Biochem Behav 1986;25:1041–49.

37. Kozlowski LT, Herman CP. The interaction of psychosocial and biological determinants of tobacco use: more on the boundary model. J Appl Soc Psychol 1984;14:244–56.

38. Rose JE, Ananda S, Jarvik ME. Cigarette smoking during anxiety-provoking and monotonous tasks. Addict Behav 1983;8:353–59.

39. Hatsukami DK, Morgan SF, Pickens RW, Champagne SE. Situational factors in cigarette smoking. Addict Behav 1990;15:1–12.

40. Lewin L. Phantastica drogues psychédéliques, stupéfiants, narcotiques, excitants, hallucinogenes. Paris: Payot, 1970.

41. Jaffe JH. Drug addiction and drug abuse. In: Gilman AG, Goodman LS, Rall TW, Murad F, eds. Goodman and Gilman's pharmacological basis of therapeutics. New York: Macmillan, 1985:532–81.

42. Schuster CR, Thompson T. Self-administration of and behavioral dependence on drugs. Annu Rev Pharmacol 1969;9:483–502.

43. Griffiths RR, Bigelow GE, Henningfield JE. Similarities in animal and human drug-taking behavior. In: Mello K, ed. Advances in substance abuse. Vol. 1. Greenwich, CT: JAI Press, 1980:1–90.

44. Cummings KM, Giovino G, Jaen CR, Emrich LJ. Reports of smoking withdrawal symptoms over a 21 day period of abstinence. Addict Behav 1985;10:373–81.

45. Hatsukami DK, Hughes JR, Pickens RW, Svikis D. Tobacco withdrawal symptoms: an experimental analysis. Psychopharmacology 1984;84:231–36.

46. Hughes JR, Hatsukami D. Signs and symptoms of tobacco withdrawal. Arch Gen Psychiatry 1986;43:289–94.

47. Pickworth WB, Herning RI, Henningfield JE. Spontaneous EEG changes during tobacco abstinence and nicotine substitution in human volunteers. J Pharmacol Exp Ther 1989;251:976–82.

48. Snyder RF, Davis FC, Henningfield JE. The tobacco withdrawal syndrome: performance decrements assessed on a computerized test battery. Drug Alcohol Depend 1989;23:259–66.

49. Pickworth WB, Herning RI, Henningfield JE. Mecamylamine reduces some EEG effects of nicotine chewing gum in humans. Pharmacol Biochem Behav 1988;30:149–53.

50. Stolerman IP, Bunker P, Jarvik ME. Nicotine tolerance in rats: role of dose and dose interval. Psychopharmacologia (Berlin) 1974;34:317–24.

51. Marks MJ, Burch JB, Collins AC. Effects of chronic nicotine infusion on tolerance development and nicotinic receptors. J Pharmacol Exp Ther 1983;226:817–25.

52. Hubbard JE, Gohd RS. Tolerance development to the arousal effects of nicotine. Pharmacol Biochem Behav 1975;3:471–76.

53. Hughes JR, Strickler G, King D, Higgins ST, Fenwick JW, Gulliver SB,

Mireault G. Smoking history, instructions and the effects of nicotine: two pilot studies. Pharmacol Biochem Behav 1989;34:149–55.

54. Jones RT, Farrell TR, III, Herning RI. Tobacco smoking and nicotine tolerance. In: Krasnegor NA, ed. Self-administration of abused substances methods for study. NIDA Research Monograph 20. DHEW Publication (ADM) 78-727. Rockville, MD: National Institute on Drug Abuse, 1978:202–8.

55. Russell MAH, Jarvis MJ, Jones G, Feyerabend C. Non-smokers show acute tolerance to subcutaneous nicotine. Psychopharmacology 1990;102:56–58.

56. Jasinski DR, Henningfield JE. Human abuse liability assessment by measurement of subjective and physiological effects. In: Fischman MW, Mello NK, eds. Testing for abuse liability of drugs in humans. NIDA Research Monograph 92. DHHS Publication (ADM) 80-1613. Washington, DC: U.S. Department of Health and Human Services, 1989:73–100.

57. Haertzen CA, Hill HE, Belleville RE. Development of the Addiction Research Center Inventory (ARCI): selection of items that are sensitive to the effects of various drugs. Psychopharmacologia 1963;4:155–66.

58. Jasinski DR, Johnson RE, Henningfield JE. Abuse liability assessment in human subjects. Trends Pharmacol Sci 1984;5:196–200.

59. Henningfield JE, Miyasoto K, Jasinski DR. Abuse liability and pharmacodynamic characteristics of intravenous and inhaled nicotine. J Pharmacol Exp Ther 1985;234:1–12.

60. Russell MAH. The smoking habit and its classification. Practitioner 1974;212:791–800.

61. Hughes JR. Distinguishing withdrawal relief and direct effects of smoking. Psychopharmacology 1991;104:409–10.

62. Russell MAH, Jarvis MJ, Sutherland G, Feyerabend C. Nicotine replacement in smoking cessation. Absorption of nicotine vapor from smoke-free cigarettes. JAMA 1987;257:3262–65.

63. Hughes JR, Hatsukami D, Pickens RW, Krahn D, Malins S, Luknic A. Effect of nicotine on the tobacco withdrawal symptom. Psychopharmacology 1984;83:82–87.

64. Ockene JK, ed. The pharmacologic treatment of tobacco dependence: Proceedings of the World Congress, November 4–5, 1985. Cambridge, MA: Institute for the Study of Smoking Behavior and Policy, 1986.

65. Jarvis MJ, Raw M, Russell MAH, Feyerabend C. Randomised controlled trial of nicotine chewing gum. Br Med J 1982;285:537–40.

66. Kato S, Wakasa Y, Yanagita T. Relationship between minimum reinforcing doses and injection speed in cocaine and pentobarbital self-administration in crab-eating monkeys. Pharmacol Biochem Behav 1987;28:407–10.

67. Ludwig AM. Pavlov's "bells" and alcohol craving. Addict Behav 1986;11:87–91.

68.  O'Brien CP, Ternes JW, Grabowski J, Ehrman R. Classically conditioned phenomena in human opiate addiction. In: Thompson T, Johanson EC, eds. Behavioral pharmacology of human drug dependence. NIDA Research Monograph 37. DHEW Publication (ADM) 81-1137. Washington, DC: U.S. Department of Public Health Services, 1981:107–15.

69.  Gritz ER. Patterns of puffing in cigarette smokers. In: Krasnegor NA, ed. Self-administration of abused substances: methods for study. NIDA Research Monograph 20. Rockville, MD: National Institute on Drug Abuse, 1978:221–35.

70.  Henningfield JE, Radzius A, Cooper TM, Clayton RR. Drinking coffee and carbonated beverages blocks absorption of nicotine from nicotine polacrilex gum. JAMA 1990;12:1560–64.

71.  Nemeth-Coslett R, Benowitz NL, Robinson N, Henningfield JE. Nicotine gum: chew rate, subjective effects and plasma nicotine. Pharmacol Biochem Behav 1988;29:747–51.

72.  Rose JE, Levin ED, Behm FM, Adivi C, Schur C. Transdermal nicotine facilitates smoking cessation. Clin Pharmacol Ther 1990;47:323–30.

73.  Hughes JR, Gust SW, Keenan RM, Fenwick JW. Effect of dose on nicotine's reinforcing withdrawal-suppression and self-reported effects. J Pharmacol Exp Ther 1990;252:1175–83.

74.  Hatsukami DK, Skoog K, Huber M, Hughes J. Signs and symptoms from nicotine gum abstinence. Psychopharmacology 1991;104:496–504.

75.  Nunn-Thompson CL, Simon PA. Therapy review. Pharmacotherapy for smoking cessation. Clin Pharm 1989;8:710–20.

76.  Prignot J. Pharmacological approach to smoking cessation. Eur Respir J 1989;2:550–60.

77.  Murphy JK, Edwards NB, Downs AD, Ackerman BJ, Rosenthal TL. Effects of doxepin on withdrawal symptoms in smoking cessation. Am J Psychiatry 1990;10:1353–57.

78.  Stolerman IP. Could nicotine antagonists be used in smoking cessation? Br J Addict 1986;81:47–53.

# 28

## Understanding Smoking Behavior and Change:
## A Key to Prevention

**KAREN SLAMA**

Hôpital Saint-Louis
Paris, France

**SERGE KARSENTY**

Centre National de la Recherche Scientifique
Paris, France

## I.  Introduction

To prevent the occurrence of most cases of lung cancer and emphysema, and to reduce the incidence of many other respiratory ailments, the number of smokers in the population must be greatly lowered. To take effective action to reduce the prevalence of tobacco use, we must first understand smoking behavior and change. Our understanding of any human behavior is enlightened by theories, but for any behavior, there are opposing theories. Views about the nature of smoking behavior and smoking cessation that have been useful in generating strategies for measurable change can be classified into four main categories.

1. Smoking is an involuntary act, due to addiction created by nicotine. Smoking cessation therefore requires external aid.
2. Smoking is a "learned" behavior. It can be "unlearned" with treatment or on one's own.
3. Smoking or not smoking are voluntary acts by individuals. Motivation and adopting new behavior are the major factors in cessation.
4. Smoking is a social trend. People who make up the trend may change, but

*559*

the social trend itself will thrive, or abate until it reaches a critical point and smoking becomes marginalized.

These categories are extremes. Environmental or dependence factors are included in the voluntary act theories, just as individual and environmental factors are acknowledged by the dependence theories. In this chapter we attempt to describe evidence that has accumulated for each of these views, their limitations, and the pro- and antismoking factors clarified by each approach which might suggest an integrated theory to explain the issues in smoking behavior change.

## II. Smoking as an Addiction: A Medical Model of Smoking

Addiction is basically identified as chronic intoxication due to an overpowering compulsive desire to consume a substance, and distress at the withdrawal of the substance [1]. Biomedical research has shown that nicotine has dependence-producing properties. It alters or mimics nerve transmitters, which interact with receptors to produce measurable biological changes [2]. The effects that are centrally mediated are defined as psychoactive (enhancing mood and feeling), euphoriant, and biologically reinforcing [3]. Patterns of self-administration and dose–response effects of nicotine are orderly, and deprivation increases drug-seeking behavior [4]. The pharmacology of nicotine can help establish emotional balance with desirable psychoactive effects (feelings of well-being and confidence) and physical effects (increased heart rate, etc.) [5], which smokers interpret as stimulating or calming, probably depending on the quantity of nicotine in the blood [6]. The physical and psychoactive impact of nicotine is swift: Nerve reactors in the body, and particularly in the brain, are stimulated quickly; self-reported effects peak within 1 min [7]. The dissipation of these effects provokes both the desire to recreate the previous state and the desire to eliminate the unpleasant effects of withdrawal. As tolerance develops, withdrawal or the threat of withdrawal become more and more powerful as stimuli to smoke. Some researchers feel that addiction to smoking is the need to smoke so as not to experience the negative symptoms and intense desire promoted by withdrawal [8]. The negative emotions a smoker wants to avoid may be caused by this response to withdrawal [9].

Addiction, conceived of as a loss of control, leads logically to a conception of cessation as a process necessitating treatment. According to proponents of this approach, because addiction takes the smoker beyond personal choice [10], responsibility for smoking is not an issue. Addiction is treated as a disorder, a sickness to be cured [11].

In the medical model of smoking cessation, the addictive substance must be combated by an extrinsic agent to combat physical dependence. Strategies consist of providing a nonharmful substitute for the desired substance, to diminish the desire provoked by withdrawal. Nicotine gum, acupuncture, and hypnosis can show success in helping smokers to endure initial withdrawal more easily. However, these aids have not shown good long-term cessation rates on their own, in the absence of behavioral treatment [12]. Although 80% of quitters suffer withdrawal, the effect of cigarette abstinence is quite mild compared to opioid or sedative addictions [2]. In fact, physical withdrawal does not appear to be the major cause of relapse back to smoking, except in the initial few weeks [13]. But many people nevertheless have great difficulty stopping and maintaining abstinence. Most researchers into dependence-producing substances do not adhere to a purely biological model of addiction [3]. Although drugs exert pharmacological influence on the body, individual perception about a drug's effects as well as expectations about pharmacological action are influential in establishing dependence as well [9]. The strategies of the medical model, however, focus on reducing withdrawal distress and have little to propose for the psychological dependence that creates conditioned craving.

## III. Smoking as Learned Behavior

Social learning or cognitive-behavior theories attempt to discover how people think, how what they think leads them to initiate, to continue, or to abandon certain maladaptive behaviors, and how those behaviors influence what people think. Successful maintenance of change is theorized by social learning theory to be the result of self-management or counterconditioning to break away from dependence.

Social learning theory suggests that people "learn" to act in a certain way because of mental associations (cognitive mediational processes) made between a situational or physiological event (a stimulus), the behavior, and a desired consequence (a reinforcement) [14]. This is known as *conditioning*. For change to occur, the behavior must be understood in its context, and dissociated with the stimulus or the reinforcer. Stopping smoking without breaking the associations results in psychological withdrawal and craving.

Craving (a totally subjective measure) appears to be a major factor in unsuccessful maintenance of abstinence from tobacco. Craving can be considered the major manifestation of conditioning, psychological dependence created by the dependence-producing properties of nicotine, but thereafter independent of it [15].

The desired physical or psychoactive states produced by smoking, the situations in which they occur, and the smoker's emotional response at the time can be perceived as belonging together. Conditioning occurs when a smoker associates a situation, thought, or feeling automatically with the act of smoking. Conditioning means that a once-unrelated event becomes a cue (stimulus) to an action (response). For example, a smoker may associate the need to smoke with events in his or her daily life, such as moments of stress, moments of pleasure, and moments of boredom; another smoker may associate smoking with certain ideas or with certain activities. These situations or feelings become cues to smoking that are as imperative as physical withdrawal. In this way, craving becomes conditioned and is independent of nicotine's presence or absence in the blood. Craving can occur initially to produce desired bodily reactions, eventually to alleviate or avoid negative physical or psychoactive deprivation symptoms, or craving can occur in the presence of situations, events, feelings, objects, and so on, that have become strongly associated with the results of smoking, be they pleasurable sensations (i.e., heightened stimulation, increased sense of control, etc.) or the alleviation or avoidance of negative sensations (negative emotions, etc.).

It has been estimated from quitting smokers' self-reported craving to smoke over time that the role of conditioning in smoking abstinence (called "nostalgia") has a half-life of 8.5 months [16]. The model of physical addiction, which emphasizes the smoker's helplessness, may discourage smokers from attempting to stop without extrinsic help [11]. The social learning model of conditioned craving places cessation within the person's control: Smoking is a learned behavior that can be unlearned. To extinguish or destroy the conditioned response, the cycle of associations must be broken. This involves disassociating smoking from desired effects (such as feeling more relaxed, or feeling better), or disassociating the cues (discriminant stimuli) from the results of smoking. In other words, if quitting smokers can understand how the environment influences their smoking, they can more easily change their environment to encourage nonsmoking. These processes do not necessarily take place in treatment but are part of a person's capacity for self-change and self-management. In fact, spontaneous cessation is the main pathway to reducing the prevalence of smoking in populations [10].

In social learning, lasting smoking cessation is theorized to be determined by the smoker's anticipation of the positive health consequences of stopping and that person's skill in dealing with smoking stimuli (withdrawal, conditioned craving, social pressure, etc.) [17]. Thus the principal elements involved are motivation and skills: skills being influenced by self-confidence and understanding of the environment, and motivation being influenced by the way people collect and use information, as explained by cognitive theories.

## IV.  Smoking or Stopping Smoking as Volitional Acts: The Role of Cognitions

Prior to stopping smoking, the decision to stop must first be made. This occurs when new choices about smoking are made possible by motivation (belief in the value of change), which is influenced by health risk assessments (awareness of the argument for change), expectancies of success, and awareness of normative antismoking pressures. *Motivation* is the term used to bring together all of the cognitive elements implicated in a desired action. This includes values, beliefs, attitudes, opinions, and so on. But only a limited relationship can be shown to exist between these general cognitive elements and specific behaviors. However, the *theory of reasoned action* (TRA) suggests that an examination of the attitudes toward a set of potential behaviors can predict behavior [18]. In other words, if we compare the amount of intention to perform each of the alternative smoking behaviors (continuing to smoke the same amount and the same brand, changing smoking behavior, or stopping smoking), we can then measure the strongest behavioral intention that is most likely to occur. The TRA proposes that behavioral intentions are the result of personal attitudes toward the behavior and perceived social pressures, called subjective norms [19]. Personal attitudes are, according to the theory, based on behavioral beliefs (What are the consequences of my smoking or not smoking?) and evaluational beliefs (How do I judge these consequences?). Subjective norms are based on normative beliefs (What do people important to me think?) and desire to comply (How much do I want to please these people?) [20]. Changing behavior is ultimately a result of changes of belief, so we need to expose the person to information that will produce those changes [19].

### A. Smokers' Health Risk Perceptions

#### Current Estimations

Information can be deflected or misunderstood. This appears to be what has happened to health risk information about smoking. Despite health information campaigns launched throughout the developed world, surveys that investigate both general knowledge and personalization of that knowledge regularly find surprising underestimations of risk.

A 1980 poll in the United States (Roper) found that 49% of smokers did not know that smoking causes most cases of lung cancer; 63% did not know that smoking causes most cases of emphysema. A 1981 Gallup poll found that 28% of smokers did not know that smoking causes cancer [21]. A survey conducted in Great Britain in the early 1980s found that only 11% of smokers believed that their smoking created an extra risk for lung cancer which could be reduced by quitting, and almost half (45%) of the smokers felt that they were incurring no added health risks by smoking [22]. A survey (unpublished) conducted in Australia in 1986 found that 50% of the smokers interviewed did not perceive themselves to be vulnerable to the health risks of smoking, and more than 75% did not believe that stopping smoking would change health risks. While just over three-fourths of final-year medical students from 14 European countries surveyed in the mid-1980s agreed that cigarette smoking is a determinant cause of lung cancer, less than 20% agreed that smoking is a determinant cause of emphysema [23].

Once the prospect of health gains is seriously believed, smoking cessation occurs [22]; therefore, it may be important to understand why health risk information is often unheeded and even disbelieved. Heuristics and cognitive consistency theories attempt to explain such results.

### Heuristics

Heuristics (cognitive simplification strategies) are the shortcuts people use to make judgments about risks, probabilities, and causes; and these judgments shape behavioral decisions. While they are tools for drawing conclusions that are often valid, they can distort judgment by diverting attention from necessary information [24]. In general, people tend to believe that their own risks for health problems are below average [25], and that they are better than average drivers, more likely to live past 80, and less likely to be harmed by what they use [26]. Risk probabilities are frequently misjudged because of cognitive errors induced by media coverage of spectacular but infrequent events such as violent catastrophic deaths. People underestimate the frequency of common but unpublicized health problems such as diabetes, stroke, asthma, emphysema, and tuberculosis [26]. Other sources of bias in judgment include an irresistible tendency to perceive sequences of events in terms of causal relations [27] (e.g., attributing a heart attack to a recent disappointment), making judgments from one source [26] (e.g., disbelieving the causal role of tobacco if one nonsmoker has lung cancer), dismissing information that does not fit into stereotypical images (once a judgment about causality and risk is established, disconfirming information is not heeded), and defensive reluctance to admit vulnerability [25]. Whatever the causes, people are often unmoved by statistical data and epidemiological risk probability data [28]. As well, belief in the relevance of life-style to one's health is dependent on one's willingness to accept responsibility for one's own health [29].

### Cognitive Consistency

Another aspect of the utilization of information pertains to theories based on the human need to resolve conflicts and contradictions between beliefs, attitudes, and behavior. Dissonancy theory, as formulated by Festinger in 1957 [30], proposes that each cognitive element (piece of knowledge, belief, or opinion about the environment or about oneself) is consonant (in accordance) or dissonant (in disaccord) in relationship with each other cognitive element and with behavior. Dissonance is psychologically unpleasant and will eventually lead to change in the least resistant of the elements or behavior [31]. But efforts will first be made to reduce dissonance by magnifying the importance of resistance opinion or behavior (e.g., exaggerating personal benefits of smoking), reducing the magnitude of rewards and punishment (e.g., minimizing health risk information), seeking information to reinforce consonance (e.g., interpreting a doctor's not asking about smoking as evidence that smoking must not be hazardous), avoiding information that increases dissonance, and distorting or disregarding information that cannot be avoided (e.g., deciding that smoking is just one more of life's little risks). Any or all of these heuristic or dissonance-reducing procedures help to explain the major underestimation of the risks of smoking made by most smokers. The implications of these theories are that health risk information about smoking has not been diffused often enough, or strikingly enough, so that minimization or disbelief is harder to achieve. Contrary to common assumption, information that is fear-producing appears consistently to motivate toward cessation. Attitude change can be mediated by the amount of fear aroused [32]. Although the commitment to attempt change can arise in a brief period of time [33], it must be acted upon before it can be eroded by pro-smoking stimuli, heuristics, or dissonance. Information that is personalized may be retained longer [17]. Physician advice is considered to hold great potential in motivating change because it provides the possibility for personal contact and consistent antitobacco information, which are the major factors in producing change among smokers in primary care [34].

### B. Expectancies

Resistance to a fear message can be aroused when people are faced with a severe threat that they perceive they are unable to avoid [35]. This may explain the importance of self-efficacy (the confidence that one can surmount any difficulties that arise because of a behavior change) in initiating smoking cessation [36]. Self-efficacy and other expectancies have been the focus of numerous studies and appear to be useful elements not only in the decision-making process [22] but also in predicting successful urge resistance after cessation has occurred [37]. The strongest barrier to developing high personal expectancies is nicotine addiction or perception of addiction.

### C. Normative Pressures

Just as smokers' evaluations are not necessarily influenced by information, or their expectancies influenced by faulty perceptions, smokers may not be aware of antismoking normative pressures, and pay more heed to pro-smoking normative pressures [22]. Many treatment programs assume that smokers, having come of their own free will, are motivated to stop smoking and are therefore fully aware of antismoking cues and normative pressures to stop smoking, although this is rarely measured. Studies of treated or spontaneous quitters who are able to maintain continuous abstinence regularly show that they have been in the presence of positive social support [38]. Whereas smoking prevention programs emphasize the need to increase awareness of antismoking norms and pressures, cessation programs do not often include such a component.

## V.  Smoking as a Social Phenomenon

The medical model of addiction does not deal with the complexities of conditioned craving. Social learning and cognition theories do not explain the evolution of smoking in the society, but attempt to indicate how maladaptive choices are influenced by the person's perception of the environment. However, an unfortunate by-product of the health education and treatment strategies evolved from social learning theory is the blame it appears to put on smokers for being "deviant." Obviously, an activity used by such a large percentage of the population cannot be named deviant [39] and an alternative explanation for smoking and smoking cessation may be needed.

The social deviancy or psychopathology associated with some types of addiction is a product of social reactions to drug use [1], depending on the current social norms. Until recently, the majority of the population conceived of smoking "in general" as voluntarily choosing to accept the possible health consequences of this act. Governmental actions to lessen the possible consequences were defined as restrictions on liberty [39]. However, changes in collective health are likely to come about, in the future as in the past, from changes in conditions that lead to disease, not by individual volitional acts. Improvements come from political, social, economic, and environmental changes [40]. A tobacco-free norm has been gaining strength in many industrialized countries. To understand the present slow social change being enacted, it may be useful to examine theories of social change.

The basic assumption behind the social movement view of smoking uptake and smoking cessation is that individual reasons pale in relation to cultural and social behavior patterns. Individual beliefs influence the decisions taken, but socioeconomic circumstances enable or proscribe enactment of these decisions. In attempting to describe community change, Green proposed that there are three essential dimensions to behavior change on a population level: (1) predisposing factors lead to an initial decision about change, both at an individual and a societal level; (2) enabling factors are those that permit the decision to be enacted initially; and (3) reinforcing factors encourage maintaining the new behavior [41]. In terms of smoking, these factors are all influenced by environment, society, and culture. People become aware of reasons to smoke or reasons to stop from their environment, from cues about appropriate behavior that they pick up from those around them, and from information about the consequences of change that they attend to. Whether the stronger messages come from pro-smoking or antismoking sources depends on the agenda of the media, the amount of liberty given to each of these forces by social norms and government regulations, the availability of tobacco products, and the extent of settings where their use is sanctioned. Finally, the way people see smokers, and whether to be a smoker is a marginal or dominant goal for young people, influences its growth or diminuation as a social movement.

Rogers has suggested that change in a social movement comes slowly by a process of diffusion of innovations [42]. In a society with a large percentage of smokers, only a few may be susceptible to change, but if opinion leaders visibly stop smoking, their change will influence others, whose quitting will in turn influence others, leading to a critical number who believe in nonsmoking as the norm, and the old "normal" behavior, smoking, becomes "unnormal" and no longer is socially approved. Thus the social movement ends, even if a marginal number of smokers remain. Smoking, previously a sign of affluence and success among Western males is now a badge of the poorer, less educated man with low prestige [43]. The pattern is less clear for women, but despite the growth of smoking with the growth of feminism, the prestige of smoking is declining. In other words, beyond individual processes, social processes influence the final outcome. This is clear if we look at social class. Today in the United States, a quitting smoker from a higher socioeconomic background has less exposure to other smokers, is given more support, has more access to outside support facilities, has a more preventive health outlook, and has greater exposure to antismoking information, all of which greatly facilitate individual effort [44].

It has been suggested that by now, nondependent smokers have probably left the ranks of active smokers and that current smokers are the dependent ones [45]. However, this suggestion does not take into account the large numbers of new, young smokers. In fact, in those countries where smoking prevalence is declining, the decrease is due more to greater numbers of smokers who are stopping than to fewer young people who are taking up smoking [46]. Unless a genetic need [47] for cigarette smoking uptake is now in operation much more than in the past, the reasons behind the greater numbers of heavy smokers may be more one of social class norms than of individual predisposition to addiction.

No society has totally reversed the smoking movement, as every advance is opposed by the manufacturers of a legally produced consumer item. But many antismoking forces are now focused on attempts to increase the legitimacy of nonsmoking [41], that is, to make smoke-free behavior the normal behavior in all public locations, unless specified otherwise. Now, even in the most progressive places, nonsmoking is the specified activity, which indicates that smoking would automatically be the norm if no specifications exist. As Marsh has said, "sociopolitical rather than health factors have been decisive in shaping the smoking controversy" about where and when smoking is acceptable [22].

For those who have abandoned the medical (physical addiction) or social learning (motivation and conditioned craving) models to act for smoking control, the social movement model has been adopted to provide strategies to bring about the "delegitimization of smoking" [22], by marginalizing tobacco use through (1) price controls to discourage young smokers who are only at an experimental stage in their smoking, (2) smoking bans in public places to redefine social norms and to reduce cues to take up or relapse to smoking, (3) advertising bans to limit the tobacco industry's possibility to strengthen pro-tobacco norms which facilitate new smoker recruitment, and (4) mass-media education campaigns to polarize public opinion so that new legislation and regulations are enforced and social norms reinforced.

Canada, which has enacted tobacco advertising bans, health warnings, and price increases as well as high-visibility public opinion campaigns, saw a 6.8% drop in per capita sales in 1989 alone [48]. The comprehensive tobacco control program enacted in Norway in the mid-1970s has had an impact on overall smoking rates [49]. Careful examination of price increases has indicated that demand for tobacco products is influenced in direct proportion to the amount of increase (elasticity), by $-0.2$ to $-0.5$. In other words, for each 10% rise in price, there will be a corresponding drop in consumption of 2 to 5%; and demand elasticity may be even higher ($-1.4$) for young people [50] and others with lower levels of disposable income and those of lower socioeconomic status [51], the very groups that hold the highest numbers of smokers. Demand elasticity also appears to be much higher in the Third World, as evidenced by research in Papua–New Guinea [52]. Research has shown small but significant increases in consumption of cigarettes due to advertising [53] and drops in consumption as tobacco advertising bans become more complete [54].

## VI. Integrating the Approaches

These seemingly opposing views of smoking can be integrated by their context within a model of the total process of an individual's smoking behavior change. Change appears to consist of stages, including awareness of reasons for change, contemplation of change, deciding to attempt change, actual attempts at change and maintenance of nonsmoking [55]. Difficulties arise at each step, and smokers may become stuck or slip back to previous steps. Key issues that are influential in a smoker's progression through the cycle are the factors that facilitate or hinder passage. Social norms and individual characteristics play a role in determining whether one thinks about stopping smoking. This creates the motivation that can facilitate a smoker's move into and through contemplation about stopping, whereas proceeding to action can be blocked by the fact of nicotine addiction and/or the perception the smoker has of his or her own addiction. If the smoker

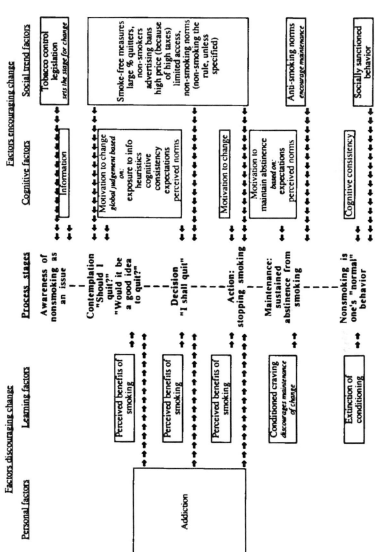

**Figure 1** Factors intervening in the process of becoming a nonsmoker.

does stop smoking, the urge to smoke (conditioned craving), even in the absence of physical withdrawal, can form a potent barrier to successful maintenance of the new behavior of not smoking. Finally, pro-smoking norms and cultural beliefs can prevent many smokers from leaving the cycle as confirmed nonsmokers by facilitating relapse, whereas antismoking norms encourage more rapid movement through all the stages. This is represented graphically in Figure 1.

If we truly want to reduce the prevalence of smoking, we must recognize the impact of the various factors included in the fight against tobacco use. Various treatments can help individuals but generally do not have an impact on social norms. The most important influences on the total prevalence of smoking in a nation appear to be strong antismoking norms (legitimization of nonsmoking and marginalization of smoking) and reduced incitations to smoke (advertising bans, restricted smoking areas, high retail price). On an individual basis, education, coupled with clear signs from important opinion leaders such as doctors and teachers that smoking is not an approved activity, can help motivate smokers, or push them toward the decision to stop smoking. Awareness of spontaneous cessation can help stimulate more spontaneous cessation and demystify the addiction barrier.

The prevention of respiratory and other smoking-related diseases may be influenced by the help provided to individual smokers through cessation treatments, and more so by consistently providing information through multiple channels to motivate smokers to stop smoking and to convince young people not to begin. These activities help lead to the development of strong antismoking norms in parts of the society that eventually discourage smoking among the whole population.

### References

1.  Fisher EB Jr, Haire-Joshu D, Morgan GD, Rehberg H, Rost K. Smoking and smoking cessation. Am Rev Respir Dis, 1990;142:702–20.
2.  Martin WR. Tobacco and health overview: a neurological approach. In: Martin WR, Van Loon GR, Iwamoto ET, Davis L, eds. Tobacco smoking and nicotine: a neurobiological approach. New York: Plenum Press, 1987:1.
3.  Nemeth-Coslett R, Henningfield JE. Rational basis for chemotherapy of tobacco dependence. In: Grabowski J, Hall SM, eds. Pharmacological adjuncts in smoking cessation. NIDA Research Monograph 53. DHHS Publication (ADM) 85-1333. Rockville, MD: National Institute on Drug Abuse, 1985:15–26.
4.  Benowitz NL. Pharmacologic aspects of cigarette smoking and nicotine addiction. N Engl J Med 1988;319:1318–30.

5. Hasenfratz M, Nil R, Bättig K. Development of central and peripheral smoking effects over time. Psychopharmacology 1990;101:359–65.
6. Marsh A. Smoking: habit or choice? Popul Trends 1984;37:14–20.
7. Henningfield JE, Nemeth-Coslett R. Nicotine dependence. Interface between tobacco and tobacco-related disease. Chest 1988;93:37S–55S.
8. Bass F. Invalidating tobacco. In: Taylor RB, ed. Health promotion: principles and clinical applications. East Norwalk, CT: Appleton-Century-Crofts, 1982:259–86.
9. Marlatt GA, Donovan DM. Alcoholism and drug dependence: cognitive social learning factors in addictive behaviors. In: Craighead WE, Kazdin AE, Mahoney MJ, eds. Behavior modification: principle, issues, and applications. 2nd ed. Boston: Houghton Mifflin, 1981.
10. Marsh A. The dying of the light. Copenhagen: WHO publication. Smoke-Free Europe 1988;7.
11. Eiser JR. Addiction as attribution: cognitive processes in giving up smoking. In: Eiser JR, ed. Social psychology and behavioral medicine. Chichester, West Sussex, England, Wiley, 1982.
12. Killen JD, Fortnam SP, Newman B, Varady A. Evaluation of a treatment approach combining nicotine gum with self-guided behavioral treatments for smoking relapse prevention. J Consult Clin Psychol 1990;58:85–92.
13. Bliss RE, Garvey AJ, Heinold JW, Hitchcock JL. The influence of situation and coping on relapse crises outcomes after smoking cessation. J Consult Clin Psychol 1989;57:443–49.
14. Kasner L. Behavior therapy: on roots, contexts, and growth. In: Wilson GT, Franks CM, eds. Contemporary behavior therapy. New York: Guilford Press, 1982.
15. Kozlowski LT, Wilkinson DA. Use and misuse of the concept of craving by alcohol, tobacco and drug researchers. Br J Addict 1987;82:31–36.
16. Fan DP, Elketroussi M. Mathematical model for addiction: application to multiple risk factor intervention trial data for smoking. J Clin Consult Psychol, 1989;57:456–59.
17. Quadrel MJ, Lau RR. Health promotion, health locus of control, and health behavior: two field experiments. J Appl Soc Psychol 1989;19:1497–1521.
18. Bettinghaus EP. Health promotion and the knowledge–attitude–behavior continuum. Prev Med 1986;15:475–91.
19. Ajzen I, Fishbein M. Understanding attitudes and predicting social behavior. Englewood Cliffs, NJ: Prentice Hall, 1980, Introduction.
20. Hill D, Rassaby J, Gardner G. Determinants of intentions to take precautions against skin cancer. Community Health Stud 1984;8:33–44.
21. State-of-the-art planning paper. Tobacco. Prepared for Phase II of the Cancer Prevention Awareness Program, Office of Cancer Communications, National Cancer Institute, 1986.

22. Marsh A, Matheson J. Smoking attitudes and behavior. An enquiry carried out on behalf of the department of Health and Social Security, London, 1983.

23. Tessier JF, Fréour P, Crofton J, Kombou L. Smoking habits and attitudes of medical students towards smoking and antismoking campaigns in fourteen European countries. Eur J Epidemiol 1989;5:311–21.

24. Moscovici S, Hewstone M. Social representations and social explanations: from the "naive" to the "amateur" scientist. In: Hewstone M, ed. Attribution theory: social and functional extentions. Oxford: Basil Blackwell, 1983.

25. Weinstein ND. Unrealistic optimism about susceptibility to health problems. J Behav Med 1982;5:441–60.

26. Slovic P, Fischhoff B, Lichtenstein S. Facts versus fears: understanding perceived risk. In: Kahneman D, Slovic P, Tversky A, eds. Judgements under uncertainty: heuristics and biases. Cambridge: Cambridge University Press, 1982.

27. Tversky A, Kahneman D. Causal schemas in judgments under uncertainty. In: Kahneman D, Slovic P, Tversky A, eds. Judgments under uncertainty: heuristics and biases. Cambridge: Cambridge University Press, 1982.

28. Nesbitt RE, Borgida E, Crandall R, Reed H. Popular induction: information is not necessarily informative. In: Kahneman D, Slovic P, Tversky A, eds. Judgements under uncertainty: heuristics and biases. Cambridge: Cambridge University Press, 1982.

29. Pill R, Stott NCH. Choice or chance: further evidence on ideas of illness and responsibility for health. Soc Sci Med 1985;20:981–91.

30. Festinger LA. Theory of cognitive dissonance. Evanston, IL: Row-Patterson, 1957.

31. Reich B, Adcock C. Values, attitudes and behavior change. London: Methuen, 1976.

32. Sutton S, Hallett R. Understanding the effects of fear-arousing communications: the role of cognitive factors and amount of fear aroused. J Behav Med, 1988;11:353–60.

33. Prochaska JO, DiClemente CC. Transtheoretical therapy: toward a more integrative model of change. Psychother Theory Res Pract 1982;19:276–88.

34. Kottke TE, Battista RN, DeFriese GH, Brekke ML. Attributes of successful smoking cessation interventions in medical practice. A meta-analysis of 39 controlled trials. JAMA 1988;259:2883–89.

35. Sutton SR. Fear arousing communications: a critical examination of theory and research. In: Eiser JR, ed. Social psychology and behavioral medicine. Chichester, West Sussex, England, Wiley, 1982.

36. Garcia ME, Schmitz JM, Doerfler LA. A fine-grained analysis of the role

of self-efficacy in self-initiated attempts to quit smoking. J Consult Clin Psychol 1990;58:317–22.

37. Condiotte MM, Lichtenstein E, Mermelstein RJ. Self-efficacy and relapse in smoking cessation programs. J Consult Clin Psychol 1982;5:983–90.
38. Cohen S, Lichtenstein E. Partner behaviors that support quitting smoking. J Consult Clin Psychol 1990;58:304–9.
39. Taylor D, Batten L. A new approach to the prevention of smoking. In: Operation smokestop. Positive Health Technical Report 2. Wessex, England: Regional Health Authority, 1983.
40. Dubos R. Man adapting. New Haven, CT: Yale University Press, 1965.
41. Calnan M. Control over health and patterns of health-related behavior. Soc Sci Med 1989;29:131–36.
42. Rogers EM. Diffusion of innovations. New York: Free Press, 1983.
43. Houston CS. The sociology of cigarette smoking. Can Med Assoc J 1986;134:878–97.
44. Kirscht JP, Janz NK, Becker MH. Psychosocial predictors of change in cigarette smoking. J Appl Soc Psychol 1989;19:298–308.
45. Glassman AH, Covey LS. Future trends in the pharmacological treatment of smoking cessation. Drugs 1990;40:1–5.
46. Chapman S. Stop smoking clinics: a case for their abandonment. Lancet 1985;1:918–20.
47. Pomerleau, OF. Underlying mechanisms in substance abuse: examples from research on smoking. Addict Behav 1981;6:187–196.
48. Mahood G. Treating the tobacco epidemic like an epidemic: the road to effective tobacco control in Canada. In: Durston B, Jamrozik K, eds. Tobacco and health 1990: the global war. Proceedings of the 7th World Conference on Tobacco and Health, 1990:88–97.
49. Bjartveit K. Fifteen years of comprehensive legislation: results and conclusions. In: Durston B, Jamrozik K, eds. Tobacco and health 1990: the global war. Proceedings of the 7th World Conference on Tobacco and Health, 1990:71–80.
50. U.S. Department of Health and Human Services. Reducing the health consequences of smoking: 25 years of progress. A report of the Surgeon General. DHHS Publication (CDC) 89-8411, 1989.
51. Townsend JL. Cigarette tax, economic welfare and social class patterns of smoking. Appl Econ 1987;19:355–65.
52. Chapman S, Richardson J. Tobacco excise and declining tobacco consumption: the case of Papua, New Guinea. Am J Public Health 1990;80:537–40.
53. Tye JB, Warner KE, Glantz SA. Tobacco advertising and consumption: evidence of a causal relationship. US J Public Health Policy, Winter 1987.
54. Laugesen M, Meads C. Advertising price, income and publicity effects

on weekly cigarette sales in New Zealand supermarkets. Br J Addict 1991;86:83–89.

55.   Prochaska JO, Crimi P, Lapsanski D, Martel L, Reid P. Self-change processes, self-efficacy and self-concept in relapse and maintenance of cessation of smoking. Psychol Rep 1982;5:983–90.

# 29

## Role of Health Professionals in Tobacco Control

**MARTIN RAW**

Kings College School of Medicine and Dentistry
London, England

## I. Introduction

"Those countries where the medical profession has been active against tobacco were often those that had been the most successful in reducing smoking prevalence and tobacco consumption. The challenge was then to try to stimulate doctors to do more, by making suggestions and providing tools for action. On a worldwide scale, doctors working together and individually have done much to combat tobacco use, and not only the medical profession but many others could benefit by sharing the stories of their successes and failures" [1].

## II. History

Historically, tobacco control advocacy had its origins in the work of the medical profession. When Alton Ochsner was a medical student in Washington in 1919, a man with lung cancer was admitted to the hospital where he worked. The professor of medicine invited students to witness the autopsy because the condition was so rare they would probably not see another case in their lifetimes.

Ochsner did not see another case until 1936, when he saw nine cases in 6 months. He was so struck by this sudden epidemic that he investigated its background. All nine were men, all heavy cigarette smokers, and all had started smoking during World war I. He also discovered that cigarette smoking was rare until that war [2].

His observations were followed by epidemiological research, by Ernst Wynder and E. A. Graham in the United States and by Richard Doll and Austin Bradford Hill in the United Kingdom. Both published their initial findings in 1950. During the 1950s, as it became clearer that smoking was the main cause of lung cancer, chronic bronchitis, and emphysema, the Royal College of Physicians in London were persuaded by Charles Fletcher to publish a report on smoking and health. In the United States, President Kennedy asked the Surgeon General to produce a report like "Smoking and Health," the result being the 1964 U.S. Surgeon General's report, and the excellent series that has continued until now. Fletcher expected that the results of the report would shock politicians into immediate action. When it became clear that this would not happen, he pressed the Royal College not only to publish a second report, but to set up a separate body to press for change. Thus was Action on Smoking and Health (London) born [3].

Action on Smoking and Health (ASH) became a campaigning body that tried to put pressure on the government for action and also directly attacked the tobacco industry. Central to its strategy was the fact that it was created by doctors and that it had influential doctors on its ruling council. It had a research committee comprised of doctors and researchers, which made sure that its campaigning activities were always based on the latest medical research. This gave it a legitimacy and authority that politicans could not easily ignore.

Tobacco use is still the major cause of lung cancer, a major cause of heart disease, and the largest single preventable cause of disease and death in countries where smoking is long established. The main method used to reduce tobacco-related disease and death is through reduction in tobacco consumption, not through treatment of the diseases. To achieve this, a vigorous and comprehensive tobacco control program must be maintained for the foreseeable future, including at least these key elements [2]:

1. Vigorous public information and education programs with the active involvement of the health care professions
2. Collection of baseline data and monitoring of tobacco prevalence, consumption, and disease trends
3. Restriction of smoking in public places, including workplaces, to protect people from involuntary exposure to tobacco smoke
4. Legal ban on *all* forms of advertising and promotion, including sponsorship and indirect advertising

5. Progressive price rises through taxation in excess of inflation
6. The setting of a good example by health professionals and in health care premises
7. Strong, unequivocal, varied health warnings on all tobacco packaging and advertising, including indirect advertising
8. Promoting economically feasible alternatives to tobacco production through carefully thought out and effective programs
9. A national focal point to stimulate, coordinate, and support these activities (e.g., a committee, an organisation, or an informal group)

## III. Role of Doctors Now

The setting of a good example by health care professionals and in the health service is crucial. Doctors are still respected figures in most cultures and people listen to their advice. People were asked in a British survey whom they respected regarding advice on health. Sixty-three percent said they completely trusted their family doctor, while only 10% trusted television, 3% a friend or neighbor, and only 2% a newspaper article [4]. We also know from the work of Michael Russell and his colleagues that smokers follow the advice of their family doctor to stop smoking if it is given simply but firmly, and followed up. However, few family doctors, even in the United Kingdom, have integrated this sort of advice into their routine work.

Many people—ordinary smokers, health professionals, even doctors—assume that smokers now know that smoking is bad for them. This is dangerously misleading. People do not make the connection between smoking (their behavior) and death (someone else's misfortune), and they do not understand the relative size of the risk. Health educators need to use images and comparison that mean something to people: for example, that smoking kills more than 20 times as many people as road accidents do. Doctors are in an especially strong position to make this point: smokers will actually listen to them. What the research in Britain shows is that even after Russell's seminal 1979 paper [5], many doctors give virtually no useful advice on smoking, and incredibly, some say nothing at all.

## IV. Role of Respiratory Health Professionals

Respiratory health professionals have an extremely important contribution to make. They should first take the trouble to learn the facts about smoking and health and understand the size of the problem. They should then learn how to counsel. There is a great deal more to this than just telling people what they should do, although that is an extremely important start. The way it is done is important, and so is the adding of constructive, practically useful information about what to do (how to stop) and how to go about it. They should then know where smokers can get further help and support and what kind of help to recommend. All these comments apply to doctors in general, but obviously due to the nature of the diseases that respiratory physicians treat, and their causes, doctors have an especially strategic role. It is probably obvious but perhaps needs restating for the record. Smoking prevalence is very high in doctors in some countries* and in these countries, probably the first thing that has to happen is that doctors must stop smoking* (Table 1). Members of the general public are hardly likely to do as doctors say and not as they do, and clearly doctors who smoke have little credibility on the subject of health.

If all this sounds like a lot—it is. But it is worthwhile. If doctors could learn to do these things, they could have a real impact in helping smokers stop and in reducing smoking-related chest diseases. Possibly the country with the most advanced training program for doctors in smoking cessation counseling at the moment is the United States, largely through the funding of the National Cancer Institute. In parallel with workers in the United Kingdom and sometimes in cooperation with them, training publications and courses are being developed and tested. In the United Kingdom at least two training courses, one for doctors in general practice and one for primary health care workers, are starting in 1992, and some useful publications are already available.

## V. Help Your Patient Stop

The British Medical Association (BMA), with the Imperial Cancer Research Fund, the World Health Organization, and International Union Against Cancer, have produced a 20-page booklet designed to give doctors (and other health professionals) the basic information and guidance they would need to help smokers stop [6], called "Help Your Patient Stop." It is part of a continuing program of work by the BMA, WHO, and European Commission (CEC) to help health professionals do more to prevent tobacco-related diseases. Other publications include a more detailed manual, "Guidelines on Smoking Cessation for the Primary Health Care Team" [7] published by WHO and UICC. "Help Your Patient Stop" is already published in French, Spanish, and Polish, and permission to translate and reprint it will always be given in return for a simple acknowl-

---

*Little information regarding the smoking habits of respiratory physicians is currently available. Two studies (Sachs DPL. Smoking habits of pulmonary physicians. N Engl J Med 1983;309:799; and Fréour P, Tessier JF. Note sur le tabagisme des pneumologues de la SPLF. Rev Mal Respir 1988;5:189–90) show smoking rates among respiratory physicians (U.S.: 12%; France: 24.5%) that are lower than those in the general population. Whether or not these two studies represent a real trend can only be indicated by international data corresponding to those gathered for general practitioners.

**Table 1**   Smoking Prevalence in Doctors in General Practice
and in the General Population in the European Community

| Country | GPs | General | Difference |
|---|---|---|---|
| Spain | 45 | 41 | +4 |
| Italy | 41 | 33 | +8 |
| Portugal | 39 | 27 | +12 |
| Greece | 39 | 42 | –3 |
| Denmark | 38 | 45 | –7 |
| Luxembourg | 36 | 33 | +3 |
| France | 31 | 35 | –4 |
| Belgium | 29 | 39 | –10 |
| Netherlands | 29 | 45 | –16 |
| Germany | 25 | 32 | –7 |
| Ireland | 20 | 37 | –17 |
| United Kingdom | 10 | 35 | –25 |

*Source*: Commission of the European Communities, 1990.

edgment (by the Public Affairs Division of the British Medical Association in London).

"Help Your Patient Stop" has six sections presented in a simple, clear design: (1) Introduction; (2) Background Information (Smoking Is Dangerous, It Is Worth Stopping, What Is Smoking?); (3) What You Can Do; (4) Questions and Answers; (5) Further Help; and (6) Three Basic Steps. The booklet does not assume that smokers understand *how* dangerous smoking is or that it is worthwhile stopping, and explains these points simply but clearly. This is important since some smokers believe that smoking is dangerous but do not try to stop because they think the damage is already done. The booklet explains the nature of smoking, particularly that it is an addiction. This should not be glossed over when counseling smokers. It can lead to underestimating the difficulty some have in stopping, or worse, being unsympathetic on the grounds that it is "just a habit."

The final section of the booklet is perhaps the most important. Not all doctors will immediately start counseling their patients to stop smoking. Indeed, the high proportion of smokers among family doctors in many European countries suggests that the doctors must stop smoking first. However, much could be achieved if more doctors followed the three simple steps at the end of the booklet:

1.   Ask about and record all patients' smoking habits in the notes.
2.   Ask all smokers to stop.
3.   Offer leaflets on stopping smoking.

These simple steps will get some smokers to think about stopping and will encourage others to stop. If the advice is given firmly and with authority, it will be listened to.

## VI. Wider Role of Doctors

Doctors can do far more than just advise patients. They began action to prevent smoking-related disease when they first discovered that smoking was dangerous. When the mere publicizing of this fact failed to persuade governments to act, they realised that they had to take more positive action—to start campaigning. Because of their respected position in society their voice will be listened to by policymakers of many kinds, including politicians. The British Medical Association formally entered the British tobacco campaign in 1984 by launching an aggressive and ongoing campaign against the tobacco industry [8]. From the beginning they worked with, and drew upon, the experience of other more seasoned organizations, including ASH, helping to develop a broad-based coalition in Britain to keep up the pressure against tobacco. Their campaign has always been based on the democratically determined official policy of their members, which means that it has had the support of thousands of ordinary (but angry) doctors. This has given the campaign power and authority.

In one instance, doctors marched in the streets to protest against the introduction into Britain of a new, dangerous product—oral snuff—known to appeal to children [2]. In others, doctors have written letters to politicians, and in yet others, have drawn attention to issues through high-profile publicity events, including press conferences at the BMA. Doctors and other health professionals played very important roles in the campaign for a tobacco act in the Australian state of Victoria. Some of the stories of these actions are told in a BMA book, "Smoking Out the Barons" [8], and a BMA/WHO/CEC book, "Clearing the Air: A Guide for Action on Tobacco" [2].

## VII. Conclusions

The prevention of tobacco-related disease requires vigorous and ceaseless action at many levels. Doctors have an enormous and crucial contribution to make. They can advise and help their patients to stop smoking. But they can do even more by acting individually and collectively through their professional association to influence those who make policy. They should not hesitate to use their status and power to fight the appalling destruction wrought by a ruthless, incredibly greedy, and amoral industry.

### References

1. Raw M. The physician's role. Three modules on tobacco for national medical associations. Copenhagen and Brussels: WHO and European Commission (CEC), 1988.
2. Raw M, White P, McNeill A. Clearing the air. A guide for action on tobacco. London: BMA, WHO, and CEC, 1990.
3. Conversation with Charles Fletcher. Br J Addict 1992;87:527–38.
4. Budd J, McCron R. Communication and health education: a preliminary study. Leicester, England: University of Leicester, 1979.
5. Russell M, Wilson C, Taylor C, Baker C. Effect of general practitioners' advice against smoking. Br Med J 1979;2:231–35.
6. Raw M. Help your patient stop. London: BMA, ICRF, UICC, and WHO, 1988.
7. Ramstrom L, Raw M, Wood M (eds.). Guidelines on smoking cessation for the primary health care team. Geneva and Copenhagen: WHO and UICC, 1988.
8. British Medical Association. Smoking out the barons. The campaign against the tobacco industry. Chichester, England: Wiley, 1986.

# 30

## Cessation Treatments for Respiratory Disease Patients

**LINDA L. PEDERSON**

University of Western Ontario
London, Ontario, Canada

## I. Introduction

Smoking cessation among patients with respiratory diseases is associated with reduction in morbidity [1–6] and prolongation of life [6–9]. In fact, the decline in lung function among this group of patients is slowed following abstinence from cigarettes for 2 or more years [10–16]. This evidence has resulted in several recent publications offering advice to both general practice and respiratory physicians concerning the importance of abstinence from cigarettes [11,12,17–19] and methods for achieving this [11,17,20–32].

Unfortunately, several factors work against attainment of this goal. First, physicians, in general, often express reluctance or hesitation in offering advice to patients because of lack of time, support staff, availability of treatment, and/or training in life-style modification [27,33], or because of apparent failure in the past [19,27,34]. Second, patients who are experiencing firsthand the effects of their smoking and yet continue to smoke are not likely to change their behavior easily. While they acknowledge the relationship of smoking to their health status, express the desire to quit, and recognize that quitting will improve their condition

[32,35–37], they admit that quitting smoking is not a very likely occurrence [36,37]. In addition, they tend to be long-term, heavy, highly addicted smokers [24,26,37–39], all factors that are not predictive of successful abstinence in the general population [3–5].

Therefore, an in-depth examination of the interventions that have been used with this patient group is warranted at this point, to provide information on effective treatment approaches and directions for future research.

### A.  Roles for Physicians

In attempting to assist patients with respiratory disease to quit smoking, the physician can adopt one or more of several roles. A hypothetical model for physician behavior [40] proposed almost 15 years ago still has relevance for practice, as evidenced by recent publications (e.g., refs. 25 and 38). These roles range from minimal involvement by acting as a role model by being a nonsmoker, to educating patients on the health risks of continued smoking, directly advising patients regarding quitting, referring individuals to smoking cessation programs, and finally, considerable involvement by personally administering specific cessation and maintenance programs. Therefore, it is not necessary that the individual physician be actively involved in the process of quitting for every patient. In the studies reviewed below, physicians have adopted a variety of roles, including minimal involvement in the actual interventions.

### B.  Scope of the Review

In this chapter we review and summarize studies of smoking cessation in patients with respiratory disease. This group includes patients who have been diagnosed with chronic obstructive pulmonary disease (COPD), emphysema, lung cancer, asthma, abnormal pulmonary function tests, allergy, industrial lung disease, and acute conditions such as pneumonia [12]. All studies with any of these patient groups have been included. The techniques reported on range from minimal interventions involving advice, to more intense ones with detailed treatment procedures, and encompass all reports whether or not the intervention occurred within the context of the practices of respiratory specialists. In addition, recommendations are made for treatment and for future research, drawing on research from other patient groups and from the smoking cessation literature in general.

## II.  Cessation Treatments

### A.  Methodological Issues

There are a several methodological criteria to consider when evaluating the studies on intervention for smoking [3,41,42]. It is desirable that studies include comparison groups, random assignment to treatment, and biochemical validation of reported smoking status; report duration of follow-up; define smoking status as continued abstinence over at least 6 months; include patients lost to follow-up as continuing smokers; have an adequate sample size for statistical analysis; and measure patient compliance with the intervention. While several of the more recent studies have been conducted in a more rigorous fashion than earlier ones, there is considerable variation in the adequacy of the methodology, making comparisons between studies difficult. In addition, some of the studies have included patients with cardiovascular disease and those from general practice or in worksite programs in addition to those with respiratory disease, with no indication of the differential effectiveness of the treatments for the various subgroups. Finally, because of the complex, multidetermined basis for smoking [34,41], some studies have utilized multifaceted interventions, thereby making conclusions about a particular intervention strategy tenuous at best.

   In the following section, six broad categories of smoking cessation strategies have been defined and the research falling under each one summarized. Details of the procedures and results can be found in Table 1. Unless otherwise specified, the subjects have been solely patients with respiratory disease, assignment to groups has been random, some measure of compliance with treatment, where relevant, has been included, success is defined as continued abstinence, and validation of reported smoking status, at least on a subsample, has occurred. In the calculation of quit rates, only the longest follow-up point has been included, and, except where indicated, individuals lost to follow-up have been counted as continuing smokers in the calculation of quit rates.

## B.  Summary of the Research Findings

### Physician Advice, Education

One of the most common interventions is for the physician to advise his or her patients that smoking cessation should occur and that improvement in symptoms would follow. This advice can range from a simple statement about quitting to more intense, repeated advice involving supportive and motivational messages, and information about positive outcomes and withdrawal symptoms. In several of the studies, physician advice serves as the control condition against which other strategies are evaluated.

   For the over 20 studies in which physician advice was the major intervention, cessation rates varied from 10.0% to over 50.0% [7,43–62], with lower rates being reported in the more recent studies. In those studies, in which variations in the strength of advice were evaluated (e.g., refs. 49, 57, 59, and 62) or information on personal risk was added [46,58,59], no overall trend in cessation rate was noted. In addition, abstinence rates for hospitalized patients vary from 63% (unvalidated) [7] to 11.5% (unvalidated) [63]. There do not

**Table 1**

| Study | Groups and settings | Quit rate[a] (%) | Duration of follow-up | Comments |
|---|---|---|---|---|
| Baker et al., 1970 [43] | Strong advice; $N$ = 134 invited, 67 joined | 25.0 (not validated) | 6 months | Part of multidimensional treatment; no control group; cannot determine if rate is sustained abstinence |
| Benton et al. 1989 [86] | Multidimensional treatment, nicotine gum optional; hospital clinic; $n$ = 195/$n$ = 148 with respiratory diseases | 32.0 | 12 months | No control group; no separation of groups; success related to fewer cigarettes smoked daily |
| Bourke et al. 1983 [87] | Nicotine gum; hospital clinic; staff and patients, $n$ = 23 nicotine gum | 17.4 (not validated) | Mean of 6.5 months | No control group; no separation of groups; small sample size |
| British Thoracic Society, 1983 [68] | Multicenter, outpatient and inpatient (1) verbal advice (2) advice and booklet (3) (2) plus placebo gum (4) (2) plus nicotine gum, respiratory $n$ = 1311 | 8.9 8.5 11.4 9.8 | 12 months | Compliance with treatment not reported; no separation of groups |
| British Thoracic Society, 1984 [88] | Multicenter, outpatients and in-patients; multidimensional treatment $n$ = 1550, respiratory $n$ = 1311, heart disease $n$ = 146, other $n$ = 193 | 9.7 | 12 months | Additional analysis of BTS (68); success related to being male, older, and those with heart disease did better than those with other diagnosis; no treatment differences |
| British Thoracic Society, 1990 [71] | Multicenter, outpatients Study A: (1) advice only $n$ = 732 (2) signed agreement, visits, letters $n$ = 730, ($n$ = 1301 respiratory disease) | 7.0 9.0 | 12 months | Study A: Success related to being male and older; those with respiratory diseases had significantly less success than those with heart disease (7.5 % vs. 14.4%). |

| | | | | |
|---|---|---|---|---|
| | **Study B:**<br>(1) advice only $n = 343$<br>(2) signed agreement $n = 347$<br>(3) letters $n = 351$<br>(4) signed agreement and letters $n = 351$ | $\left.\begin{array}{c}5.2\\4.9\end{array}\right\}5.1*$<br>$\left.\begin{array}{c}8.5\\8.8\end{array}\right\}8.7*$ | | **Study B:** Success related to being male and older; disease not a factor |
| Burns, 1969 [44] | Private, $n = 94$<br>Physician advice | 47.0<br>(not validated) | 3 months | No control group; success related to fewer withdrawal symptoms, lower neuroticism, and being male |
| Burnum, 1974 [45] | Private, $n = 94$<br>Physician advice | 25.0<br>(not validated) | Average of 5 years | No control group; patients who had harmed themselves with tobacco, alcohol, food, drugs; no separation of groups |
| Campbell et al., 1986 [65] | Chest clinic<br>(1) control $n = 535$<br>(2) booklet $n = 671$ | 2.7<br>3.9 | 12 months | Patients referred for chest radiography; success related to increasing age, and being male |
| Campbell et al. 1987 [64] | General practice<br>(1) usual advice, $n = 149$<br>(2a) placebo gum, $n = 138$<br>(b) plus letter, $n = 137$<br>(c) plus letter/follow-up warning, $n = 137$<br>(3a) nicotine gum, $n = 138$<br>(b) plus letter, $n = 142$<br>(c) plus letter/follow-up warning, $n = 144$<br>25% respiratory problems | 1.3<br>3.6<br>$\left.\begin{array}{c}1.5\\1.5\end{array}\right\}2.2$<br>5.1<br>$\left.\begin{array}{c}2.8\\1.4\end{array}\right\}3.1$ | 12 months | Compliance with treatment not reported; success related to increasing age; N.S. trend for greater success in respiratory patients |

*(continued)*

587

**Table 1** Continued

| Study | Groups and settings | Quit rate[a] (%) | Duration of follow-up | Comments |
|---|---|---|---|---|
| Campbell et al., 1991 [89] | Hospital chest unit<br>(1) placebo gum<br>(2) nicotine gum<br>Lung disease, $n = 111$<br>Heart disease, $n = 85$<br>Other, $n = 16$ | 20.0<br>20.0 | 12 months | Dependency score not related to success but moderate, older smokers were more likely to quit; heart disease patients more likely to quit |
| Carmody et al., 1988 [90] | VA smoking cessation clinic<br>Nicotine gum plus<br>(1) behavioral skills<br>(2) minimal contact | 41.0<br>50.0 | 3 months | No separation of groups; more highly addicted smokers less likely to quit |
| Copperstock and Thom, 1982, [46] | Respiratory, $n = 33$<br>Interviews | 36.0<br>(not validated) | Cross-sectional | Quit rates compared for patients with circulatory and musculoskeletal diagnosis; reason for quitting provided |
| Crowley et al., 1989 [74] | Chest clinic, $n = 8$<br>Lottery ticket as reinforcement for reduced CO levels | 0.0 | < 3 weeks | CO levels significantly lower but was because patients refraining on test afternoons; small sample size |
| Crowley et al., 1991 [75] | VA hospital<br>Study 1:<br>(1) lottery ticket (LT) reinforcement for reduced CO levels, $n = 10$<br>(2) yoked control, $n = 10$<br>Study 2:<br>LT reinforcement for nonsmoking levels with nicotine gum, $n = 12$ | 0.0<br><br>0.0 | Average of 3 months<br><br>14 days | Small sample size; no reduction in CO levels; nonquitters proceeded to Study 2<br><br>Quit rate not reported; reduction in number of cigarettes smoked, inhalation of CO, and increase in time since last cigarette smoked; nonquitters proceeded to Study 3 |

| Study | Sample | % Quit | Follow-up/Design | Comments |
|---|---|---|---|---|
| Daughton et al., 1980 [7] | Study 3: Multipath LT reinforcement of non-smoker CO levels, n = 14 Hospitalized, n = 107 | 63.0 (not validated) | 10 days | Small sample size; results same as above; overall quit rate for all studies - 16.7% |
| Davison and Duffy, 1982 [47] | Lung cancer patients who survived for at least 5 years, n = 52 (50% advised to quit) | 25.0 (not validated) | Cross-sectional | No control groups, retrospective; ex-smokers and smokers differed in psychosocial factors |
| Devins and Edwards, 1988 [48] | GP referred, n = 48 No intervention | 10.4 (not validated) | 3 months | Retrospective reports; no control group; no patients smoked post-operatively; 75% resumed smoking Self-efficacy related to reduced smoking |
| Dudley et al., 1977 [49] | Chest clinic Never smokers, n = 66 Smokers, n = 42 Quitters, n = 132 | 76.0 (not validated) | Cross-sectional | No control group; retrospective; ex-smokers and smokers differed in psychosocial assets, stability, and expression of depression |
| Erbland and Blessing, 1991 [63] | VA Hospital (1) advice, n = 26 (2) education, n = 25 (3) education plus nicotine gum, n = 58 COPD, n = 18/CVD, n =25 | 11.5 4.0 8.0 | 12 months | No separation of COPD and CVD patients |
| Guzman, 1978 [76] | Chest clinic, n = 36 Individual and group therapy Cardiopulmonary | 5.0 (not validated) | 24 months | No control group; 20% decreased amount smoked |
| Hall et al., 1983 [62] | Health motivation, n = 19 Aversive conditioning, n = 16 | 10.0 30.0 | 6 months | Mood states related to reduction; no separation of groups |

*(continued)*

**Table 1** Continued

| Study | Groups and settings | Quit rate[a] (%) | Duration of follow-up | Comments |
|---|---|---|---|---|
| Hall et al., 1984 [72] | Cardiopulmonary<br>(1) rapid smoking, $n = 28$<br>(2) waiting list control, $n = 86$ | 50.0<br>0.0 }** | 24 months | Nonrandomized assignment to groups; no separation of groups |
| Kilburn and Warshaw, 1990 [77] | Asbestos exposure, $n = 2,689$<br>(1) feedback of medical exam responder, $n = 504$; nonresponders interviewed by phone, $n = 101$<br>(2) historical control, $n = 870$ | 29.8 }<br>17.0 } 26.7 }**<br>4.7 }<br>(not validated) | Average of 6 to 25 months | Nonrandom (self-selection); calculated $\chi^2$ for group 1 vs. group 2, $p < 0.001$ |
| Knudsen et al., 1985 [50] | Lung cancer patients<br>$n = 57$ (75% respiratory rate)<br>Current, $n = 16$<br>Former, $n = 41$ | 58.6 with losses to follow-up<br>85.0 without losses<br>(not validated) | Retrospective | Quit rate for those who quit at the time of their cancer diagnosis; reasons for quitting and experiences provided |
| Kozak, 1990 [94] | Healthy, $n = 38$<br>COPD, $n = 32$<br>CVD, $n = 26$ | 42.0<br>42.0<br>63.0<br>(not validated) | 12 months | Nicotine gum and control, but differences not reported by intervention |
| Mausner, 1970 [51]<br>Peabody, 1972 [52] | Private patients<br>Eight physicians, $n = 136$<br>Not given | 51.0<br>(not validated)<br>25.0<br>(not validated) | 3 to 12 months<br>Not given | No control group; ex-smokers and smokers differed in severity of disease<br>Only quit rate reported |
| Pederson et al., 1980 [53] | Private, $n = 137$ | 27.4<br>(not validated) | Retrospective<br>6 months to 7 years | No control group; multivariate analysis; ex-smokers and smokers differed on diagnosis, age, and sex |
| Pederson et al., 1982, 1983 [54,55] | Newly diagnosed pulmonary, $n = 308$ | 12.9<br>(not validated) | 6 months | No control group; multivariate predictive model developed, 92% accuracy |

| Study | Setting / groups | Success rate (%) | Follow-up | Comments |
|---|---|---|---|---|
| Pederson et al., 1983 [66] | Private, respiratory<br>(1) advice plus self-help manual, n = 35<br>(2) advice, n = 40 | 16.7<br><br>25.6<br>(not validated) | 6 months | Alternate week assignment to groups; success related to duration of habit |
| Pederson et al., 1988 [56] | Respiratory, n = 160 | 17.5 with losses to follow-up 39.1 without losses<br>(not validated) | 4 to 7 years | Test of long-term usage of multivariate predictive model, developed in [54,55], 70% accuracy |
| Pederson et al., 1991 [91] | Respiratory clinics<br>(1) nicotine gum, n = 25<br>(2) self-help manual, n = 29<br>(3) nicotine gum and manual, n = 36<br>(4) control, n = 30 | 13.4<br>11.6<br>11.7<br>12.1 | 12 months | Manual designed for respiratory patients; compliance poor; more addicted smokers less likely to quit |
| Pederson et al., 1991 [67] | Hospitalized patients<br>(1) advice plus self-help manual plus alternate day counselling, n = 37<br>(2) advice, n = 37 | 33.3<br><br>21.4 | 6 months | Compliance poor |
| Raw, 1976 [57] | Motivating advice—"white coat"<br>Motivating advice—"no white coat"<br>Interview—"white coat"<br>Interview—"no white coat"<br>n = 10 per group | Overall 12.5<br>(not validated) | 3 months | 4 of 5 quitters in "white coat" condition, not clear if rate is sustained abstinence |

*(continued)*

**Table 1** Continued

| Study | Groups and settings | Quit rate[a] (%) | Duration of follow-up | Comments |
|---|---|---|---|---|
| Risser and Belcher, 1990 [58] | Outpatient clinic VA hospital (1) control-educational intervention, $n$ = 45 (2) plus motivation CO message, $n$ = 45 (five active medical conditions) | 6.7  20.0 with losses to follow up | 12 months | Not clear what medical conditions are; not clear whether smoking status is sustained abstinence; significant difference in quit rates exists only with non responders excluded |
| Rose and Hamilton, 1978 [59] | Normal care, $n$ = 731 Intervention using individualization of risks, $n$ = 714 | 14.0 36.0 (not validated) | 3 years | High risk for cardiorespiratory disease; not clear if rate is sustained abstinence |
| Rose and Udechuku, 1971 [60] | Hospitalized with chronic bronchitis, $n$ = 40 | 25.0 (not validated) | Not given | No control group; among all patients including those with atherosclerosis and hypertension 69% recalled advice |
| Sachs et al., 1981 [73] | Cardiopulmonary, hardcore smokers, $n$ = 16 Rapid smoking | 37.5 with losses to follow-up 50.0 without losses to follow-up | 12 months | Not clear whether smoking status is sustained abstinence; no control group; success related to spouse not smoking and milder disease |
| Sachs et al., 1987 [92] | Restrictive ventilatory defect (1) nicotine gum, $n$ = 44 (2) waiting list control, $n$ = 27 | $\left.\begin{matrix}27.0 \\ 0.0\end{matrix}\right\}**$ | 24 months | Compliance high among successful abstainers |

| Study | Setting/Sample | Quit rate (%) | Follow-up | Comments |
|---|---|---|---|---|
| Sirota et al., 1985 [69] | Cardiopulmonary, VA medical center Behavioral program, n = 8 | 50.0 | 5 years | No control group; small sample size; chemical quit rate verification vague; no separation of groups; smoking reduction rates reported |
| Tonnesen et al., 1988 [93] | Clinic (1) healthy, n = 134 (2) self-reported COPD, n = 38 control, n = 56 2 or 4 mg nicotine gum, n = 116 | 33.3 } 16.2 } ** 5.7 } 27.2 } ** | 22 months | Not blinded; no difference in dose of gum; low dependent smokers more likely to quit |
| Turner et al., 1985 [70] | Pulmonary Brand fading, n = 4 | 25.0 | 6 months | No control group; small sample size; reduction in smoking rate reported |
| Williams, 1969 [61] | Chest clinic, n = 204 Advice | 18.5 with losses to follow-up 23.0 without losses to follow-up (not validated) | 6 months | No control group |

*, $p < 0.05$; **, $p < 0.01$

appear to be any trends toward absolute levels of cessation being associated with specific methodological features, such as the inclusion of a biochemical measure to validate reported smoking. In several more recent evaluations involving other techniques, when advice served as the control or "usual care" condition, rates as low as 1.3% have been reported (e.g., ref. 64).

It appears as if many people who have respiratory symptoms quit smoking on their own before being examined by a respirologist, and those who continue to smoke are those for whom advice alone is not likely to lead to behavior change.

### Behavioral Approaches and Self-Help Manuals

Interventions falling into this category are based on theoretical models concerning the habitual nature of smoking and the process of quitting [4,24,41]. Included here are various strategies, such as gradual reduction of number of cigarettes or nicotine/tar levels (brand fading), setting a target date, substitution behavior, contracting, reinforcement schedules, aversive conditioning (e.g., rapid smoking), coping skills, and covert sensitization (e.g., imagining smoking situations). These strategies can be used in the context of either a group or an individualized format, with or without assistance from a health professional. The group setting provides the inclusion of social support (see below), while the individualized, self-help approach is based on the premise that most people who have successfully quit smoking have done so on their own [66]. Fairly detailed programs/manuals are followed, with specific tasks to be performed at various points in time.

A variety of behavioral treatments have been assessed and for the most part have proven to be no more effective than a range of control conditions. The use of manuals on quitting has been found to be ineffective [65–68], as have behavioral programs [69] and brand fading [70]. Two techniques that might offer some promise are the inclusion of follow-up letters [71] and rapid smoking [72], although in two studies [62,73] using the latter technique, no differences were found in comparison to control conditions. One interesting approach has been the use of lottery tickets as reinforcement for reduction of carbon monoxide levels [74,75]; however, the achievement of abstinence was not a primary outcome of the relatively short follow-ups (3 months).

### Clinics and Support Groups

Included in this category are those interventions sponsored in many instances by nonprofit community agencies (e.g., Cancer Society, Lung Association, YM/YWCA) or commercial organizations. One of the most important aspects of these programs is the social support offered by both the group leader and the other members [76]. As noted above, these programs frequently include a behavioral component, but this is not necessary. No formal evaluations were found in the literature that have focused on this category of techniques.

Presumably, at least some unknown number of patients who are advised to quit smoking seek out assistance from the wide variety of programs that are offered.

### Disease-Related Feedback

Some of the interventions have involved providing feedback on pulmonary function tests results, based on providing individual, personalized information on the detrimental effects of smoking, in contrast to more generalized information on the ill effects of smoking often incorporated into physician advice. In addition, improvement in lung function and potential improvement in symptomatology is considered to provide reinforcement for continued abstinence from smoking. Disease-related feedback and information is often incorporated into advice to quit smoking (e.g., refs. 46 and 59). One study [77] evaluated this approach formally, with encouraging results. Approximately five times more successful abstainers were found in the group receiving this information than in a historical control; however, concurrent control and validation of reports would have provided stronger evidence for the effect. It should also be noted that this evaluation was not confined to patients with diagnosed respiratory conditions, but included those who were at risk of disease. A second study [58] using feedback on spirometry, carbon monoxide, and PFTs, also reported a significant increase in cessation over a control condition; however, when losses to follow-up were included as continuing smokers (a conservative approach), the groups did not differ statistically.

### Pharmacological Treatments

Procedures that fall into this category can be classified into three general groupings: (1) treatment of specific withdrawal symptoms using drugs such as clonidine, (2) nicotine antagonists for central and peripheral blocking, and (3) nicotine replacement therapies [24]. The rationale for these approaches is based on the psychoactive and addictive properties of nicotine [78], and those in the third category have been the focus of considerable research. No studies were located in which treatments in categories 1 and 2 were assessed; however, recommendations for their use appear in the literature.

Nicotine gum has been used as an aid to smoking cessation in a wide variety of settings. There is some evidence to indicate that it may be useful for "healthy smokers" when combined with behavior therapy or group counseling (e.g., ref. 79) and comprehensive physician training in its use (e.g., ref. 80). There is reason to believe that nicotine gum may provide help for smokers whose major reason for smoking is that of nicotine dependence or addiction, as compared to habit, tension reduction, or stimulation [81–84], and that strength of the gum is an important consideration for these individuals (e.g., ref. 85). Patients with respiratory disease report that they are highly addicted to smoking (e.g., refs. 24, 26, 37, and 38); therefore, it might be anticipated that this intervention would prove to be effective with this group.

The studies that have focused on this group of patients, however, have not found such an advantage for nicotine gum when evaluated against other treatments, placebo gum, or in combination with other interventions [63,64,68,86–91], with two exceptions [92,93]. No differences between the 2- and 4-mg gum have emerged. In one study [94] over 40% of a group who used the gum ad lib reported success, but differences between treated and control conditions were not reported. It has been noted that compliance with prescribed use of the gum has not been great (e.g., ref. 91), probably due to some unpleasant side effects. It appears that the gum is effective among those who do comply [92].

### Others

Included in this category are such treatments as hypnosis, acupuncture, and laser therapy, and mass media campaigns, among others [41]. As with some of the other treatments, noted above, no formal evaluations of these approaches were found in the literature.

## III. Synthesis and Discussion

### A. Variables Related to Abstinence

Overall, it does not appear that there are many treatment variables or interventions consistently leading to improvement in levels of abstinence for this group of patients. However, some treatment approaches might be worth pursuing, among them those that include specific disease-related feedback in the form of PFTs or spirometry, and those in which compliance with nicotine gum is achieved.

In addition, some trends can be noted in patient and physician variables as they relate to successful abstinence. In terms of patient variables, older patients [53,64,65,71,88,89] and males [53,64,65,71,89] are more likely to be success- ful, as are those who report lower dependence and smoke fewer cigarettes [44,86,90]. In addition, self-efficacy, defined as patients' predicted probability of quitting, has been found to be related to cessation (e.g., refs. 48, 54, and 55), as were some measures indicative of better psychological adjustment (e.g., refs. 7, 44, 49, and 62). Among the physician characteristics investigated have been intensity of advice, use of follow-ups, and physician smoking. But overall, very little attention has been paid to these kinds of variables in most of the studies. More in-depth research is needed, possibly including qualitative assess- ment [94,95], as well as more traditional quantitative approaches.

## B. Research Recommendations

There are several lines of research that might profitably be pursued in this area. First, as noted above, some attention should be paid to physician variables, specifically those that have been demonstrated to be effective both with other patient groups and with other types of life-style change. Among these are the impact of the "caringness" of the physician, qualitative assessment of the "barriers" to physicians adopting this role with their patients [95,96], development of educational material on the variety of roles and levels of involvement that the physician can utilize, and provision of information regarding the availability and use of referrals to community resources and to other health professionals, such as health educators, nurses, pharmacists, and dentists [97–99]. In addition, research is needed on repetition and consistency of the advice/information, additional training in life-style modification, the potential of treatment tailoring/individualization for a particular patient (possibly in continuing medical education courses), and the utility of a sequence of progressively active interventions [33,38,100]. At another level, research on whether training in life-style modification in medical schools might be used to better prepare the next generation of physicians for dealing with these issues is recommended [101].

With regard to specific treatments, additional research is needed on the effectiveness of disease-related feedback given the promising findings reported in the literature [58,77]. Further, the reasons for the use of pharmacological interventions remain to be further examined given the fact that some studies on the effectiveness of nicotine gum have reported promising results [92–94,102]. Particular emphasis might be made on methods for improving compliance with treatment and/or patient characteristics that are related to compliance. In addition, the recently developed transdermal nicotine patch with this patient group might prove to be an effective technique [103–105].

Among the patient characteristics that merit further investigation are stages of change along the dimension of readiness to quit smoking [106–109] and the types or levels of intervention that are appropriate for the given stages, relationships between categories of patient characteristics (such as psychosocial and/or motivational ones) and achievement of abstinence, and the utility of matching patients to treatments [106].

Needless to say, any research in this area should incorporate appropriate controls, randomization, objective validation, follow-ups of sufficient duration, and report on outcomes for all patients initiated into the study, including losses to follow-up, dropouts, and deaths. The development and use of theoretical frames of reference, such as suggested with regard to other areas (e.g., refs. 108, 110, and 111), should serve as the basis for at least some of the research. Finally, given the multifaceted nature of the behavior, the interaction between patient and physician, and psychological and physical adjustment to disease, the use of complex research designs, incorporating multivariate statistical procedures, is strongly recommended. The physician can participate at many levels in future research by collaborating or consulting with investigators and/or assuming an active role as a principal investigator.

## C.  Treatment Recommendations

While several areas of investigation are worth pursuing, definitive answers will not be available in the near future. The entire process of conducting useful investigations is a time-consuming one. Therefore, the question about what the physician who is involved in treatment of patients with respiratory disease should do in the meantime remains. There are several recent publications that provide advice to physicans in this regard [11,17,20–32]. All of the interventions reviewed above have received some attention.

There are several issues that need to be considered in recommending a specific treatment to a given patient. First is the question of whether the patient wants to try to quit smoking. If the patient is in one of the stages that precede active attempts, the most profitable approach is probably to provide information about smoking and its impact on health. Repeat advice would appear to be warranted until the patient is ready to quit, as it has been suggested that such advice may provide the impetus for the patient to progress from one stage to the next [106]. There are instruments available that provide the information necessary to determine the patients readiness to quit [107–109].

Second, when the person decides that he or she is prepared to attempt to quit, matching or tailoring the particular cessation intervention recommended to the patient's reasons for smoking is suggested. As noted above, the individual techniques have been developed based on a variety of assumptions concerning the underlying mechanisms for smoking. Again, there are instruments available for assessing smoking motivation (e.g., ref. 84), to help guide the physician and the patient in this regard. Given the results of such assessments, it might be reasonable for the physician to suggest that more than one technique be used.

Third, working with the patient to develop a plan for cessation is recommended, based on the notion that no one technique will appeal to all patients. This approach means that the physician should be acquainted with a variety of techniques and be able to provide the patient with a list of techniques and community resources, so that educated decisions can be made.

Finally, cessation of smoking is a process, not an event. In other words, continued support is essential; the physician should not assume that once the patient has quit smoking it is no longer necessary to reinforce abstinence [112]. Recidivism is high in the first 3 to 6 months [41] and some evidence suggests that the process can be a continuing one over several years [109].

## IV. Summary

Patients with respiratory diseases who continue to smoke offer a challenge and a source of frustration to the physician, in both terms of treatment for their progressive disease and assistance in the achievement of abstinence from smoking. Although many strategies are available for the physician to use, no obviously effective treatment has emerged from the research available. More carefully conducted research is needed on patient, treatment, and physician variables, incorporating both quantitative and qualitative methods. The physician can participate in such endeavors by collaborating and consulting with other investigators and/or assuming an active role as a principal investigator. Before definitive answers become available, it is recommended that physicians attempt to assess the individual patient's readiness to change, become informed about the range of treatments available, tailor his or her advice and guidance to the individual, and work with the patient to develop a treatment package.

## Acknowledgments

Personnel support for the author is provided by a National Health Research Scholar Award, Health and Welfare Canada. The author wishes to acknowledge Marion Merrell Dow, Canada, who provided funds for the writing of this chapter, Julie McWhinney for assistance in collecting and summarizing the literature, and S. B. Bull, N. M. Lefcoe, and J. M. Wanklin for their critical reading of the manuscript.

## References

1. Holland WW. Chronic obstructive lung disease prevention. Br J Dis Chest 1988;82(1):32–44.
2. Peat JK, Woolcock AJ, Cullen K. Decline of lung function and development of chronic airflow limitation: a longitudinal study of non-smokers and smokers in Busselton, Western Australia. Thorax 1990;45:32–37.
3. U.S. Department of Health and Human Services. The health consequences of smoking: chronic obstructive lung disease. A report of the Surgeon General. DHHS (PHS) 84-50205. U.S. Department of Health and Human Services, Public Health Service, Office on Smoking and Health, 1984.
4. U.S. Department of Health and Human Services. Reducing the health consequences of smoking: 25 years of progress. A report of the Surgeon General. DHHS (CDC) 89-8411. U.S. Department of Health and Human Services, Public Health Service, Centers for Disease Control, 1989.
5. U.S. Department of Health and Human Services. The health benefits of smoking cessation. A report of the Surgeon General. DHHS (CDC)

90-8416. U.S. Department of Health and Human Services, Public Health Service, Center for Chronic Disease Prevention and Health Promotion, 1990.

6. Vollmer WM, McCamant LE, Johnson LR, Buist AS. Respiratory symptoms, lung function, and mortality in a screening center cohort. Am J Epidemiol 1989;129(6):1157–69.

7. Daughton DM, Fix AJ, Kass I, Patil KD. Smoking cessation among patients with chronic obstructive pulmonary disease (COPD). Addict Behav 1980;5(2):125–28.

8. Daughton DM, Fix AJ, Kass I, Patil KD. Three-year survival rates of pulmonary rehabilitation patients with chronic obstructive pulmonary disease. J Natl Med Assoc 1984;76(3):265–68.

9. Kuller LH, Ockene JK, Townsend M, Browner W, Meilahn E, Wentworth DN. The epidemiology of pulmonary function and COPD mortality in the multiple risk factor intervention trial. Am Rev Respir Dis 1989;140:S72–S81.

10. Brown CA, Crombie IK, Smith WCS, Tunstall-Pedoe H. The impact of quitting smoking on symptoms of chronic bronchitis: results of the Scottish Heart Health Study. Thorax 1991;46:112–16.

11. Kesten S, Rebuck AS. Management of chronic obstructive pulmonary disease. Drugs 1989;38(1):160–74.

12. Kutty K, Varkey B. Chronic obstructive pulmonary disease. Reversing airflow obstruction from chronic bronchitis and emphysema. Postgrad Med 1988;84(4):60–67,70,74,77.

13. Kuller LH, Ockene JK, Meilahn E, Wentworth DN, Svenson KH, Neaton JD, for MRFIT. Cigarette smoking and mortality. Prev Med 1991;20:638–54.

14. Postma DX, Sluiter HJ. Prognosis of chronic obstructive pulmonary disease: the dutch experience. Am Rev Respir Dis 1989;140:S100–S105.

15. Tashkin DP, Clark VA, Coulson AH, Simmons M, Bourque LB, Reems C, Detels R, Sayre JW, Rokaw SN. The UCLA population studies of chronic obstructive respiratory disease. VII. Effects of smoking cessation on lung function: a prospective study of a free-living population. Am Rev Respir Dis 1984;130:707–15.

16. Townsend MC, Duchene AG, Morgan J, Browner WS, for MRFIT. Pulmonary function in relation to cigarette smoking and smoking cessation. Prev Med 1991;20:624–37.

17. American College of Chest Physicians. Smoking cessation intervention: how to help your patients quit. A postgraduate review. Dallas: American College of Chest Physicians, 1984.

18. Gross NJ. Chronic obstructive pulmonary disease: current concepts and therapeutic approaches. Chest 1990;97(2);19S–23S.

19. Vial WC. Southwestern International Medicine Conference: cigarette smoking and lung disease. Am J Med Sci 1986;291(2):130–42.
20. American College of Physicians. Methods for stopping cigarette smoking. Ann Intern Med 1986;105:281–91.
21. Anthonisen, NR. Chronic obstructive pulmonary disease. Can Med Assoc J 1988;138:503–10.
22. Campbell IA. Stopping patients smoking. Br J Dis Chest 1988;82(2):9–15.
23. Francis PB Jr, Petty TL, Winterbauer RH. Pulmonary disease: helping the COPD patient help himself. Patient Care 1984;June:177–87.
24. Fisher EB, Haire-Joshu D, Morgan GD, Rehberg H, Rost K. State of the art: smoking and smoking cessation. Am Rev Respir Dis 1990;142(3):702–20.
25. Hill D. The role of the doctor in patient smoking cessation. Cancer Forum 1983;7:5–8.
26. Moody PM, Haley JV. Quantified human smoking behavior among various disease categories. Int J Addict 1985;20(5):751–61.
27. Orleans CT. Understanding and promoting smoking cessation: overview and guidelines for physician intervention. Annu Rev Med 1985;36:51–61.
28. Petty TL. Chronic obstructive pulmonary disease: can we do better? Chest 1990;97(2):2S–5S.
29. Raw M, Friend J. The role of chest physicians as smoking cessation counsellors. Paper presented at the 5th World Conference on Smoking and Health, Winnipeg, Manitoba, Canada, 1983.
30. Sachs DPL. Clinical challenge in cardiopulmonary medicine: self-assessment. J Am Coll Chest Physicians 1985;6(1):1–3,6–8.
31. Sachs DPL. Advances in smoking cessation treatment. Curr Pulmonol 1991;12:139–98.
32. Sly RM. The role of physicians in smoking cessation (editorial). Ann Allergy 1989;63:163–64.
33. Duncan C, Stein MJ, Cummings SR. Staff involvement and special follow-up time increase physicians' counseling about smoking cessation: a controlled trial. Am J Public Health 1991;81(7):899–901.
34. Cummings KM, Giovino G, Sciandra R, Koeningsberg M, Emont SL. Physician advice to quit smoking: who gets it and who doesn't. Am J Prev Med 1987;3(2):69–75.
35. Biener L, O'Donnell CR, Galuska E, Sherman CB. Effect of pulmonary screening feedback and pulmonary limitation simulation on motivation to quit smoking. Paper presented at the World Conference on Lung Health, Boston, May 1990.
36. Lefcoe NM, Pederson LL, Blennerhassett G. Attitudes of patients with chronic respiratory disease toward smoking cessation. Can Family Physician 1988;34:1041–44.

37. Tay SC, McLean S, Parton R. Smoking habits and related beliefs among hospital patients (letter). Med J Aust 1989;151:423–24.
38. Fisher EB, Rost K. Smoking cessation: a practical guide for the physician. Clin Chest Med 1986;7(4):551–65.
39. Sachs DPL. Treatment of cigarette dependency: what American pulmonary physicians do. Am Rev Respir Dis 1984;129(6):1010–13.
40. Lichtenstein E, Danaher BG. What can the physician do to assist the patient to stop smoking? In: Brashear RE, Rhoades ML, eds. Chronic obstructive lung disease: clinical treatment and management. St. Louis, MO: CV Mosby, 1978:227–41.
41. Schwartz JL. Review and evaluation of smoking cessation methods: the United States and Canada, 1975–1985. NIH 87-2940. U.S. Department of Health and Human Services, Public Health Service, National Institutes of Health, 1987.
42. Ockene JK, Shaten J, for MRFIT. Introduction, overview, method and conclusions. Prev Med 1991;20:552–63.
43. Baker TR, Oscherwitz M, Corlin R, Jarboe T, Teisch J, Nichaman MZ. Screening and treatment program for mild chronic obstructive pulmonary disease. JAMA 1970;214(8):1448–55.
44. Burns BH. Chronic chest disease, personality and success in stopping cigarette smoking. Br J Prev Soc Med 1969;23(1):23–27.
45. Burnum JF. Outlook for treating patients with self-destructive habits. Ann Intern Med 1974;81(3):387–93.
46. Cooperstock R, Thom B. Health, smoking and doctors' advice. J R Coll Gen Pract 1982;32(236):174–78.
47. Davison G, Duffy M. Smoking habits of long-term survivors of surgery for lung cancer. Thorax 1982;37(5):331–33.
48. Devins GM, Edwards PJ. Self-efficacy and smoking reduction in chronic obstructive pulmonary disease. Behav Res Ther 1988;26(2):127–35.
49. Dudley PL, Aickin M, Martin CJ. Cigarette smoking in a chest clinic population: psychophysiologic variables. J Psychosom Res 1977;21:367–75.
50. Knudsen N, Schulman S, Van Den Hoek J, Fowler R. Insights on how to quit smoking: a survey of patients with lung cancer. Cancer Nurs 1985;8(3):145–50.
51. Mausner JS. Cigarette smoking among patients with respiratory disease. Am Rev Respir Dis 1970;102(5):704–13.
52. Peabody HD Jr. A practical approach to the office management of cessation of cigarette smoking. In: Richardson RG, ed. 2nd World Conference on Smoking and Health. London: Pitman Medical, 1972:185–89.
53. Pederson LL, Williams JI, Lefcoe NM. Smoking cessation among

pulmonary patients as related to type of respiratory disease and demographic variables. Can J Public Health 1980;71(3):191–94.

54. Pederson LL, Baskerville JC, Wanklin JM. Multivariate statistical models for predicting change in smoking behavior following physician advice to quit smoking. Prev Med 1982;11(5):536–49.

55. Pederson LL, Baskerville JC. Multivariate prediction of smoking cessation following physician advice to quit smoking: a validation study. Prev Med 1983;12(3):430–36.

56. Pederson LL, Wanklin JM, Lefcoe NM. Self-reported long-term smoking cessation in patients with respiratory disease: prediction of success and perception of health effects. Int J Epidemiol 1988;17(4):804–9.

57. Raw M. Persuading people to stop smoking. Behav Res Ther 1976;14(2):97–101.

58. Risser NL, Belcher DW. Adding spirometry, carbon monoxide and pulmonary symptom results to smoking cessation counseling: a randomized trial. J Gen Intern Med 1990;5:16–22.

59. Rose G, Hamilton PJS. A randomized controlled trial of the effect on middle-aged men of advice to stop smoking. J Epidemiol Community Health 1978;32(4):275–81.

60. Rose G, Udechuku JC. Cigarette smoking by hospital patients. Br J Prev Soc Med 1971;25(3):160–61.

61. Williams HO. Routine advice against smoking. A chest clinic pilot study. Practitioner 1969;202(1211):672–76.

62. Hall SM, Bachman J, Henderson JB, Barstow R, Jones RT. Smoking cessation in patients with cardiopulmonary disease: an initial study. Addict Behav 1983;8:33–42.

63. Erbland ML, Blessing ML. Smoking cessation methods in veterans with smoking-induced illness. Paper presented at the International Conference of the American Thoracic Society, Anaheim, CA, May 1991.

64. Campbell IA, Lyons E, Prescott RJ. Stopping smoking: do nicotine chewing-gum and postal encouragement add to doctor's advice? Practitioner 1987;23:114–17.

65. Campbell IA, Hansford M, Prescott RJ. Effect of a "stop smoking" booklet on smokers attending for chest radiography: a controlled study. Thorax 1986;41:369–71.

66. Pederson LL, Wood T, Lefcoe NM. Use of a self-help smoking cessation manual as an adjunct to advice from a respiratory specialist. Int J Addict 1983;18(6):777–82.

67. Pederson LL, Wanklin JM, Lefcoe NM. The effects of counseling on smoking cessation among patients hospitalized with chronic obstructive pulmonary disease: a randomized clinical trial. Int J Addict 1991;26(1):107–19.

68. British Thoracic Society. Comparison of four methods of smoking withdrawal in patients with smoking related diseases. Br Med J 1983;286:595–97.
69. Sirota AD, Curran JP, Habif V. Smoking cessation in chronically ill medical patients. J Consult Clin Psychol 1985;41(4):575–79.
70. Turner SA, Daniels JL, Hollandsworth JG. The effects of a multicomponent smoking cessation program with chronic obstructive pulmonary disease outpatients. Addict Behav 1985;10:87–90.
71. British Thoracic Society. Smoking cessation in patients: two further studies by the British Thoracic Society. Thorax 1990;45:835–40.
72. Hall RG, Hall SM, Sachs DPL, Benowitz NL. Two-year efficacy and safety of rapid smoking therapy in patients with cardiac and pulmonary disease. J Consult Clin Psychol 1984;52:574–81.
73. Sachs DPL, Hall RG, Sachs BL, Hall SM. Success of rapid smoking therapy in smokers with pulmonary and coronary heart disease. Am Rev Respir Dis 1981;123:111.
74. Crowley TJ, Andrews AE, Cheney J, Zerbe G, Petty TL. Carbon monoxide assessment of smoking in chronic obstructive pulmonary disease. Addict Behav 1989;14:493–502.
75. Crowley TJ, MacDonald MJ, Zerbe GO, Petty TL. Reinforcing breath carbon monoxide reductions in chronic obstructive pulmonary disease. Drug Alcohol Depend 1991;29(1):47–62.
76. Guzman C. Quit smoking rate in the Ottawa out-patient rehabilitation programme for patients with chronic lung disease. Personal communication, 1978.
77. Kilburn KH, Warshaw RH. Effects of individually motivating smoking cessation in male blue collar workers. Am J Public Health 1990;80(11):1334–37.
78. The health consequences of smoking: nicotine addiction. A report of the Surgeon General. DHHS (CDC) 88-406. U.S. Department of Health and Human Services, Public Health Service, Centers for Disease Control, Office on Smoking and Health, 1988.
79. Killen JD, Fortmann SP, Newman B, Varady A. Evaluation of a treatment approach combining nicotine gum with selfguided behavioral treatments for smoking relapse prevention. J Consult Clin Psychol 1990;58:85–92.
80. Wilson DM, Taylor DW, Gilbert JR, Best JA, Lindsay EA, Willms DG, Singer J. A randomized trial of a family physician intervention for smoking cessation. JAMA 1988;260:1570–74.
81. Jarvis MJ, Russell MAH. Smoking withdrawal in patients with smoking related diseases (correspondence). Br Med J 1983;286:976–77.
82. Sachs DPL. Pharmacologic, neuroendocrine and biobehavioral basis for tobacco dependence. Curr Pulmonol 1987;8:371–406.

83. Sachs DPL. Nicotine polacrilex: practical use requirements. Curr Pulmonol 1989;10:141–58.

84. Fagerstrom DO. Efficacy of nicotine chewing gum: a review. Prog Clin Biol Res 1988;261:109–28.

85. Kornitzer M, Kittel F, Dramaix M, Bourdoux PA. A double blind study of 2 mg. versus 4 mg. nicotine-gum in an industrial setting. J Psychosom Res 1987;31:171–76.

86. Benton BE, Robinson GM., Martin PD. The Wellington Hospital smoking cessation clinic. NZ Med J 1989;102:613–15.

87. Bourke J, Callaghan B. Experiences with nicotine chewing-gum in resistant smokers (letter to the editor). Ir Med J 1983;76(2):112.

88. British Thoracic Society. Smoking withdrawal in hospital patients: factors associated with outcome. Thorax 1984;39:651–56.

89. Campbell IA, Prescott RJ, Tjeder-Burton SM. Smoking cessation in hospital patients given repeated advice plus nicotine or placebo gum. Respir Med 1991;85:155–57.

90. Carmody TP, Loew DE, Hall RG, Breckenridge JS, Breckenridge JN, Hall SM. Nicotine polacrilex: clinic-based strategies with chronically ill smokers. J Psychoactive Drugs 1988;20:269–74.

91. Pederson LL, Bull SB, Lefcoe NM. The effectiveness of nicotine gum and a self-help smoking cessation manual for patients with diagnosed pulmonary disease. Unpublished manuscript, 1991.

92. Sachs DPL, Benowitz NL, Silver KJ. Effective use of nicotine polacrilex in patients with chronic obstructive pulmonary disease. In: Aoki M, et al., eds. Smoking and health 1987. New York: Elsevier Science Publishers, 1987:793–95.

93. Tonnesen P, Fryd V, Hansen M, Helsted J, Gunnersen AB, Forchammer H, Stockner M. Two and four mg nicotine chewing gum and group counselling in smoking cessation: an open, randomized, controlled trial with a 22 month follow-up. Addict Behav 1988;13(1):17–27.

94. Kozak JT. Nicotine chewing gum therapy in diseased smokers. Paper presented at the World Meeting on Lung Health, Boston, May 1990.

95. Willms DG, Best JA, Wilson DMC, Gilbert JR, Taylor DW, Lindsay E, Singer J, Johnson NA. Patients' perspectives of a physician-delivered smoking cessation intervention. Am J Prev Med 1991;7(2):95–100.

96. Willms DG, Best JA, Taylor DW, Wilson DMC, Lindsay E. A systematic approach for using qualitative methods in primary prevention research: a focus on smoking. Med Anthropol Q 1990;4:391–409.

97. American Pharmacy. Helping your patients stop smoking: new resources, new approaches. Am J Pharm 1984;NS24(4):46–48.

98. Rose MA. Intervention strategies for smoking cessation: the role of oncology nursing. Cancer Nurs 1991;14(5):225–31.

99. Knudsen N, Schulman S, Fowler R, Van Den Hoek J. Why bother with stop-smoking education for lung cancer patients. World Smoking Health 1985;10(3):21–22.

100. Ebert RV, McNabb ME. Cessation of smoking in prevention and treatment of cardiac and pulmonary disease. Arch Intern Med 1984;144:1558–59.

101. Kenney RD, Lyles MF, Turner RC, White ST, Gonzalez JJ, Irons TG, Sanchez CJ, Rogers CS, Campbell EE, Villagra VG, Strecher VJ, O'Malley MS, Stritter FT, Fletcher SW. Smoking cessation counseling by resident physicians in internal medicine, family practice and pediatrics. Arch Intern Med 1988;148:2469–73.

102. Kottke TE, Batista RN, DeFriese GH, Brekke ML. Attributes of successful smoking cessation interventions in medical practice: a meta-analysis of 39 controlled trials. J Am Med Assoc 1988;259(19):2883–89.

103. Abelin T, Buehler A, Muller P, Vesamin K, Imhof PK. Controlled trial of transdermal nicotine patch in tobacco withdrawal. Lancet 1989;1:7–10.

104. Hurt RD, Laugher GC, Offord KP, Kottke TE, Dale LC. Nicotine replacement therapy with use of a transdermal nicotine patch: a randomized double-blind placebo-controlled trial. Mayo Clin Proc 1990;65:1529–37.

105. Tonnesen P, Norregaard J, Simonsen K, Sauve V. A double blind trial of a 16-hour transdermal nicotine patch in smoking cessation. N Engl J Med 1991;325:311–15.

106. Bass F. Helping patients quit smoking. Can Fam Phys 1989;35:1497–1502.

107. DiClemente CC, Prochaska JO. Self-change and therapy change of smoking behavior: a comparison of processes of change in cessation and maintenance. Addict Behav 1982;7:133–42.

108. Prochaska JO. A transtheoretical model of behavior change: learning from mistakes with majority populations. Paper presented at the Prevent Chronic Disease Conference, Washington, DC, October 1991.

109. Prochaska JO, DiClemente CC, Velicer WF, Ginpil S, Norcrosss JC. Predicting change in smoking status for self-changers. Addict Behav 1985;10:395–406.

110. Gallagher EB. Chronic illness management: a focus for future research applications. In: Gochman DS, ed. Health behavior: emerging research perspectives. New York: Plenum Press, 1988:397–408.

111. Pederson LL, Wanklin JM, Bull SB, Ashley MJ. A conceptual framework for the roles of legislation and education in reducing exposure to environmental tobacco smoke. Am J Health Promot 1991;6(2):105–11.

112. National Working Conference on Smoking Relapse. Health Psychol 1986;5(Suppl):1–68.

# 31

## Principles of an Antitobacco Policy for the Prevention of Respiratory and Nonrespiratory Diseases

**ALBERT HIRSCH**

Hôpital Saint-Louis
Paris, France

**KJELL BJARTVEIT**

National Council on Tobacco and Health
National Health Screening Service
Oslo, Norway

## I. Introduction

On May 20, 1984, U.S. Surgeon General C. Everett Koop issued a call for a smoke-free society by the year 2000 [1]. The potential redistribution of economic resources of a tobacco-free society would be of far less consequence than a significantly enriched quality and quantity of life [2]. In consequence, the challenge is to reach this goal in the most efficient way.

The fight against tobacco consumption is different from one country to another, depending on many parameters, such as style of life, the existence of tobacco farming and nationalized cigarette production, the system of taxation, the way of distribution, and the legislation in the country. In this chapter we review the health consequences of tobacco, the need for a comprehensive antitobacco program, the WHO and EC antitobacco programs, and the principles of a comprehensive and international antitobacco policy.

## II. Health Consequences of Tobacco

At the end of World War II very little attention had been paid to the possible health effects of smoking. While tobacco had been used for over 300 years as snuff, chewed, and smoked in pipes, very little had been smoked in the form of cigarettes prior to the advent of their industrial production. As the other ways in which tobacco had been used were much less hazardous because smoke was not inhaled, the massive uptake of tobacco cigarettes escaped close scrutiny in terms of health effects.

Cigarettes become common at the beginning of the twentieth century, and lung cancers and myocardial infarctions took many years to appear. But by 1950, five large case-control studies of tobacco use in relation to cancer were reported from Great Britain and the United States. The results were so striking that by 1954 the conclusion that smoking was a major cause of lung cancer was amply confirmed [3,4]. Lung cancer mortality for ex-smokers is related to the number of years since cessation. After 15 years without smoking, ex-smokers have a mortality rate only slightly greater than that of nonsmokers [5].

As time passed, cigarette smoking was shown to be associated with other diseases, in particular myocardial infarction, chronic obstructive lung disease, and cancers of the respiratory and upper digestive tracts. The International Agency for Research on Cancer [6] and the 1989 U.S. Surgeon General's report, *Reducing the Health Consequences of Smoking* [7], have identified cancers of the lung, larynx, and esophagus, as well as oral cancers as causally smoking related. Cancers of bladder, pancreas, stomach, liver, nasal sinuses, cervix uteri, adenocarcinoma of kidney, and leukemia are probably causally related to smoking.

Despite the recognition of smokers cough, chronic bronchitis and emphysema were not attributed to smoking until the mid-1950s, when cohort studies began to show that the mortality from these diseases was closely related to the amount smoked. Now we know that the risk of developing a chronic obstructive lung disease is increased 20- to 30-fold when smoking is regular and heavy. This disease becomes severe in about one-fifth of cigarette smokers. The causal relationship in that case is demonstrated by the change in the rate of deterioration of lung function from the moment that smoking stops [8].

Other health effects have been found to be causally related to tobacco: coronary heart disease, atherosclerotic peripheral vascular disease, and stroke [7]. Although the risk increase is not as great for coronary heart disease as for lung cancer, tobacco-related deaths from ischaemic heart diseases are more frequent, due to the high prevalence of this disease in industrialized countries. Tobacco is also causally related to intrauterine growth retardation and to low-birth-weight babies [7]. Table 1 presents estimates of the prevalence of some of the diseases due to smoking.

Stopping smoking reduces the health risks caused by tobacco. Mortality from coronary heart disease decreases rapidly after cessation, and within a few years, the mortality of ex-smokers is the same as for nonsmokers. This, and the decrease in frequency of both lung carcinoma and chronic obstructive lung disease after smoking cessation, justifies undertaking cessation programs for smokers.

**Table 1** Smoking-Related Diseases and Estimated Percentages Due to Smoking

| Disease category | Estimated percentage of total incidence caused by smoking |
|---|---|
| Coronary heart disease | Males 43%, females 25% |
| Peripheral vascular disease | 90–98% |
| | |
| Cancer | 27% |
|   Lung cancer | 80–85% |
|   Laryngeal cancer | 84% |
|   Oral cavity cancer | 87% (snuff) |
|   Bladder cancer | Males 40–60%, females 25–35% |
| | |
| Respiratory diseases | 80–90% |

*Source:* Data from ref. 21, first of two parts.

During the 1990s, 3 million deaths per year will be tobacco related, and if current worldwide smoking patterns were to persist, 10 million deaths per year from tobacco could be observed in the 2020s. About half a billion of the world's population today could be killed by tobacco and about one-fourth of a billion while still in middle age (35 to 69), losing, on average, 20 years of life [9]. These dramatic figures, which are due primarily to the very long delay between increased smoking and increases in death rates, emphasize the urgency of initiating efficient worldwide antitobacco control.

## III. Emergence of the Concept of a Comprehensive Antitobacco Policy

Even with the publication in 1962 of the British Royal College of Physicians report [10] and in 1964 of the U.S. Surgeon General's Report on Smoking and Health [11] and although health education campaigns were provided, political action against tobacco consumption was limited in the 1960s. By the mid-1970s, Sweden had began tobacco control measures, and Finland, Iceland, and Norway had comprehensive governmental programs, including advertising bans. In the rest of Europe, North America, and Australasia, under the influence of voluntary health organizations and sometimes through governmental input, measures were taken to create an antismoking environment to varying degrees. Even today, laws to make tobacco use illegal cannot be passed, and it is left largely to each individual to determine whether or not to smoke. This creates a wide range of smoking habits, depending largely on socioeconomic, cultural, and psychological characteristics of the populations.

The principal feature of the smoking habit in a given population is its diffusion, which resembles the spreading of an epidemic. In some countries where tobacco is grown, such as France, Italy, or Spain, production of tobacco products is nationalized. Until the 1970s, this national production furnished the majority of the national market. Now, however, even in these countries, the cigarette market is in quasi-totality furnished by the six giant multinational companies: Philip Morris, R.J. Reynolds Industries, and American Brands from the United States, British-American Tobacco (BAT) Industries and the Imperial Group from the United Kingdom, and the Rembrandt Group of South Africa [12].

In the European Community, tobacco control has developed according to the characteristics of the tobacco issue in the state members, which were identified in the early 1980s [13]. The French–Italian system (also in operation in Spain, Portugal, and Greece) is characterized by high tobacco cultivation, weak industrial manufacturing by an old state monopoly, and relatively low tobacco consumption despite low price. In these countries, tobacco health effects are largely unknown to the public and governmental antitobacco programs are based mainly on banning tobacco advertising. The northern countries of the EC (Belgium, Denmark, Germany, Luxembourg, the Netherlands, and the United Kingdom) are characterized by multinational tobacco production and/or manufacturing, high consumption, and a population aware of tobacco health effects. Germany, Luxembourg, and the Netherlands impose high taxation but few other governmental control measures. In Belgium, many tobacco control laws have been enacted. In the United Kingdom, a strong tobacco industry is opposed by a strong antismoking lobby. Advertising policy is generally based on voluntary agreements with the industry. In Denmark there is almost no tobacco control legislation.

Undoubtedly, the tobacco industry has profitted by the lack of coherence in the antitobacco programs, which either did not exist or were independent of each other, subverting regulations in stricter countries with procedures developed in less strict countries. To coordinate tobacco control in Europe, the European office of WHO (Copenhagen) and the EC created a unified tobacco policy in Europe in the mid-1980s.

## IV. Europe Without Tobacco (WHO) and Europe Against Cancer (EC) Programs

In 1984, the 32 state members of the European region of WHO adopted a unique policy to assure health for all Europeans in 2000 [14]. In 1987, the European regional committee of WHO adopted an action plan against tobacco [15] to encourage and help the governments to adopt and enforce antitobacco legislation. This action plan includes six aims: the development and implementation in each country of a comprehensive policy against tobacco, increasing collaboration with nongovernmental organizations, facilitation of knowledge by the public of the health consequences of tobacco use, help of the different planned actions, the collection and diffusion of the data concerning the projects, and monitoring and evaluation of the action plan.

Similarly, the Europe Against Cancer program was launched at the initiative of heads of state and governments of the European Community at the European councils held in June and November 1985 in Milan and Luxembourg [16] to reduce the number of deaths from cancer by 15% for the year 2000. The 10-point European code that was developed by the European cancer experts is central to the Europe Against Cancer campaign. This code places smoking prevention in the European Community at the top of the list of preventive actions. In the framework of its Europe Against Cancer program the commission has set up a series of 14 measures to be taken [17]. The proposed actions are as follows: (1) upward alignment of taxation on tobacco manufactured in the European Community; (2) financing of preventive actions at the national level by the use of increased fiscal measures on tobacco; (3) publication of tobacco price indexes by the statistical office of the European communities; (4) harmonization of cigarette labeling in the European Community; (5) prohibition of cigarettes with a high tar content; (6) harmonization of the standards for the components of tobacco smoke; (7) prohibition of tax-free sales of tobacco in the European Community; (8) protection of children from tobacco sales; (9) reorientation of tobacco production toward less toxic varieties and study of the possibilities of reconversion; (10) information and public awareness campaigns in the fight against tobacco; (11) study of national provisions, and development of proposed community regulations on tobacco smoking in public places; (12) study of national provisions, and development of proposed community regulations on the limitation of tobacco publicity; (13) comparative analysis of antismoking campaigns; and (14) information exchange in the fight against smoking.

The European Commission created a European Bureau for Action on Smoking Prevention (BASP), which maintains relations with all European organizations of smoking prevention. In addition, the European Commission maintains contact with WHO, with whom it organized the first European Conference on smoking policies in Madrid in November 1988. The results of these coordinated efforts are already present. Smoking prevalence has decreased dramatically, and the public health impact is being felt in the United Kingdom, Finland, Iceland, Ireland, Norway, and Sweden, countries which were, in Europe, the leaders in the fight against tobacco. The percentage of smokers in Belgium and the Netherlands has also decreased sharply over the past 20 years.

Now, other countries, such as France, Italy, and Portugal, are engaged in tobacco control.

## V.  Principles of a Comprehensive and International Antitobacco Policy

The health consequences of tobacco smoking are not inevitable, and countries such as the United Kingdom and the United States, which adopted antitobacco campaigns in the 1960s, are beginning to profit from the continuous trend of tobacco consumption decrease: in these countries tobacco-related mortality has recently stabilized or even declined [7]. This is due both to a decrease of new smokers and to a decrease of mortality in male ex-smokers; decreases having been measured for mortality from coronary heart disease, lung carcinoma, and chronic obstructive lung disease.

As mentioned before, there is a redistribution of the world market for tobacco products. The major risk is the insidious invasion of the territory of national tobacco monopolies by the international commercial industry. The new markets for tobacco use are in the Third World, mainly in Asia [18], with two examples: (1) the establishment of joint ventures between the Chinese tobacco monopoly and an international commercial industry (Philip Morris), and (2) the aggressive invasion by the international industry of countries such as Japan, Korea, Taiwan, and Thailand, whose tobacco supplies are traditionally provided by national monopolies [19]. When considering Figure 1, showing balanced world tobacco production and use in 1990, and excess U.S. tobacco production and national use in 1990, it is clear that new markets are being found. Besides Asia, two other markets have been opened by multinational companies: Africa and, recently, Eastern and Central Europe. On September 13, 1990, the two largest U.S. companies, Philip Morris and R.J. Reynolds agreed to sell 34 billion cigarettes to Russia, and in early September, BAT gave a price quotation to supply 4 billion cigarettes to the Russian Republic for US $1.9 billion, to be paid in cash and countertrade items—items that can easily be sold on international markets [20].

A comprehensive and global tobacco control policy must associate all control measures in all parts of the world. Whatever their individual strengths, they are inefficient if they are not all implemented together, then monitored and sustained for a very long time [21]. These measures are as follow:

1.   Legislation in two fields: (a) protection of nonsmokers' rights and health, with the establishment by law of a clean indoor air policy in public places and public transport, as well as at premises of work, and (b) protection of young people and quitting smokers in the establishment by law of freedom from all forms of tobacco promotion.

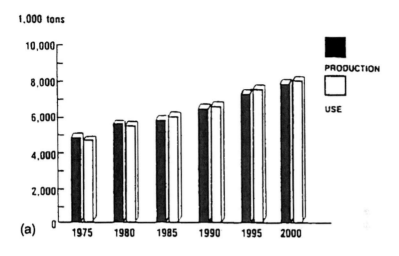

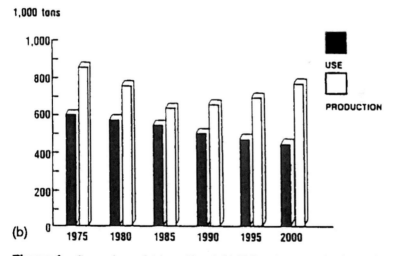

**Figure 1** Comparison of (a) world and (b) U.S. tobacco production and use. (From ref. 19.)

2. Increased price and higher taxes on tobacco products are very dissuasive to teenagers. An increase of 10% a year on cigarette price decreases the consumption among adolescents by up to 14% or more (7).

3. Smoking cessation with clinical interventions and community intervention programs, with the help of all the health professionals, especially general practioners and nurses, as well as voluntary health organizations.

4. Reducing the tar (carcinogen) and nicotine (addictive) contents of cigarettes. But there is no threshold value and no safe cigarette, and low-tar cigarettes are harmful to vascular and respiratory systems, so the final aim must be a tobacco-free world;

5. Heightened public awareness, encouraged by voluntary associations, health professionals, health warnings, media, and so on, to eliminate the primary avoidable cause of death and impairment.

### References

1. Koop CE. A smoke-free society by the year 2000. Presented as the Julia M. Jones Lecture at the Annual Meeting of the American Lung Association, Miami Beach, FL, May 20, 1984.
2. Warner KE. Health and economic implications of a tobacco free society. JAMA 1987;258:2080–86.
3. Hammond EC, Horn D. The relationship between human smoking habits and death rates: a follow-up study of 1,987,766 men. JAMA 1954;154:1316–28.
4. Doll R, Hill AB. The mortality of doctors in relation to their smoking habits. A preliminary report. Br Med J 1954;1:1451–55.
5. Doll R, Hill AB. Lung cancer and other causes of death in relation to smoking: a second report on the mortality of British doctors. Br Med J 1956;2:1071–81.
6. IARC monographs on the evaluation of the carcinogenic risk of chemicals to humans. Vol. 38. Tobacco smoking. Lyon, France: IARC, 1986.
7. U.S. Surgeon General's Report. Reducing the health consequences of smoking: 25 years of progress. A report of the Surgeon General. DHHS Publication (CDC) 89-8411, 1989.
8. Fletcher CM, Peto R. The natural history of chronic airflow obstruction. Br Med J 1977;1:1645–48.
9. Peto R, Lopez AD. World-wide mortality from current smoking patterns. In: Proceedings of the 7th World Conference on Tobacco and Health, Perth, Western Australia, April 1–5, 1990:66–68.
10. Royal College of Physicians. Smoking and health. London: Pitman Medical, 1962.
11. U.S. Department of Health, Education and Welfare. Smoking and health. A report of the advisory committee to the Surgeon General of the U.S. Public Health Service, 1964. PHS Publication 1103. Washington, DC: U.S. Government Printing Office, 1964.
12. Taylor P. The smoke ring: tobacco, money and multinational politics. London: Sphere Books, 1985.

13. Levy E. Analyse des stratégies actuelles ou envisageables de la lutte antitabagique dans les pays de la Communauté Européenne. Commission des Communautés Européennes, November 1981.
14. Les Buts de la Santé pour Tous. Organisation Mondiale de la Santé. Bureau Régional de l'Europe, Copenhagen, 1985.
15. Plan d'Action Contre le Tabagisme. EUR/RC37/7. Organisation Mondiale de la Santé, Bureau Régional de l'Europe.
16. Christopoulos S. Smoking prevention in the context of "Europe Against Cancer" programme of the EC. In: Proceedings of the 7th World Conference on Tobacco and Health, Perth, Western Australia, April 1–5, 1990:135–138.
17. Official Journal of the European Communities, C50, February 26, 1987.
18. Mackay J. Tobacco: the third world war. Thorax 1991;46:153–56.
19. Gray N. Global overview of the tobacco problem. In: Proceedings of the 7th World Conference on Tobacco and Health, Perth, Western Australia, April 1–5, 1990:19–25.
20. Joossens L. Test the East: the tobacco industry and Eastern Europe. Brussels: European Bureau for Action on Smoking Prevention, November 1990.
21. Fielding JE. Smoking: health effects and control. N Engl J Med 1985;313:491–498, 555–561.

# AUTHOR INDEX

*Italic numbers give the page on which the complete references is listed.*

## A

Aalberse, R. C., 243, 244, 246, 247, 249, *254*
Aamodt, T., 25, *35*, 46, *57*
Aasen, A. J., 499, *524*
Abbat, J. D., 201, *206*
Abbey, D. E., 419, 420, 423, 426, *436*
Abboud, R., *146*, 326, *338*, 486, *495*
Abd El-Hafez, S. A., 314, *316*
Abe, T., 380, *391*
Abelin, T., 597, *606*
Abenhaim, L., 417, 418, 419, 432, *435*
Abraham, P. A., 357, *369*
Abrahamson, M., 332, *342*
Abrams, W. R., 337, *343*, 359, *370*
Acheson, E. D., 46, 52, *57*, *63*, 87, 91, *95*, 98, 99, 100, 101, 103, 104, 105, 106, 110, *112*, *113*, *114*, 176, 179, 180, *187*, *190*, *191*
Acheson, R. E. D., 139, *148*
Ackad, M., 74, 75, *79*
Ackerman, B. J., 552, *558*
Adams, J. D., 417, *435*, 503, *525*

Adams, M. J., Jr., 154, 156, *164*
Adams, R. M., 268, *275*
Adcock, C., 564, *572*
Adelberg, S., 376, *386*, *387*
Adelmann-Grill, B. C., 353, *368*
Adesnick, M., 152, *163*
Adivi, C., 551, *558*
Adkinson, N. F., Jr., 270, *275*
Aerts, C., 328, *339*
Afford, S. C., 330, *340*
Agabiti, N., 465, 476, 479, 480, *491*
Aggarwal, A., 74, *79*
Agostini, R., 104, 105, *114*
Ahlbom, A., 99, 100, *113*
Ahlborg, G., 92, *96*
Ahlmark, A., 13, *30*
Ahrens, W., 84, 87, 90, 91, *93*, 183, *192*
Aiache, J. M., 232, 233, 234, 235, *240*, *241*
Aickin, M., 585, 589, 596, *602*
Aisner, S., 382, *391*
Aitio, A., 38, *53*
Ajzen, I., 563, *571*
Akers, S., 357, 358, 359, *370*
Akiba, S., 432, *439*

# SUBJECT INDEX

## A

$\alpha$1-antitrypsin (A1AT), 317, 318, 319,
320–321
Abstinence (*see* Smoking cessation)
Acetaldehyde:
in mainstream smoke, 500, 507
as a respiratory carcinogen, 508
in tobacco, 507
Acetic acid, in cigarette smoke, 500
Acetone
in cigarette smoke, 500
in polluted air, 514
Acetonitrile, in cigarette smoke, 500
Acetyline, in cigarette smoke, 500
Acid pollution:
acid rain, 293
as aerosols, 282, 284, 285, 286
and health effects, 284
Acridine, 41
Acrolein:
in cigarette smoke, 500, 508
in environmental tobacco smoke, 514
as a tumor enhancer, 508
Acrylonatrile, 44
in tobacco smoke, 507

Actinomycetes:
and contamination due to air con-
ditioning (Thermoactinomy-
cetes), 226, 230, 231
and hypersensitivity pneumonitis,
264
Acupuncture, in smoking cessation,
561
Acute respiratory illness, 449–452
Addiction (*see* Nicotine dependence)
Adduct (*see also* Cellular macro-
molecules), 47, 49–50, 173
Adenocarcinoma, 37, 97, 517
Aeroallergens, 137
Africa, market for tobacco, 612
Age, airway responsiveness and, 475
Agricultural chemicals, use on tobacco
crops, 499, 502
Agricultural workers, 86, 110
Air cleaner:
air cleaning and mites, 248, 249
filtration and SBS, 237
HEPA, 249, 270
negative ion generators and mites,
249
Air conditioner (*see* HVAC)